ACE Lifestyle &

Management Consultant Manual

The Ultimate Resource for Fitness Professionals

Second Edition

American Council on Exercise®

Editors

Cedric X. Bryant, Ph.D.

Daniel J. Green

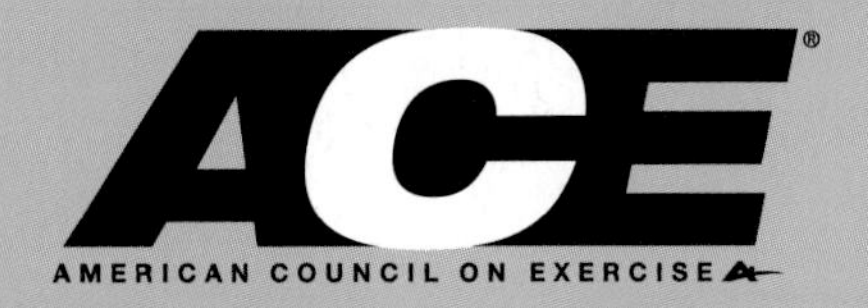

Library of Congress Catalog Card Number: 2007943258

ISBN 9781890720254

B C D E

Distributed by:
American Council on Exercise
P.O. Box 910449
San Diego, CA 92191-0449
(858) 279-8227
(858) 279-8064 FAX
www.acefitness.org

Project Editor: Daniel J. Green
Technical Editor: Cedric X. Bryant, Ph.D.
Cover Design & Art Direction: Karen McGuire
Associate Editor: Marion Webb
Special Contributor & Proofreader: Kim Summers
Production: Nancy Garcia
Photography: Dennis Dal Covey
Anatomical Illustrations: James Staunton
Index: Kathi Unger
Chapter Models: Angel Chelik, Brian Friedman, Todd Galati, Kim Lehman, Kristie Spalding

Acknowledgments:
Thanks to the entire American Council on Exercise staff for their support and guidance through the process of creating this manual.

P09-014

Table of Contents

Reviewers

Liz Applegate, Ph.D., is the director of sports nutrition and a faculty member for the Nutrition Department at the University of California, Davis. She is the author of several books, including *Nutrition Basics for Better Health and Performance* and *Encyclopedia of Sports and Fitness Nutrition*. She has written more than 300 articles for national magazines and is nutrition editor and columnist for *Runner's World* magazine. She frequently serves as a keynote speaker at industry, athletic, and scientific meetings, and as a consultant to professional athletes.

Barbara A. Brehm, Ed.D., is professor of exercise and sport studies at Smith College, Northampton, Mass., where she teaches courses in nutrition, health, and stress management. She is also director of the Smith Fitness Program for Faculty and Staff and an instructor for the Smith College Executive Education Programs. She is the author of several books, including *Successful Fitness Motivation Strategies,* and is a contributing editor for *Fitness Management* magazine.

Fabio Comana, M.A., M.S., is an exercise physiologist, research scientist, and spokesperson for the American Council on Exercise. He also currently teaches courses in exercise science and nutrition at the University of California, San Diego and San Diego State University. Comana regularly presents and writes on many topics related to exercise, fitness, and nutrition, and has authored or co-authored more than three dozen articles and chapters in various publications. He has master's degrees in exercise physiology and nutrition, and currently holds certifications from ACE, the American College of Sports Medicine (ACSM), the National Strength and Conditioning Association (NSCA), and the International Society of Sports Nutrition (ISSN).

Richard T. Cotton, M.A., is the national director of certification for the American College of Sports Medicine (ACSM). Before joining ACSM, he was the chief exercise physiologist at MyExercisePlan.com. Cotton is the former chief exercise physiologist for the Scripps Clinic & Research Foundation as well as for the American Council on exercise, where he also served as a media spokesperson and technical editor. He is certified by ACSM as both a Preventive and Rehabilitative Program Director and Exercise Specialist.

Tara Coghlin Dickson, M.S., R.D., C.S.S.D., is the sports dietitian for Stanford University Hospital and Clinics' Sports Medicine Program at Stanford University Medical Center, St. Francis Memorial Hospital's Center for Sports Medicine, and the University of San Francisco Athletic Department. She is a board certified specialist in sports dietetics, an active member of the Sports Cardiovascular and Wellness Practice Group of the American Dietetic Association, and co-author of *The Stanford Life Plan for a Healthy Heart.*

Natalie Digate-Muth, M.P.H., R.D., L.D.N., is currently pursuing a medical doctor degree at the University of North Carolina at Chapel Hill. In addition to being a registered dietitian, she is an ACE-certified Personal Trainer and Group Fitness Instructor, an American College of Sports Medicine Health and Fitness Instructor, and a National Strength and Conditioning Association Certified Strength and Conditioning Specialist. She is also an ACE Master Trainer and a freelance nutrition and fitness author.

Marilyn A. Guthrie has spent more than 25 years developing and implementing employee health-management programs designed to improve the health and productivity of employees and their family members. She is the manager of health promotion for Washington Mutual, where she oversees the organization's strategic health-management approaches and programs. A recognized expert and speaker on health promotion and innovative health-management interventions, she has presented at numerous conferences and contributed to several books on health promotion.

Tracie Rogers, Ph.D., is a sport and exercise psychology specialist and owner of the BAR Fitness Studio located in Phoenix, Arizona. She teaches, speaks, and writes on psychological constructs related to physical-activity participation and adherence. She is also a faculty associate at Arizona State University in the department of kinesiology.

Randal Schober, Ed.D., is the executive director of the HeadNorth Foundation, which was formed to support the needs of spinal cord injury survivors. Schober formerly held positions as a professor of exercise science and health at the University of North Carolina, and as an exercise physiologist with the world-renowned cardiac program at Sharp Memorial Hospital in San Diego. He has more than 15 years of experience in health and wellness initiatives and coaching.

Dixie Stanforth, M.S., has been a lecturer at The University of Texas at Austin in the Department of Kinesiology since 1985 and serves as a consultant to many organizations, corporations, and certifying boards. Stanforth, who received her master's degree in exercise science from the University of Arizona, continues to be involved in the research of current fitness topics while emphasizing her commitment to teaching and training others.

Philip R. Stanforth, M.S., is a lecturer and director of the Fitness Institute of Texas in the Department of Kinesiology and Health Education at The University of Texas at Austin. While at Texas he also served as the Local Project Coordinator for the HERITAGE Family Study.

David K. Stotlar, Ed.D., serves as the director of the School of Kinesiology & Physical Education at the University of Northern Colorado. He teaches on the faculty in the areas of sport management and sport marketing, has had more than 70 articles published in professional journals, and has written more than 40 chapters in various textbooks and books on sport, fitness, and physical education.

Robyn Stuhr, M.S., is the executive vice president for the American Council on Exercise and has more than 20 years experience in health promotion, sports medicine, and cardiac rehabilitation. Stuhr has lectured extensively about a variety of fitness and health topics, including exercise for bone and cardiovascular health, weight management, body image, the female athlete triad, exercise and menopause, and motivational strategies to enhance exercise adherence. She also has written several book chapters and articles on exercise and fitness.

Jenny R. Susser, Ph.D., has a doctoral degree in clinical health psychology and specializes in sport psychology. She works with athletes dealing with injury, disordered eating, transition from sport and personal issues, and those who want to improve performance, using tools like mental imagery, relaxation, goal-setting, intensity control, self-talk, and counseling. She also has conducted research on athletic injury recovery, investigating the use of mental imagery on recovery.

Kara A. Witzke, Ph.D., is an associate professor and department chair of kinesiology at California State University San Marcos in San Diego County. She has worked in industry and various wellness venues around the country and has promoted wellness and lifestyle management to children and adults of all ages through education, research, and community involvement. She is active in the ACE exam development process and is an ACE media spokesperson. Her current research focuses on the effects of exercise on both diabetes and bone health.

Foreword

The American Council on Exercise published its first *Lifestyle & Weight Management Consultant Manual* in 1996 and much in our understanding of the multifaceted approach needed to implement true weight management has changed since that time. A quick perusal of the table of contents provides ample evidence, as this second edition contains 19 chapters (as opposed to 11 in that first edition) and the book is approximately 200 pages longer than the first edition. This dramatic increase in content stems from a new focus on the psychological aspects of weight management, as well as more in-depth coverage of the physiology of obesity and the techniques of lifestyle coaching.

The fitness industry is at the center of a great paradox: Americans are spending more and more money each year on diet books, fitness club memberships, and pricey home gym equipment, while at the same time becoming more obese and less healthy. In other words, people are motivated enough to take the first step toward improving their health and quality of life, but inevitably fail when it comes time to truly commit to making meaningful lifestyle changes. The primary role of an LWMC is to help individuals bridge that gap and live healthier lives over the long haul. Much attention and research has focused on correct form during strength-training exercises, appropriate exercise intensities during cardiovascular workouts, and whether to stretch before or after an exercise session, but none of that matters very much if the individual quits the routine within the first six months—as the majority of exercisers do.

While our understanding of these behavioral issues has increased in the past decade, the obesity trends in the United States continue to head in the wrong direction. The great challenge for all fitness professionals, and specifically for LWMCs, is to individualize the program for each client to match his or her interests, goals, needs, and readiness for change. Diets don't work. Exercise alone isn't enough. It is up to you to educate your clients on the need for a lifelong commitment to overall lifestyle change. And while that can seem to be an intimidating notion, the changes made can be simple and, with persistence and practice, become as much a habit as eating buttery popcorn in a movie theater or snacking on chips before bed.

Yes, much has changed in the fitness industry since 1996, but one thing remains constant: it is up to fitness professionals and the fitness industry as a whole to find ways to reach and motivate the millions of Americans who don't get enough exercise, eat unhealthfully, and have a less-than-optimal quality of life. And, in a theme you will encounter throughout this book, motivating them to take the first step is not enough. We have to enable them to make these important lifestyle changes a new permanent way of living.

Scott Goudeseune
President and CEO

Introduction

From as far back as 1993, when the ideas behind this certification were first being brainstormed, ACE's Lifestyle & Weight Management Consultant certification program has focused on using an integrated approach to tackle the issues of behavioral change and weight management. Helping a client lose weight and then maintain that weight loss through lifestyle change requires knowledge of exercise science, nutritional science, and behavioral science, as well as an ability to turn that knowledge into practical tips and individualized programs.

The exam content outline, which appears as Appendix B of this manual, was created by a team of top experts who represent each branch of required knowledge and also actively work in the health and fitness industry. The creation of this document is not an academic exercise, but rather an attempt to precisely define the roles and responsibilities of an LWMC, as well as delineate the knowledge and skills needed to meet those responsibilities on a day-to-day basis.

The *ACE Lifestyle & Weight Management Consultant Manual,* Second Edition, presents the most current, complete picture of the knowledge, instructional and counseling techniques, and professional responsibilities that LWMCs need to safely and effectively help clients make appropriate lifestyle changes. It is designed to serve as a comprehensive resource to help you in your daily practice and as a study aid for candidates preparing for the ACE LWMC certification exam. Each chapter is a building block of knowledge, arranged logically to give you an understanding of the basic principles and skills inherent to effective lifestyle and weight management.

The foundation upon which all exercise programs must be built is found in the three chapters that make up Part I: Exercise Science. This section of the manual is new to this edition and includes discussions of anatomy, the fundamentals of applied kinesiology, and exercise physiology. Chapter 1 covers the body's systems—cardiovascular, respiratory, digestive, skeletal, neuromuscular, muscular, and endocrine—detailing their functions and explaining how each is affected by physical activity. Chapter 2 presents the various regions of the human body and explains the kinesiology of the various muscle groups. It also covers the following topics that are of special interest to LWMCs: posture and balance, core stability, and obesity-related biomechanics. Chapter 3 details the benefits of physical activity and how it impacts the body's various systems.

The two chapters that comprise Part II cover the topics of health behavior psychology and communication, counseling, and group dynamics. Together these chapters address the all-important topic of behavioral science. Chapter 4 introduces various models of behavioral theory (many of which are covered more completely later in the manual) and discusses the issues of motivation and adherence. Chapter 5 teaches the reader how to build rapport with clients and develop positive group dynamics and camaraderie.

Part III: Nutritional Science includes three chapters that cover the following: basic nutrition and digestion, application of nutrition, and current concepts in weight management. Chapter 6 introduces the various macro- and micronutrients and details the processes of digestion and absorption. Chapter 7 explains how to apply nutritional theories and help clients adhere to eating plans. This chapter also covers the nutritional requirements for various populations, from very active adults to individuals struggling with specific conditions. Chapter 8 reviews popular diets and pharmacological agents and explains the benefits and drawbacks of each. In addition, this chapter covers eating disorders and their associated health risks.

The next three chapters comprise Part IV: Screening, Assessment, and Referral. Chapter 9 explains the importance of a proper health screening and covers various assessment issues, including a client's readiness to change. Chapter 10 reviews body-composition assessment techniques and approaches to sharing results with clients. Chapter 11 explains the importance of making referrals when appropriate and staying within the LWMC's scope of practice.

Part V is where all of the previous knowledge is put together into practical application. Chapter 12 covers weight-management programming and details the transtheoretical model of change and the importance of understanding a client's current stage of readiness before trying to implement a program. This chapter also teaches the reader how to track progress and overcome obstacles. Chapter 13 covers the various components of a well-designed exercise program, beginning with goal-setting and continuing on through appropriate progressions and modifications. Chapter 14 teaches the LWMC how to implement an eating plan while staying within the scope of practice. It also explains how to interview clients and use various tracking tools. The next chapter presents lifestyle-modification strategies and teaches the reader how to implement a lifestyle-modification program. This chapter also covers the all-important topic of knowing when to refer a client. Chapter 16 stresses the importance of moving beyond weight loss to weight maintenance and presents the correlates and methods of this behavior. This chapter also covers counseling skills and professional ethics.

Part VI delves more deeply into the physiology of obesity and covers exercise for individuals with medical or health limitations. Chapter 17 discusses the prevalence of overweight and obesity, as well as the health consequences of those conditions. Chapter 18 provides exercise guidelines and recommendations for several common conditions, including hypertension, asthma, and diabetes.

Finally, Part VII covers the legal, professional, and ethical responsibilities of an LWMC. Chapter 19 presents such topics as employee vs. independent contractor, scope of practice, insurance needs, and legal concepts and defenses. It is essential that LWMCs not neglect this aspect of the profession.

We are confident that the information provided in this manual will enhance the quality of service provided by LWMCs. Ultimately, the true goal—which we share with each of our certified professionals—is to improve the overall health and quality of life of all people. We sincerely hope that this book serves you well in your efforts.

Cedric X. Bryant, Ph.D.
Chief Science Officer

Daniel J. Green
Project Editor

Part I

Exercise Science

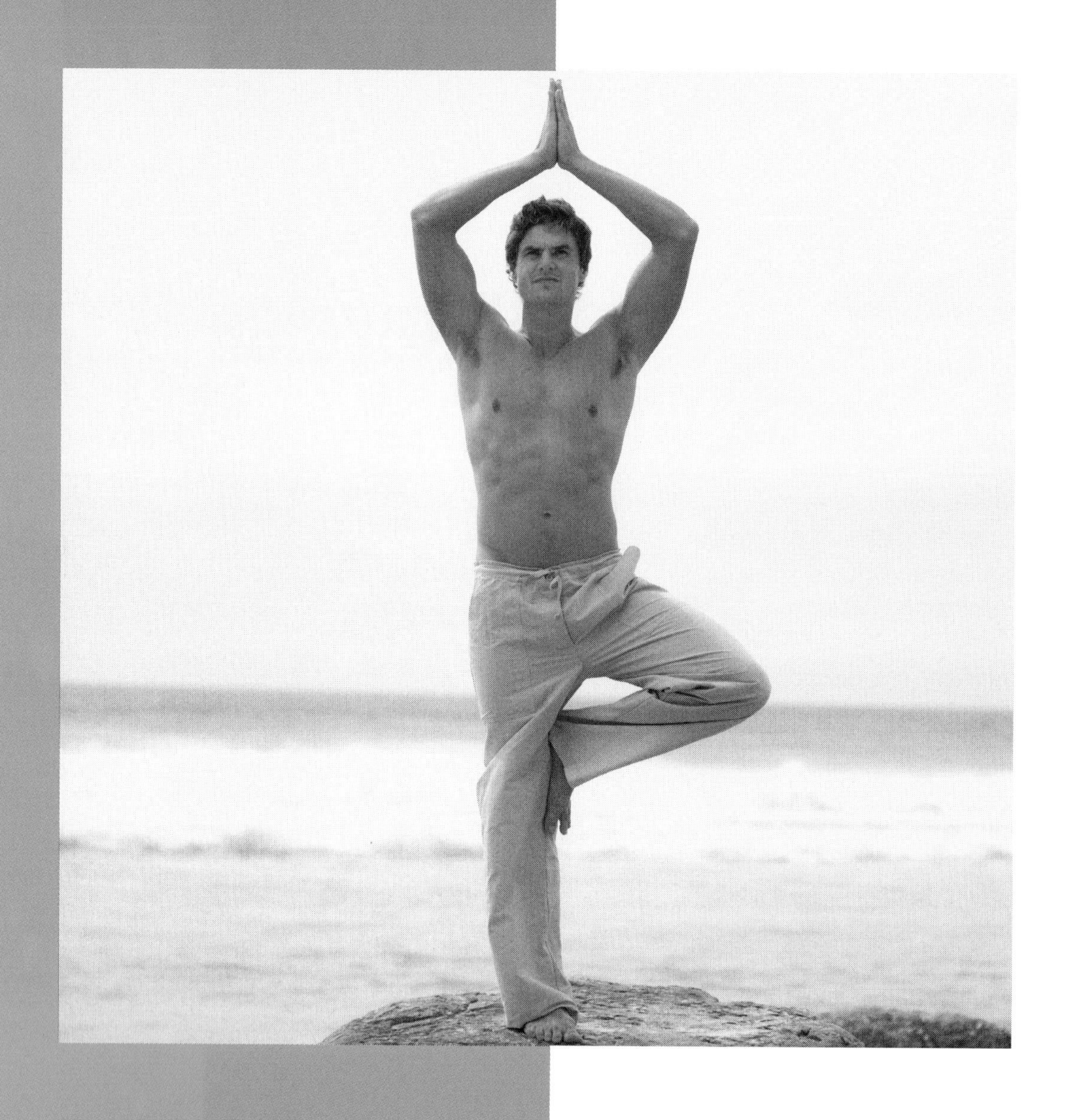

Sabrena Merrill

Sabrena Merrill, M.S., has been actively involved in the fitness industry since 1987, focusing on teaching group exercise, owning and operating her own personal training business, and managing fitness departments in commercial fitness facilities. Merrill is a former full-time faculty member in the Kinesiology and Physical Education Department at California State University, Long Beach. She has a bachelor's degree in exercise science as well as a master's degree in physical education/biomechanics from the University of Kansas, and has numerous certifications in exercise instruction. Merrill, an ACE-certified Personal Trainer and Group Fitness Instructor and ACE Faculty Member, educates other fitness professionals about current industry topics through speaking engagements at local establishments and national conferences, as well as through educational videos. She is a spokesperson for ACE and is involved in curriculum development for ACE continuing education programs.

Chapter 1

Anatomy

IN THIS CHAPTER:

The study of the human body has its origins in prehistoric times, making it one of the oldest known sciences. The term anatomy comes from the Greek word *anatomē,* which means "dissection" or "to cut apart." Originally, anatomical understanding came largely from observations of dissected plants and animals. The proper understanding of a structure, however, must include knowledge of function in the living organism (i.e., physiology). Therefore, anatomy is almost inseparable from physiology, which is sometimes called functional anatomy. In this chapter, human anatomy is presented as the science of studying the body's structures and how these structures operate through various systems.

Anatomical structures were originally named in Greek, Latin, and Arabic. With a knowledge of the important anatomical, directional, and regional terms associated with the structures of the body, people often find that most tissues are named quite descriptively (Table 1-1). A good example is the comparison between the biceps brachii and biceps femoris muscles. Biceps refers to a "two-headed muscle." Therefore, both muscles are composed of two heads. The location of each muscle, however, is quite different. The word brachii comes from the root term "brachium," which means muscle of the arm, whereas the word femoris comes from "femur," which is the large bone of the thigh. The biceps brachii is a muscle of the front, upper arm and the biceps femoris is a muscle found in the back of the thigh. Table 1-2 provides a list of common anatomical terminology, which will help individuals to decipher the root words, and thus, the meaning of bodily structures.

Naming the various parts of the human body required anatomists to develop a reference position, so that structures and areas of the body could be described in relation to each other. This **anatomical position** refers to a person standing erect with the head, eyes, and palms facing forward. Feet are together with the toes pointing forward and the arms are hanging by the sides. A representation of anatomical position is given in Figure 1-1, along with the anatomical planes of motion.

There are four structural levels in the body: cells, tissues, organs, and systems. The most basic structures are the cells. They make up the tissues, which are the next most complex level. Fitness professionals should gain a basic understanding of the structure and function of muscular, nervous, and connective tissues. In terms of complexity, the next structural level in the body consists of the

Table 1-1
Anatomical, Directional, and Regional Terms

Anterior (ventral)	Toward the front
Posterior (dorsal)	Toward the back
Superior	Toward the head
Inferior	Away from the head
Medial	Toward the midline of the body
Lateral	Away from the midline of the body
Proximal	Toward the attached end of the limb, origin of the structure, or midline of the body
Distal	Away from the attached end of the limb, origin of the structure, or midline of the body
Superficial	External; located close to or on the body surface
Deep	Internal; located further beneath the body surface than the superficial structures
Cervical	Regional term referring to the neck
Thoracic	Regional term referring to the portion of the body between the neck and the abdomen; also known as the chest (thorax)
Lumbar	Regional term referring to the portion of the back between the abdomen and the pelvis
Plantar	The sole or bottom of the feet
Dorsal	The top surface of the feet and hands
Palmar	The anterior or ventral surface of the hands
Sagittal Plane	A longitudinal (imaginary) line that divides the body or any of its parts into right and left sections
Frontal Plane	A longitudinal (imaginary) section that divides the body into anterior and posterior parts; lies at a right angle to the sagittal plane
Transverse Plane	Also known as the horizontal plane; an imaginary line that divides the body or any of its parts into superior and inferior sections

Table 1-2
Common Anatomical (Medical) Terminology

Root	Meaning	Term	Definition
arthro	joint	arthritis	inflammation in a joint
bi	two	biceps	two-headed muscle
brachium	arm	brachialis	muscle of the arm
cardio	heart	cardiology	the study of the heart
cephalo	head	cephalic	pertaining to the head
chondro	cartilage	chondro-ectomy	excision of a cartilage
costo	rib	costo-chondral	pertaining to a rib and its cartilage
dermo	skin	dermatitis	inflammation of the skin
hemo, hemat	blood	hemorrhage	internal or external bleeding
ilio	ilium	ilium	the wide, upper part of the pelvic bone
myo	muscle	myocitis	inflammation of a muscle
os, osteo	bone	osteomalacia	softening of the bone
pulmo	lung	pulmonary artery	vessel that brings blood to the lungs
thoraco	chest	thorax	chest
tri	three	triceps	three-headed muscle

Figure 1-1
Anatomical position and planes of motion

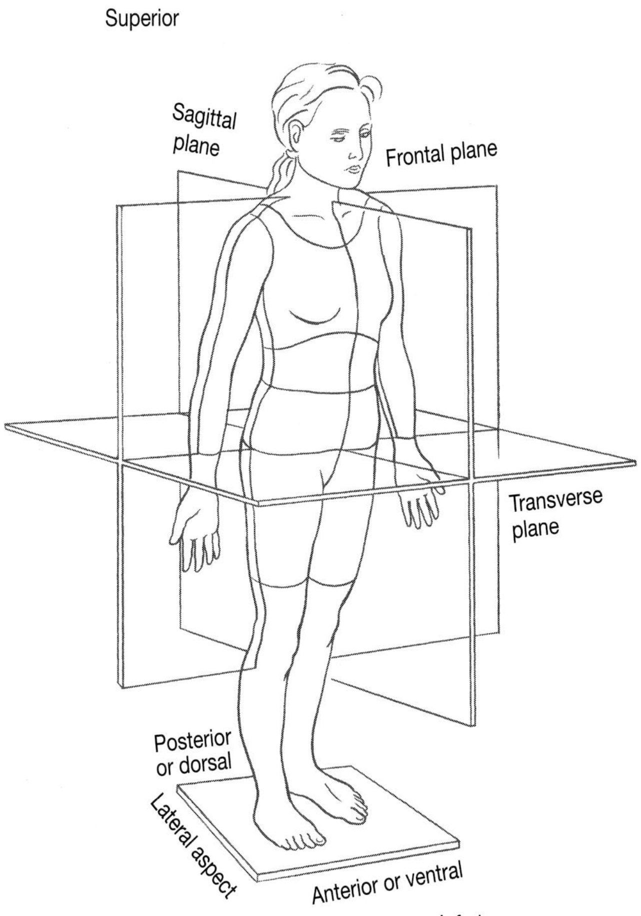

organs. An organ is formed by two or more tissues combining to serve as a specialized physiologic center for the body. The stomach, for example, is an organ lined with **epithelial tissue** (a tissue that lines various body cavities), and its walls are formed by muscle tissue. Its specific physiological function is to prepare ingested food for digestion.

At the highest structural level, the body is composed of systems. Organs that function cooperatively and have a common purpose (such as the digestion and absorption of food) are said to be part of a body system. For instance, the mouth, **esophagus,** stomach, and intestines are all part of the digestive system. Fitness professionals should be familiar with the following systems: cardiovascular, respiratory, digestive, skeletal, neuromuscular, muscular, and endocrine.

Cardiovascular System

The cardiovascular, or circulatory, system is a closed-circuit system composed of the heart, blood vessels, and blood. Blood continuously travels a circular route through the heart into the **arteries,** then to the **capillaries,** into the **veins,** and back to the heart. Together with the respiratory system, the heart and blood vessels deliver oxygen and nutrients to the body's tissues while also removing waste, such as carbon dioxide and metabolic by-products.

Blood, the fluid component of the cardiovascular system, links the internal environment of the body to the external environment by transporting materials between the two environments as well as among the various cells and tissues. The liquid component of blood, called **plasma,** is responsible for carrying **hormones,** plasma proteins, food materials (e.g., carbohydrates, amino acids, lipids), **ions** (e.g., sodium, chloride, bicarbonate), and gases (e.g., oxygen, nitrogen, carbon dioxide) throughout the body. The portion of the blood that is not plasma contains the formed elements, which include red blood cells, various types of white blood cells, and **platelets.** Given that blood "feeds" virtually all tissues, its primary function is transportation. In addition, the cardiovascular system plays an important role in temperature regulation and acid–base balance.

Blood is transported throughout the body via blood vessels. The categories of blood vessels include the following:

- Arteries and **arterioles,** which carry oxygen-rich blood away from the heart
- Veins and **venules,** which return oxygen-poor blood to the heart
- Capillaries, which provide sites for gas, nutrient, and waste exchange between the blood and tissues

As blood leaves the heart to nourish the body, it is carried by the arteries (Figure 1-2a). Large arteries, such as the **aorta** and its major branches, are thick and elastic and are passively stretched as the blood is ejected from the heart. **Arteriosclerosis** (i.e., hardening of the arteries and narrowing of the arteries due to plaque accumulation), which is commonly seen in older adults, contributes to arterial rigidity and decreases the arteries' ability to expand. This condition gives way to an increase in blood pressure, which is commonly associated with aging. As arteries lead away from the heart, they branch extensively to form a "tree" of smaller, microscopic vessels called arterioles. Eventually, the arterioles develop into "beds" of much smaller structures, the capillaries. Capillaries have extremely thin walls, and, consequently, allow the exchange of materials between the blood and the **interstitial fluid** between the cells. Blood passes from the capillary beds to small venous vessels called venules. As venules lead back to the heart, they increase in size and become veins (Figure 1-2b). The walls of veins are thinner and less elastic than arterial walls. Commonly found inside the veins of the lower limbs are valves that allow blood to flow in only one direction—toward the heart. Blood leaving the major veins—the superior and inferior vena cava—empties directly into the heart, where it is transported to the lungs to pick up a fresh supply of oxygen.

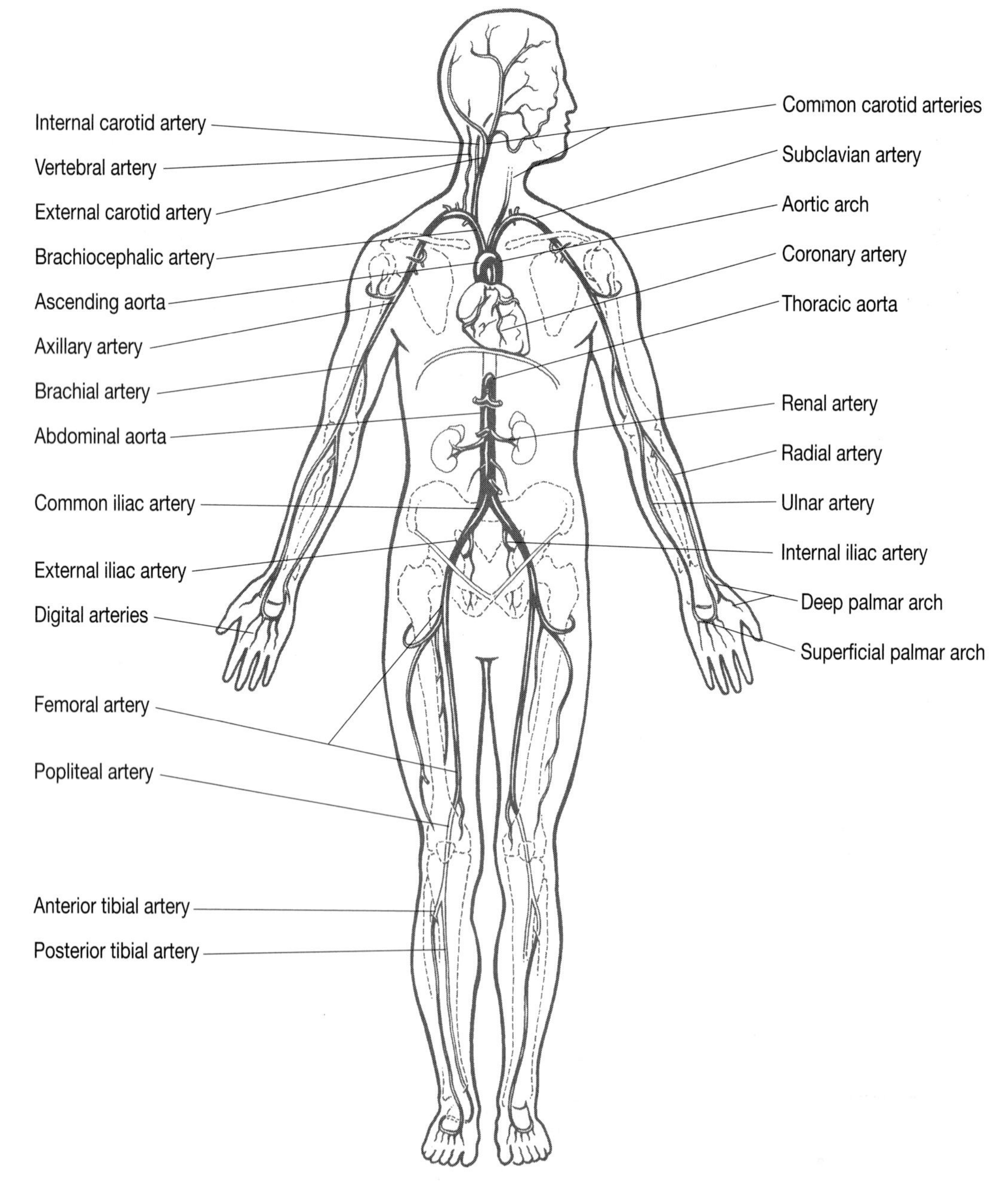

Figure 1-2a
Major arteries of the body (anterior view)

The heart serves as a pump, pushing the blood throughout the body. It is located between the lungs and lies just left of center, behind the sternum. The adult heart is approximately the size of a closed fist. It is divided into four chambers and is often considered two pumps in one, as the right two chambers are responsible for pulmonary circulation and the left two chambers are responsible for systemic circulation. The chambers of the heart consist of two atria and two ventricles. The atria are small and located superior to the ventricles, which make up the bulk of the heart. The right atrium and the right ventricle form the right pump, while the left atrium and left ventricle combine to form the left pump (Figure 1-3). The right and left sides of the heart are separated by a muscular wall, called the interventricular septum, which prevents the mixing of blood from the two sides of the heart.

To function as a pump, the heart must have both receiving and propulsion chambers and valves, which direct blood flow through the heart. Blood movement within the heart is from the atria (the receiving chambers) to

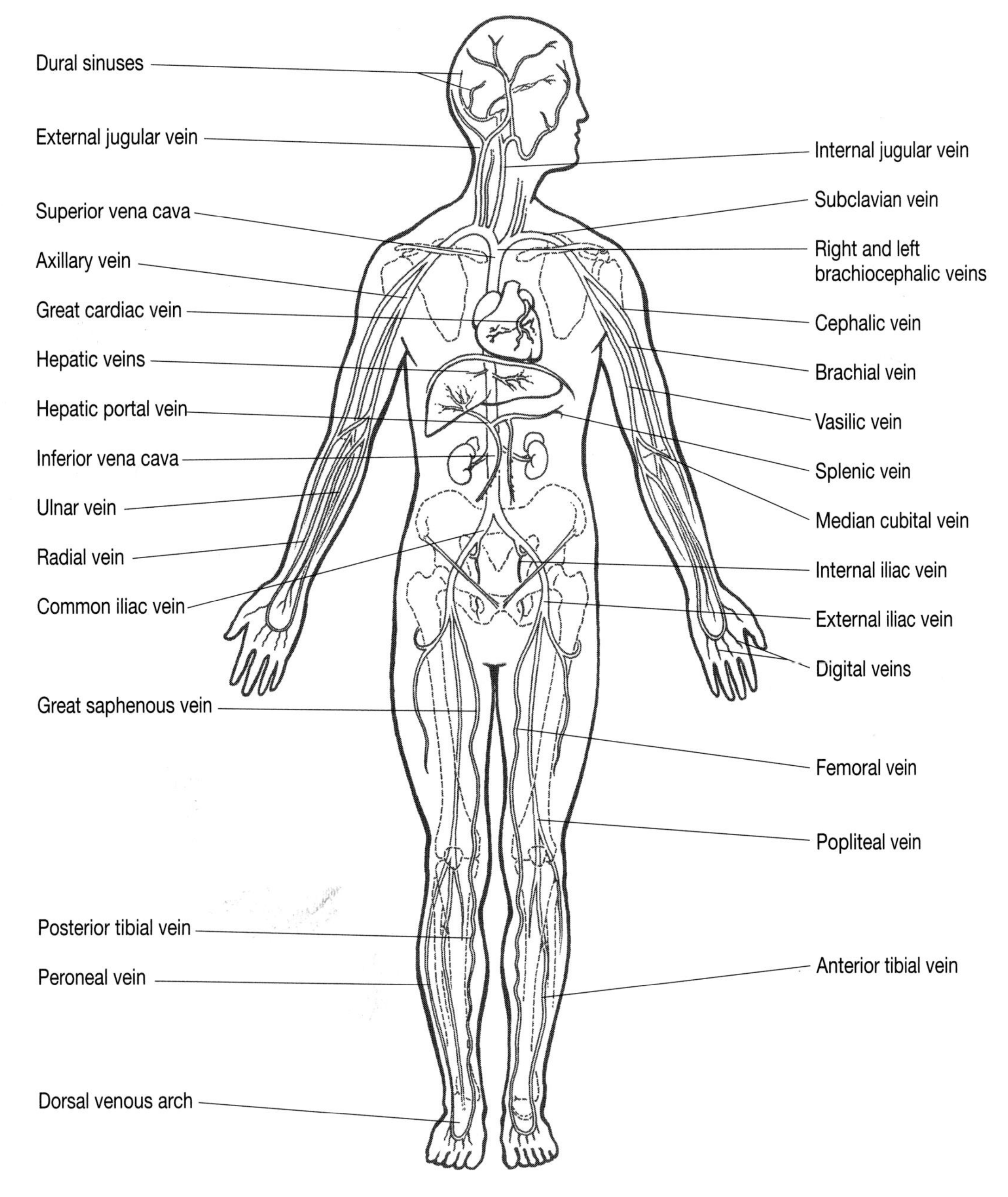

Figure 1-2b
Major veins of the body (anterior view)

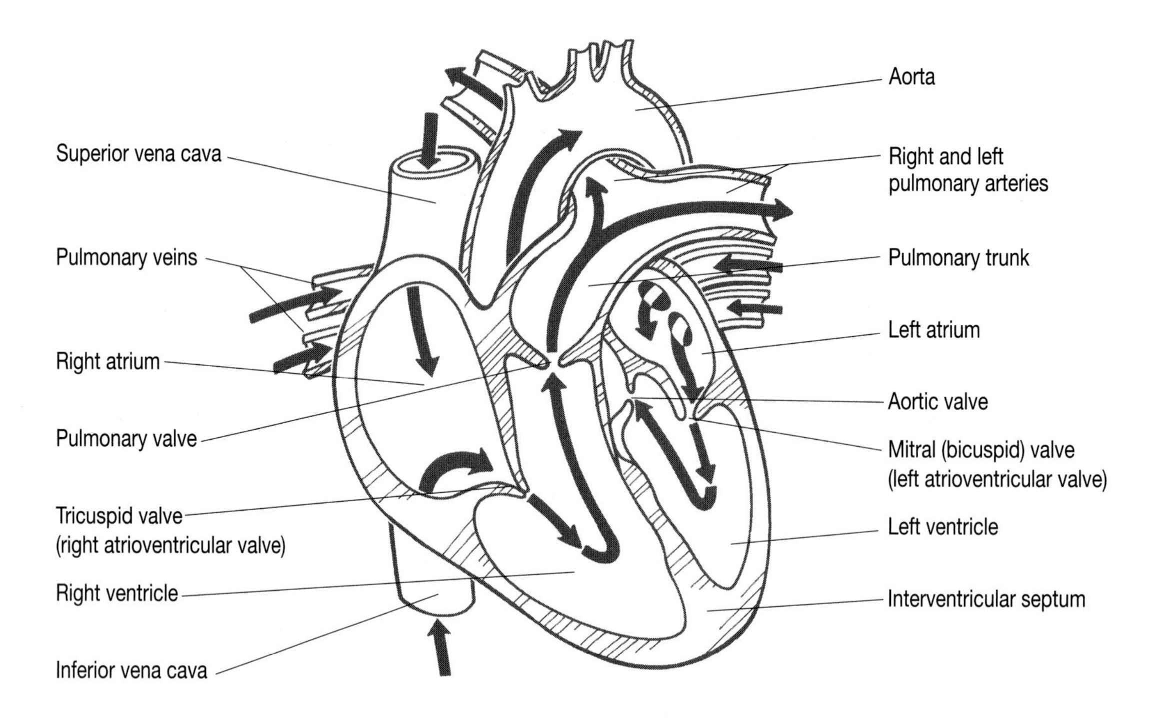

Figure 1-3
Structure of the heart and flow of blood within it

the ventricles (the propulsion chambers) and from the ventricles to the arteries. Backward movement of blood within the heart is prevented by four one-way valves. The right and left atrioventricular valves connect the atria with the right and left ventricles, respectively. Backflow from the arteries into the ventricles is prevented by the pulmonary semilunar valve (right ventricle) and the aortic semilunar valve (left ventricle).

The right side of the heart receives blood that is partially depleted of its oxygen content and contains an elevated level of carbon dioxide after having passed through the cells. This blood is then pushed into the lungs, where it releases its carbon dioxide in exchange for oxygen. This is called the **pulmonary circuit.** The left side of the heart receives newly oxygenated blood from the lungs and pumps it to the various tissues of the body through the **systemic circuit.** The specific pathway of blood through the heart starts as venous blood (blood coming back to the heart through the veins). All the blood from the venous system enters the right atrium first. From there, blood enters the right ventricle, which pumps it to the lungs through the pulmonary arteries (the exception to arteries carrying oxygen-rich blood). In the lungs, the blood picks up a fresh supply of oxygen and gives off carbon dioxide. The oxygenated blood returns from the lungs to the left atrium through the pulmonary veins (the exception to veins carrying oxygen-poor blood). From the left atrium, blood enters the left ventricle, and is then pumped through the aorta to the rest of the body (except for the lungs).

The **cardiac cycle** is the period from the beginning of one heartbeat to the beginning of the next. The right and left sides of the heart perform their pumping actions simultaneously. In other words, when the heart beats, both atria contract together to empty the blood into the ventricles. Approximately 0.1 second after the atria contract, both ventricles contract to deliver blood to the pulmonary and systemic circuits. The repeating phases of contraction and relaxation are called **systole** and **diastole.** Systole refers to the contraction phase of the cardiac cycle, during which blood leaves the ventricles, while diastole refers to the relaxation phase of the cardiac cycle, during which blood fills the ventricles.

Respiratory System

The structures of the respiratory system make it possible for the body to exchange gases between the external environment and the tissues. Specifically, the respiratory system provides a means to replace oxygen and remove carbon dioxide from the blood. In addition, it makes vocalization possible and plays an important role in the regulation of the acid–base balance during exercise. The respiratory system is made up of the nose, nasal cavity, **pharynx, larynx, trachea, bronchi,** and lungs. Together, these structures form a group of passages that filter air and transport it into the lungs, where gas exchange occurs within microscopic air sacs called **alveoli** (Figure 1-4).

Air enters the respiratory system through both, the nostrils and the mouth. The air is warmed and passed through the pharynx (throat), and then the larynx (the area of the "Adam's apple"). Humans normally breathe approximately 5 to 6 liters of air per minute through the nose when at rest, but use the mouth as the primary passageway for air when ventilation is increased to approximately 20 to 30 liters per minute during exercise. From the larynx, air travels through the trachea (windpipe), which extends to the fifth or sixth thoracic vertebrae, where it divides into two smaller branches: the right and left primary bronchi. The primary bronchi divide into smaller secondary bronchi, one for each lobe of the lung. The secondary bronchi then branch into many tertiary bronchi that repeatedly branch further, resulting in tiny bronchioles. The bronchioles continue to branch to form terminal bronchioles, which ultimately divide into even smaller respiratory bronchioles that end in clusters of alveoli (i.e., thin-walled air sacs).

The lungs contain approximately 300 million alveoli, which provide an enormous surface area for gas exchange. It is estimated that the total surface area available for diffu-

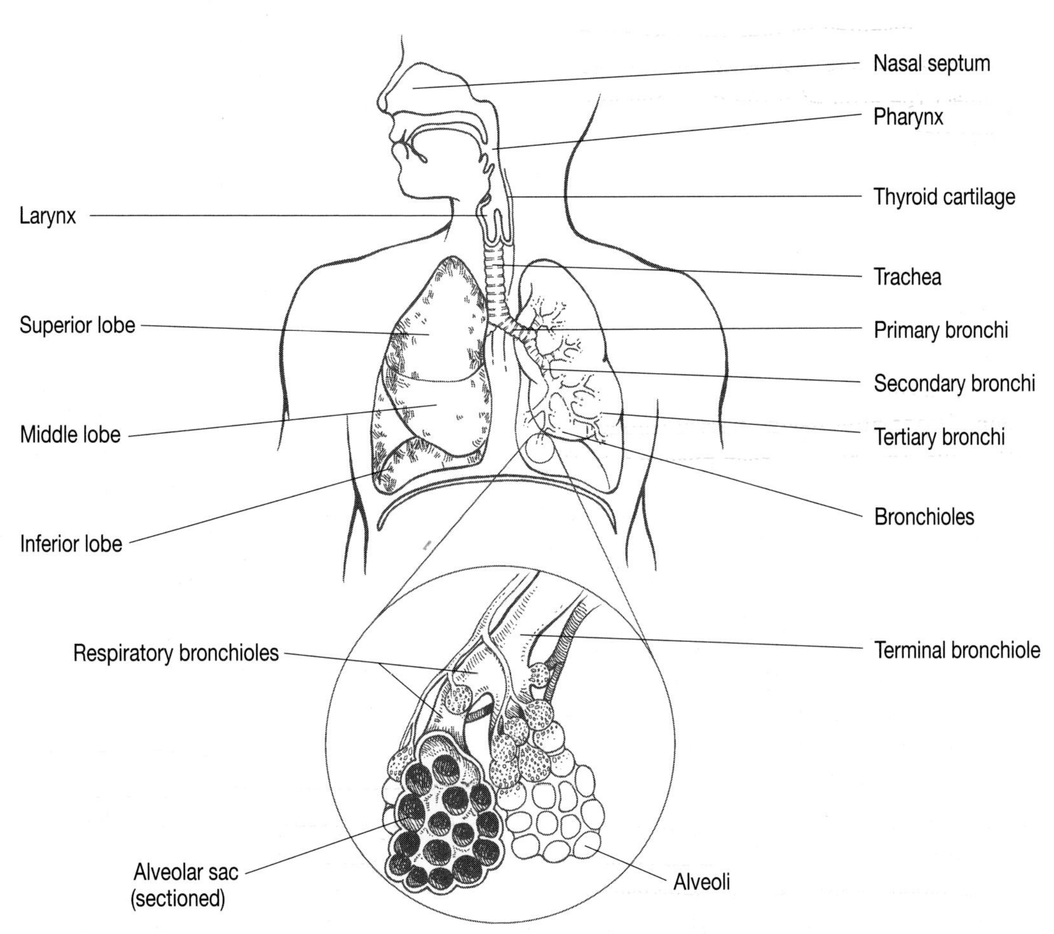

Figure 1-4
Upper and lower respiratory pathways

sion in the human lung is about the size of a tennis court.

The lungs are encased within the rib cage. These paired, cone-shaped structures house the primary, secondary, and tertiary bronchi, as well as the various bronchioles and alveoli. The two lungs are separated by a space called the **mediastinum,** which contains several important organs, including the heart, aorta, esophagus, and part of the trachea. The lungs rest on top of the most important muscle of **inspiration,** the diaphragm, which is the only skeletal muscle considered essential for life. When the diaphragm contracts, it forces the abdominal contents downward and forward while the external intercostals (groups of muscles that run between the ribs) lift the ribs outward. This action reduces the pressure in the membranes surrounding the lungs and, in turn, causes the lungs to expand. This expansion allows airflow into the lungs. At rest, the diaphragm and external intercostals perform most of the work of inspiration. However, during physical activity, accessory muscles of inspiration are recruited, including the pectoralis minor, scalenes, and sternocleidomastoid. By assisting the diaphragm and external intercostals in the effort to further increase the volume of the **thorax,** these muscles aid in inspiration. **Expiration** occurs passively during normal, quiet breathing, requiring no assistance from muscle action. However, during exercise, expiration becomes active. Important muscles of expiration, such as the rectus abdominis, internal obliques, serratus posterior, and internal intercostals, are activated to help pull the rib cage downward and force air from the lungs by squeezing the abdominal organs upward against the diaphragm.

The muscles of respiration adapt to regular exercise training, as do the locomotor skeletal muscles. Regular endurance exercise increases the oxidative capacity of respiratory muscles, which improves respiratory muscle endurance. This is important because respiratory muscles have been shown to fatigue with exercise, adversely affecting the ability to breathe during both moderate- and high-intensity activities. Improving respiratory muscle endurance enhances exercise performance at various intensities.

Digestive System

Each cell in the body requires a constant source of energy to perform its specific function. People obtain energy from ingested food that has been mechanically or chemically processed by the body so that it can ultimately pass through the wall of the **gastrointestinal (GI) tract** and enter the bloodstream. The vascular system carries food molecules through the hepatic portal vein to the liver before distributing them throughout the body. After entering the cells, the digested food molecules may be reassembled into proteins, carbohydrates, and fats, or may be used in the production of energy to support body activity. The digestive system carries out six basic processes:

- Ingestion of food into the mouth
- Movement of food along the digestive tract
- Mechanical preparation of food for digestion
- Chemical digestion of food
- Absorption of digested food into the circulatory and **lymphatic systems**
- Elimination of indigestible substances and waste products from the body by defecation

The Lymphatic System

The lymphatic system is composed of an extensive network of capillaries, collecting vessels, lymph nodes, and lymphoid organs, and serves to return excess fluid from between the cells (interstitial fluid) back to the bloodstream, thus preventing swelling of the intercellular spaces (edema). Lymph fluid is very similar to blood, except that it contains no red blood cells or platelets, as these components cannot escape through the blood-vessel walls. Once **lymph** enters the blood through specialized vessels called lymphatic capillaries, it circulates through the arteries, blood capillaries, and veins. There are four important functions of the lymphatic system:

- Destruction of bacteria and other foreign substances that are present in lymph nodes
- Specific immune responses that aid in manufacturing antibodies to destroy bacteria and foreign substances
- The return of interstitial fluid to the bloodstream
- Prevention of excessive accumulation of tissue fluid and filtered proteins by drainage into highly permeable lymphatic capillaries in the connective tissues

At its most basic structural level, the digestive system consists of a tube—called the GI tract—that extends from the mouth to the **anus.** When food is in the GI tract, it is considered to be outside of the body. To enter the body, the ingested food must cross the cells that line the wall of the digestive tract; many substances pass through the GI tract without being absorbed. Although the GI tract is one continuous tube, it is divided into several separate regions, each of which performs specialized functions in the digestive process. These regions include the mouth, pharynx, esophagus, stomach, small intestine, and large intestine (Figure 1-5).

Food enters the body through the mouth, where the mechanical process of chewing breaks large pieces of food into smaller ones. Saliva blends with these pieces to ease swallowing and dissolve some of the food particles, thus allowing the food to be tasted by the taste buds on the tongue. Furthermore, secretions from the salivary glands contain an enzyme that initiates carbohydrate digestion. Food that is swallowed passes through the mouth to the pharynx, which serves as a common passageway for both the respiratory and digestive systems. The act of swallowing causes food to slide across the **epiglottis,** bypassing the entrance to the lungs. This is important because the epiglottis closes off the trachea to prevent choking when swallowing. After a

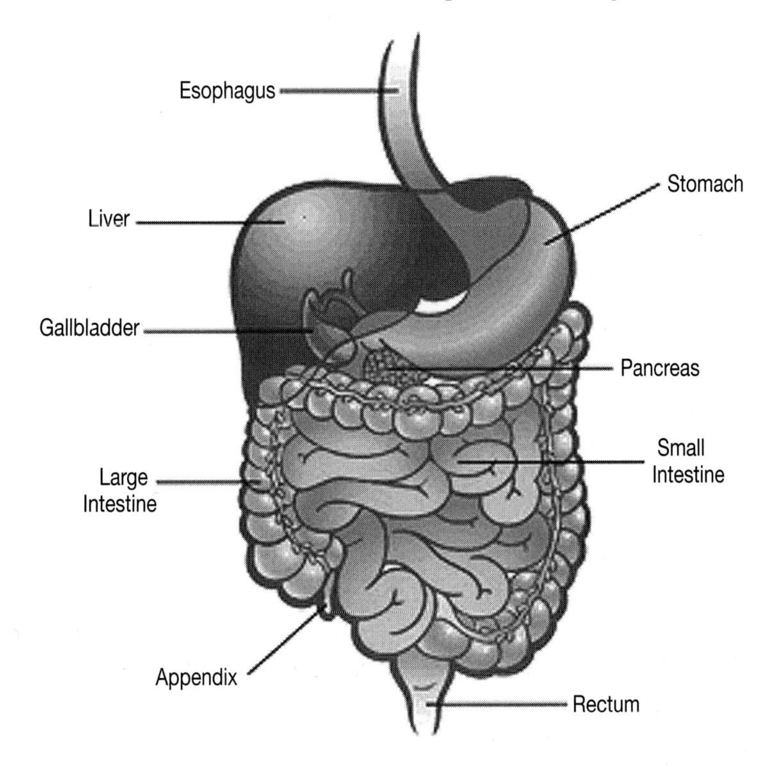

Figure 1-5
The gastrointestinal (GI) tract

Source: This image was provided by KidsHealth, one of the largest resources online for medically reviewed health information written for parents, kids, and teens. www.KidsHealth.org; www.TeensHealth.org.

mouthful of food has been swallowed, it is called a **bolus.**

Next, the bolus slides down the esophagus—a muscular tube that connects the pharynx with the stomach. Located behind the trachea, the esophagus passes through the mediastinum of the thorax and passes through the diaphragm, where it ultimately empties into the stomach. Waves of contractions, called peristalses (singular = **peristalsis**), move the food through the esophagus, where it enters the stomach through the **cardiac sphincter,** which sits at the upper portion of the stomach. The stomach prepares ingested food by chemical and mechanical means for passage into the small intestine. The chemical action consists of specialized stomach cells that produce secretions to break down food particles; these secretions also protect the stomach cells from being broken down. The mechanical action occurs when the stomach grinds the food into a suspension of particles to create a thick liquid mixture known as **chyme.** The stomach stores chyme until it can be emptied into the small intestine at a rate appropriate for optimal digestion and absorption. Chyme leaves the stomach and enters the small intestine through the **pyloric sphincter.**

The small intestine is the primary site for digestion and absorption of food, including the energy-providing nutrients (protein, carbohydrate, and fat), vitamins, minerals, and water. Therefore, it is important for the stomach to store food and pass it into the small intestine at a rate that does not exceed the small intestine's capacity. In general, it takes hours to digest and absorb a meal that took only minutes to consume. Measuring a length of approximately 21 feet (6.4 meters), the small intestine is divided into three segments—the **duodenum** [the first 8 inches (20.3 cm)], the **jejunum** [8 feet (2.4 meters)], and the **ileum** [12 feet (3.7 meters)].

As it passes through the duodenum, chyme is exposed to **bile** from the liver and gallbladder (which aids in the digestion of fat), and pancreatic enzymes from the pancreas (which aid in the digestion of protein, carbohydrate, and fat). In the small intestine, a process similar to peristalsis, called segmentation, not only pushes the chyme, but also periodically squeezes it momentarily, thereby forcing the intestinal contents backward a few inches and allowing the digestive juices and absorbing cells to make better contact with the nutrients. Most absorption of food molecules occurs in the duodenum and the jejunum through the surfaces of microscopic, hair-like projections called **villi** and **microvilli.** Each projection has its own capillary network and lymph vessel, so as food molecules move across them, the nutrients can immediately pass through into the bloodstream and body fluids.

By the time chyme reaches the large intestine (sometimes called the **colon**), digestion and absorption are mostly complete. The large intestine, which is approximately 5 feet (1.5 meters) long, is called "large" because its diameter is greater than that of the small intestine. The final absorption of water and salt occurs in the large intestine, leaving semisolid waste that is passed out of the body through the anus. Fiber and other indigestible substances in the diet provide bulk against which the muscles of the colon can work to expel the waste. Transit time of a meal through the digestive system (from mouth to colon) can take several hours and depends on the nutrient composition of the meal.

The kidney is another organ related to digestion, but it is actually part of its own distinct system (the urinary system). The kidneys are located on each side of the vertebral column in the posterior abdominal cavity. They are the body's main excretory organs and are critically important for maintaining the body's internal environment within a range that is optimal for survival of the cells. The kidneys carry out their functions by eliminating from the body a variety of metabolic products, such as urea, uric acid, and creatinine and by excreting or conserving water and **electrolytes.** As blood flows through the kidneys, some of the plasma is filtered out. As the filtrate flows along, water, electrolytes, **glucose, amino acids**, and other important substances are reabsorbed and returned to the blood. Hormones regulate the reabsorption and secretion processes within the kidneys and allow them to exert a high degree of control over which materials get excreted or reabsorbed. When the reabsorption and secretion processes are completed, the remaining fluid in the kidneys is transported to the bladder and excreted as urine.

Skeletal System

The human skeleton is an active, living tissue that performs several important functions: support, movement, protection, storage, and formation of blood cells (**hemopoiesis**). The body has a total of 206 bones, most of which are paired (e.g., right and left femurs, right and left tibias) (Figure 1-6). The structural functions of bone include giving support to the soft tissues of the body and providing attachment

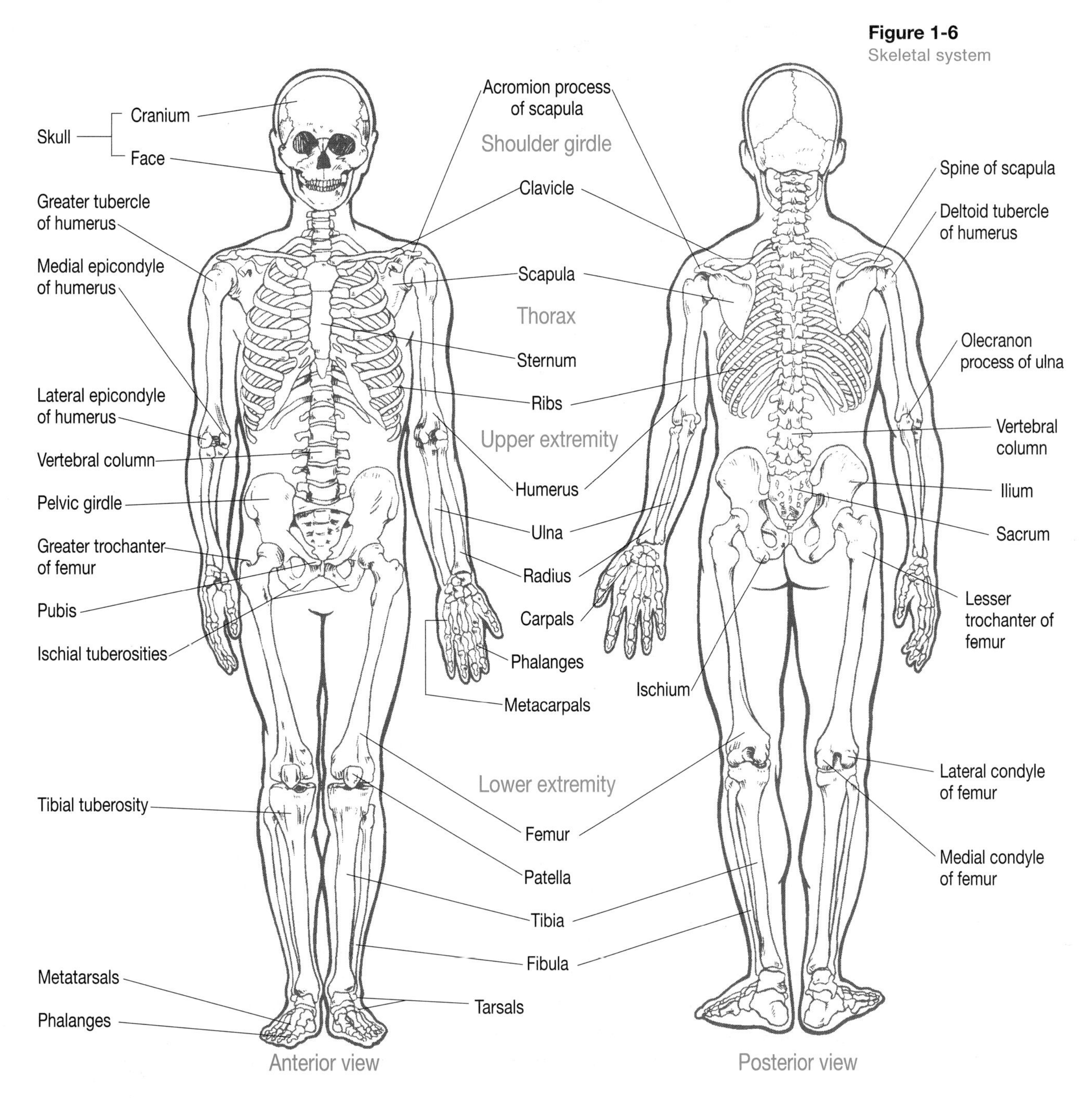

Figure 1-6
Skeletal system

sites for most muscles, which play an important role in movement. Many of the body's muscles attach to bone, and when the muscles contract, the bones move at their **articulations** (joints). The skeleton also provides protection for many of the body's organs. For example, the skull encases the brain, the vertebrae form a canal around the spinal cord, the rib cage protects the heart and lungs, and the bony pelvis guards the urinary bladder and internal reproductive organs. The skeleton is also a storehouse for two essential minerals—calcium and phosphorous—that are necessary for the proper functioning of other body systems. In addition, fat, sodium, potassium, and other minerals are stored in the bones. Recall that bones are not static structures. They are constantly breaking down to release minerals and other substances into the blood, while simultaneously rebuilding to provide the body with flexible, yet sturdy, structural support. After birth, the skeleton is a production site for blood cells found within the circulatory system (e.g., red blood cells, certain white blood cells, platelets).

The various shapes of bones determine how they are classified (i.e., long, short, flat, irregular). Long bones are so named because they are longer than they are wide, which means that they have a long axis. Most of the bones of the limbs are classified as long bones (e.g., humerus, radius, ulna, femur, tibia, fibula, phalanges). Bones that are approximately the same length and width are called short bones (e.g., carpals, tarsals). Flat bones are thin and typically curved. They include some of the bones of the skull, the ribs, and the sternum. Bones that do not fit into the previous categories are classified as irregular bones because of their diverse shapes (e.g., hip bones, vertebrae, certain skull bones).

Bones are composed of a dense outer layer, called compact or **cortical bone,** and a honeycomb-like inner structure, called spongy or **trabecular bone.** The cortical shell makes up roughly 75% of the skeleton, whereas the trabecular network makes up the remaining 25%. Cortical bone is essential, because it provides strength, **tendon** attachment sites for muscles, and organ protection without excessive weight. Trabecular bone serves two vital purposes. It provides a large surface area for mineral exchange and helps to maintain skeletal strength and integrity. It is particularly abundant in the vertebrae and at the ends of long bones, sites that are under continuous stress from motion and weightbearing. Areas containing a large percentage of trabecular tissue are most likely to fracture when the bone is weakened due to a disease such as **osteoporosis.**

A closer look at a typical long bone reveals its many structures (Figure 1-7). The shaft, called the **diaphysis,** is located between the two ends, which are named the proximal and distal epiphyses (singular = **epiphysis**). The hollow space inside the diaphysis is called the medullary cavity, which is used as a storage site for fat and is sometimes called the yellow bone marrow cavity. It is lined by a thin connective-tissue layer called the **endosteum.** The diaphysis and outer layers of the epiphyses are made of cortical bone, whereas trabecular bone is concentrated in the central regions of the epiphyses. Certain long bones contain red marrow—which is essential in the manufacture and maturation of red blood cells, most white blood cells, and platelets—in the trabecular tissue of their epiphyses. An **epiphyseal cartilage,** also called a "growth plate," separates the diaphysis and epiphysis in children and young adults, providing a means for the bone to increase in length. In adults, when skeletal growth has been completed, the epiphyseal cartilage is replaced by bone and the area is called the epiphyseal line. A dense connective-tissue layer called the **periosteum** covers the outer surface of bone and is well supplied with blood vessels and nerves, some of which enter the bone.

Throughout life, the human skeleton is continuously being broken down while simultaneously being restored. In fact, most

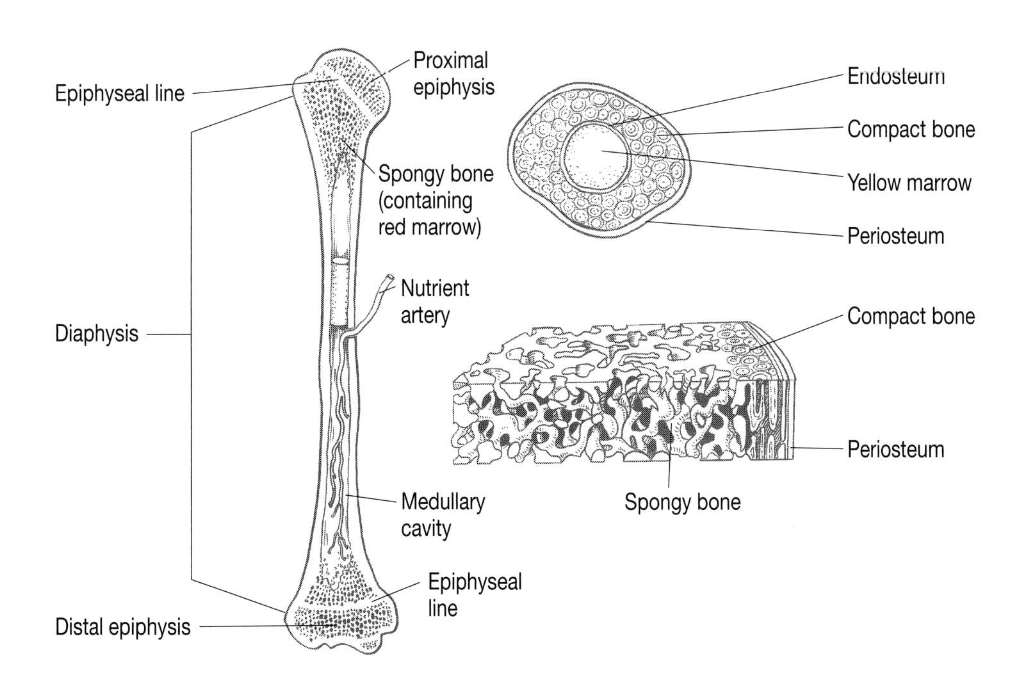

Figure 1-7
Long bone gross anatomy

of the adult skeleton is replaced approximately every 10 years. In adults, a process called remodeling is responsible for the continual reshaping and rebuilding of the skeleton in response to internal and external signals from specialized bone cells that either build bone (**osteoblasts**) or break it down (**osteoclasts**). Remodeling is vital for bone health for several reasons. First, the remodeling process repairs damage to the skeleton that can result from repeated stresses. It also prevents the accumulation of too much old bone, which can lose its resilience and become brittle. Furthermore, remodeling plays an important role in removing calcium and phosphorous from the bones when these minerals are deficient in the diet or when an increased need exists due to pregnancy or lactation.

Although the size and shape of the skeleton is genetically determined, it can be greatly affected by loading or impact from physical activity. Ultimately, a bone's size and shape fits best with its function. In other words, "form follows function." **Wolff's law** indicates that changes in bone structure coincide with changes in bone function. That is, when the skeleton is subjected to stressful forces, such as those that occur with exercise, it responds by laying down more bone tissue, thereby increasing its density. Conversely, when individuals experience prolonged periods of bed rest due to illness or injury, their bones lose mineral and become less dense. Maintaining adequate bone density is an important issue for all adults. Fitness professionals can play a crucial role in helping clients preserve bone tissue by educating them about the importance of exercise and proper nutrition.

Axial Skeleton

Of the 206 bones that make up the skeleton, 80 are categorized as the axial skeleton (Table 1-3). Consisting of the skull, vertebral column, sternum, and ribs, the axial skeleton's most important functions are to provide the main axial support for the body and protect the central nervous system and the organs of the thorax. Fitness professionals should have a fundamental knowledge of the structure of the vertebral column, since the mechanics of the spine affect all exercise performance. The vertebral column consists of 33 vertebrae, which are categorized by regions (Figure 1-8). The upper region (neck area) of the spine contains seven cervical vertebrae, which are the smallest and most delicate. The mid-region, below the cervical vertebrae, contains 12 thoracic vertebrae that are each attached to a rib. The lower region consists of five lumbar vertebrae, the sacrum (five fused vertebrae), and the coccyx (four fused vertebrae). The lumbar vertebrae are the largest and heaviest vertebrae due to their role in continuously receiving ground reaction forces and axial compression forces.

Appendicular Skeleton

The remaining 126 bones are categorized as the appendicular skeleton, which includes the bones of the upper and lower limbs and the pectoral (shoulder) and pelvic (hip) girdles (see Table 1-3). The pectoral and pelvic girdles represent the means by which the appendicular skeleton articulates (joins together) with the axial skeleton. Although the pectoral girdle (clavicle and scapula) attaches to the axial skeleton only at the sternum and provides little support for the upper-body structures, the support is sufficient because the upper limbs do not bear the body's weight. This minimal connection with the axial skeleton allows the pectoral girdle to express a wide range of movements at the shoulder. In contrast, the pelvic girdle (ilium, ischium, and pubis—known collectively as the os coxae) does support the body's weight and therefore has more extensive attachments to the axial skeleton through its articulation with the sacrum (see Figure 1-6). Furthermore, each side of the pelvic girdle is united by a strong joint made of cartilage called the pubic symphysis.

Articulations

The bones of the skeleton come together at articulations (joints.) When two bones meet at a junction, they are said to "articulate" with each other (e.g., the femur articulates inferiorly with the tibia). While most joints allow movement between two bones, some permit little, if any, movement. The three main types of joints are fibrous, cartilaginous, and synovial. Fibrous joints are held tightly together by fibrous connective tissue and allow little or no movement. They are classified as synarthroidal (syn = together; arthron = joint). In other words, synarthroidal joints are considered immovable joints and include the

Table 1-3
Bones in the Axial and Appendicular Skeletons

Axial Skeleton	Number of Bones
Skull	
Cranium	8
Face	14
Hyoid	1
Vertebral Column	26
Thorax	
Sternum	1
Ribs	24
(Auditory ossicles)*	6
	80

Appendicular Skeleton	Number of Bones
Lower Extremity	
Phalanges	28
Metatarsals	10
Tarsals	14
Patella	2
Tibia	2
Fibula	2
Femur	2
Pelvic Girdle	
Hip or pelvis (os coxae = ilium, ischium, pubis)	2
Shoulder Girdle	
Clavicle	2
Scapula	2
Upper Extremity	
Phalanges	28
Metacarpals	10
Carpals	16
Radius	2
Ulna	2
Humerus	2
	126

* The auditory ossicles, three per ear, are not considered part of the axial or appendicular skeletons, but rather a separate group of bones. They were placed in the axial skeleton group for convenience.

sutures of the skull and the joint between the distal ends of the tibia and fibula (Figure 1-9). In cartilaginous joints, the bones are connected by cartilage and little or no movement is allowed. A characteristic of one type of cartilaginous joint, a symphysis, is the fibrocartilaginous pad, or disc, that separates the two bones. The junction of the two pubic bones (pubic symphysis) and the junctions between the bodies of adjacent vertebrae (see Figure 1-8) are examples of symphyses.

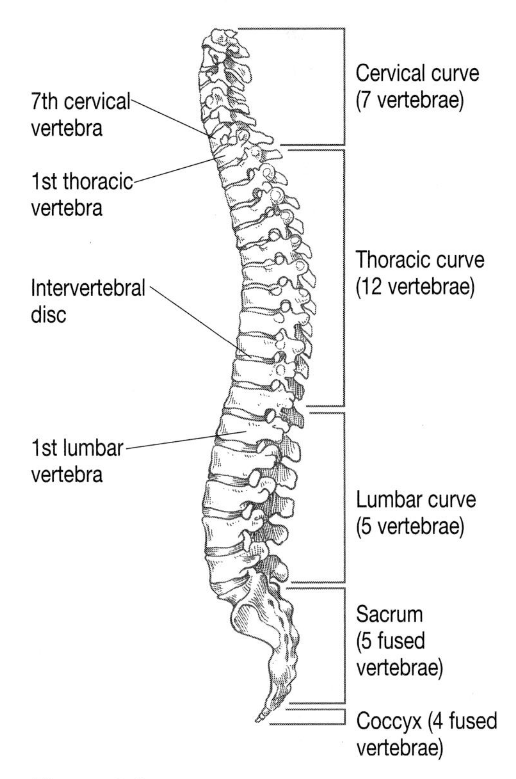

Figure 1-8
Vertebral column (lateral view)

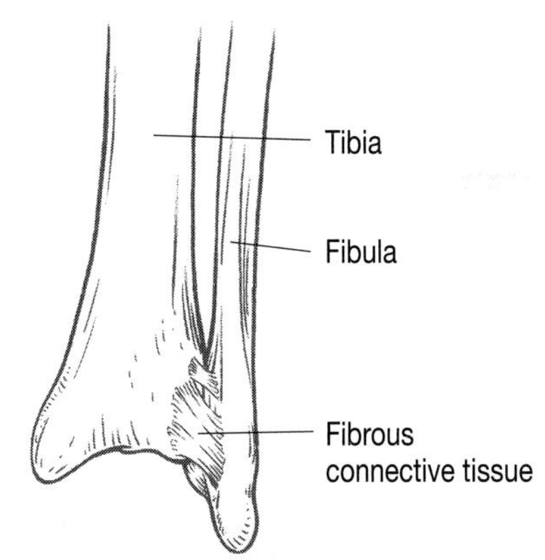

Figure 1-9
Example of a fibrous joint

The most common type of joint in the body is the synovial joint, which is freely moveable. Because of this freedom, synovial joints are classified as diarthroses (diarthrosis means "through joint"). Synovial joints have four characteristic traits: an articular cartilage, an articular capsule, a synovial membrane, and synovial fluid. Articular cartilage refers to the hyaline cartilage (from the Greek word *hyalos,* meaning glass) that covers the end surfaces of long bones. The articular capsule encloses the joint with a double-layered membrane. The outer layer is composed of a dense fibrous tissue that forms **ligaments** to strengthen the joint. The inner layer is the synovial membrane, which is well supplied with capillaries and produces a thick fluid called synovial fluid. The fluid nourishes the articular cartilages and lubricates the joint surfaces. Some synovial joints also have articular discs made of fibrocartilage, such as the menisci in the knee. The medial and lateral meniscus help absorb shock in the knee, increase joint stability, direct synovial fluid to aid in nourishment of the knee, and increase joint contact surface area, thereby decreasing overall pressure on the joint.

Movements of Synovial Joints

Synovial joints move depending on the shapes of their bony structures and their articular surfaces. A joint's **axis of rotation** allows it to move in various planes, where the plane of movement is generally perpendicular to the axis. The axis of rotation is an imaginary line that forms a right angle to the plane of movement about which a joint rotates. For example, the bones of the elbow allow the forearm to move anteriorly and posteriorly (**sagittal plane**) around an imaginary horizontal line that passes through it from side to side (transverse axis of rotation) (Figure 1-10). To review which planes of movement are perpendicular to each other, see Figure 1-1. Some joints have more than one axis of rotation, allowing them to move in various planes. Joints that move in one plane only and have one axis of rotation are called uniaxial joints. These joints are also called "hinge" joints, because hinges (like those on a door) allow movement in only one plane. The ankles and elbows are examples of uniaxial joints.

Joints that allow movement in two planes that are perpendicular to each other are called biaxial joints. Examples of biaxial joints are the foot, knee, hand, and wrist. Biaxial joint movement can be observed when the index finger (first phalanx) moves anteriorly and posteriorly (sagittal plane movement around a transverse axis) and laterally and medially (**frontal plane** movement around a sagittal axis) (see Figure 1-10). Still other joints permit movement in three axes of rotation. These are called triaxial joints and include the hip, thumb, and shoulder. The shoulder, for example, allows the humerus to move anteriorly and posteriorly; laterally and medially; and rotate internally and externally (**transverse plane** movement around a longitudinal axis) (see Figure 1-10). A summary of the major joints in the body, classified by type and movements, is presented in Table 1-4.

Figure 1-10
Movement of synovial (diarthrodial) joints

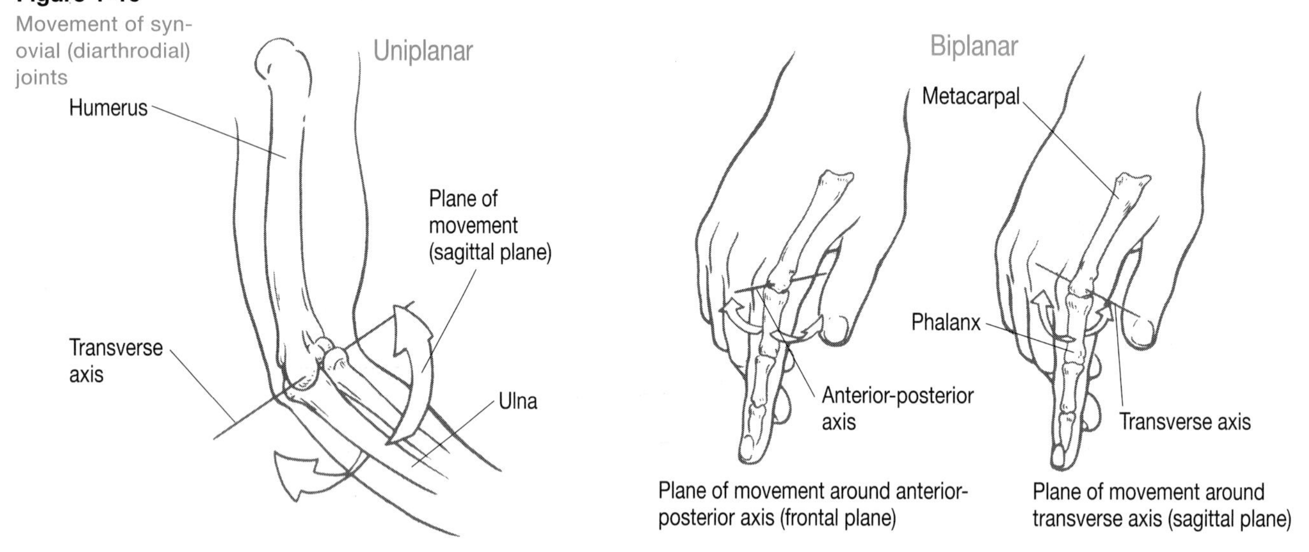

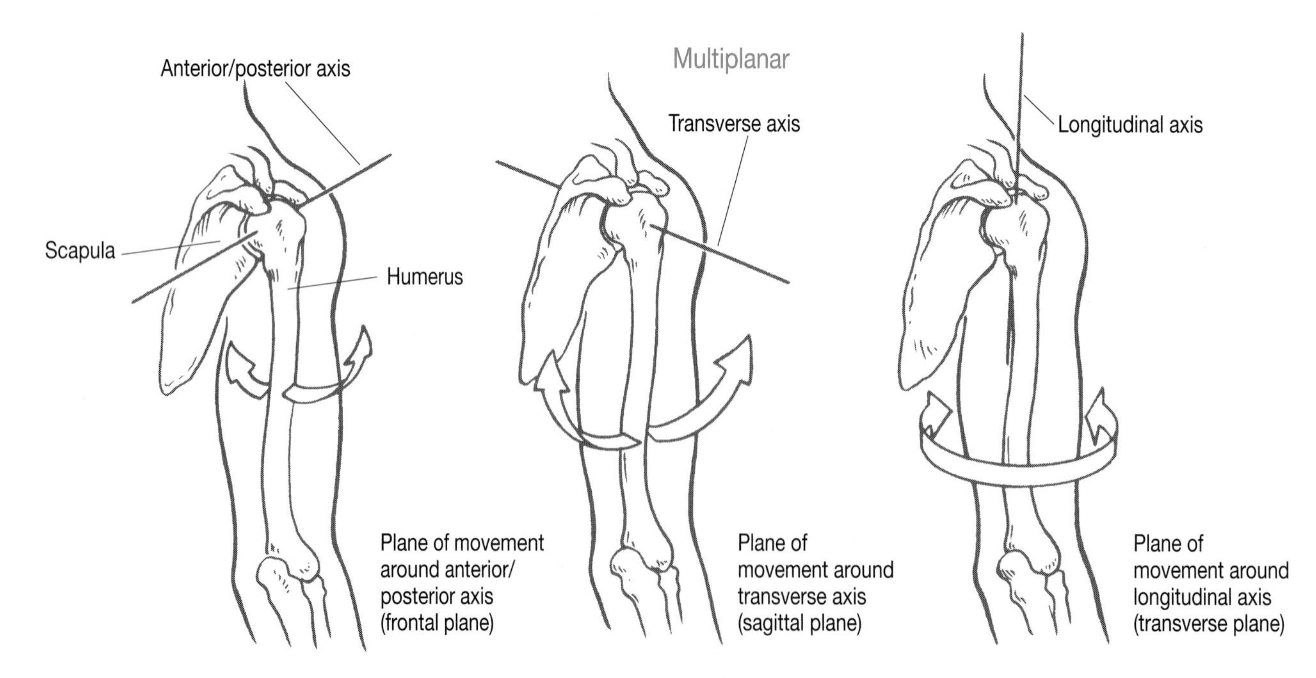

There are four general groups of movements that occur in synovial joints throughout the body: gliding, angular, **circumduction,** and rotation. In gliding, the surfaces of two adjoining bones move back and forth upon each other. An example of a gliding joint is the articulation between the head of a rib and the body of its associated vertebra. Angular movement describes an increase or decrease in the angle between two adjoining bones. There are four angular movements defined for synovial joints: flexion, extension, abduction, and adduction. Flexion describes movement in which the bones comprising a joint move toward each other in the sagittal plane, decreasing the joint angle between them. An example is bringing the forearm upward toward the upper arm, as in elbow flexion. Extension is the opposite of flexion and causes the angle between two adjoining bones to increase in the sagittal plane. An example is starting with the calf upward toward the back of the thigh and moving it downward away from the thigh, as in knee extension (Figure 1-11).

Abduction occurs when a part of the body is moved away from the midline of the body, such as lifting an arm or leg away from the side of the body. Adduction is the opposite of abduction and refers to movement of a body part toward the midline of the body, such as lowering an arm or leg from an abducted position downward toward the side of the body (Figure 1-12).

Table 1-4
Major Joints in the Body

Region/Joint	Type	Number of Axes of Rotation	Movement(s) Possible
Lower Extremity			
Foot (metatarsophalangeal)	Synovial (condyloid)	2	Flexion & extension; abduction & adduction; circumduction
Ankle (talocrural)	Synovial (hinge)	1	Plantarflexion & dorsiflexion
Between distal tibia & fibula	Fibrous	0	Slight movement possible
Knee (tibia & femur)	Synovial (modified hinge)	2	Flexion & extension; internal & external rotation
Hip	Synovial (ball & socket)	3	Flexion & extension; abduction & adduction; circumduction; internal & external rotation
Upper Extremity			
Hand (metacarpophalangeal)	Synovial (condyloid)	2	Flexion & extension; abduction & adduction; circumduction
Thumb	Synovial (saddle)	3	Flexion & extension; abduction & adduction; circumduction; opposition
Wrist (radiocarpal)	Synovial	2	Flexion & extension; abduction & adduction; circumduction
Proximal radioulnar	Synovial (pivot)	1	Pronation & supination
Elbow (ulna & humerus)	Synovial (hinge)	1	Flexion & extension
Shoulder	Synovial (ball & socket)	3	Flexion & extension; abduction & adduction; circumduction; internal & external rotation
Ribs & sternum	Cartilaginous	0	Slight movement possible

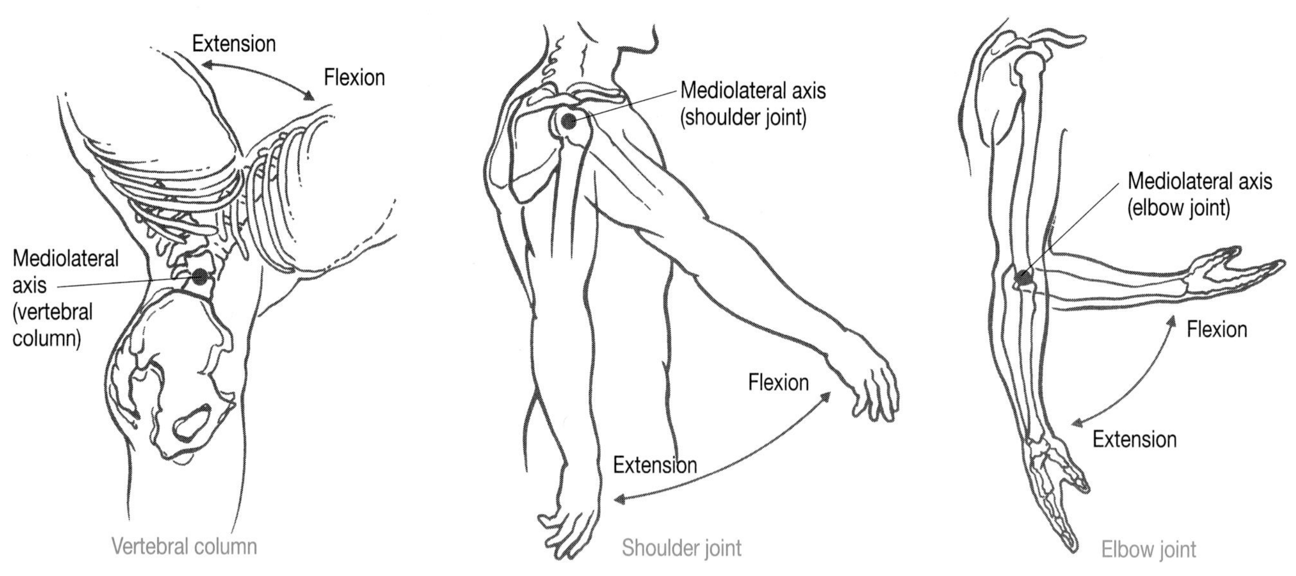

Figure 1-11
Segmental movements in the sagittal plane

Redrawn from *Biomechanics,* 3rd ed., Kreighbaum, E. & Barthels, K. Copyright 1990 by Macmillan Publishing Company. Reprinted by permission of Pearson Education, Inc.

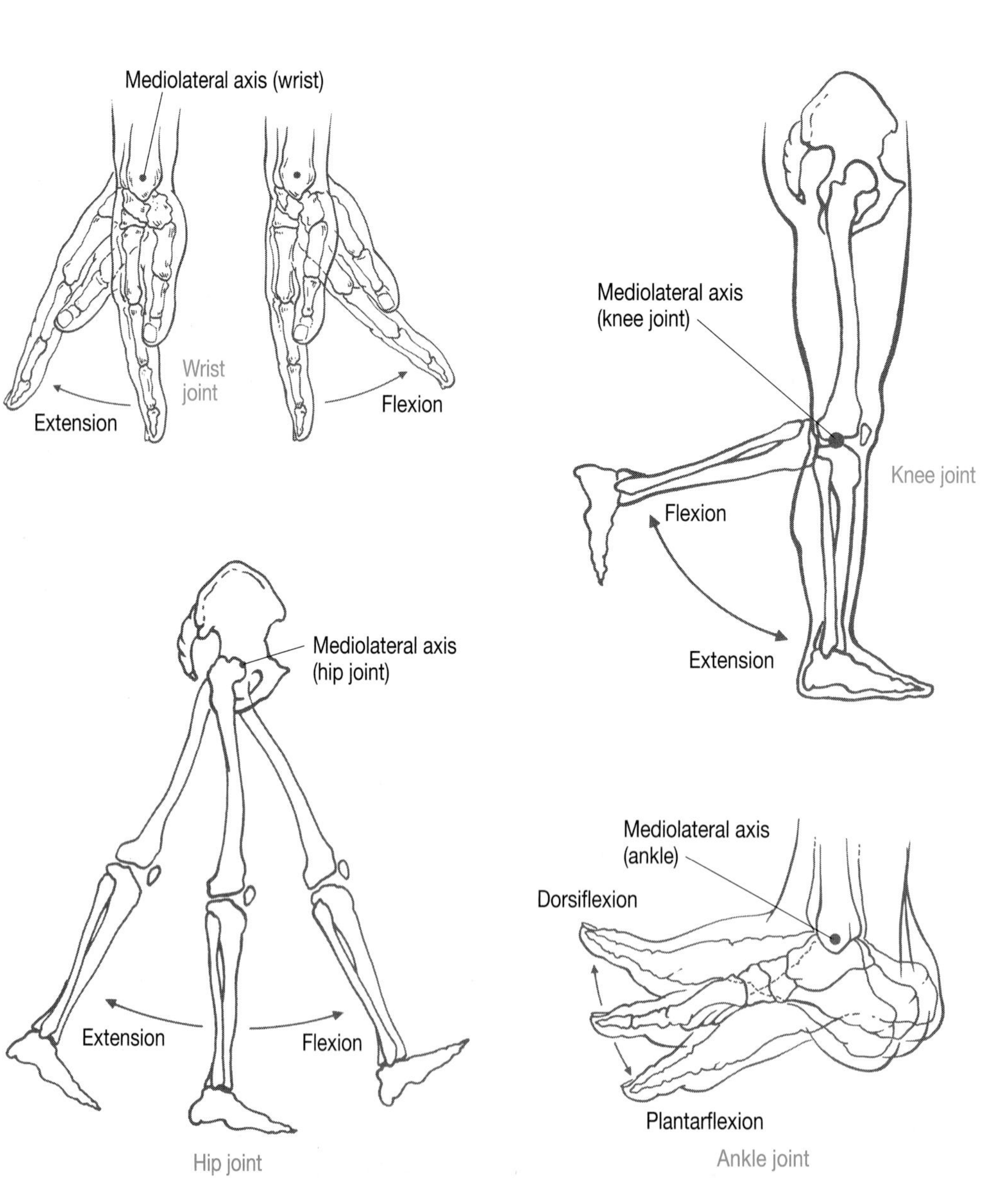

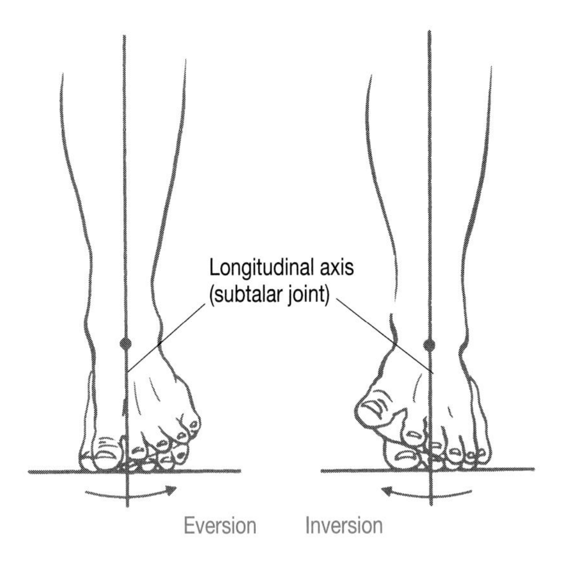

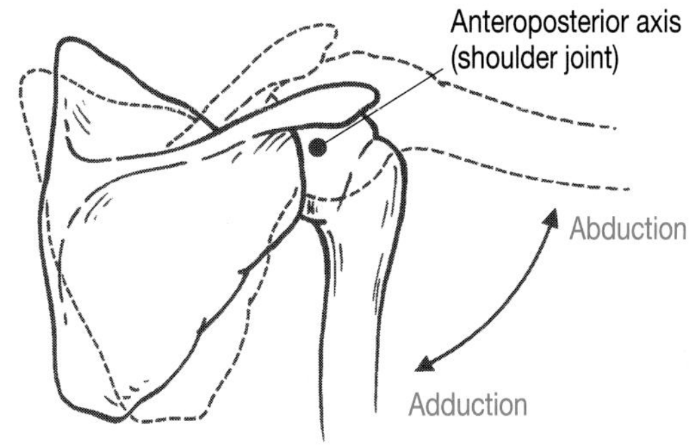

Figure 1-12
Segmental movements in the frontal plane

Redrawn from *Biomechanics,* 3rd ed., Kreighbaum, E. & Barthels, K. Copyright 1990 by Macmillan Publishing Company. Reprinted by permission of Pearson Education, Inc.

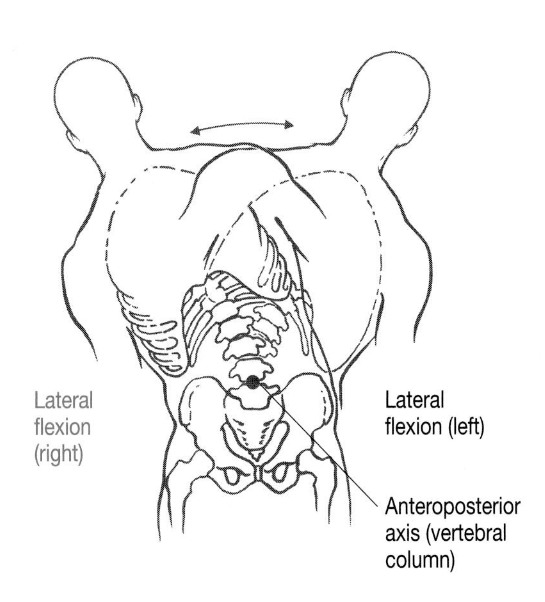

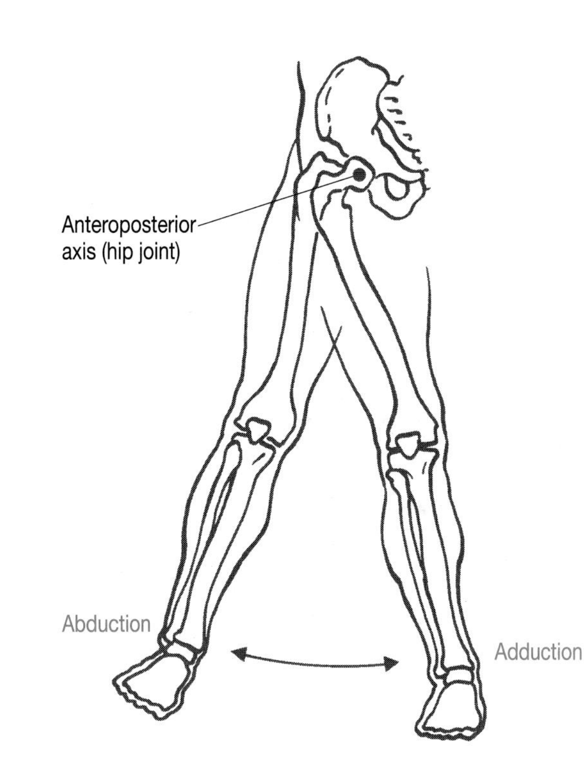

In the case of the fingers and toes, the reference point for abduction and adduction is the midline of the hand and foot, respectively. For example, abduction of the fingers occurs when they move away from the third digit of the hand (i.e., spreading the fingers apart). Conversely, adduction of the fingers refers to the digits moving out of abduction toward the third digit. Abduction of the toes is accomplished by moving them away from the second toe (i.e., spreading the toes apart) and adduction occurs when the toes move out of abduction toward the second toe. All abduction and adduction movements occur in the frontal plane.

Certain joints, such as the shoulder and hip, are capable of incorporating all four angular movements to create one motion called circumduction. That is, the movement is actually a sequential combination of flexion, extension, abduction, and adduction. An easy way to remember circumduction is to picture a swimmer performing arm circles as a warm-up prior to diving in the pool. The circular motion represents circumduction of the shoulder joints.

Rotation describes motion of a bone around a central (longitudinal) axis. From an anatomical position, movement of the anterior surface of the humerus or femur inward is called internal (medial) rotation. Conversely, movement of the anterior surface of humerus or femur outward is called external (lateral) rotation. A specific type of rotation, called pronation and supination, occurs at the radioulnar joint. Rotating the forearm outward so the palm faces anteriorly is supination, whereas rotation of the forearm inward so the palm faces posteriorly is pronation. Anatomical position, therefore, requires supination of the forearm (see Figure 1-1). Rotation around a longitudinal axis occurs in the transverse plane. This also includes rotation of the spine and inversion and eversion of the foot (Figure 1-13). A summary of all the synovial joint fundamental movements is presented in Table 1-5.

Neuromuscular System

The overall function of the nervous system is to collect information about external conditions in relation to the body's external state, analyze this information, and initialize appropriate responses to fulfill specific needs. In other words, the nervous system gathers information, stores it, and controls various bodily systems in response to this input. The muscular system, which is composed of more than 600 individual muscles, is responsible for movement of various body parts. The neuromuscular system is the connection of the muscles to the brain and spinal cord through a network of nerve circuits that direct the ebb and flow of muscular energy.

Neural Organization

The nervous system is separated into various divisions based on either structural or

Table 1-5
Fundamental Movements (From Anatomical Position)

Plane	Action	Definition
Sagittal	Flexion	Decreasing the angle between two bones
	Extension	Increasing the angle between two bones
	Dorsiflexion	Moving the top of the foot toward the shin (only at the ankle joint)
	Plantarflexion	Moving the sole of the foot downward; "pointing the toes" (only at the ankle)
Frontal	Abduction	Motion away from the midline of the body (or part)
	Adduction	Motion toward the midline of the body (or part)
	Elevation	Moving to a superior position (only at the scapula)
	Depression	Moving to an inferior position (only at the scapula)
	Inversion	Lifting the medial border of the foot (only at the subtalar joint)
	Eversion	Lifting the lateral border of the foot (only at the subtalar joint)
Transverse	Rotation	Internal (inward) or external (outward) turning about the vertical axis of bone
	Pronation	Rotating the hand and wrist medially from the elbow
	Supination	Rotating the hand and wrist laterally from the elbow
	Horizontal flexion	From a 90-degree abducted arm position, the humerus is flexed in toward the midline of the body in the transverse plane
	Horizontal extension	The return of the humerus from horizontal flexion
Multiplanar	Circumduction	Motion that describes a "cone"; combines flexion, extension, abduction, and adduction in sequence
	Opposition	Thumb movement unique to humans and primates

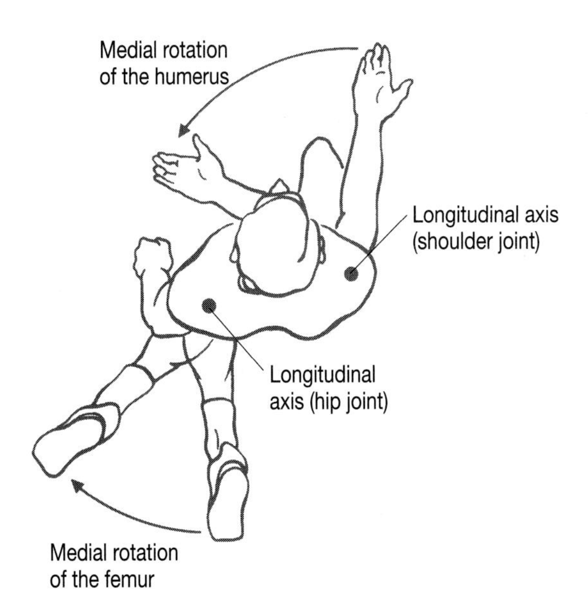

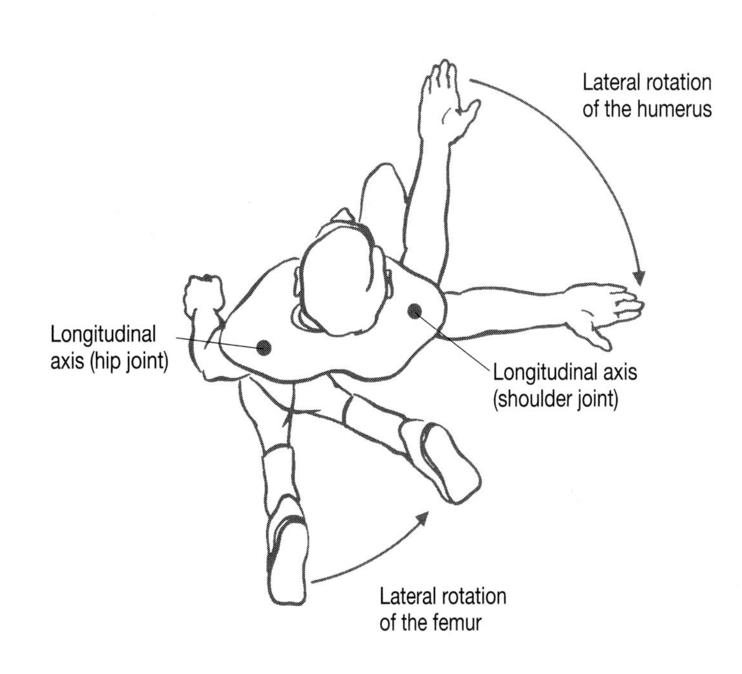

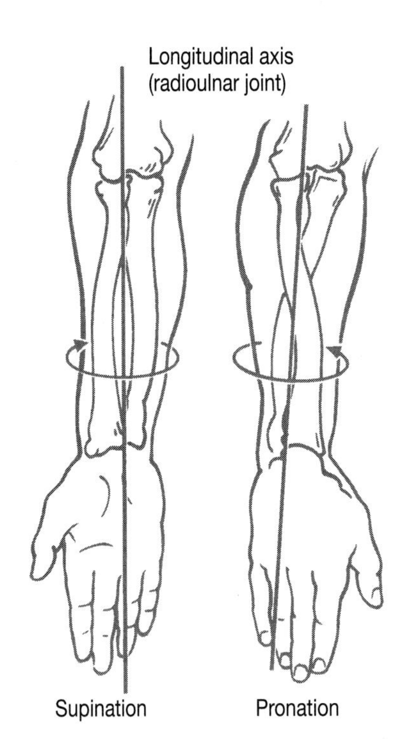

Figure 1-13
Segmental movements in the transverse plane

Redrawn from *Biomechanics,* 3rd ed., Kreighbaum, E. & Barthels, K. Copyright 1990 by Macmillan Publishing Company. Reprinted by permission of Pearson Education, Inc.

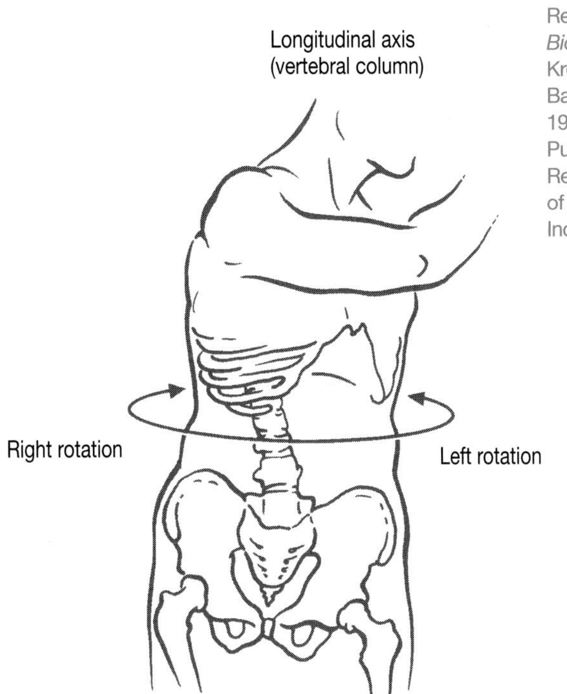

functional characteristics. Keep in mind that these divisions—which are called nervous systems themselves—are still part of a single, overall nervous system. In terms of structure, the nervous system is divided into two parts: the **central nervous system (CNS)** and the **peripheral nervous system (PNS).** The CNS consists of the brain and spinal cord, which are both encased and protected by bony structures—the skull and the vertebral column, respectively. The CNS is responsible for receiving sensory input from the PNS and formulating responses to this input. This makes the CNS the integrative and control center of the nervous system. The PNS is composed of all the nervous structures located outside of the CNS, namely the nerves and **ganglia** (nerve cell bodies associated with the nerves). In part, the PNS is made up of pairings of nerves that branch out from the brain and spinal cord from different regions. Twelve pairs of cranial nerves, which arise from the brain and brain stem, exit the cranial cavity through **foramina** (small holes) in the skull. Thirty-one pairs of spinal nerves, which arise from the spinal cord, exit the vertebral column through intervertebral foramina. Named for the region of the spine where they originate and the vertebral level from which they emerge, the paired spinal nerves are classified as eight cervical, 12 thoracic, five lumbar, five sacral, and one coccygeal (Figure 1-14). A list of the spinal nerve roots and the muscles they innervate is presented in Table 1-6.

In terms of function, the PNS is separated into two categories: the afferent (sensory)

Figure 1-14
Spinal cord and spinal nerves (posterior view)

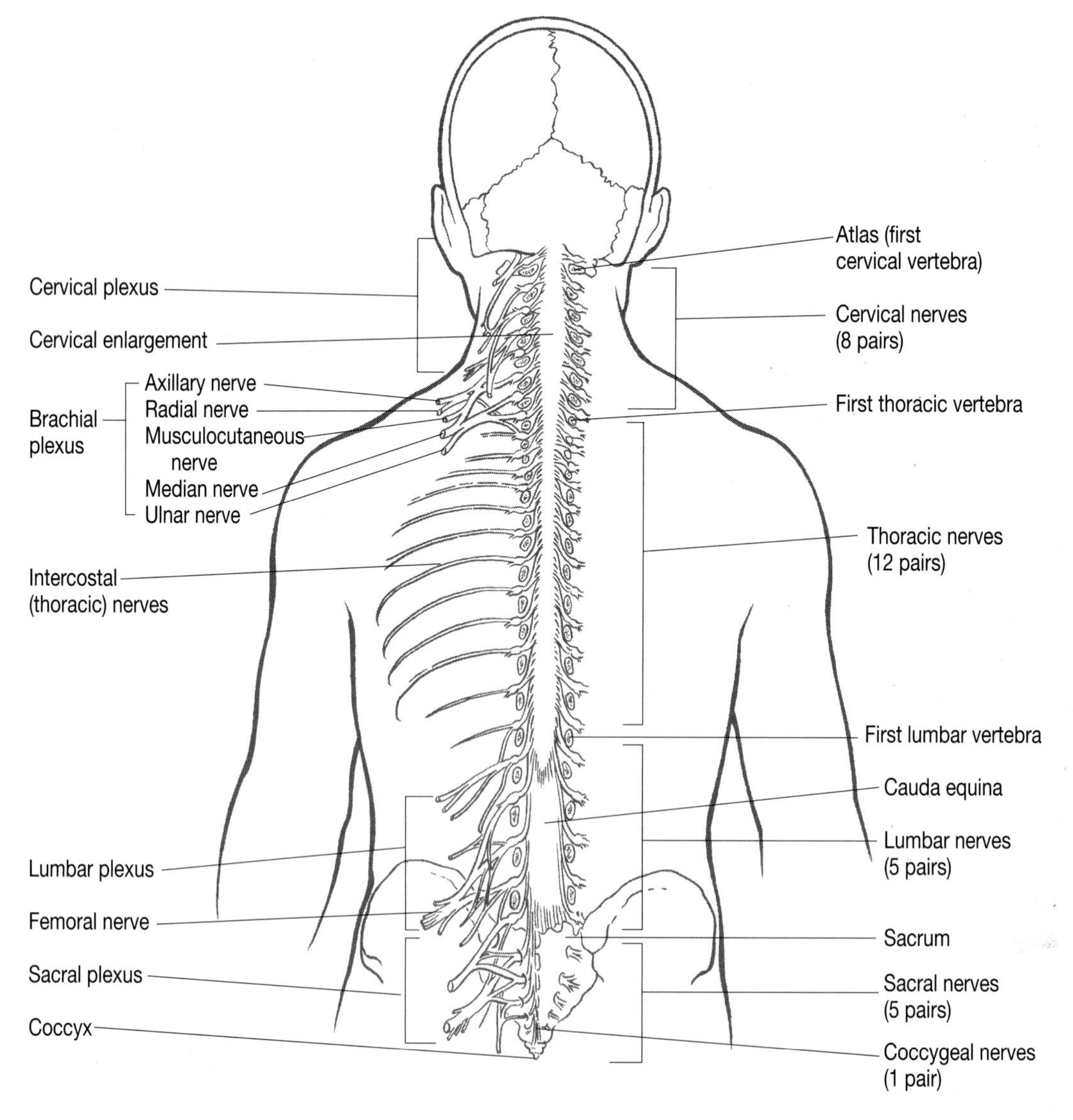

Table 1-6
Selected Spinal Nerve Roots and Major Muscles Innervated

Nerve Root	Muscles Innervated
C5	Biceps brachii, deltoid, supraspinatus, infraspinatus
C6	Brachioradialis, supinator, extensor carpi radialis longus and brevis, extensor carpi ulnaris
C7	Triceps brachii, flexor carpi radialis, flexor carpi ulnaris
C8	Extensor pollicis longus and brevis, adductor pollicis longus
T1	Intrinsic muscles of the hand (lumbricals, interossei)
L2	Psoas major and minor, adductor magnus, adductor longus, adductor brevis
L3	Rectus femoris, vastus lateralis, vastus medialis, vastus intermedius, psoas major and minor
L4	Tibialis anterior, tibialis posterior
L5	Extensor hallucis longus, extensor digitorum longus, peroneus longus and brevis, gluteus maximus, gluteus medius
S1	Gastrocnemius, soleus, biceps femoris, semitendinosus, semimembranosus, gluteus maximus
S2	Gluteus maximus, flexor hallucis longus, flexor digitorum longus
S4	Bladder, rectum

division and the efferent (motor) division. The afferent division carries nerve impulses to the CNS from receptors located in the skin, **fascia,** joints, and visceral organs. In other words, afferent sensory data is incoming information. In contrast, the efferent division handles outgoing information and can be divided into the somatic and autonomic nervous systems. The somatic nervous system is mostly under conscious control and carries nerve impulses from the CNS to the skeletal muscles. In some instances, muscle contractions brought on by the somatic nervous system are not consciously controlled, such as in the case of a reflex response. The autonomic nervous system is made up of nerves that transmit impulses to the smooth muscles, cardiac muscle, and glands. These visceral motor impulses generally cannot be consciously controlled. The autonomic nervous system is further divided into the sympathetic and parasympathetic divisions. The sympathetic nervous system is activated when there is a stressor or an emergency, such as severe pain, anger, or fear. Called the "fight or flight" response, this activation affects nearly every organ to enable the body to stop storing energy and mobilize all resources to respond to the stressful event or activity. The **parasympathetic nervous system** aids in controlling normal functions when the body is relaxed; it aids in digesting food, storing energy, and promoting growth.

Structures of the Nervous System

The most basic structural and functional component of the nervous system is the neuron (nerve cell). The neuron is composed of a cell body (soma) and one or more processes—fibrous extensions called **dendrites** and **axons** (Figure 1-15). Dendrites conduct electrical impulses toward the cell body, while axons transmit electrical signals away from the cell body. Neurons may have hundreds of the branching dendrites, depending on the neuron type, but each neuron has only one axon. For an electrical impulse to travel through

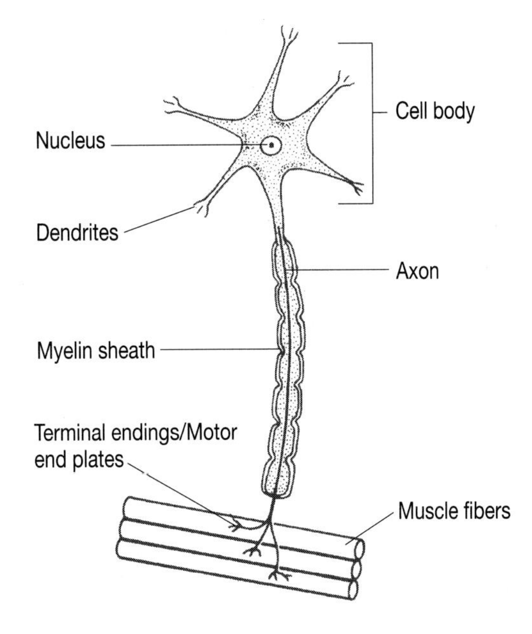

Figure 1-15
Basic anatomical structure of a motor neuron (or nerve cell) and motor end plate

the nervous system, it must be passed from one neuron to the next. Most neurons do not have direct contact with each other. Instead, neurons remain separated from each other by a small space called a **synapse.** To carry the impulse across the synapse from one neuron to the other, the first neuron releases a chemical transmitter substance that attaches to receptors located on the membrane of the second neuron. Most axons are covered with a fatty substance called **myelin,** which insulates the axon and keeps the electrical current from migrating outside of the neuron. A nerve is made up of the processes of many neurons held together by connective tissue sheaths. Sensory nerves carry impulses to the CNS, whereas motor nerves carry nerve impulses from the CNS to the PNS. Motor neurons form a **neuromuscular junction** with the skeletal muscles they supply.

Proprioception

The sense of knowing where the body is in relation to its various segments and the external environment is called **proprioception.** The sensory information gathered to achieve this kinesthetic awareness comes from structures called **proprioceptors,** which are internal receptors located in the skin, in and around the joints and muscles, and in the inner ear. Cutaneous receptors are located in the skin and send sensory information regarding pressure, touch, and movement of the hairs on the skin. Joint receptors are located in the joint capsules and the surrounding ligaments. They transmit sensory information relating to positions, velocities, and accelerations occurring at the joints. In addition, pressure receptors within the joints provide added information about pressure changes that is used for important postural adjustments and normal gait.

Another type of proprioceptor, the musculotendinous receptor, is involved in muscular control and coordination. There are two such types of receptors—the **Golgi tendon organ (GTO)** and the **muscle spindle.** Connected to approximately 15 to 20 muscle fibers and located between the muscle belly and its tendon, the GTO senses increased tension within its associated muscle when the muscle contracts or is stretched. One of the GTO's functions when it senses muscle contraction is to cause an inhibition of the contraction (**autogenic inhibition**). It has been theorized that this function adjusts muscle output in response to fatigue. That is, when muscle tension is reduced due to fatigue, GTO output is also reduced, which lowers its inhibitory effect in its own muscle and allows the muscle to increase its contractile ability. Furthermore, GTO activation results in an enhanced contraction of the opposing (**antagonist**) muscle group. Both of these properties have important implications in flexibility because a muscle can be stretched more fully and easily when the GTOs have inhibited the muscle's contraction and allowed the antagonistic muscle group to contract more readily.

A second type of musculotendinous receptor, the muscle spindle, is located mostly in the muscle belly and lies parallel to the muscle fibers. This arrangement causes the muscle spindle to stretch when the muscle itself experiences a stretch force, thereby exciting the muscle spindle and causing a reflexive contraction in the muscle known as the stretch reflex. The muscle spindle's reflex contraction of its associated muscle simultaneously causes the antagonist muscle group to relax (**reciprocal inhibition**). For example, if the gastrocnemius is stretched rapidly, the muscle spindles within the muscle belly cause it to contract. At the same time, if the opposing muscle group (tibialis anterior) is contracting, the muscle spindle reflex causes it to relax. The muscle spindles and the GTOs work together through their reflexive actions to regulate muscle stiffness, and therefore, contribute largely to the body's sense of postural control (Figure 1-16).

The body relies on the vestibular system for sensory information related to the position of the head in space and sudden changes in the directional movement of the head. Located in the inner ear, the vestibular system is composed of three fluid-containing semicircular canals that lie at right angles to each other.

Each canal contains sensory hair cells that detect the movement of the fluid in the canals. When the angular position of the head changes, fluid rushes over the hair cells and causes them to bend. This response signals to the CNS the direction of the head's rotation and the position of the head during movement. The vestibular system functions to coordinate many motor responses and helps stabilize the eyes to maintain postural stability during stance and locomotion.

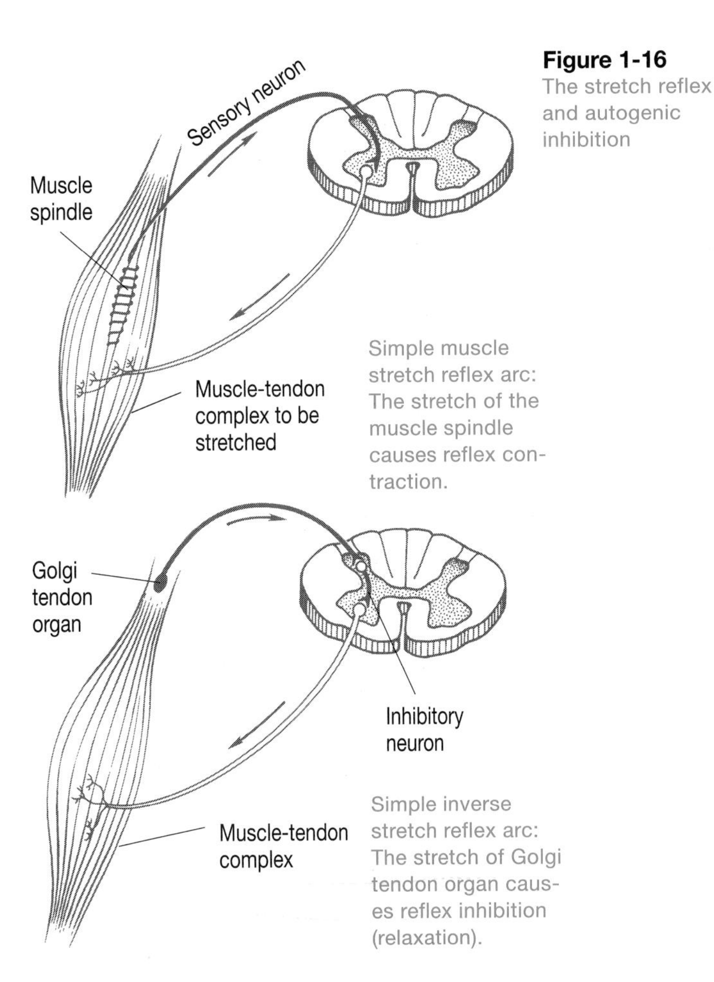

Figure 1-16
The stretch reflex and autogenic inhibition

Muscular System

Muscle tissue is categorized into different types based on its function, is controlled both voluntarily and involuntarily, and is able to produce various levels of force based on its size and shape. One property that all muscle tissue has in common is its ability to contract and develop tension. There are three types of muscle tissue—skeletal muscle, smooth muscle, and cardiac muscle. Skeletal muscle attaches to the skeleton and, through contraction, exerts force on the bones and moves them. Skeletal muscle is considered voluntary muscle because it is normally under the conscious control of the individual. When viewed under a microscope, skeletal muscle tissue exhibits alternating light and dark bands, giving it a striped appearance. This characteristic is the reason skeletal muscle is also called striated muscle.

Smooth muscle is found in the walls of hollow organs and tubes, such as the stomach, intestines, and blood vessels, and functions to regulate the movement of materials through the body. It is named smooth muscle because it lacks the striated appearance of skeletal muscle. Because it is not under conscious control, it is considered involuntary. Cardiac muscle forms the wall of the heart and is a very specialized tissue that functions to maintain the constant pumping action of the heart. Cardiac tissue is involuntary, like smooth muscle, and is striated in appearance, just like skeletal muscle.

Muscle Function

Because of skeletal muscle's role in movement and physical activity, it is the main focus of this section. Before going into detail about skeletal muscle structure and function, a brief discussion about certain connective tissues is necessary. At each end of the belly of most skeletal muscles, a specialized form of connective tissue, called a tendon, attaches the muscle to the bones. Tendons are typically defined as either tendons of **origin** or tendons of **insertion.** The tendon of origin is usually attached to the proximal bone of a joint, which is typically the less mobile of the two bones that make up the joint. In contrast, the tendon of insertion is typically attached to the more distal bone of a joint, which is usually the more moveable of the two bones that make up the joint. When describing the attachment sites of muscles, it is common to state the origin and insertion of the muscle. For example, the brachialis muscle originates on the anterior humerus and inserts on the ulnar tuberosity and coronoid process of the ulna.

Understanding the origins and insertions of the major muscle groups is important for all fitness professionals. Fundamentally, skeletal muscles perform their required tasks by pulling on bones to create joint movement. That is, when a muscle contracts, its origin and insertion attachments move closer together. In contrast, when a muscle is stretched, its origin and insertion points move farther apart. Correct anatomical knowledge of muscle attachments is crucial when designing safe and effective exercise programs, but there is more to consider. Each joint movement incorporates all of the supporting structures surrounding it. Pairings of muscles called **agonists** and antagonists help to illustrate this point. A muscle that creates a major movement is called a primary mover, or agonist. The muscle on the opposite side of the joint is called an opposing muscle, or antagonist. For example, the quadriceps muscle group in the front of the thigh produces knee extension. When the quadriceps contracts to extend the knee, it is considered the agonist muscle group, whereas on the opposite side of the joint, the hamstrings (antagonist) is being stretched. This type of functional pairing of muscle groups is found throughout the body.

When visually comparing the various skeletal muscles, it is evident that they come in different shapes and muscle-fiber arrangements (Figure 1-17). These characteristics vary from muscle to muscle because of functionality. In some muscles, the muscle fibers run parallel to the long axis of the muscle, forming a long, strap-like arrangement. This type of muscle is classified as a longitudinal muscle, and although it is capable of producing considerable movement, it is relatively weak compared to other muscle-fiber arrangements. The sartorius muscle of the thigh is an example of a longitudinal muscle. Other muscles have a tendon that runs the entire length of the muscle, with the muscle fibers inserting diagonally into the tendon. In some muscles of this type, all of the muscle fibers insert onto one side of the tendon (unipennate), and in others, the muscle fibers insert obliquely onto each side of the tendon (bipennate). Unipennate (e.g., tibialis anterior) and bipennate (e.g., rectus femoris) muscles typically produce less movement than longitudinal muscles, but are capable of creating greater force during contraction. In multipennate muscles, the muscle fibers have a complex arrangement that involves the convergence of several tendons. The deltoid muscle of the shoulder is a multipennate muscle.

Muscle-fiber Types

Skeletal muscle can be divided into two general categories based on how quickly they contract: **fast-twitch muscle fibers** and **slow-twitch muscle fibers.** Slow-twitch fibers (also called slow-oxidative or type I fibers) contain relatively large amounts of mitochondria and are surrounded by more capillaries than fast-

Figure 1-17
Muscle fiber arrangements

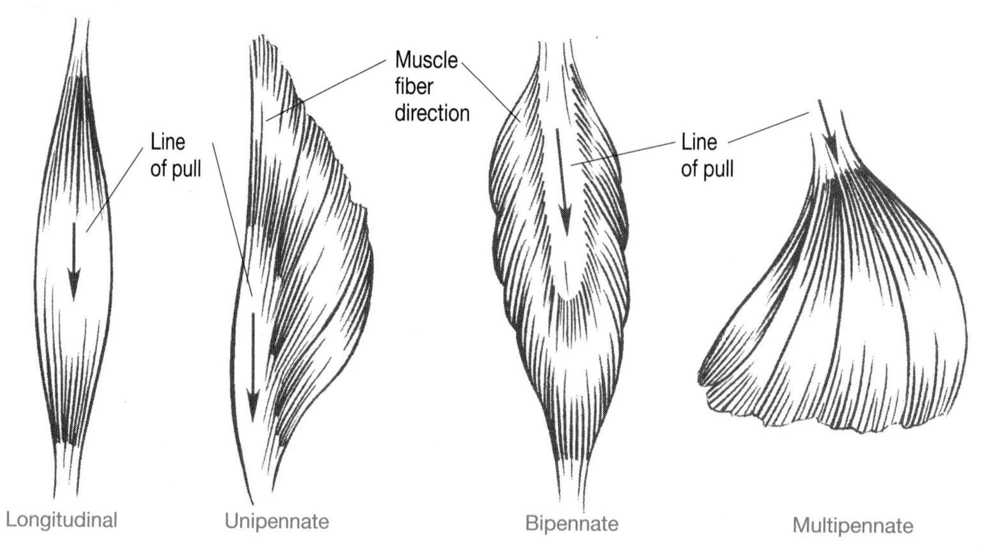

twitch fibers. Additionally, slow-twitch fibers contain higher concentrations of myoglobin than do fast-twitch fibers. The high concentration of myoglobin, the large number of capillaries, and the high mitochondrial content make slow-twitch fibers resistant to fatigue and capable of sustaining aerobic metabolism. As the name implies, slow-twitch fibers contract more slowly than fast-twitch fibers. Furthermore, slow-twitch fibers create lower force outputs and are more efficient than fast-twitch fibers.

It is generally agreed that there are two subtypes of fast-twitch fibers—identified as type IIx and IIa. Traditionally, the fastest type of skeletal muscle fiber in humans has been called the type IIb fiber. However, research in the late 1980s led to the discovery of new properties in the skeletal fast-twitch muscle fibers of both rodents and humans, which has prompted scientists to re-label these fibers as type IIx (Pette, 2001). Type IIx muscle fibers (sometimes called fast-glycolytic fibers) contain a relatively small amount of mitochondria, have a limited capacity for aerobic metabolism, and fatigue more easily than slow-twitch fibers. In fact, these fibers cannot sustain their effort for more than a few seconds. However, they possess a high number of glycolytic enzymes, which provide them with a considerable anaerobic capacity. Type IIx fibers are the largest and fastest, and are capable of producing the most force of all the skeletal muscle fibers, but are notably less efficient than slow-twitch fibers (Shoepe et al., 2003). A second subtype of fast-twitch muscle fibers is the type IIa fiber (also called intermediate or fast-oxidative glycolytic fibers). These fibers possess speed, fatigue, and force-production capabilities somewhere between slow-twitch and type IIx fibers. They are also used for strength and power activities, but can sustain an effort for longer than the type IIx fibers—up to three minutes in highly trained athletes. Type IIa fibers are unique in that they are highly adaptable. That is, with endurance training, they can increase their oxidative capacity to levels similar to those observed in slow-twitch fibers.

A muscle's fiber-type composition is typically an equal mixture of both fast- and slow-twitch fibers, though some muscle groups are known to be made up of primarily fast- or slow-twitch fibers. The percentage of specific fiber types contained in skeletal muscle may be influenced by genetics, hormones, and the activity and exercise habits of the individual. Fiber composition of skeletal muscles is thought to play an important role in sport and exercise performance. It is commonly believed that successful power athletes possess a relatively large percentage of fast-twitch fibers, whereas endurance athletes generally possess a large percentage of slow-twitch fibers. However, it should be noted that muscle-fiber composition is only one variable that determines success in overall physical performance.

Muscle Contraction

Skeletal muscle is composed of tiny, individual muscle cells, called muscle fibers. Muscle fibers are held in place by thin sheets of connective tissue membranes called fasciae (singular = fascia). The fascia that encases the entire muscle is known as the epimysium. Within the epimysium are bundles of muscle fibers that are individually wrapped in a fibrous sheath of fascia known as the perimysium. Within the perimysium are muscle fibers, which are in turn wrapped in a fascia, called endomysium (Figure 1-18).

Muscle-fiber Microanatomy

As noted earlier, when highly magnified with a microscope, skeletal muscle fibers have a cross-striated appearance with alternating light and dark bands. Each muscle fiber contains several hundred to several thousand threadlike **myofibrils** (protein filaments) that run parallel to each other and extend lengthwise throughout the cell. The dark bands, called A bands, contain the protein filament myosin. The light bands, or I bands, is where the protein filament actin is located. Actin filaments also extend into the A bands, where they overlap with the myosin filaments. Crossing the center of each I band is a dense Z line that divides the myofibrils into a series

Figure 1-18
Organization of muscle

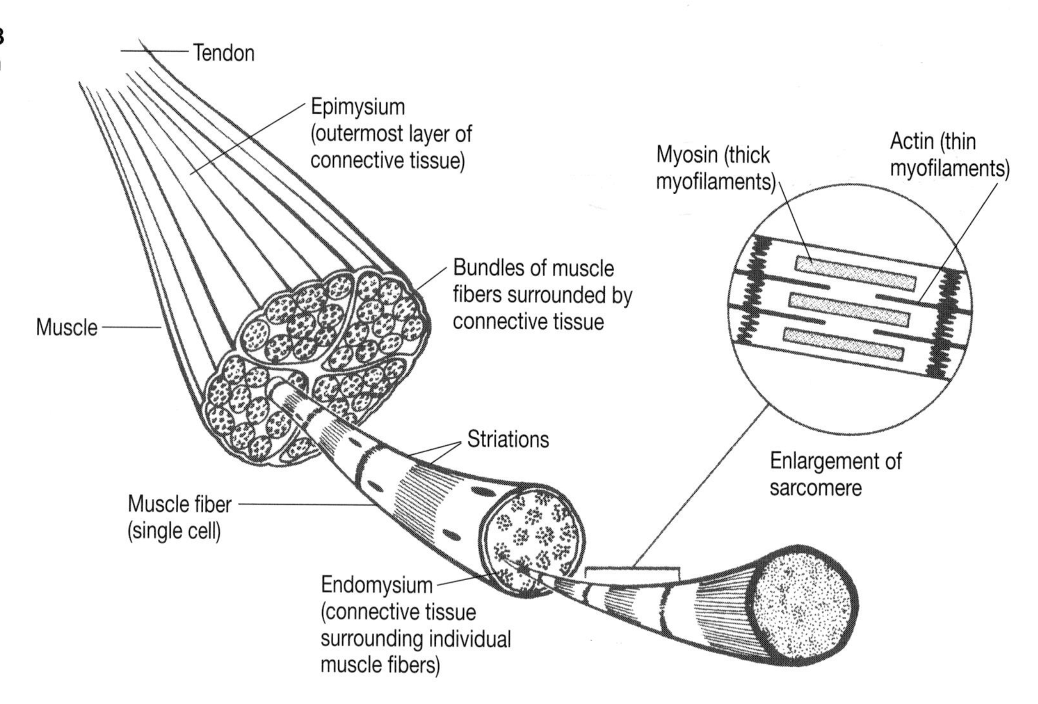

of repeating segments called **sarcomeres.** The sarcomere is considered the functional contracting unit of skeletal muscle, and is the portion of a myofibril that is found between two Z lines. In the center of a sarcomere is a lighter, somewhat less dense area called the H zone. This region is lighter in color, because actin does not extend into this area and the myosin filament becomes thinner in this middle region. A thin, darker M line crosses the center of the H zone. The H zone contains only myosin filaments. Actin filaments are found in the I band and in the part of the A band, up to the H zone. Actin filaments attach directly to the Z lines. The myosin filaments have tiny projections called cross-bridges that reach out at an angle toward the actin filaments.

Sliding Filament Model

When a muscle fiber contracts, the energy used to drive the contraction comes primarily from a substance within the cell called **adenosine triphosphate (ATP).** Muscle contraction occurs when the brain and spinal cord direct motor neurons to release a neurotransmitter called **acetylcholine** at the neuromuscular junction. Once the acetylcholine is detected, calcium is released into the area surrounding the fiber. The calcium exposes binding sites along the actin filament for the myosin filament. As long as there is sufficient ATP, the myosin filaments bind with receptor sites on the actin filaments and cross-bridges are formed. The myosin pulls the actin toward the center and the sarcomere shortens (i.e., the Z lines are pulled closer together) (Figure 1-19). Because all of the sarcomeres shorten simultaneously, the overall length of the muscle fiber is shortened. If multiple muscle fibers are stimulated to contract at the same time, the entire muscle will contract.

Naming Skeletal Muscles

Certain criteria are used in the naming of a muscle, such as its shape, size, and location in the body. These criteria facilitate finding muscles and learning about their specific locations:

- *Shape:* The names of certain muscles include references to their shape (e.g., the rhomboid muscles resemble the geometric shape of a rhomboid).
- *Action:* Some muscle names include references to their actions in the body (e.g., the extensor digitorum longus muscle extends the toes).

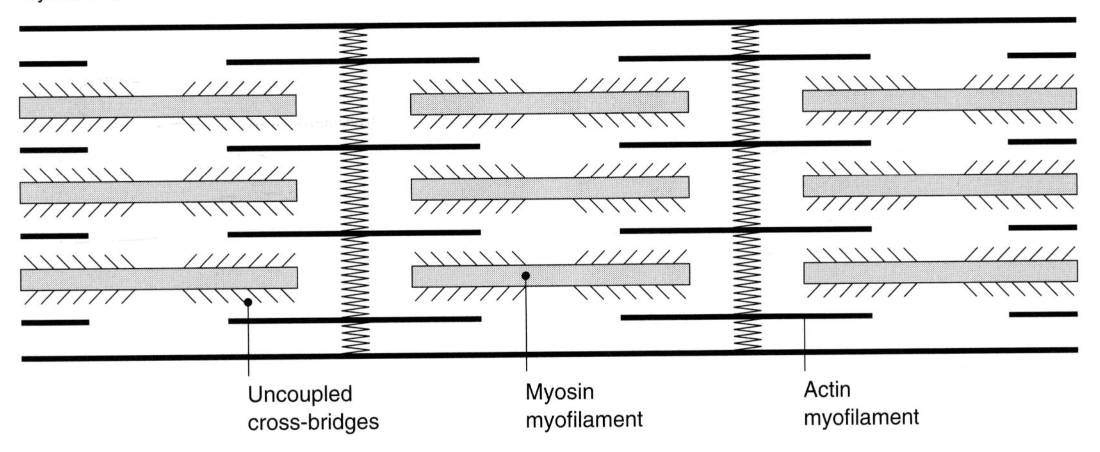

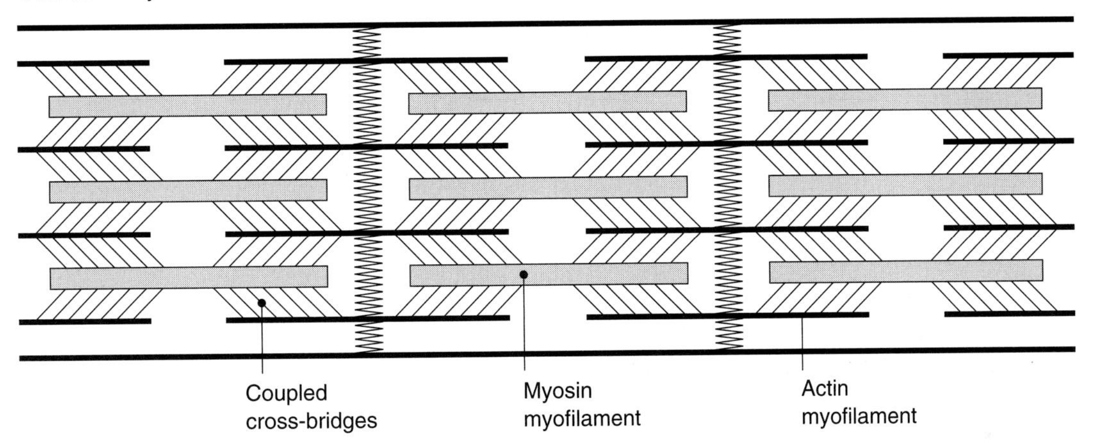

Figure 1-19
The sliding filament theory

- *Location:* Certain muscles can be located by a reference to location in their names (e.g., the posterior tibialis muscle is located on the back side of the tibia).
- *Attachments:* The points of origin and insertion of some muscles can be deciphered in their names (e.g., the coracobrachialis muscle originates on the coracoid process of the scapula and inserts on the brachium, which means arm).
- *Number of divisions:* Muscle names sometimes refer to the number of divisions that make up their structure [e.g., the triceps brachii muscle is an arm muscle consisting of three (tri) heads].
- *Size relationships:* Sometimes muscle names describe a muscle's size in relation to others (e.g., the gluteus maximus is a larger muscle than the gluteus minimus).

Muscles of the Upper Extremity

Although not a complete review of every muscle in the upper extremity, this section covers the most commonly used major muscle groups contributing to movement at the scapula, shoulder, elbow, and wrist.

Major Muscles That Act at the Shoulder Girdle

The shoulder girdle consists of the articulations between the medial end of each clavicle with the sternum, the lateral end of each clavicle with the scapula, the scapula with the soft tissues of the thorax, and the scapula with the head of the humerus. The muscles that act on the scapula are those of the shoulder girdle. Since the scapulae have no bony articulation with the rib cage, the scapulothoracic "joint" is supported with soft tissues. Thus, the main function of shoulder-girdle muscles is to fixate the scapula. When the scapula is immobilized, it serves as a stable point of origin for the muscles that move the humerus. There are four posterior muscles that anchor the scapula (trapezius, rhomboid major, rhomboid minor, and levator scapulae) and two anterior muscles (pectoralis minor and serratus anterior).

The shape of the trapezius allows it to perform several distinct actions. If the upper portion contracts, the scapula is elevated, as in shrugging the shoulders. In contrast, if the lower portion contracts, **depression** of the scapula occurs. When all parts of the trapezius are working together, they tend to pull upward and adduct the scapula at the same time. If the scapula is fixed, the trapezius assists in neck extension. Additionally, the trapezius fixates the scapula for deltoid action as it is used in preventing the glenoid fossa from being pulled downward during the lifting of objects or when carrying an object on the tip of the shoulder, such as the strap of a purse. The rhomboid muscles are responsible for adducting and downwardly rotating the scapula. Further, from a more functional perspective, both rhomboid major and minor muscles are used in pull-up movements. As an individual hangs from a horizontal bar, suspended by the hands, the scapulae tend to be pulled away from the top of the chest. When the

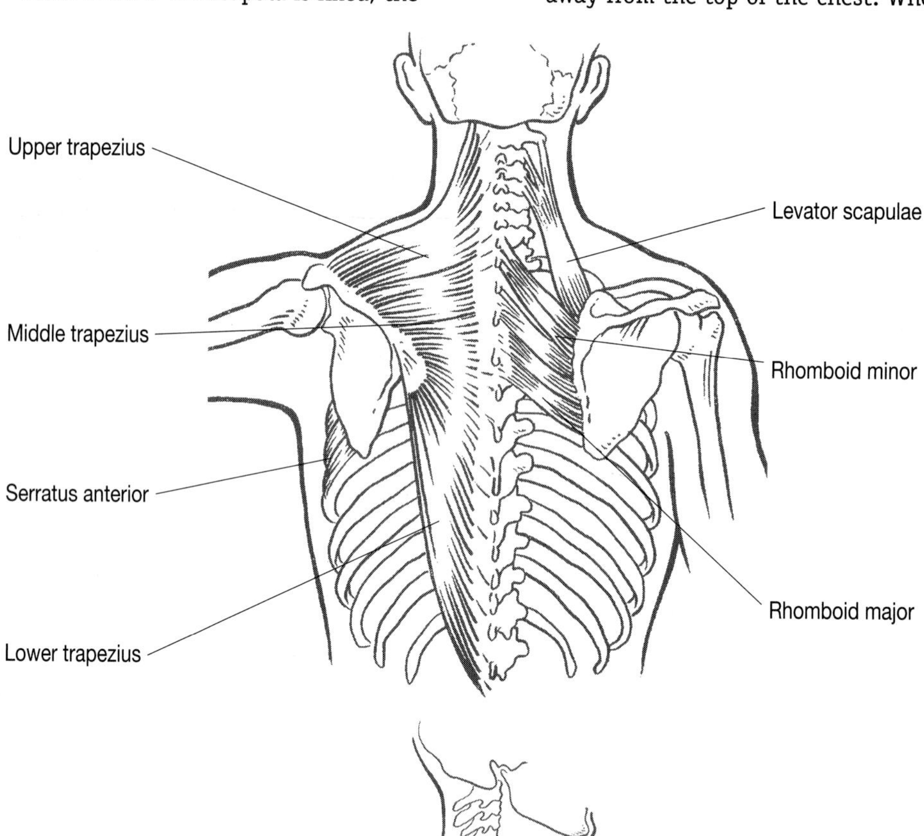

Figure 1-20
Superficial and deep muscles that act at the scapulothoracic articulation

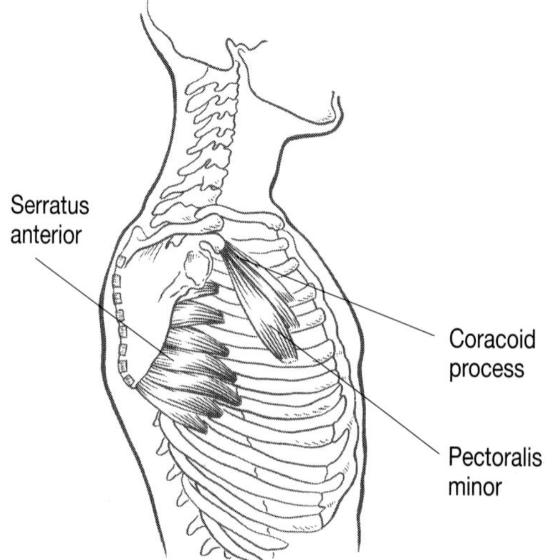

Figure 1-21
Anterior shoulder-girdle muscles

pull-up movement begins, the rhomboids draw the medial border of the scapulae down and back toward the spinal column.

The levator scapulae muscle is so named because of its primary function of elevating the superior medial portion of the scapula. In addition to assisting the upper trapezius during elevation of the scapula, the levator scapulae muscles bilaterally extend the neck or unilaterally flex the neck to one side when the scapulae are anchored by the pectoralis minor (Figure 1-20). The two anterior muscles of the shoulder girdle also work to stabilize the scapula. Additionally, the pectoralis minor and serratus anterior function to abduct the scapulae during pushing movements with the hands. The pectoralis minor acts as an antagonist to the trapezius, rhomboids, and levator scapulae, whereas the serratus anterior acts as an antagonist to the rhomboids (Figure 1-21). The origins, insertions, primary functions, and examples of exercises to develop the muscles of the shoulder girdle are presented in Table 1-7.

Major Muscles That Act at the Shoulder

The most mobile joint in the body, the shoulder joint consists of the articulation of the head of the humerus with the glenoid fossa and the associated cartilage of the scapula. Nine muscles cross the shoulder joint and insert on the humerus, with seven of the nine muscles arising from the scapulae (supraspinatus, infraspinatus, subscapularis, teres minor, deltoid, teres major, and coracobrachialis). Two arise from the axial skeleton and have no attachments on the scapulae (pectoralis major and latissimus dorsi). The supraspinatus, infraspinatus, subscapularis, and teres minor derive their names from the portion of the scapula from which they originate. This group of four muscles is called the rotator cuff, which can be remembered using the acronym **SITS** (Figure 1-22).

The rotator-cuff muscles surround the head of the humerus, with the primary stabilizing function of holding the humeral head in the glenoid fossa. The lack of bone supporting the shoulder joint requires that these muscles and their associated tendons work as stabilizers to prevent subluxation or dislocation of the humeral head from the glenoid fossa. The supraspinatus holds the head of the humerus in the glenoid fossa from a superior position and can be easily injured, especially with throwing movements. It crosses the upper

Table 1-7
Major Muscles That Act at the Shoulder Girdle

Muscle	Origin	Insertion	Primary Function(s)	Selected Exercises
Trapezius	Occipital bone, spines of cervical and thoracic vertebrae	Acromion process and spine of scapula	Upper: elevation of scapula Middle: adduction of scapula Lower: depression of scapula	Upright rowing, shoulder shrugs with resistance
Levator scapulae	Upper four or five cervical vertebrae	Vertebral border of scapula	Elevation of scapula	Shoulder shrugs with resistance
Rhomboid major and minor	Spines of 7th cervical through 5th thoracic vertebrae	Vertebral border of scapula	Adduction and elevation of scapula	Chin-ups, supported dumbbell bent-over rows
Pectoralis minor	Anterior surface of ribs 3 through 5	Coracoid process of scapula	Stabilization, depression, and anterior movement of the scapula	Push-ups, incline bench press, regular bench press, cable crossover flys
Serratus anterior	Outer surface of ribs 1 through 9	Ventral surface of vertebral border of scapula	Stabilization, abduction, and upward rotation of the scapula	Push-ups, incline bench press, pull-overs

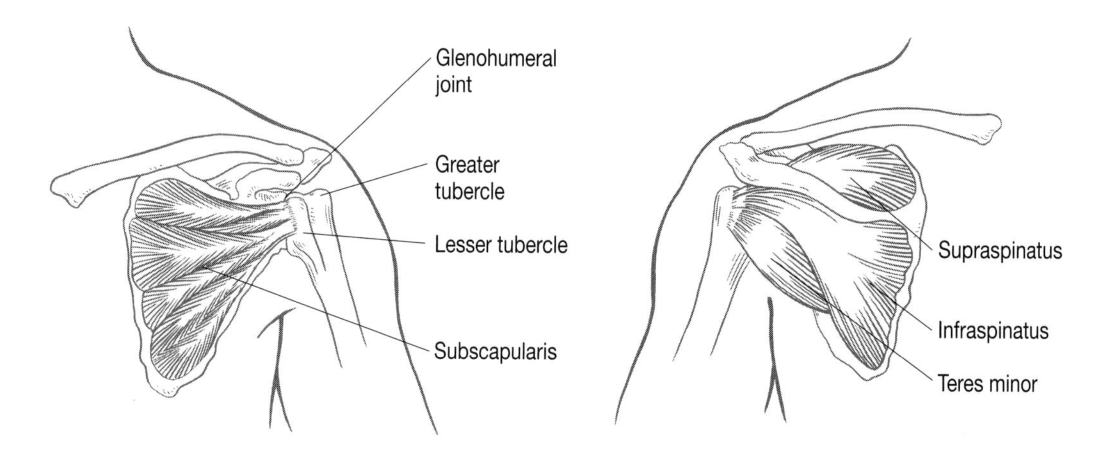

Figure 1-22
Rotator cuff muscles

part of the shoulder joint and assists the deltoid during abduction of the arm. The infraspinatus works with another rotator-cuff muscle, the teres minor, when the rhomboids stabilize the scapula by flattening it to the back so that the humerus may be externally rotated. Both muscles help hold the head of the humerus in the glenoid cavity in addition to externally rotating it. The subscapularis is the only rotator cuff muscle to originate on the anterior portion of the scapula. In addition to its function of helping to stabilize the shoulder joint, it acts as a medial rotator of the arm. The subscapularis also requires help from the rhomboids in stabilizing the scapulae to make it effective in its actions.

The deltoid is a large muscle that forms a cap over and around the shoulder (Figure 1-23). Because its fibers pass in front of, directly over, and in the back of the shoulder, the deltoid's actions are varied, with some of the actions being antagonistic to each other. The anterior fibers flex and internally rotate the humerus, whereas the posterior fibers extend and laterally rotate the humerus. For proper functioning, the trapezius fixes the scapula as the deltoid pulls on the humerus. Thus, any movement of the humerus on the scapula will involve all or part of the deltoid.

The teres major arises from the lower medial portion of the scapula and primarily acts to internally rotate the humerus (Figure 1-24).

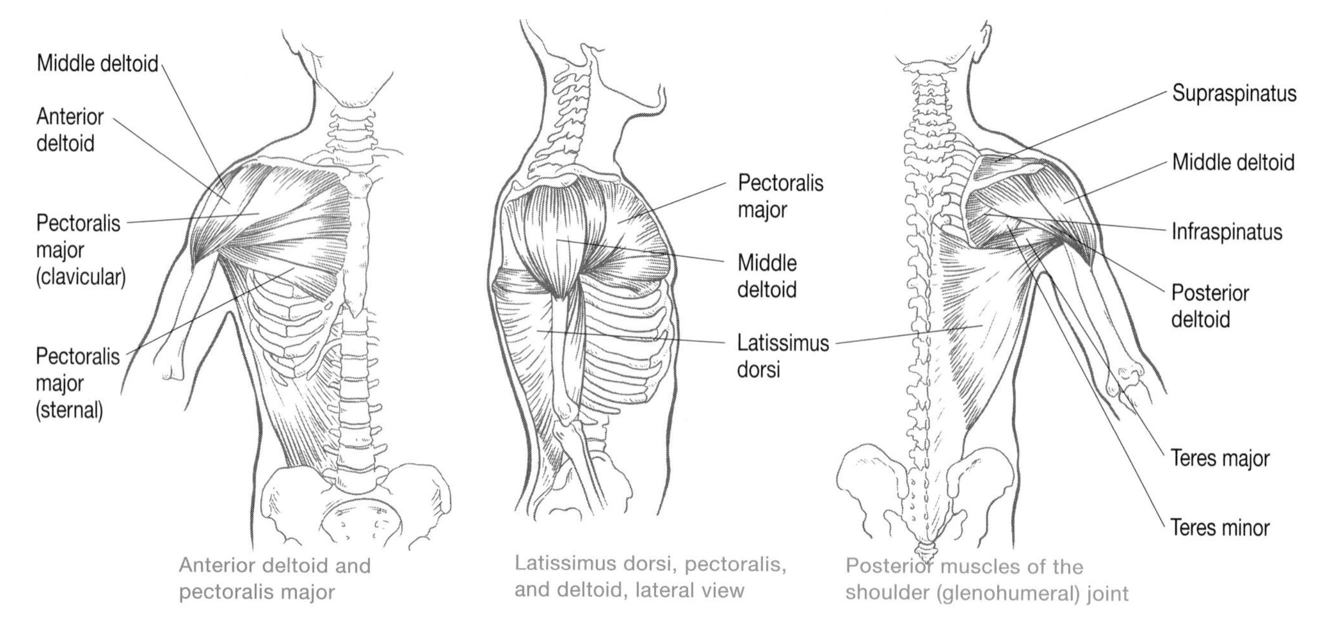

Figure 1-23
Superficial shoulder muscles

This muscle is effective only when the rhomboids stabilize the scapula. Otherwise, the scapula would move forward to meet the arm when the teres major contracts. The teres major works with the latissimus dorsi and is sometimes called the "little lat." The coracobrachialis is the remaining muscle that originates on the scapula. Its location in front of the shoulder allows it to assist in flexion and adduction of the humerus (Figure 1-25).

The remaining two muscles that act at the shoulder joint, latissimus dorsi and pectoralis major, originate from the axial skeleton. Located in the mid- to lower-back, the latissimus dorsi is the widest muscle of the posterior trunk (see Figure 1-24). It is one of the most important, powerful extensor muscles of the humerus. Additionally, it acts to adduct and internally rotate the humerus. When the insertion is fixed, such as when hanging by the arms, the latissimus dorsi can anteriorly tilt the pelvis as well as assist in lateral flexion of the spine. The pectoralis major is a large, fan-shaped muscle that lies on top of the smaller pectoralis minor (Figure 1-26). Its position on the anterior chest wall allows it to effectively work together with the latissimus dorsi to adduct the humerus from a raised, abducted position. It also works to internally rotate the humerus. Because its tendon of insertion twists such that the fibers of the clavicular portion insert below those of its sternocostal portion, the pectoralis major can also extend and flex the shoulder. The clavicular portion flexes an extended shoulder, whereas the sternocostal portion extends a flexed shoulder. The origins, insertions,

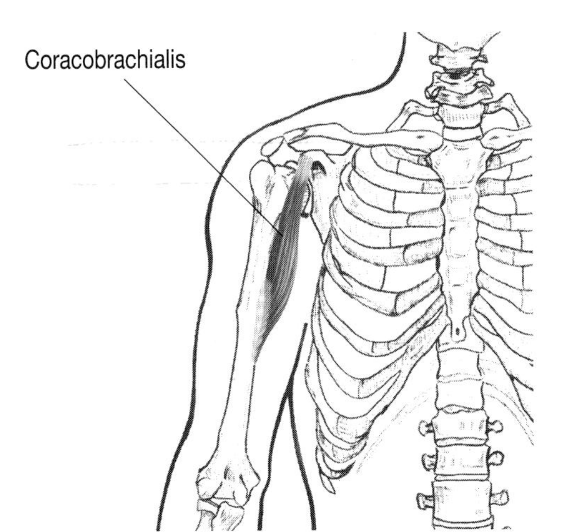

Figure 1-25
Deep muscle that originates on the shoulder blade (scapula) and assists in flexion and adduction of the arm

Reprinted with permission from Golding, L. & Golding, S. (2003). *Fitness Professional's Guide to Musculoskeletal Anatomy and Human Movement.* Monterey, Calif.: Healthy Learning.

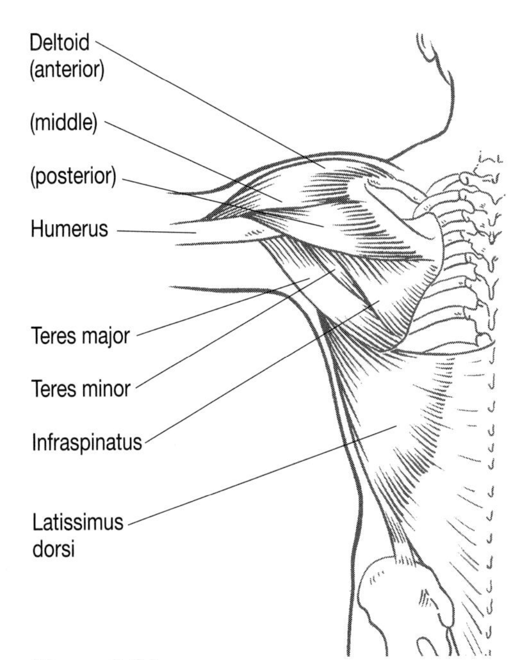

Figure 1-24
Superficial musculature of the superior and inferior shoulder joint, prime movers for shoulder abduction (deltoid) and adduction (latissimus dorsi and teres major)

Redrawn from Luttgens, K., Deutsch, H., & Hamilton, N. (1992). *Kinesiology* (8th ed.). Madison, Wis.: Brown & Benchmark. Reprinted with permission from The McGraw-Hill Companies.

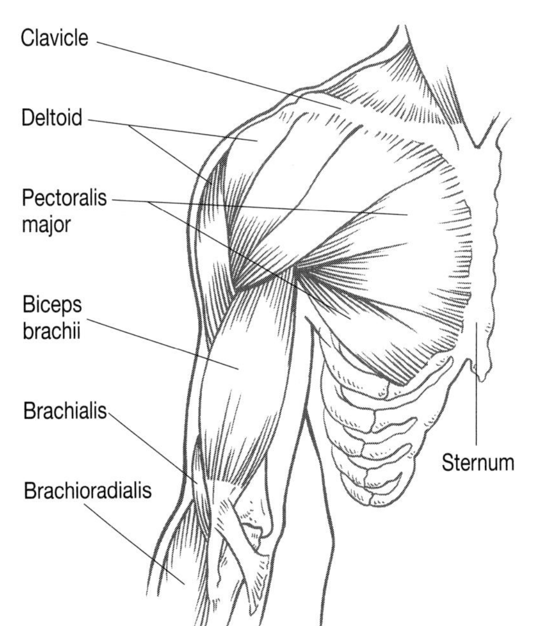

Figure 1-26
Superficial musculature of the anterior chest, shoulder, and arm

primary functions, and examples of exercises to develop the muscles that act at the shoulder are presented in Table 1-8.

Major Muscles That Act at the Elbow

The articulations of the distal end of the humerus with the proximal ends of the radius and ulna comprise the elbow joint. Additionally, the articulation of the radius and ulna with each other must be considered, since these two bones are responsible for pronation and supination of the forearm. Actions that occur at the elbow joint primarily come from contractions of muscles located in the upper arm. Two upper-arm anterior muscles (biceps brachii and brachialis) and one posterior upper-arm muscle (triceps brachii) are responsible for the most powerful forearm movements. As the name implies, the biceps brachii has two heads, both of which originate on the scapula. Because of its scapular attachments, it can assist as a weak flexor of the shoulder. When the forearm is supinated, the biceps brachii acts as a strong flexor of the elbow. However, because of its insertion on the radius, the biceps brachii also acts to supinate the forearm when the forearm is pronated. Lying deep to the biceps brachii, the brachialis is another strong flexor of the forearm. The brachialis pulls on the ulna, which does not rotate, making it the only pure flexor of the elbow (see Figure 1-26). The brachioradialis, the bulk of which is located in the forearm, also acts to flex the elbow. This action of flexion by the brachioradialis is favored when the mid-position between pronation and supination of the forearm is assumed. The triceps brachii muscle is a three-headed structure that is the only muscle located in the posterior compartment of the upper arm (Figure 1-27). One of its portions—the long head—originates from the scapula, allowing

Table 1-8
Major Muscles That Act at the Shoulder

Muscle	Origin	Insertion	Primary Function(s)	Selected Exercises
Pectoralis major	Clavicle, sternum, and first six costal cartilages	Greater tubercle of humerus	Flexion, adduction, and internal rotation	Push-ups, pull-ups, incline bench press, regular bench press, climbing a rope, all types of throwing, tennis serve
Deltoid	Anterolateral clavicle, border of the acromion, and lower edge of spine of the scapula	Deltoid tubercle of humerus on mid-lateral surface	Entire muscle: abduction Anterior fibers: flexion, internal rotation Posterior fibers: extension, external rotation	Lateral "butterfly" (abduction) exercises with dumbbells; anterior deltoid has similar functions to the pectoralis major
Latissimus dorsi	Lower six thoracic vertebrae, all lumbar vertebrae, crests of ilium and sacrum, lower four ribs	Medial side of intertubercular groove of humerus	Extension, adduction, and internal rotation	Chin-ups, rope climbing, dips on parallel bars, rowing, any exercise that involves pulling the arms downward against resistance (e.g.,"lat" pull-downs on exercise machine)
Rotator cuff	Various aspects of scapula	All insert on greater tubercle of humerus except for the subscapularis, which inserts on the lesser tubercle of the humerus	Infraspinatus and teres minor: external rotation Subscapularis: internal rotation Supraspinatus: abduction	Exercises that involve internal and external rotation (e.g., tennis serve, throwing a baseball), internal and external rotation exercises from prone position with dumbbells
Coracobrachialis	Coracoid process of scapula	Middle, medial surface of the humerus	Weak assister in flexion and adduction	Arm front raise, machine pec deck

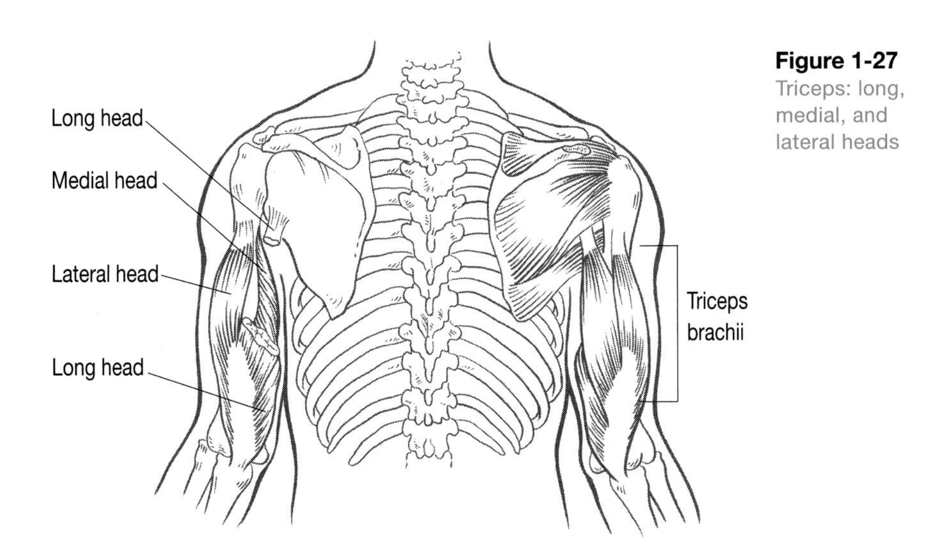

Figure 1-27
Triceps: long, medial, and lateral heads

Table 1-9
Major Muscles That Act at the Elbow and Forearm

Muscle	Origin	Insertion	Primary Function(s)	Selected Exercises
Biceps brachii	Long head from tubercle above glenoid cavity; short head from coracoid process of scapula	Radial tuberosity and bicipital aponeurosis	Flexion at elbow and supination at forearm	"Curling" with barbell, chin-ups, rock climbing, upright "rowing" with barbell
Brachialis	Anterior humerus	Ulnar tuberosity and coronoid process of ulna	Flexion at elbow	Same as for biceps brachii
Brachioradialis	Distal ⅔ of lateral condyloid ridge of humerus	Radial styloid process	Flexion at elbow	Same as for biceps brachii
Triceps brachii	Long head from lower edge of glenoid cavity of scapula; lateral head from posterior humerus; short head from distal ⅔ of posterior humerus	Olecranon process of ulna	Extension at elbow	Push-ups, dips on parallel bars, bench press, military press
Pronator teres	Distal end of medial humerus and medial aspect of ulna	Middle ⅓ of lateral radius	Flexion at elbow and pronation at forearm	Pronation of forearm with dumbbell
Pronator quadratus	Distal ventral surface of ulna	Distal ventral surface of radius	Pronation	Resisted pronation of the forearm
Supinator	Lateral epicondyle of humerus	Proximal, lateral surface of radius	Supination	Resisted supination of the forearm

it to act as a weak extensor of the shoulder. All three heads converge into one tendon that inserts on the olecranon process of the ulna. The triceps brachii acts as the primary extensor of the elbow. The origins, insertions, primary functions, and examples of exercises to develop the muscles that act at the elbow are presented in Table 1-9.

Major Muscles That Act at the Wrist

The articulations of the distal ends of the radius and ulna with the carpal bones of the hand comprise the wrist joint. Most of the muscles that function at the wrist have their origins on the humerus, thereby making the bulk of their structures toward the proximal end of the forearm. Although these muscles cross the elbow joint, they have only very slight actions at the elbow. The muscles that act at the wrist can be divided into two main groups based on location and function (Figure 1-28). The muscles of the anterior group serve as flexors of the wrist and pronators of the forearm and originate mostly on the medial epicondyle of the humerus. They include the flexor carpi radialis, flexor carpi ulnaris, palmaris longus, pronator teres, and pronator quadratus. The

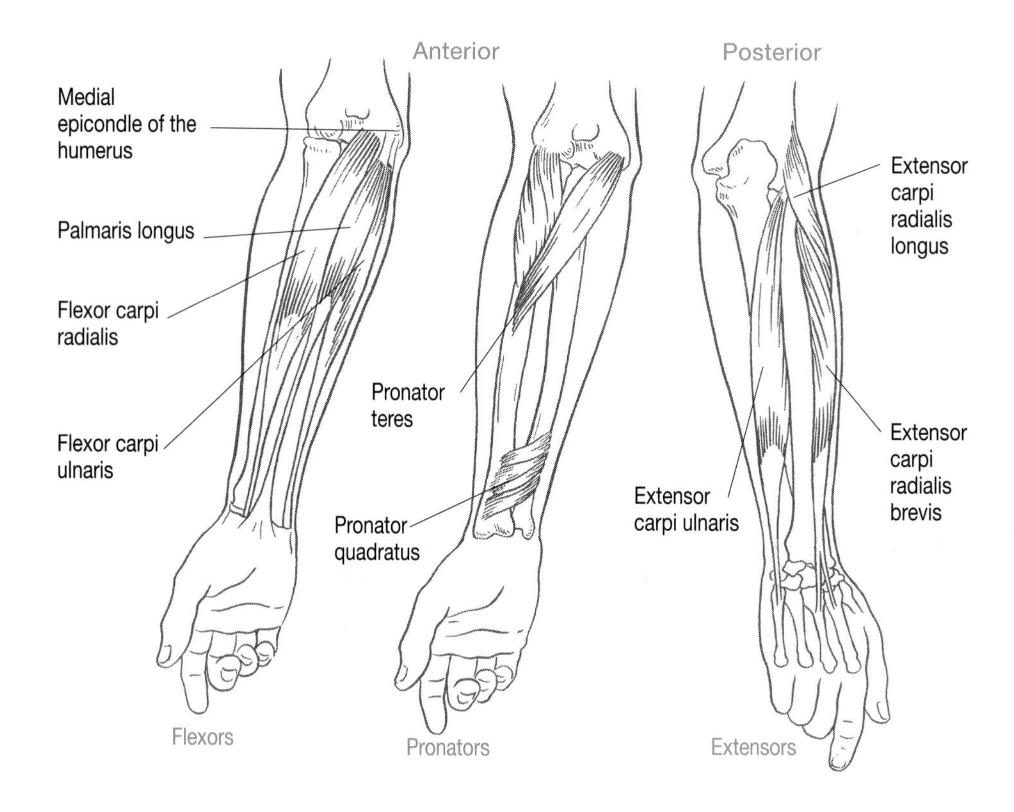

Figure 1-28
Muscles of the wrist

Table 1-10
Major Muscles That Act at the Wrist

Muscle	Origin	Insertion	Primary Function(s)	Selected Exercises
Flexor carpi radialis	Medial epicondyle of humerus	2nd and 3rd metacarpals	Flexion	Wrist curls against resistance; grip-strengthening exercises for humerus; baseball and softball; racquet sports, particularly racquetball and badminton
Flexor carpi ulnaris	Medial epicondyle of humerus	5th metacarpal	Flexion	Same as flexor carpi radialis
Extensor carpi radialis longus	Lateral epicondyle of humerus	2nd metacarpal	Extension	"Reverse" wrist curls; racquet sports, particularly tennis
Extensor carpi ulnaris	Lateral epicondyle of humerus	5th metacarpal	Extension	Same as extensor carpi radialis longus
Palmaris longus	Medial epicondyle of humerus	Palmar aponeurosis	Flexion	Wrist curls

muscles of the posterior group of the forearm serve as extensors of the wrist and supinators of the forearm and originate mostly on the lateral epicondyle of the humerus. They include the extensor carpi radialis longus, extensor carpi ulnaris, and supinator. The origins, insertions, primary functions, and examples of exercises to develop the muscles that act at the wrist are presented in Table 1-10.

Muscles of the Torso

Muscles That Act at the Trunk

The major muscles of the trunk that support, stabilize, and move the spine are presented in this section. These include the muscles of the abdominal wall (rectus abdominis, external obliques, internal obliques, and transverse abdominis) and the muscles that are located on the posterior surface of the spine (erector spinae). The abdominal wall has no skeletal structures to support it and therefore must rely on strength from the multidirectional layers of muscles comprising it. The rectus abdominis is a superficial, flat muscle that is located on the anterior aspect of the abdominal wall (Figure 1-29). It runs vertically from the pubis to the ribcage and functions mainly as a flexor of the spine. Additionally, the rectus abdominis controls the tilt of the pelvis by pulling the pubis upward, preventing anterior pelvic tilt. The external oblique makes up the outermost layer of the abdominal wall and primarily serves to rotate and assist in bilaterally flexing the spine. Its fibers run medially and downward in the same direction as the hands when an individual puts the hands into his or her front coat pockets. The internal oblique lies beneath the external oblique and acts to rotate and assist in bilaterally flexing the spine. Its fibers run upward and medially, opposing those of the external oblique (Figure 1-30). The oblique muscles work together to rotate the trunk. Rotation of the trunk to the right involves simultaneous contraction of the right internal oblique and the left external oblique. The deepest muscle of the abdominal wall is the transverse abdominis, which has fibers that run horizontally, encircling the abdominal cavity (see Figure 1-29). The transverse abdominis acts to compress the abdominal cavity, stabilize the lumbar and pelvic regions, and assist in forced

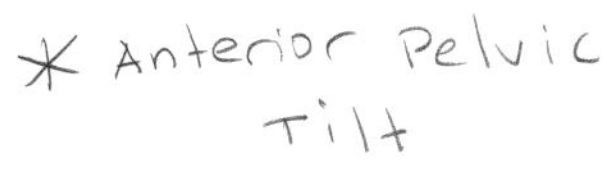

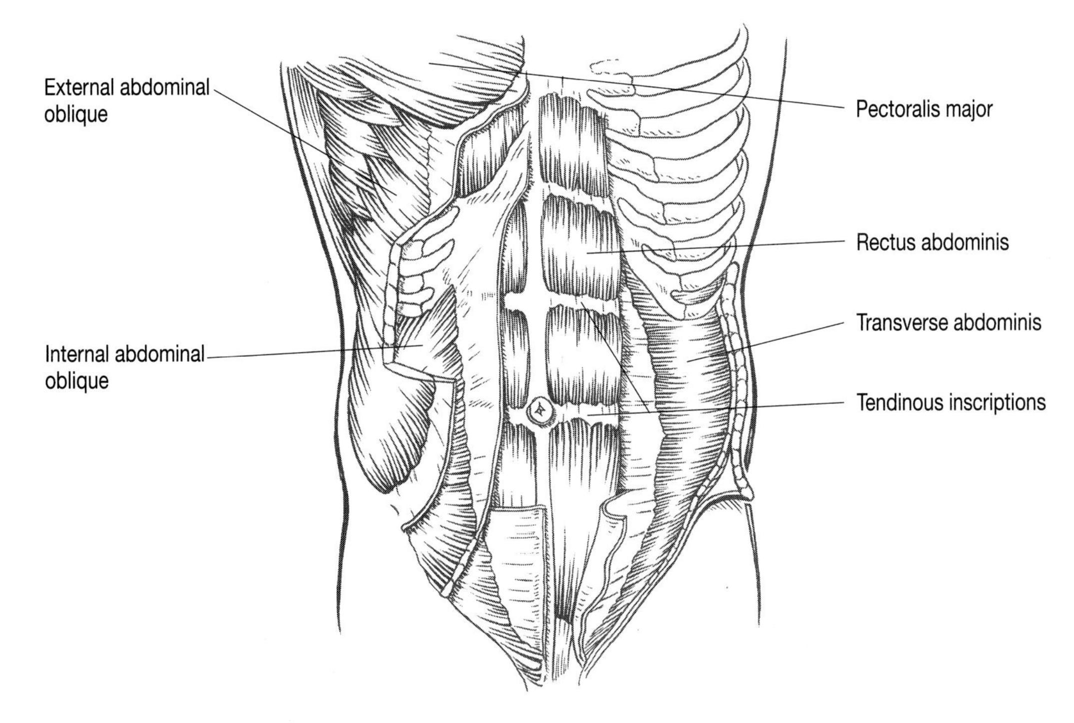

Figure 1-29
Muscles of the abdominal wall

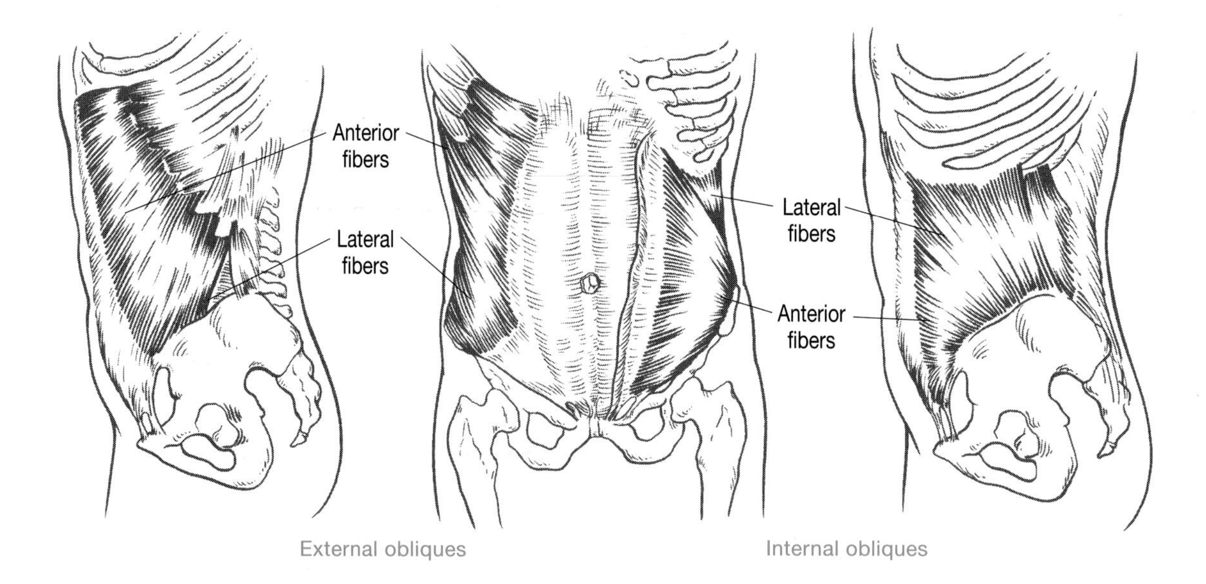

Figure 1-30
External and internal obliques

expiration. This muscle tightens the thoracolumbar fascia and helps stabilize the sacroiliac joints. Because its fibers are oriented horizontally, their contraction reduces the diameter of the abdomen (i.e., "sucking in the gut"). Collectively, the muscles of the abdominal wall aid in forced expiration during heavy breathing by exerting pressure on the abdominal contents, thereby forcing the diaphragm upward.

The posterior longitudinal muscle that runs vertically from the sacrum to the skull is known as the erector spinae and has three subdivisions that form separate columns along the back—the iliocostalis, the spinalis, and the longissimus (Figure 1-31). The most lateral column, the iliocostalis, inserts on the ribs. The most medial column, the spinalis, inserts on the vertebrae. The column of the longissimus is located between the iliocostalis and the spinalis. The erector spinae muscle groups are further divided into lumborum, thoracis, cervicis, and capitis portions, which derive their names from their points of insertion on or near certain vertebrae. The erector spinae act to extend the spine when they act bilaterally. If they contract unilaterally, they act as lateral flexors of the spine. The origins, insertions, primary functions, and examples of exercises to develop the muscles that act at the trunk are presented in Table 1-11.

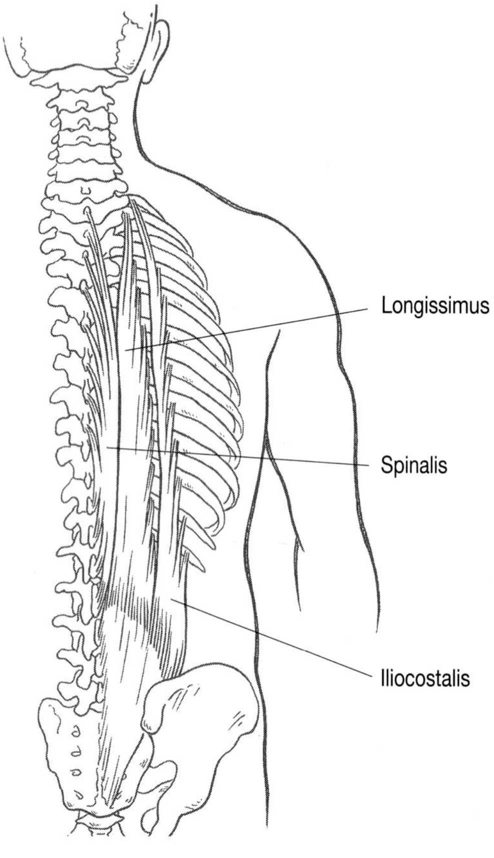

Figure 1-31
The erector spinae muscles (posterior view)

Redrawn from Daniels, L. & Worthingham, C. (1986). *Muscle Testing* (5th ed.). Philadelphia: Elsevier Inc. Reprinted with permission from Elsevier Science.

Longissimus
Spinalis
Iliocostalis

Muscles of the Lower Extremity

Compared to the musculature of the upper limbs, the muscles of the lower extremity tend to be bulkier and more powerful to serve their function in locomotion. The muscles of the lower limbs create somewhat less movement than those of the upper limbs, but they provide relatively

Table 1-11
Major Muscles That Act at the Trunk

Muscle	Origin	Insertion	Primary Function(s)	Selected Exercises
Rectus abdominis	Pubic crest	Cartilage of 5th through 7th ribs and xiphoid process	Flexion and lateral flexion of the trunk	Bent-knee sit-ups, partial curl-ups, good posture, pelvic tilts
External oblique	Anteriolateral borders of lower 8 ribs	Anterior half of ilium, pubic crest, and anterior fascia	Lateral flexion of the trunk	Twisting bent-knee sit-ups (rotation opposite) and curl-ups
Internal oblique	Iliac crest	Cartilage of last 3 to 4 ribs	Lateral flexion of the trunk	Twisting bent-knee sit-ups (rotation same side) and curl-ups
Transverse abdominis	Iliac crest, lumbar fascia, and cartilages of last 6 ribs	Xiphoid process of sternum, anterior fascia, and pubis	Compresses abdomen	No motor function
Erector spinae	Posterior iliac crest and sacrum	Angles of ribs, transverse processes of all ribs	Extension of trunk	Squat, dead lift, prone back extension exercises, good standing posture

more strength and stability. Additionally, the pelvis is fully supported by the skeleton, whereas the shoulder girdle relies more on soft-tissue structures for stability and strength. Although this section does not offer a complete review of every muscle in the lower extremity, it covers the most commonly used major muscle groups that contribute to movement at the hip, knee, and ankle.

Muscles That Act at the Hip

The hip joint is made up of the articulation of the head of the femur with the acetabulum (the cup-shaped space created by the adjoining of the three pelvic bones—the ilium, ischium, and pubis). An anterior view of the hips and pelvis reveals nine muscle groups—iliopsoas, sartorius, rectus femoris, tensor fascia latae, pectineus, adductor brevis, adductor longus, adductor magnus, and gracilis. A posterior viewpoint shows 12 muscle groups—gluteus maximus, gluteus medius, gluteus minimus, six deep lateral rotators, and three hamstrings muscles.

Most of the muscles that act at the hip arise from the pelvis. One muscle, the psoas major, originates from the lumbar vertebrae and shares a tendon with the iliacus muscle, which arises from the ilium. Because these two muscles converge and insert on the femur with the same tendon, they are often referred to as the iliopsoas muscle (Figure 1-32). The main actions of the iliopsoas are flexion and external rotation of the femur. When the thigh is fixed, such as when rising from a supine position to a sitting position, the iliopsoas pulls on the lumbar vertebrae and flexes the spine and pelvis on the femur. When the trunk is fixed, such as when an individual is lying supine and lifting the legs up from the floor, the iliopsoas flexes the femur on the pelvis. In this position, the lumbar attachments of the psoas pull on the vertebrae and can create excessive lordosis and low-back pain in individuals who do not have enough abdominal strength to counterbalance this force. The abdominals can be used to prevent this low-back discomfort by pulling upward on the pelvis and thus "flattening" the back.

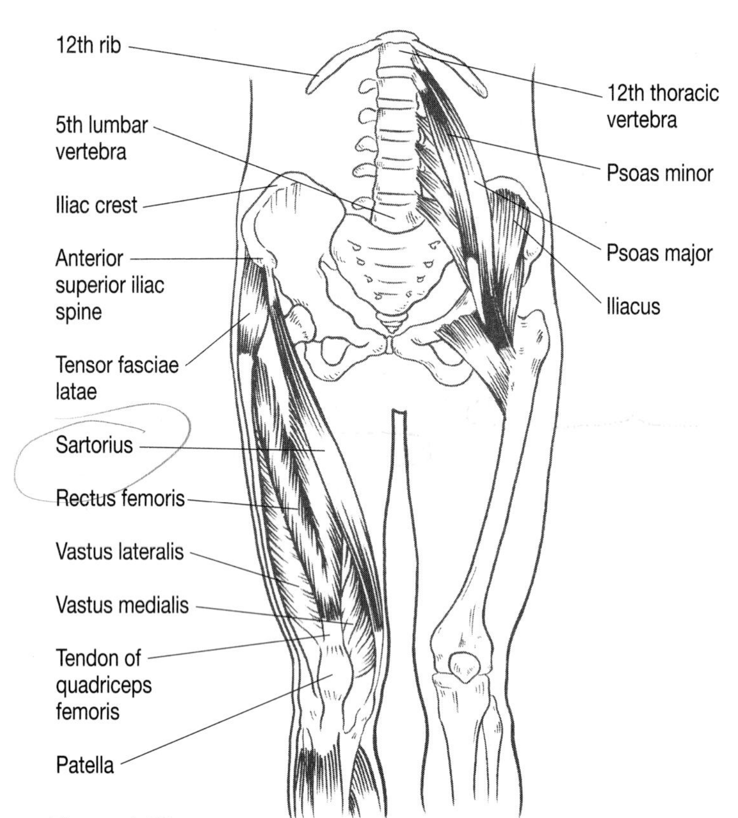

Figure 1-32
Anterior musculature of the hip and knee, prime movers for hip flexion (iliacus, psoas major and minor) and knee extension

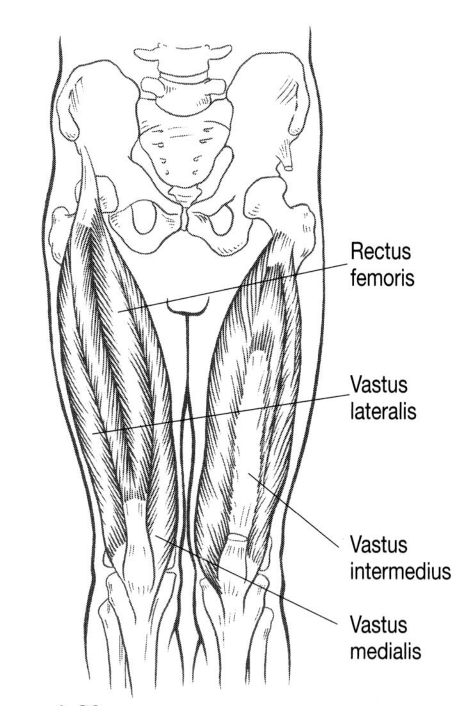

Figure 1-33
Quadriceps muscles

Arising from the anterior ilium and inserting on the medial tibia, the sartorius is the longest muscle in the body (see Figure 1-32). It crosses both the hip and the knee and produces flexion at both joints when activated. This muscle is sometimes referred to as the "tailor" muscle because it is very much involved in sitting cross-legged, which at one time was considered the tailor's position. In fact, sartorius is Latin for "tailor." The rectus femoris originates just below the sartorius on the anterior ilium and inserts into the patellar tendon (Figure 1-33). This muscle is part of the quadriceps femoris muscle group and is the only one that acts at both the hip and the knee; the other quadriceps muscles act only at the knee. The rectus femoris produces flexion at the hip and extension at the knee. Although the tensor fasciae latae is a lateral hip muscle, it can be viewed while looking at the pelvis anteriorly (see Figure 1-32). It inserts on the iliotibial tract, which is a strong band of connective tissue that extends from the lateral hip downward to the lateral knee. The tensor fasciae latae primarily serves to stabilize the knee by tightening the iliotibial tract. From the supine position, raising the leg with the thigh internally rotated calls it into action. The pectineus is a short muscle that crosses the anterior hip (Figure 1-34). Due to its angle of pull, it is a flexor, strong

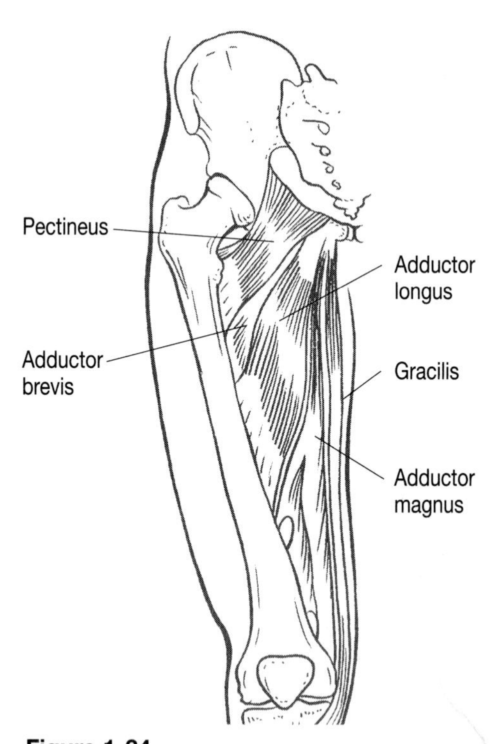

Figure 1-34
Medial muscles of the hip that are responsible for adduction

adductor, and external rotator of the hip. Another group of muscles that can be viewed anteriorly that act on the hip is the adductor group. As their names indicate, the adductor brevis, longus, and magnus act to adduct the hip. Another hip adductor, the gracilis, also assists in flexing the knee (see Figure 1-34).

The muscles that are observed when looking at the pelvis posteriorly mainly act to extend the hip and externally rotate the femur. Three gluteal muscles serve to give shape to the buttocks and provide a powerful means for movement. The gluteus maximus is the largest and most superficial posterior hip muscle (Figure 1-35). Because its tendon of insertion passes behind the hip, the gluteus maximus acts as an extensor and external rotator of the hip. When movement between the pelvis and femur approaches and goes beyond 15 degrees of extension, the gluteus maximus acts an extensor and rotator of the hip. It is not used extensively in ordinary walking. However, a strong action of the gluteus maximus occurs in running, hopping, and jumping.

Deep to the gluteus maximus is the smaller gluteus medius. Its tendon of insertion crosses over the top of the hip joint, making it a hip abductor. Deep to the gluteus medius is the still smaller gluteus minimus. Its tendon of insertion passes in front of the hip joint, thereby allowing it to internally rotate the femur (Figure 1-36). In terms of function, both the gluteus medius and minimus have important roles in walking. As the weight of the body is suspended on one leg, these muscles prevent the opposite hip from sagging. As the body ages, these muscles tend to lose their effectiveness, but they may be strengthened by activities that require an individual to transfer weight from one foot to the other.

A group of six posterior hip muscles called the deep lateral rotators is responsible for externally rotating the femur in the acetabulum. They are the piriformis, gemellus inferior, gemellus superior, obturator internus, obturator externus, and quadratus femoris (Figure 1-37). Of interest is the

Figure 1-35
Posterior musculature of the hip and knee, prime movers for hip extension (gluteus maximus and hamstrings) and knee flexion (hamstrings and gastrocnemius)

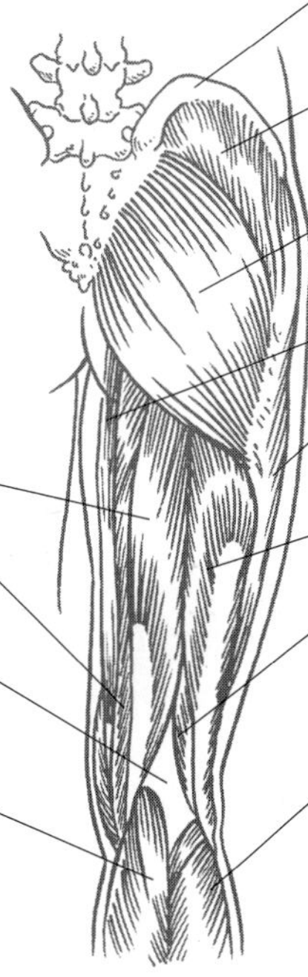

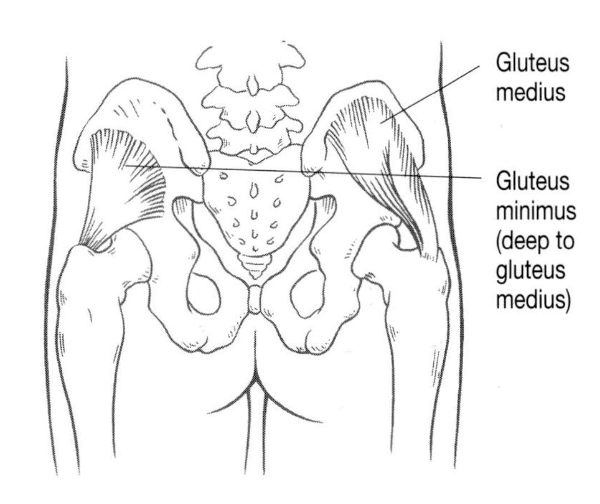

Figure 1-36
Abductors of the posterior hip

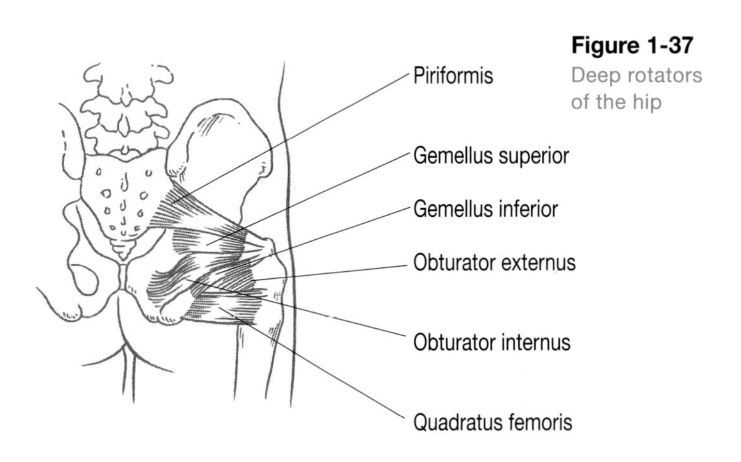

Figure 1-37
Deep rotators of the hip

most superior of the lateral rotators, the piriformis. The sciatic nerve may pass through or just inferior to the piriformis and in some individuals is associated with "sciatica," an irritation of the sciatic nerve that causes pain, tingling, or weakness in the lower extremity.

Three muscles in the posterior thigh are responsible for extending the hip. They are referred to as the hamstring muscle group and consist of the biceps femoris, semimembranosus, and semitendinosus (see Figure 1-35). The origins, insertions, primary functions, and examples of exercises to develop the muscles that act at the hip are presented in Table 1-12.

Muscles That Act at the Knee

The articulation of the distal femur with the proximal tibia and fibula comprise the knee joint. The muscles located in the thigh are responsible for movement at the knee. The thigh muscles are grouped by fasciae into anterior, posterior, and medial compartments. The anterior compartment is also called the extensor compartment, because the muscles in this location primarily extend the knee. There are five muscles in the anterior compartment of the thigh. Four of them (rectus femoris, vastus intermedius, vastus lateralis, and vastus medialis) are collectively called the quadriceps femoris (see Figure 1-33). They are individually named and originate from different areas, but they all converge and share one tendon of insertion, the patellar tendon. The quadriceps femoris is responsible for extending the knee. As mentioned earlier, one of the muscles, the rectus femoris, also crosses the hip joint and contributes to hip flexion. The fifth muscle of the anterior compartment is the sartorius, which was mentioned earlier for its action at the hip. Recall that because of its position as it crosses the knee, it assists in knee flexion.

The posterior, or flexor, compartment consists of the hamstring muscles. These muscles were mentioned earlier for their action of extension at the hip. They are also the primary flexors of the knee. The tendons of insertion of the semimembranosus and semitendinosus pass medially behind the knee, whereas the biceps femoris tendon passes laterally behind the knee. The triangular space created between these tendons on the posterior aspect of the knee is called the popliteal space (see Figure 1-35).

The medial compartment of the thigh is also referred to as the adductor compartment. Five muscles comprise the adductor compartment (adductors magnus, longus, and brevis; pectineus; and gracilis). These muscles were mentioned earlier for their role in adducting the hip joint. In addition to adduction of the hip, the gracilis contributes to flexion at the knee. The origins, insertions, primary functions, and examples of exercises to develop the muscles that act at the knee are presented in Table 1-13.

Muscles That Act at the Ankle and Foot

The ankle joint, which is composed of the articulations between the distal tibia, distal fibula, and proximal talus, acts as a hinge, allowing only dorsiflexion and plantarflexion. The articulation of the talus and the calcaneus is referred to as the subtalar joint, which allows inversion and eversion of the foot. The muscles contained in the lower leg control movements at the ankle and foot. Like the thigh, the lower leg has three separate compartments that are divided by connective tissue. The anterior compartment contains muscles that extend the toes and dorsiflex and/or invert the foot. The posterior compartment consists of muscles that plantarflex the foot and/or flex the toes. The lateral compartment is made up of muscles that act to plantarflex and/or evert the foot.

The anterior compartment, which is made up of muscles including the anterior tibialis, extensor hallucis longus, extensor digitorum longus, and peroneus tertius, is located just lateral to the thick shaft of the tibia (Figure 1-38). The structures of the posterior compartment include the superficial gastrocnemius, soleus, and plantaris

Table 1-12
Major Muscles That Act at the Hip Joint

Muscle	Origin	Insertion	Primary Function(s)	Selected Exercises
Iliacus	Inner surface of the ilium and base of sacrum	Lesser trochanter of femur	Flexion and external rotation	Straight-leg sit-ups, running with knees lifted up high, leg raises
Psoas major and minor	Transverse processes of all 5 lumbar vertebrae	Lesser trochanter of femur	Flexion and external rotation	Essentially same as iliacus
Rectus femoris	Anterior-inferior spine of ilium	Superior aspect of patella and patellar tendon	Flexion	Running, leg press, squat, jumping rope
Gluteus maximus	Posterior ¼ of iliac crest and sacrum	Gluteal line of femur and iliotibial band	Extension and external rotation	Cycling, plyometrics, jumping rope, squats, stair-climbing machine
Biceps femoris	Ischial tuberosity	Lateral condyle of tibia and head of fibula	Extension	Cycling, hamstring curls with knee in external rotation
Semitendinosus	Ischial tuberosity	Proximal anterior-medial aspect of tibia	Extension	Cycling, hamstring curls with knee in internal rotation
Semimembranosus	Ischial tuberosity	Posterior aspect of medial tibial condyle	Extension	Same as semitendinosus
Gluteus medius and minimus	Lateral surface of ilium	Greater trochanter of femur	Abduction	Side-lying leg raises, walking, running
Adductor magnus	Pubic ramus and ischial tuberosity	Medial aspects of femur	Adduction	Side-lying bottom-leg raises; manual-resistance adduction exercises
Adductor brevis and longus	Pubic ramus and ischial tuberosity	Medial aspects of femur	Adduction	Side-lying bottom-leg raises, resisted adduction
Piriformis	Anterior surface of the sacrum	Greater trochanter of the femur	External rotation	Resisted external rotation of the thigh
Obturator internus	Inner rim of the obturator foramen	Greater trochanter of the femur	External rotation	Resisted external rotation of the thigh
Obturator externus	Outer rim of the obturator foramen at the pubis and ischium	Trochanteric fossa of the femur	External rotation	Resisted external rotation of the thigh
Superior gemellus	Ischial spine	Greater trochanter of the femur	External rotation	Resisted external rotation of the thigh
Inferior gemellus	Ischial tuberosity	Greater trochanter of the femur	External rotation	Resisted external rotation of the thigh
Quadratus femoris	Ischial tuberosity	Just below the greater trochanter of the femur	External rotation	Resisted external rotation of the thigh
Iliopsoas	Transverse processes of T12 and L1 through L5; iliac crest and fossa	Lesser trochanter of the femur	Flexion and external of the hip	Hanging knee raise; raising the legs from the floor in a supine position
Gracilis	Pubic symphysis and arch	Medial tibia just below the condyle	Adduction	Side-lying bottom-leg raises; resisted adduction exercises

Table 1-13
Major Muscles That Act at the Knee Joint

Muscle	Origin	Insertion	Primary Function(s)	Selected Exercises
Rectus femoris	Anterior-inferior spine of ilium	Superior aspect of patella and patellar tendon	Extension (most effective when the hip is extended)	Cycling, leg press machine, squats, vertical jumping, stair climbing, jumping rope, plyometrics
Vastus lateralis, intermedius, and medialis	Proximal ⅔ of anterior femur at midline	Patella and tibial tuberosity via the patellar tendon	Extension (particularly when the hip is flexed)	Same as for rectus femoris, resisted knee extension, in-line skating, cross-country skiing
Biceps femoris	Ischial tuberosity	Lateral condyle of tibia and head of fibula	Flexion and external rotation	Jumping rope, hamstring curls with knee in external rotation
Semitendinosus	Ischial tuberosity	Proximal anterior medial aspect of tibia	Flexion and internal rotation	Jumping rope, hamstring curls with knee in internal rotation
Semimembranosus	Ischial tuberosity	Posterior aspect of medial tibial condyle	Flexion and internal rotation	Same as semitendinosus
Gracilis	Pubic symphysis and arch	Medial tibia just below the condyle	Adduction and flexion	Side-lying bottom-leg raises; resisted adduction exercises
Sartorius	Anterior superior iliac spine	Proximal medial tibia just below the tuberosity	Flexion and external rotation of the hip; flexion of the knee	Knee lift with hip external rotation, wide stance onto bench

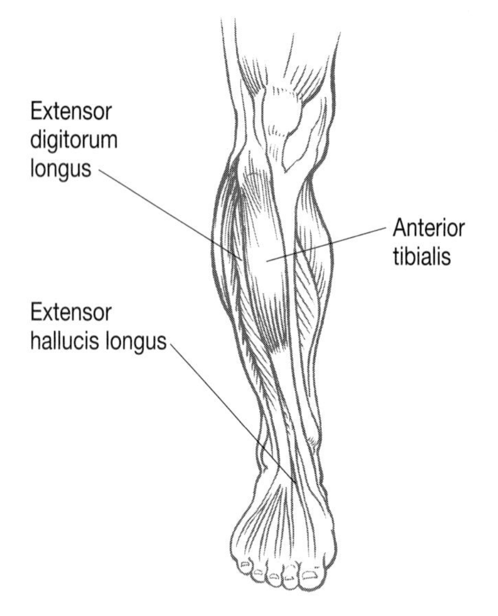

Figure 1-38
Anterior tibial compartment muscles—prime movers for dorsiflexion and inversion

muscles, and the deep popliteus, flexor hallucis longus, flexor digitorum longus, and tibialis posterior muscles (Figure 1-39). The gastrocnemius and soleus make up the bulk of the calf and share a common insertion, the Achilles tendon. In addition to plantarflexion of the ankle, the gastrocnemius is responsible for flexing the knee because of its origins on the femur. This muscle is more effective as a knee flexor, however, if the foot is elevated, such as when performing a supine lying hamstring curl. Additionally, the gastrocnemius is more effective as a plantarflexor if the knee is held in extension, which can be experienced when sitting too close to the wheel when driving a car. When the knees are flexed, the gastrocnemius becomes an ineffective plantarflexor and it becomes more difficult to depress the brakes. The gastrocnemius is the primary focus during standing calf work, whereas the soleus is the primary focus of seated calf exercises. The lateral compartment of the leg contains the peroneus longus and brevis (Figure 1-40). The origins, insertions, primary functions, and examples of exercises to develop the muscles that act at the ankle and foot are presented in Table 1-14.

Endocrine System

The endocrine system, which is made up of various glands throughout the body, is responsible for regulating bodily activities through the production of hor-

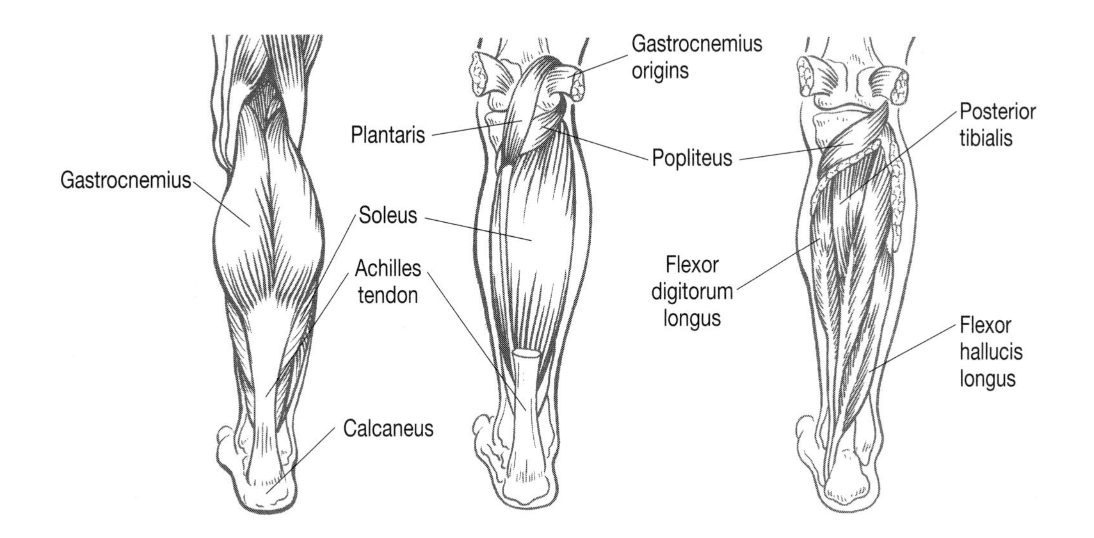

Figure 1-39
Posterior tibial compartment muscles primarily responsible for plantarflexion of the ankle

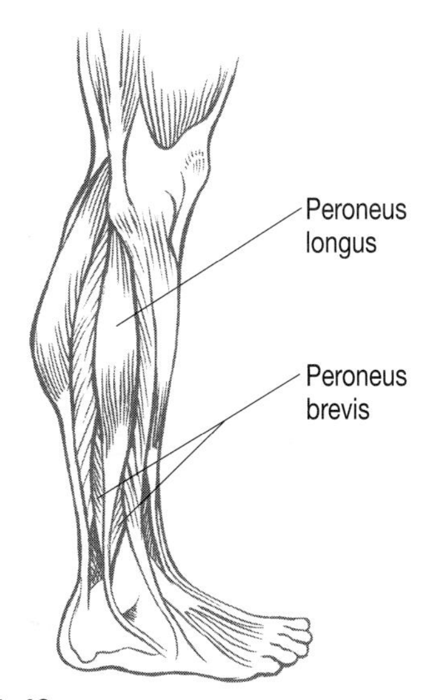

Figure 1-40
Lateral tibial compartment muscles, prime movers for eversion

mones. Hormones are chemical substances that generally fit into one of two categories: steroid-derived hormones and hormones synthesized from amino acids. The cells of the endocrine glands release their hormones directly into the bloodstream, where they are delivered to target organs. The principle endocrine glands are the pituitary, thyroid, parathyroids, adrenals, pancreas, and gonads.

The pituitary gland is often referred to as the "master gland," because of its regulatory effect on several other endocrine glands and its importance in controlling a number of diverse bodily functions. It is located beneath the brain and divided into anterior and posterior lobes. The posterior lobe releases a hormone called vasopressin, which acts on the kidneys and is considered an antidiuretic (i.e., a substance that inhibits urine production, thus aiding in the retention of bodily fluid). The posterior portion also releases oxytocin, a hormone that stimulates the smooth muscles of the reproductive organs and intestines.

The anterior portion of the pituitary gland releases six hormones that affect various important bodily functions: follicle-stimulating hormone (FSH), luteinizing hormone (LH), thyroid-stimulating hormone (TSH), **adrenocorticotropin hormone (ACTH),** growth hormone (GH), and prolactin. FSH and LH are called gonadotropins because of their effects on the gonads (ovaries and testes). These substances control the secretion of **estrogen** and **progesterone** in the ovaries and the production of **testosterone** in the testicles. TSH stimulates the synthesis and release of thyroxine from the thyroid gland, which helps control the rate at which all cells utilize oxygen. ACTH controls the secretion in the adrenal gland of hormones that influence the metabolism of carbohydrates, sodium, and potassium. ACTH also controls the rate at which substances are exchanged between the blood and tissues. GH specifically stimulates growth of the skeletal system, but also general growth.

Table 1-14
Major Muscles That Act at the Ankle and Foot

Muscle	Origin	Insertion	Primary Function(s)	Selected Exercises
Anterior tibialis	Proximal ⅔ of lateral tibia	Medial aspect of 1st cuneiform and 1st metatarsal	Dorsiflexion at ankle; inversion at foot	Cycling with toe clips, resisted inversion (with dorsiflexion)
Peroneus longus	Head of fibula and proximal ⅔ of lateral fibula	Inferior aspects of medial tarsal (1st cuneiform) and 1st metatarsal	Plantarflexion at ankle; eversion at foot	Resisted eversion of foot, walking on inside of foot
Peroneus brevis	Distal ⅔ of lateral fibula	Base of the 5th metatarsal	Plantarflexion at ankle; eversion at foot	Resisted eversion of foot with rubber tubing, walking on inside of foot
Gastrocnemius	Posterior surfaces of femoral condyles	Posterior surface of calcaneus via Achilles tendon	Plantarflexion at ankle	Hill running, jumping rope, calf raises with barbell on shoulders, cycling, stair-climber machine, in-line skating
Soleus	Proximal ⅔ of posterior surfaces of tibia and fibula	Posterior surface of calcaneus via Achilles tendon	Plantarflexion at ankle	Virtually the same as for gastrocnemius; bent-knee toe raises with resistance
Posterior tibialis	Posterior surface of tibia-fibular interosseous membrane	Lower medial surfaces of medial tarsals and metatarsals	Plantarflexion at ankle; inversion at foot	Resisted inversion of foot with surgical tubing, with plantarflexion
Extensor hallucis longus	Anterior middle fibula and interosseous membrane	Dorsal surface of the distal phalanx of the great toe	Dorsiflexion and inversion of the foot; extension of the great toe	Resisted inversion with dorsiflexion
Extensor digitorum longus	Lateral condyle of tibia, proximal ¾ of the fibula, and interosseous membrane	Dorsal surface of the phalanges of toes 2 through 5	Dorsiflexion and eversion of foot; extension of toes 2 through 5	Resisted eversion with dorsiflexion
Peroneus tertius	Distal ⅓ of the fibula and interosseous membrane	Dorsal surface of the base of the 5th metatarsal	Dorsiflexion and eversion of the foot	Resisted eversion with dorsiflexion
Plantaris	Posterior surface of the femur above the lateral condyle	Calcaneus	Flexion of the knee; plantarflexion of the foot	Same as gastrocnemius
Popliteus	Lateral condyle of the femur	Proximal tibia	Knee flexion; internal rotation of the lower leg	Same as semitendinosus and semimembranosus (see Table 1-13)
Flexor hallucis longus	Lower ⅔ of the fibula	Distal phalanx of the great toe	Flexion of the great toe; plantarflexion and inversion of the foot	Resisted inversion with plantarflexion
Flexor digitorum longus	Posterior tibia	Distal phalanges of toes 2 through 5	Flexion of toes 2 through 5; plantarflexion and inversion of the foot	Resisted inversion with plantarflexion

Additionally, GH promotes the entrance of amino acids into the body's cells for their incorporation into protein and releases fatty acids into the blood for use as energy. GH has also been shown to promote the formation of glucose and its release into the blood. Another anterior pituitary hormone, prolactin, is involved in the initiation and maintenance of breast-milk production and secretion in females.

The thyroid gland is located anterior to the upper part of the trachea and is among the largest endocrine organs in the body. Mentioned earlier for its functions controlled by the pituitary gland, the thyroid gland releases three hormones: thyroxine, triiodothyronine, and calcitonin.

Thyroxine and triiodothyronine are iodine-containing hormones that are released by the thyroid to regulate the metabolism of carbohydrates, proteins, and lipids, thereby increasing the body's oxygen consumption and heat production. The third hormone, calcitonin, lowers blood calcium and phosphate levels by accelerating the absorption of calcium by the bones. The parathyroid glands are four structures located on the posterior surface of the thyroid gland. These glands release parathyroid hormone (PTH), which is primarily responsible for controlling the levels of calcium and phosphorus in the blood through its actions on the kidneys and the skeleton. PTH increases bone resorption, which functions to break down bone calcium for its release into the blood. Further, PTH works synergistically with vitamin D to maintain the body's calcium levels.

The adrenal glands appear as two pyramid-shaped organs located close to the superior border of each kidney. Each gland consists of two distinct parts: the medulla (inner portion) and the cortex (outer portion). The adrenal medulla and the adrenal cortex are so distinct that each portion is, in effect, its own distinct endocrine organ. The adrenal medulla produces two hormones: **epinephrine** (adrenaline) and **norepinephrine** (noradrenaline). These substances function cooperatively to prepare the body for emergencies or stressful events. Epinephrine acts to elevate blood glucose levels; increase the rate, force, and amplitude of the heartbeat; and dilate blood vessels that feed the heart, lungs, and skeletal muscles. The release of norepinephrine causes an increase in heart rate and in the force of contraction of the cardiac muscle. It also contributes to constriction of blood vessels in most areas of the body. The adrenal cortex secretes mineralocorticoids associated with sodium and potassium metabolism, glucocorticoids that aid in the utilization of glucose and mobilization of fatty acids, and gonadocorticoids, including testosterone, estrogen, and progesterone.

The pancreas lies just below the stomach and, in addition to its role in producing digestive enzymes, functions as an endocrine gland that produces hormones involved in regulating carbohydrate metabolism. The pancreas secretes **insulin,** which acts to facilitate the uptake and utilization of glucose (blood sugar) by cells and prevent the breakdown of **glycogen** (the storage form of glucose) in the liver and muscle. This function makes insulin a powerful hypoglycemic agent—that is, it decreases the blood sugar level. Insulin also plays a role in lipid and protein metabolism, as it favors lipid formation and storage and facilitates the movement of amino acids into cells. The pancreas secretes another hormone, **glucagon,** which generally opposes the actions of insulin. Glucagon decreases glucose oxidation and increases the blood sugar level (hyperglycemia). Its main action appears to be stimulation of the breakdown of glycogen in the liver for its release into the bloodstream.

The gonads are the endocrine glands that produce hormones that promote sex-specific physical characteristics and regulate reproductive function. The sex hormones testosterone and estrogen are found in both males and females, but in varying concentrations. In the male, testosterone is produced in the testes and acts to initiate sperm production, stimulate the development of male secondary sex characteristics, and promote tissue building. The ovaries in the female are the primary source for the production of estrogen, which regulates ovulation, menstruation, the physiological adjustments during pregnancy, and the appearance of female secondary sex characteristics. Furthermore, estrogen affects the blood vessels, bones, lungs, liver, intestines, prostate, and testes. Table 1-15 summarizes the major endocrine glands and some selected effects of their associated hormones.

Summary

A thorough knowledge of human anatomy is essential for any fitness professional. LWMCs must know how the body's various systems—cardiovascular, respiratory, digestive, skeletal, neuromuscular, muscular, and endocrine—are affected by both exercise and a lack of exercise. Subsequent chapters expand upon some of the topics covered here, specifically on the effects that overweight and obesity have on the body's physiological systems.

Table 1-15
Major Endocrine Glands and Their Hormones

Gland	Hormones	Selected Effects
Pituitary	Antidiuretic hormone	Promotes reabsorption of water in the kidneys
	Oxytocin	Stimulates the contraction of the smooth muscle of the uterus and intestines
	Follicle stimulating hormone (FSH) and luteinizing hormone (LH)	Stimulates gonads to secrete sex hormones
	Thyroid stimulating hormone (TSH)	Stimulates thyroid gland to secrete thyroid hormones
	Adrencocorticotropin hormone (ACTH)	Stimulates adrenal glands to secrete glucocorticoids
	Growth hormone (GH)	Stimulates general growth and skeletal growth, and promotes metabolic functions
	Prolactin	Initiates and maintains breast-milk secretion in females
Thyroid	Thyroxine and triiodothyronine	Increases oxygen consumption and heat production, and affects many metabolic functions
	Calcitonin	Decreases blood calcium and phosphate levels
Parathyroids	Parathyroid hormone (PTH)	Raises plasma calcium levels and lowers plasma phosphate levels
Adrenals	Epinephrine	Affects carbohydrate metabolism, generally promoting hyperglycemia. Constricts vessels in the skin, mucous membranes, and kidneys, but dilates vessels in skeletal muscle
	Norepinephrine	Increases heart rate and force of contraction of the heart beat, and constricts blood vessels in most areas of the body
	Mineralocorticoids	Promote reabsorption of sodium and excretion of potassium in the kidneys
Pancreas	Insulin	Causes liver and muscle cells to take up glucose and store it in the form of glycogen; encourages fat cells to take on blood lipids and turn them into triglycerides; also has several other anabolic effects throughout the body
	Glucagon	Causes the liver to convert stored glycogen into glucose and release it into the bloodstream

References

Pette, D. (2001). Historical perspectives: Plasticity of mammalian skeletal muscle. *Journal of Applied Physiology,* 90, 3, 1119–1124.

Shoepe, T. et al. (2003). Functional adaptability of muscle fibers to long-term resistance exercise. *Medicine & Science in Sports & Exercise,* 35, 6, 944–951.

Suggested Reading

Behnke, R.S. (2006). *Kinetic Anatomy.* Champaign, Ill.: Human Kinetics.

Calais-Germain, B. (1993). *Anatomy of Movement.* Seattle, Wa: Eastland Press, Inc.

Chikly, B. (2006). *Silent Waves: Theory and Practice of Lymph Drainage Therapy*. Scottsdale, Ariz.: I.H.H. Publishers.

Delavier, F. (2006). *Strength Training Anatomy.* Champaign, Ill.: Human Kinetics.

Golding, L.A. & Golding, M.G. (2003). *Musculoskeletal Anatomy and Human Movement.* Monterey, Calif.: Healthy Learning.

Travell, J.G. & Simons, D.G. (1999). *Myofascial Pain and Dysfunction: The Trigger Point Manual.* (2nd ed.). Baltimore, Md.: Williams & Wilkins.

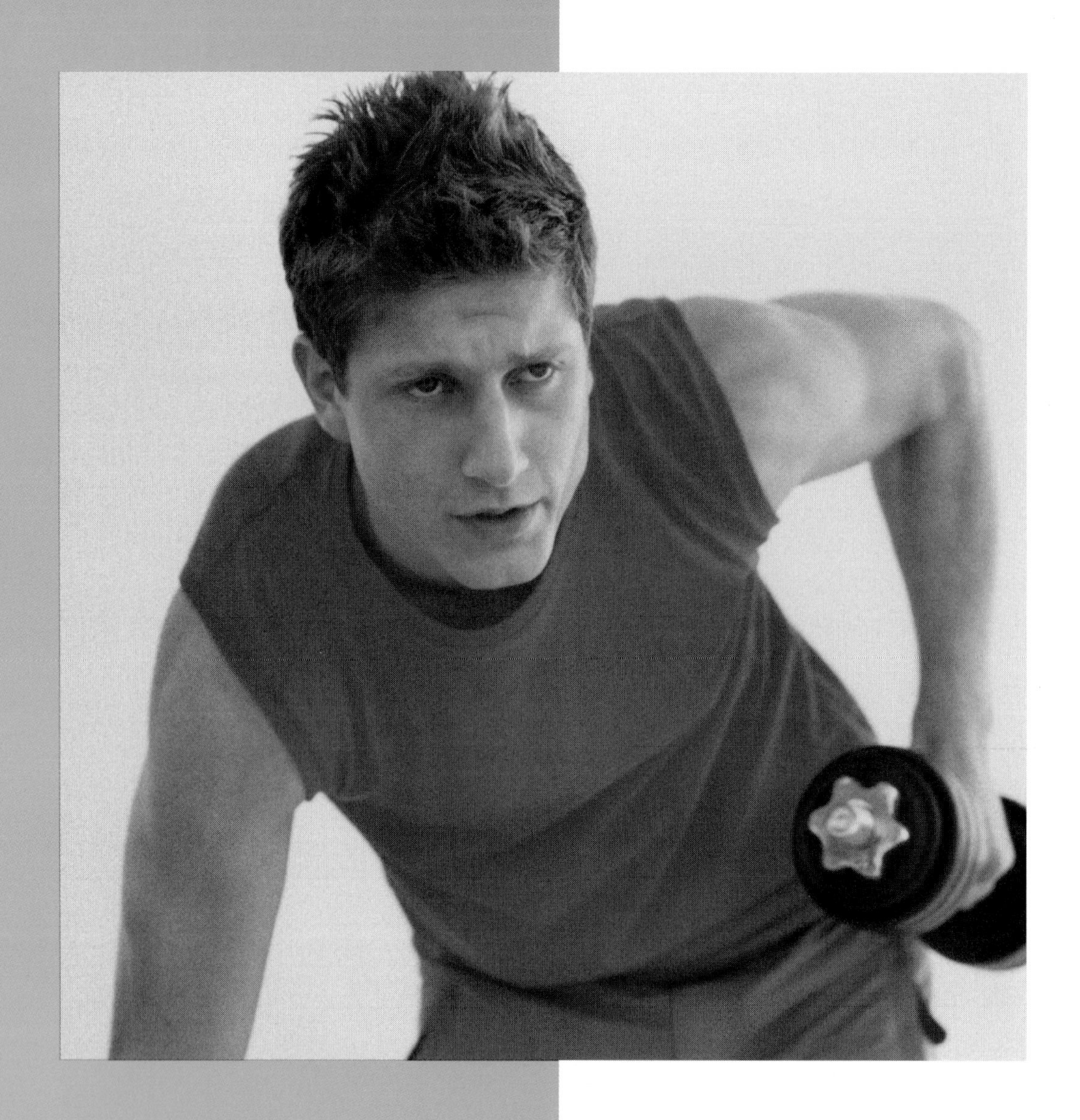

Rod A. Harter

Rod A. Harter, Ph.D., A.T.,C., FACSM, is an associate professor in the Department of Nutrition and Exercise Sciences at Oregon State University in Corvallis. Dr. Harter is a certified athletic trainer and a fellow of the American College of Sports Medicine. His areas of specialization include kinesiology, biomechanics, and sports medicine.

ACE would like to acknowledge the contributions to this chapter made by Sabrena Merrill, M.S., fitness industry consultant, author, and educator.

Chapter 2

Fundamentals of Applied Kinesiology

IN THIS CHAPTER:

Kinesiology involves the study of human movement from biological and physical science perspectives. A common way for professors to describe kinesiology to their students is to have them imagine the human body as a living machine designed for the performance of work. To accomplish this work, there must be meaningful and purposeful integration of the anatomical, neurological, and physiological systems in accordance with the physical laws of nature. Understanding the principles and concepts of kinesiology will provide a framework with which to analyze the vast multitude of human movements, and to make decisions and judgments regarding the safety and effectiveness of a particular movement sequence or sport skill and its role in the accomplishment of a specific fitness or personal goal of a client.

In this context, expertise in kinesiology will provide the tools to analyze common **activities of daily living (ADL)**, as well as the specialized movements associated with exercise performance. To use these tools, consider the body's daily activities, postures, and the mechanical stresses that it undergoes in these positions. Next, identify possible areas of weakness or tightness caused by those habitual positions and activities. Then, design activities to improve the body's function under those specific conditions. The result will be balanced fitness programs for clients that not only include cardiovascular endurance, but also proper body mechanics, neutral postural alignment, and **muscular balance.**

Biomechanical Principles Applied to Human Movement

As an area of study, **biomechanics** involves the application of mechanics to living organisms (chiefly human beings) and the study of the effects of the forces applied. Within the study of mechanics, there are two major areas of interest to the Lifestyle & Weight Management Consultant (LWMC): **kinematics** and **kinetics.** Kinematics involves the study of the form, pattern, or sequence of movement without regard for the forces that may produce that motion. Kinetics is the branch of mechanics that describes the effects of forces on the body. From a kinesiology viewpoint, a force can be either internal (e.g., produced by muscles) or external (e.g., produced by gravity's pull on a barbell), and cause, modify, or oppose motion.

The analytical process within kinesiology can either be quantitative (mathematically derived) or qualitative (subjective). Biomechanics research laboratories at major universities, medical schools, and hospitals use state-of-the art equipment costing hundreds of thousands of dollars to perform precise quantitative analyses of movement. In contrast, current digital camera technology is relatively inexpensive and will allow a fitness professional to create a record of a client's movement pattern at the beginning and later stages of learning a new skill or task (e.g., exercising on a stability ball). Sharing this visual record with the participant, along with a critique of the movement, allows for self-analysis and improvement. A more common example of a "low-tech" kinesiological qualitative analysis is the real-time use of a mastery of kinesiological principles when training in an exercise facility with mirrored walls to give clients verbal cues for immediate self-correction when necessary.

Even though an LWMC will use the naked eye rather than expensive digital cameras and computers to analyze human movement, he or she will still need to understand the physical laws that apply to the motion of all objects. While Sir Isaac Newton, a 17th century English mathematician, is perhaps best known for his conceptualization of the **law of gravity** after observing an apple falling from a tree to the ground, his formulation of three important natural laws that govern motion represents his greatest contribution to science. When taken together, Newton's laws of motion provide a better understanding of the interrelationships among forces, mass, and human movement—at individual joints or of the body as a whole.

Law of Inertia

Newton's first law of motion, known as the **law of inertia,** states that a body at rest will stay at rest and that a body in motion will stay in motion (with the same direction and velocity) unless acted upon by an external force. A body's inertial characteristics are proportional to its mass. Therefore, it is more difficult to start moving a heavy object than a light one. Similarly, if two objects are moving at the same velocity, it requires more effort to stop or slow the heavier object than the lighter one. For LWMCs, resistance-training programs probably have the greatest association with Newton's first law. For example, the "sticking point" at the beginning of a biceps curl occurs in part due to the difficulty of overcoming the dumbbell's inertial property of being at rest, and in part due to the mechanical disadvantage of the human body to generate internal forces when the elbow is fully extended.

Law of Acceleration

The **law of acceleration,** Newton's second law, states that the force (F) acting on a body in a given direction is equal to the body's mass (m) multiplied by the body's acceleration (a) in that direction ($F = ma$). Newton's second law also relates to a moving body's momentum (M), in that a body's linear momentum is equal to its mass multiplied by its velocity (v) ($M = mv$). For a given mass, the application of additional force will accelerate the body to a higher velocity, thus creating greater momentum. For a given velocity, linear momentum will be increased if the mass of the body is increased. Angular momentum is governed by similar principles, but the motion performed is about an axis. If a participant is using a 10-pound (4.5-kg) dumbbell to slowly perform biceps curls, there will be less momentum produced than when moving that same weight at a faster rate. If the velocity of movement is held constant, but the participant switches to a 15-pound (6.8-kg) dumbbell (greater mass, m), then momentum (M = mv) will increase proportionally.

Law of Reaction

Newton's third law, commonly referred to as the **law of reaction,** states that every **applied force** is accompanied by an equal and opposite reaction force. Said differently, for every action there is an equal and opposite reaction. This law has bearing on the ground-reaction forces (impact forces) that the body must absorb during activities such as step training, **plyometrics,** and jogging. According to Newton's principles, the ground exerts a force against the body equal to the force that the body applies to the ground as a person walks, jogs, or sprints. Step training and martial arts–derived exercise programs remain popular activities even though the magnitude of the ground-reaction forces associated with each may place clients at risk for a variety of overuse injuries. Athletic shoes designed specifically for step training have additional cushioning in the metatarsal region of the foot for injury prevention, as the forefoot is where much of the vertically directed ground-reaction force is concentrated. A biomechanical analysis of step aerobic exercise reported that significantly smaller-magnitude ground-reaction forces occurred with a 6-inch (15-cm) step when compared to 8-inch (20-cm) and 10-inch (25-cm) step heights (Maybury & Waterfield, 1997). Little difference in ground-reaction forces existed between the 8-inch (20-cm) and 10-inch (25-cm) step heights; these findings suggest that participants should use a lower step height to reduce the risk of an overuse injury to the lower limb.

An understanding of the anatomical and biomechanical factors that affect muscles and create movement is crucial for effective exercise design and program implementation. The next step in this process is to apply these principles to identify the individual and collective contributions of muscles through an analytical process. Leonardo da Vinci, perhaps the premier anatomist in all of history, simplified the study of functional anatomy when he likened human tendons to "cords attached to skeletons." Remembering a muscle's location, the attachment sites of its tendons, and its lines of action (i.e., the orientation of the muscle fibers in relation to a particular joint) will provide a clear understanding of the anatomical motions that muscle produces.

A helpful analogy is to view the production of human movement similar to how a puppeteer manipulates the strings of a puppet to make it move; the "strings" that produce motion are the tendons connected to the muscles that have been activated by the **central nervous system (CNS).** The following sections contain numerous examples of common movements produced during exercise by the muscles of the lower and upper extremities.

Kinesiology of the Lower Extremity

In this chapter, movements of the lower extremity are defined as those that occur at the hip, knee, and ankle joints. The normal ranges of motion for these joints are presented in Figure 2-1. The subsequent sections provide details regarding the functions of the primary muscles in the lower extremity and examples of exercises to develop strength and improve flexibility.

Anterior Hip Muscles: Hip Flexors

The most important muscles, or **prime movers,** for hip flexion are the iliopsoas, rectus femoris, sartorius, and tensor fasciae latae. These muscles act synergistically to

Figure 2-1
Lower-extremity movements and active ranges of motion

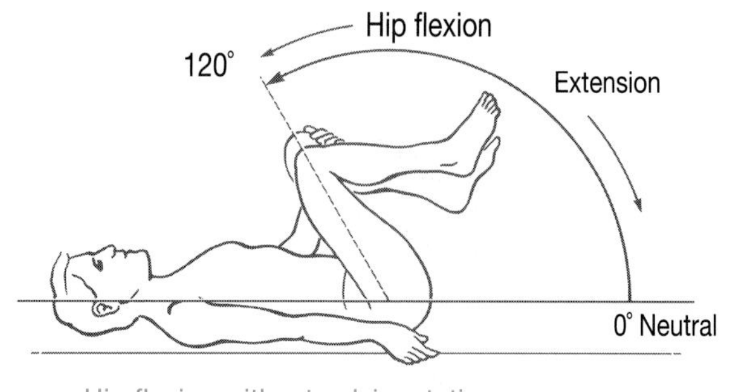

Hip flexion without pelvic rotation

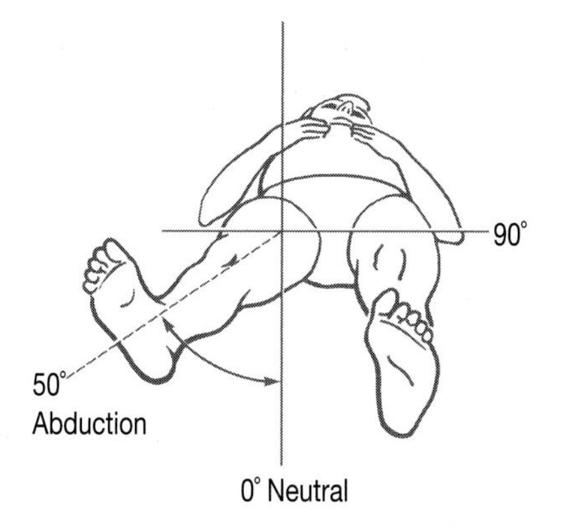

Range of motion for hip abduction

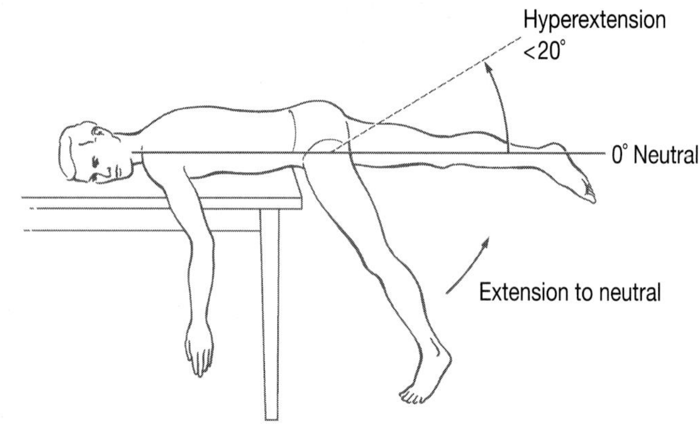

Hip extension and hyperextension (<20°)

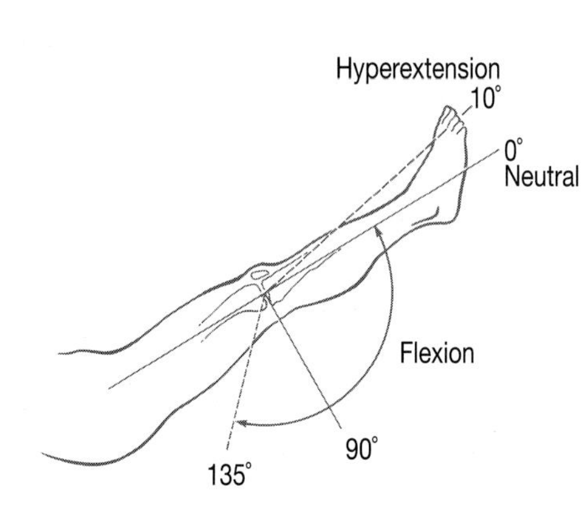

Range of motion of the knee: flexion-extension and hyperextension

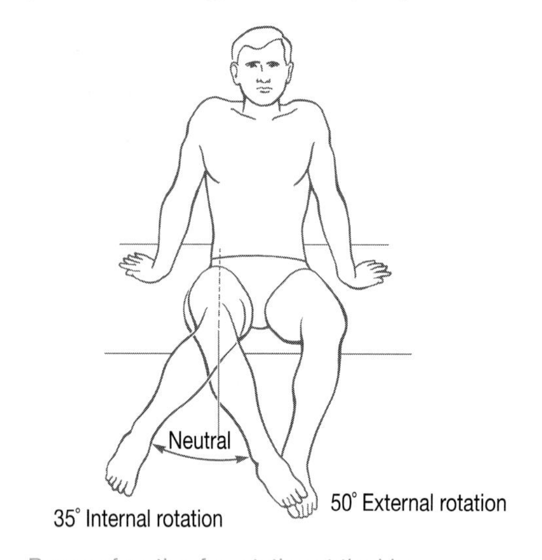

Range of motion for rotation at the hip

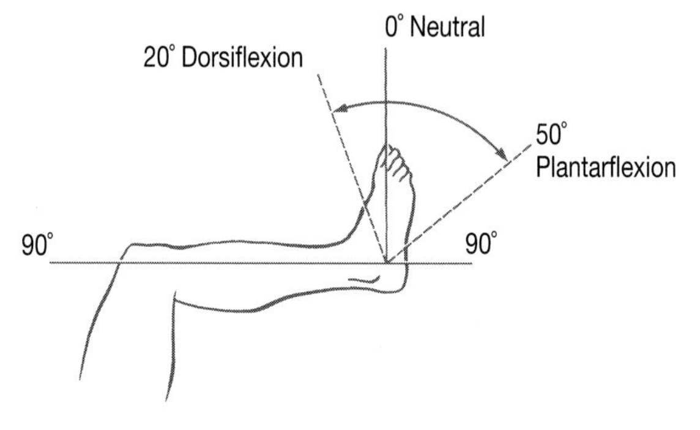

Ankle range of motion with the knee flexed

cause hip flexion, as in a straight-leg raise or knee lift. They also act eccentrically to control hip extension, such as in the downward phases of a straight-leg raise or knee lift.

The iliopsoas is actually three muscles—the iliacus, psoas major, and psoas minor (absent in about 40% of people)—that function together as one unit. The iliacus gets its name from the Latin root ilium, meaning groin or flank. The iliacus has its origin on the inner surface of the ilium bone of the hip (near the sacroiliac joint) and inserts into the lesser trochanter of the femur. The psoas major and psoas minor originate on the transverse processes of the five lumbar vertebrae and attach to the femur at the lesser trochanter. Given the origin of the psoas muscles in the low back and attachment to the proximal femur, they have poor mechanical efficiency (leverage) when recruited to raise or lower the mass of a straight leg. In most people, the abdominals are not strong enough to balance the large force created by the psoas to keep the spine in neutral position during a straight-leg lift. This is one reason why straight-leg sit-ups and leg-lowering exercises are not recommended. Because of its origin at the lumbar spine, psoas tightness (inflexibility) or **hypertrophy** can result in passive hyperextension of the lumbar spine, a condition known as **lordosis.** Tightness in the iliopsoas can also be attributed to a lack of stretching exercises and poor standing and sitting postures.

To stretch the iliopsoas, have clients stand in a forward lunge position with the front knee flexed and the back leg straight with the foot flat on the floor (Figure 2-2). Instruct them to activate their abdominal muscles to slightly flex the lumbar spine and hold this position for at least 15 seconds. Careful supervision of this activity is important, as the tendency is to hyperextend the lumbar spine during this stretch, putting unwanted compressive loads on the joints of the lumbar spine. To strengthen the iliopsoas, clients can perform a resisted knee lift (Figure 2-3). Most healthy active people have adequate strength in their hip flexors through ADL such as walking and stair climbing. As people age, there is a tendency to become less active, and the decreased stride length and hip flexion range of motion observed in many older adults during walking is the direct result of the loss of hip flexor muscular strength.

The rectus femoris is the only one of the four muscles of the quadriceps femoris that crosses the hip joint. This muscle works at both the knee and hip; concentric action of the rectus femoris results in hip flexion, knee extension, or both simultaneously. An effective exercise to strengthen this muscle is the standing straight-leg raise, producing an overload in both hip flexion and knee extension. To stretch the rectus femoris, perform the

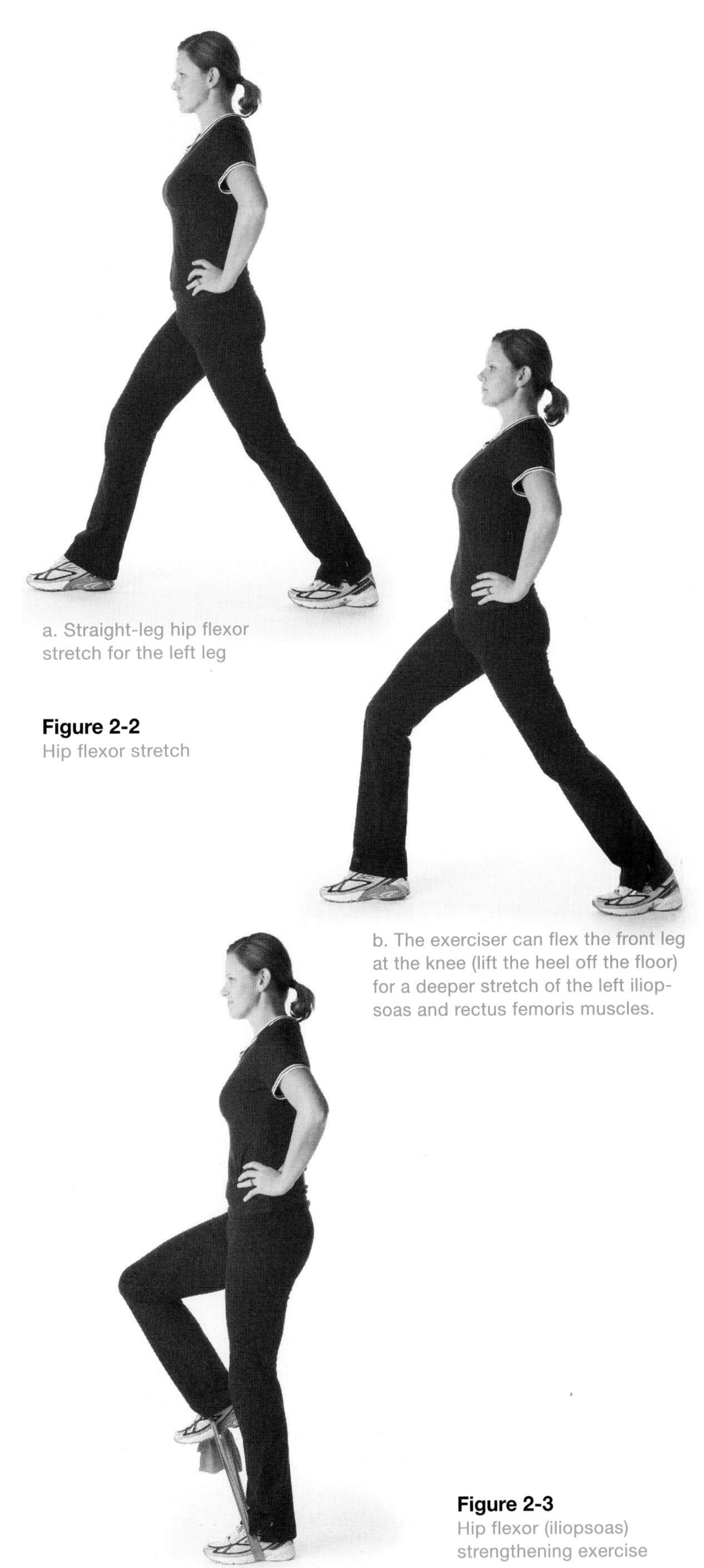

a. Straight-leg hip flexor stretch for the left leg

b. The exerciser can flex the front leg at the knee (lift the heel off the floor) for a deeper stretch of the left iliopsoas and rectus femoris muscles.

Figure 2-2
Hip flexor stretch

Figure 2-3
Hip flexor (iliopsoas) strengthening exercise

iliopsoas lunge stretch, then lower the body so that the back knee bends.

The sartorius is the longest muscle in the body, originating from the anterior superior iliac spine (ASIS) and inserting onto the medial tibia, just below the knee. This multijoint muscle flexes, abducts, and externally rotates the hip while flexing and internally rotating the knee. Just lateral to the sartorius is the tensor fasciae latae (TFL), a short muscle with a very long tendon that combines with tendon fibers from the lower fibers of the gluteus maximus to form the **iliotibial band.** The TFL originates on the ASIS and inserts on the lateral tibia just below the knee. Sprinters typically have highly developed TFL muscles from the explosive hip flexion action required when coming out the starting blocks at the beginning of a race.

Posterior Hip Muscles: Hip Extensors

The primary hip extensors are the hamstrings (biceps femoris, semitendinosus, and semimembranosus) and the gluteus maximus. Working concentrically, these muscles extend the hip joint against gravity, such as during a prone leg lift. They are also activated eccentrically to control hip flexion (e.g., motion during the downward phase of a squat or lunge) (Figure 2-4).

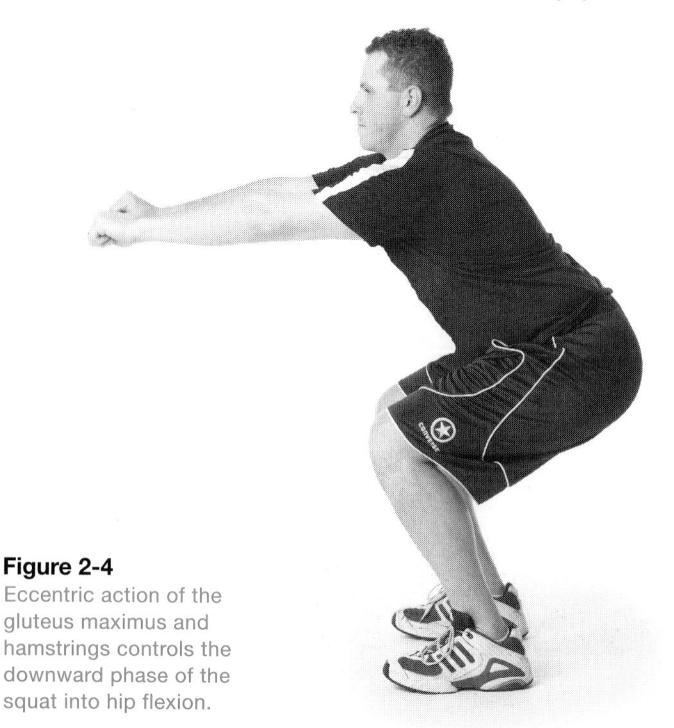

Figure 2-4
Eccentric action of the gluteus maximus and hamstrings controls the downward phase of the squat into hip flexion.

Electromyographic studies show that during normal walking and other low-intensity movements, the hamstrings act as prime movers for hip extension. There also is some electrical activity in the gluteus maximus muscle. During higher-intensity activities such as stationary cycling, stair climbing, and sprinting, in which greater hip ranges of motion and more powerful hip extension are required, the gluteus maximus plays the primary role. Other activities, such as indoor cycling classes, jumping rope, and power walking on hilly terrain, also recruit the gluteus. If a client lists "buns of steel" as a fitness goal, be sure to include moderate- to higher-intensity activities that extend and hyperextend the hip. One guideline for choosing activities that involve the gluteus maximus is to select exercises that require at least 90 degrees of hip flexion. These activities tend to be more vigorous and require firing of the gluteus maximus to provide the extra force needed to help the hamstrings accomplish the task of extending the hip through such a large range of motion.

Lateral Hip Muscles: Hip Abductors and External Rotators

The abductors and external rotators of the hip are found posterior and lateral to the hip joint in an area commonly referred to as the buttocks. The three gluteal muscles—gluteus medius, gluteus minimus, and the superior fibers of the gluteus maximus—are the primary hip abductors and are assisted by the TFL (Figures 2-5 and 2-6). The gluteus medius is the largest of the hip abductor muscles, two times larger than the gluteus minimus; the TFL is the smallest (Clark & Haynor, 1987).

The origins of these muscles are superior to the joint; therefore, when these muscles act concentrically (remember da Vinci's analogy of "cords attached to skeletons"), the hip is pulled away from the midline of the body into **abduction.** Recall that the function of a muscle depends on the orientation (line of pull) of its fibers in relation to the

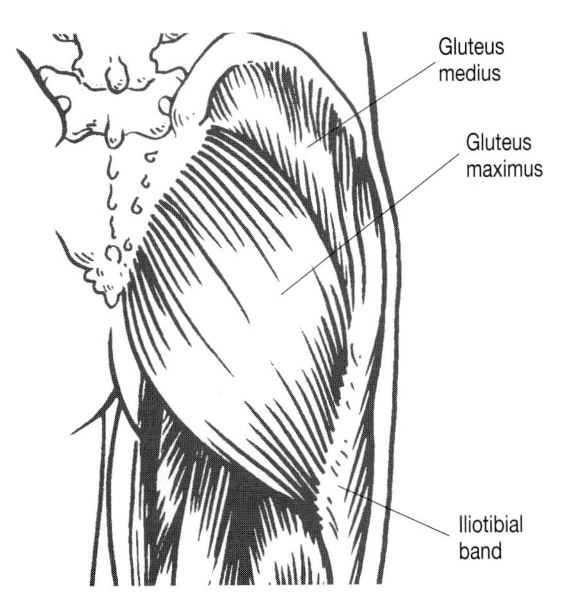

Figure 2-5
Superficial gluteal muscles of the hip

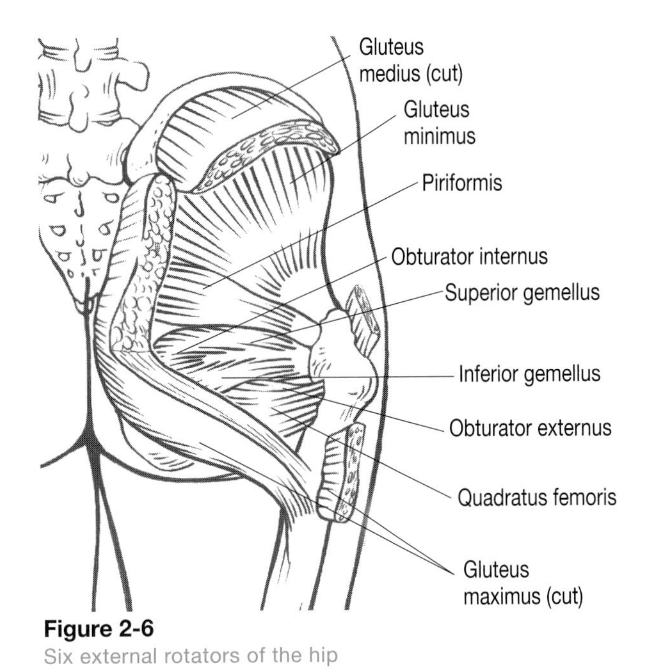

Figure 2-6
Six external rotators of the hip

joint at which it is acting. The primary function of the gluteus maximus is hip extension, while the main action of the gluteus medius is hip abduction. However, about one-third of the fibers of the gluteus maximus cross the hip superior to the functional axis of the joint, while the other two-thirds of the muscle fibers cross inferior to the joint axis for abduction and **adduction.** This means that concentric activation of those fibers of the gluteus maximus superior to the joint axis will produce abduction, while the inferior fibers will cause adduction. In a similar anatomical paradigm, the anterior fibers of the gluteus medius attach medially to the hip joint axis for rotation, and produce internal rotation when acting concentrically. The posterior fibers of the gluteus medius insert lateral to the hip's axis for rotation and thus will create external rotation when activated concentrically.

There are six external rotators of the hip located deep to the gluteus maximus. From superior to inferior, these muscles are the piriformis, superior gemellus, obturator internus, obturator externus, inferior gemellus, and the quadratus femoris (see Figure 2-6). The orientation of the muscle fibers in this group is horizontal and this, coupled with their position posterior to the joint, makes them highly efficient external rotators of the hip. When the hip is extended, the gluteus maximus also functions as an external rotator.

The optimal arc of motion for the gluteus medius to produce hip abduction is between 0 and 40 degrees of hip flexion, as its mechanical efficiency as an abductor diminishes beyond that range. When abduction exercises are performed with the hip flexed more than 40 degrees, the six small external rotators of the hip take on the role of prime movers (Lundy, 2006).

To stretch the external rotator muscles, have the participant lie flat on his or her back and pull the flexed knee and hip diagonally across the body (Figure 2-7). This position involves adduction and internal rotation, which effectively stretches these muscles.

An understanding of concentric and eccentric muscle actions is critical for the proper

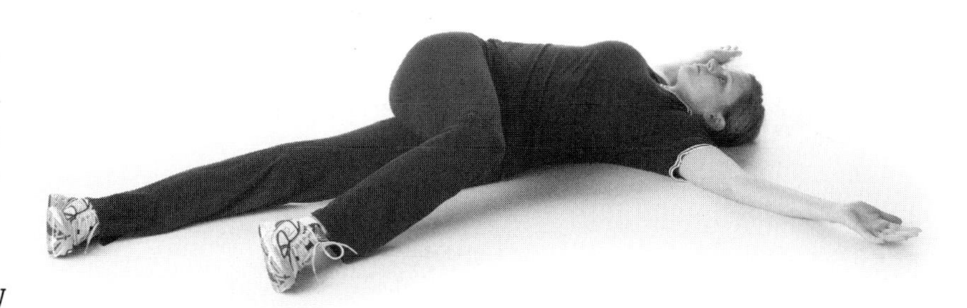

Figure 2-7
Stretching of the deep external rotators of the left hip. The exerciser should keep the shoulders and back flat; pull the flexed hip and knee across the torso.

design of exercise programs. If the movement direction is opposite the pull of gravity, the active muscle is working concentrically; if the direction of movement is the same as the pull of gravity, then the muscle is working eccentrically. However, when gravity is "eliminated" during movements that occur perpendicular to the pull of gravity or parallel to the mat, each muscle group acts concentrically to produce the desired motion. When resistance is added through the use of elastic bands or stability balls, the same principles apply in all planes of motion; concentric muscle actions occur if the movement increases the resistance in the elastic tubing, and eccentric muscle actions occur if the motion decreases the resistance offered by the elastic tubing.

Figure 2-8 employs a series of hip abduction and adduction exercises to provide examples of how body position can modify the influence of gravity. In Figure 2-8a, side-lying leg lifts are depicted. The initial action is hip abduction upward against gravity's downward pull. No motion will occur until sufficient internal muscle forces are created. Therefore, the hip abductors are acting concentrically as agonists. In the downward phase of the leg lift, the hip joint action is adduction. This joint motion occurs slowly in the same direction as gravity's pull; therefore, the hip abductors are working eccentrically as agonists to control

Figure 2-8
Concentric and eccentric hip muscle actions

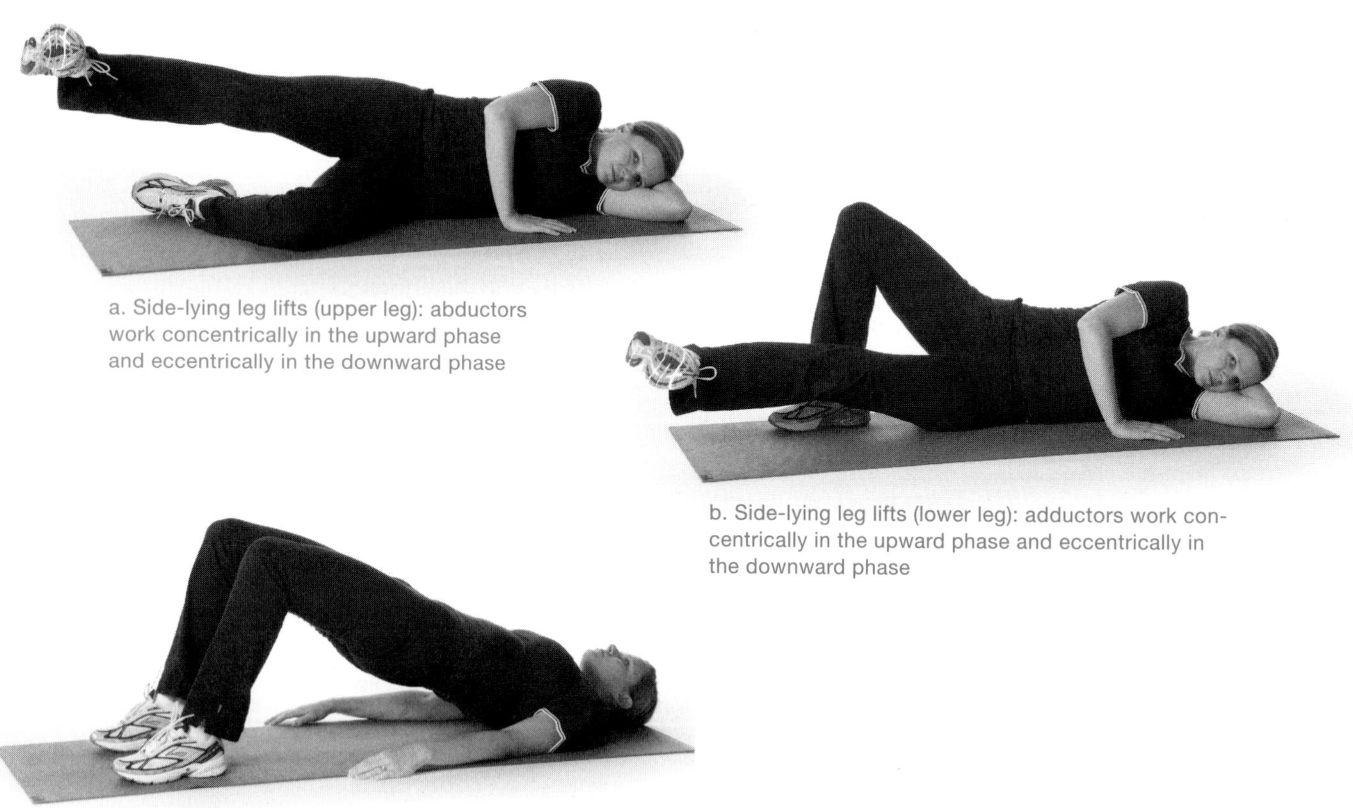

a. Side-lying leg lifts (upper leg): abductors work concentrically in the upward phase and eccentrically in the downward phase

b. Side-lying leg lifts (lower leg): adductors work concentrically in the upward phase and eccentrically in the downward phase

c. Supine hip abduction/adduction with the hips extended: abduction of the hip joints occurs as the legs move further apart, while the adductors control the movement of the legs together

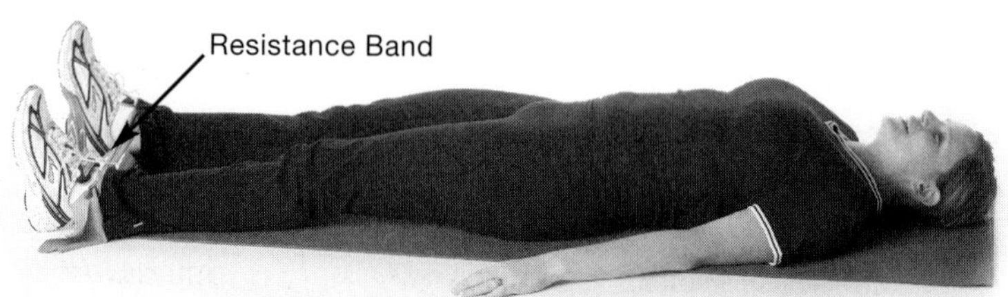

d. Concentric (legs apart) and eccentric (legs together) actions of the hip abductors with elastic resistance

hip adduction. The hip abductors are the prime movers for the hip abduction and adduction motions seen in this activity. The hip adductors serve as the prime movers for the hip adduction and abduction motions when the lower leg is extended and raised against the force of gravity (Figure 2-8b).

Figure 2-8c shows a supine hip abduction/adduction exercise with the hips extended, knees flexed, and feet on the floor; abduction of the hip joints occurs as the legs move further apart. Since the movement occurs perpendicular to the force of gravity, the hip adductors control the movement of the legs together via eccentric muscle action. To move the legs apart, the hip abductor muscles work concentrically. The hip adductors are the prime movers for the hip adduction and the hip abductors serve as the prime movers for the abduction motions observed in this exercise.

In the final example (Figure 2-8d), elastic tubing is utilized so that concentric muscle actions of the hip abductors occur when the exerciser moves her legs away from midline, increasing the resistance in the elastic tubing. Conversely, eccentric muscle actions occur in the hip abductors during the return to the starting position (adduction), against the force supplied by the elastic band at the lower leg.

Medial Hip Muscles: Hip Adductors and Internal Rotators

The muscles that produce adduction and internal rotation are located anterior, inferior, and medial to the hip joint. In this case, the muscle names clearly indicate their function—the primary adductors are the adductor magnus, adductor longus, and adductor brevis. See Figure 2-8 for several good examples of exercises that recruit the adductors of the hip.

Because of the anatomical configuration of the hip, there are no true primary internal rotators of the hip for movements starting from the anatomical position because no single muscle has a superior mechanical advantage over another to produce internal rotation torque (Neumann, 2002). As the hip joint is increasingly flexed toward 90 degrees, the most important internal rotators of the hip are the adductor longus and brevis muscles, gluteus medius and minimus, pectineus, and tensor fasciae latae. Lindsay et al. (1992) point out that the changes in the mechanical advantage (leverage) of the internal rotators improves dramatically when strength is tested in a flexed-hip versus an extended-hip position, increasing maximum internal rotation torque by as much as 50%.

The inner thigh is an area of concern for many clients. Many people want to lose the fat that has accumulated along the medial thigh and improve both the muscle tone and strength of their adductors. It is important to educate clients that spot reduction of fat does not work, regardless of what they see on television infomercials. To decrease body-fat stores along the inner thigh or anywhere else in the body, daily caloric expenditure must consistently exceed daily caloric intake. Irrespective of gender, participation in physical activity for 30 minutes a day on most days of the week will most effectively help with weight loss and help decrease body-fat percentage.

Anterior Knee Muscles: Knee Extensors

The large muscle on the front of the thigh, the quadriceps femoris, is the prime mover for knee extension when acting concentrically. As the Latin roots of its name implies, the quadriceps femoris is composed of four different muscles located on the femur that work together to extend the knee. Three of the four muscles—the vastus lateralis, vastus medialis, and vastus intermedius—originate on the proximal femur. The rectus femoris is the only one of the quadriceps that crosses the hip joint and produces hip flexion when acting concentrically, a function made possible by its origin on the anterior inferior iliac spine. The quadriceps muscles combine distally to form the patellar tendon, the second largest tendon in the body. The patella, the largest sesamoid ("seed-like") bone in the body, is found within the patellar tendon and acts like a pulley to increase the mechanical advantage of the quadriceps by as much as 30% at some knee-joint angles.

During relaxed standing, there is little activity in the quadriceps to keep the knees extended, as most of the body weight is borne statically on the joint surfaces of the lower extremity. When moving from a standing position to a seated position, the quadriceps act eccentrically to allow knee flexion, thereby permitting a controlled (safe) descent of the body into the chair. When getting up from a chair, the quadriceps muscles act concentrically as prime movers to extend the knee. In the varied ADL, strong quadriceps femoris muscles are needed for lifting heavy objects, walking, and climbing stairs. Squats, lunges, and stepping are important exercises in preparing the quadriceps for most ADL. Many experts agree that the safest approach in exercise programming is to limit knee flexion to no more than 90 degrees during weightbearing exercises.

Posterior Knee Muscles: Knee Flexors and Rotators

The primary knee flexors are the hamstrings muscle group: semitendinosus, semimembranosus, and biceps femoris. The hamstrings are referred to as a biarticular group of muscles, producing knee flexion as well as hip extension when acting concentrically. Additionally, the two medial hamstrings—semimembranosus and semitendinosus—are internal rotators of the knee. The lateral hamstring, the biceps femoris, is an external rotator of the knee. Knee-joint rotation is only possible in flexed-joint positions, as a phenomenon known as the **screw-home mechanism** increases knee-joint stability by locking the femur on the tibia (or vice-versa) when the knee is fully extended.

The sartorius, popliteus, gastrocnemius, and gracilis are secondary knee flexors (Figure 2-9) (also see Figure 1-39, page 45). The popliteus plays a very unique role in that it is responsible for initiating knee flexion and "unlocking" the knee from its extended position.

Figure 2-9
Pes anserine muscles: sartorius, gracilis, and semitendinosus

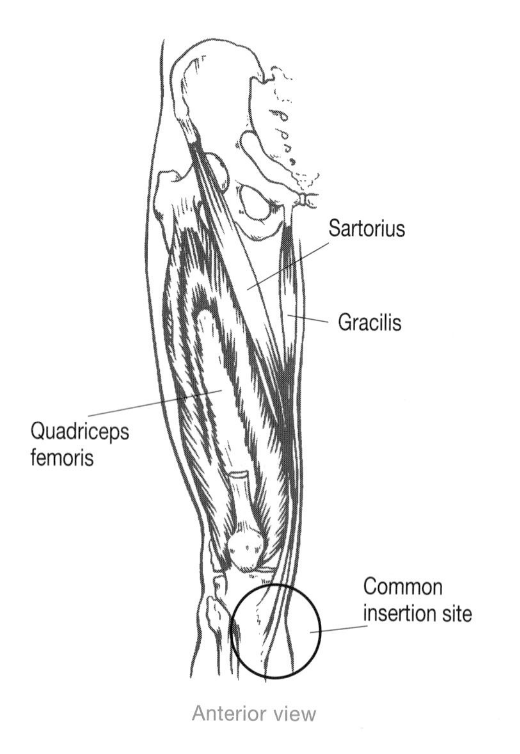

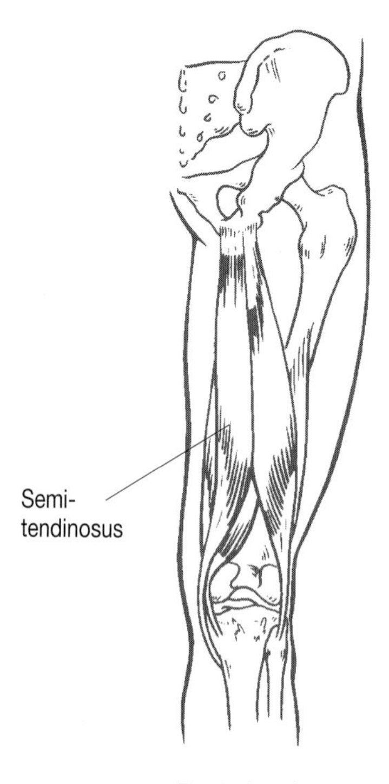

To stretch the hamstrings effectively, have clients assume a position that places the targeted limb in hip flexion and knee extension (Figure 2-10). From a standing position, the client will put the foot of the leg to be stretched on a step and slowly bend forward at the waist, keeping a flat back (**neutral spine position**). This stretch can also be performed while sitting on a stability ball. Both of these positions isolate the stretch to the hamstrings group and avoid overstressing the erector spinae muscles. To increase the intensity of this stretch, have the client flex the knee and hip of the limb not being stretched.

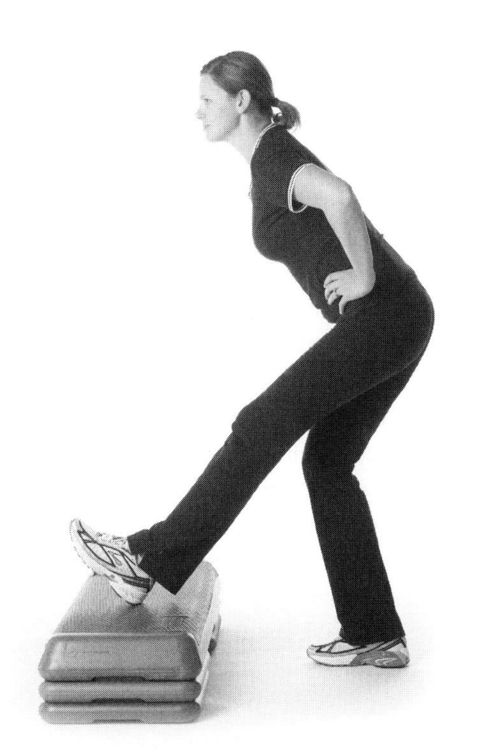

Figure 2-10
Standing hamstring stretch; hands should be used for balance—the exerciser should not apply pressure on the knee

Anterior Leg Muscles: Dorsiflexors

The muscles below the knee are organized into four finite compartments. The muscles in the anterior compartment of the lower leg are the anterior tibialis, extensor hallucis longus, and extensor digitorum longus (Figure 2-11) (also see Figure 1-38, page 44). When acting concentrically, these muscles produce dorsiflexion of the ankle. These muscles also work together during locomotor activities, such as walking and running, to eccentrically lower the foot to the ground with control. Without the vital eccentric action of the dorsiflexor muscles as dynamic shock absorbers, the foot would slap the ground with each stride or impact. Given that the ground-reaction forces during running are three to five times one's body weight with each stride and that there are approximately 1,500 to 1,800 strides (ground impacts) per mile (1.6 km), the importance of the shock-absorption role of these muscles cannot be overstated.

The anterior tibialis inserts on the medial aspect of the foot and combines with the posterior tibialis to serve as the prime movers for inversion of the foot. A common method of warming these muscles prior to impact activities is to perform toe tapping, stepping either straight ahead or side-to-side. Having clients walk for short distances with only their heels touching the ground is also a good warm-up activity for these anterior-compartment muscles.

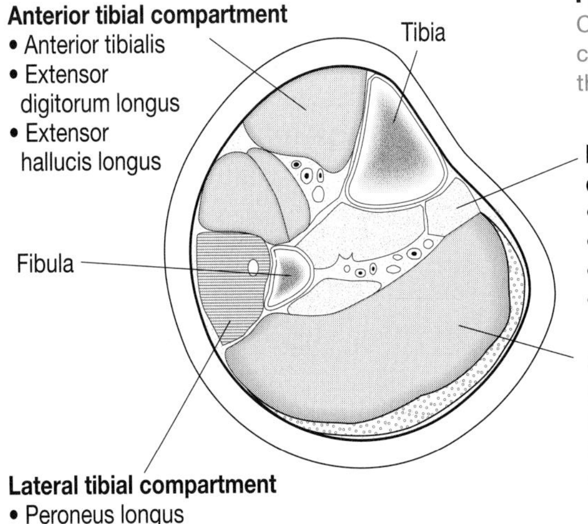

Figure 2-11
Contents of the muscular compartments of the lower leg

Posterior Leg Muscles: Plantarflexors

The large muscles of the superficial posterior tibial compartment (see Figures 1-39 and 2-11) are the primary plantarflexors of the ankle joint. While more easily palpated and more visible than the underlying soleus muscle, the gastrocnemius is actually the smaller of the two. These muscles combine distally to form the Achilles tendon, the largest tendon in the body, which attaches posteriorly to the calcaneus. The gastrocnemius, as mentioned previously, acts at both the knee and the ankle; the soleus only works at the ankle joint. Indeed, there are eight muscles that act as **synergists** for plantarflexion, evidence of the adaptive importance of plantarflexion force production (e.g., "fight or flight" mechanism). The remaining six muscles of the lower leg—the posterior tibialis, flexor hallucis longus, flexor digitorum longus, plantaris, peroneus longus, and peroneus brevis—play secondary functional roles in producing the propulsion force required for human locomotion.

The gastrocnemius and soleus muscles are often inflexible, particularly among clients who regularly wear high-heeled shoes. To stretch the two-joint gastrocnemius, the hip and knee should be extended and the ankle should be in a dorsiflexed position while the heel remains on the ground. To stretch the soleus, a similar posture is assumed, except that the knee is flexed to about 20 degrees to isolate the soleus. These stretches can be performed while seated or lying down, but more commonly are performed against a real or imagined wall or by utilizing a step aerobics bench (Figure 2-12).

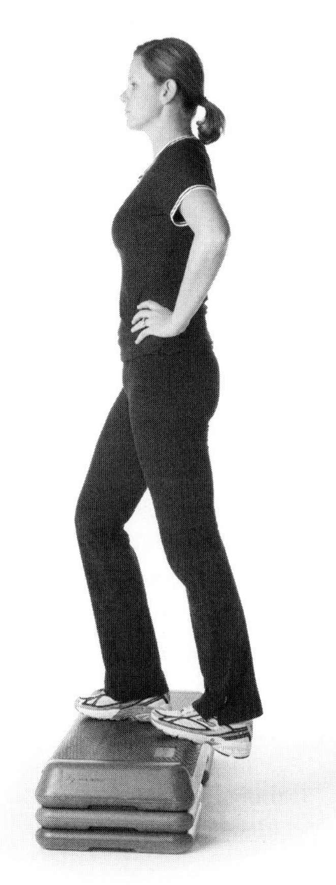

Figure 2-12
Stretching of the gastrocnemius (rear leg) and soleus (front leg) muscles

Lateral Leg Muscles: Evertors

The peroneus longus and peroneus brevis are muscles found in the lateral tibial compartment (see Figure 2-11 and Figure 1-40, page 45) that are responsible for eversion of the foot (i.e., pulling the foot laterally in the frontal plane). The tendons of these muscles curve around behind the lateral malleolus and attach on the foot. Both muscles play secondary roles as plantarflexors at the ankle due to their posterior location relative to the axis of motion of the talocrural (ankle) joint. These muscles are active during virtually all locomotor activities to provide dynamic stability at the subtalar joint, acting eccentrically to prevent the joint from rolling too far into inversion and overloading the lateral ankle ligaments, possibly causing a sprain.

Medial Leg Muscles: Invertors

There are two muscles that are primarily responsible for concentric inversion (i.e., pulling the foot toward the midline in the **frontal plane**): the tibialis anterior and tibialis posterior. A key anatomical point is to focus on the insertion sites of the distal tendons of these muscles. As their names suggest, the tibialis anterior muscle is located on the front of the tibia and is a key muscle for dorsiflexion in the **sagittal plane.** Its antagonist muscle in the sagittal plane is the tibialis posterior, found on the posterior aspect of the tibia and acting as a plantarflexor. While the functions of these muscles are opposite in the sagittal plane, they function as synergists in the frontal plane to produce inversion when they act concentrically. Similar to the evertors, these muscles are active during most weightbearing activities as **dynamic stabilizers** of the ankle joint.

Kinesiology of the Spine and Pelvis

Posture and Balance

Posture refers to the biomechanical alignment of the individual body parts and the orientation of the body to the environment. In human activities, the body is always experiencing some kind of movement change. Because of the body's dynamic nature, people are constantly performing muscle contractions in an effort to maintain **balance.** The term balance is often used synonymously with equilibrium and implies movement control. Balance is the ability to maintain the body's position over its base of support within **stability limits,** both statically and dynamically. Stability limits are boundaries of an area of space in which the body can maintain its position without changing the base of support (i.e., without taking a step).

The maintenance of balance is related to a body's **center of gravity (COG).** COG is a location where the body's mass is distributed evenly in all planes. In most individuals, it is located just anterior to, and in line with, the second sacral vertebrae, but it changes from person to person depending on their build. For example, a pregnant or obese exerciser has a COG that is displaced more anteriorly than a person of average size, due to the increased abdominal mass associated with each condition. COG is not a tangible place and is not necessarily always located within the body. COG is an abstract concept that is used to define movement of body segments relative to one another. A person's COG changes during movement depending on movement patterns and additional loads. (Figure 2-13).

Recall that balance is the ability to maintain the body's position over its base of support within stability limits. In the standing position, a person's base of support is the contact between the feet and the floor, and his or her stability limits are defined by the length of the feet and the distance between them. Efficient standing balance requires that the body's COG be kept within stability limits (i.e., between the feet). A large, wide base of support is more stable than a small, narrow one because the stability limits encompass a larger space for one's COG to move within, resulting in a lesser likelihood that the COG will move outside of the feet. Therefore, standing with the feet apart provides more stability than standing with the feet close together. This is one reason why individuals with balance problems prefer to stand and walk with their feet further apart. If a

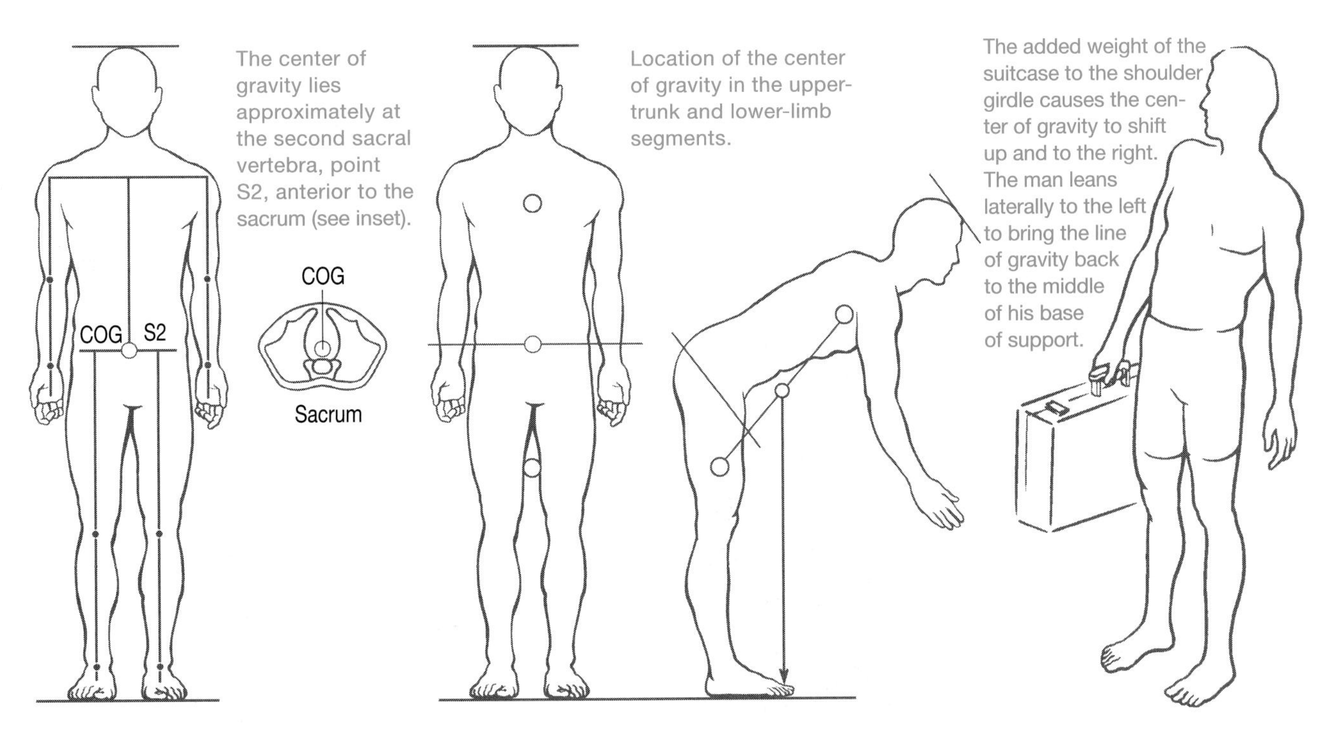

Figure 2-13
Center of gravity

person's COG shifts beyond the limits defined by the feet, it is likely that a fall will occur unless he or she takes a step to recover balance, thereby shifting the COG to its original position between the feet. To prepare for real world conditions associated with COG changes, weight-shifting exercises can be utilized (e.g., forward or backward lunges).

Posture and the Neutral Spine

Given the wide variation of human body shapes, sizes, and types, there are few people who actually have what can be called an "ideal" posture. Muscularity, flexibility, and pattern of fat deposition are just three of many factors that influence real (versus idealized) posture (Neumann, 2002). The spine of a fully grown healthy adult has 24 movable vertebrae and three normal curves: the cervical and lumbar regions are naturally convex anteriorly and concave posteriorly, referred to as a lordotic curvature. In contrast, the thoracic region possesses a curve that first develops in utero from the fetal position—concave anteriorly and convex posteriorly—known as a **kyphotic** curve (Figure 2-14).

This idealized neutral spine position requires the mathematical balance of 12 vertebrae that are curved in an anterior direction (seven cervical vertebrae plus five lumbar vertebrae) with the 12 thoracic region vertebrae that are curved in a posterior direction. The normal active ranges of motion of the thoracic and lumbar regions of the spine are presented in Figure 2-15.

An LWMC can assess muscular balance by having a participant stand in the anatomical position and observing him or her from the back and from the side. If a person stands in this neutral alignment and is viewed from the rear, the line of gravity (envision a plumb bob suspended from above) would pass through the midline of the skull, the center of the vertebral column over the spinous processes, the vertical crease between the buttocks, and touch the ground midway between the feet. Fitness professionals can promote good posture and muscular balance by having clients perform all activities with as close to a neutral spine alignment as possible. Effective cueing and correction techniques, combined with verbal and visual feedback, will help clients become more aware of their posture. Good posture is a neuromuscular skill that can be achieved or reacquired through repetition and practice.

The position of the pelvis plays a major role in the determination of the forces applied at the lumbar spine. If the lumbar spine is correctly aligned with regard to the pelvis, and the pelvis is properly balanced in relation to the legs, the forces applied to the low back can be reduced. Achieving this balance requires excellent muscle strength and flexibil-

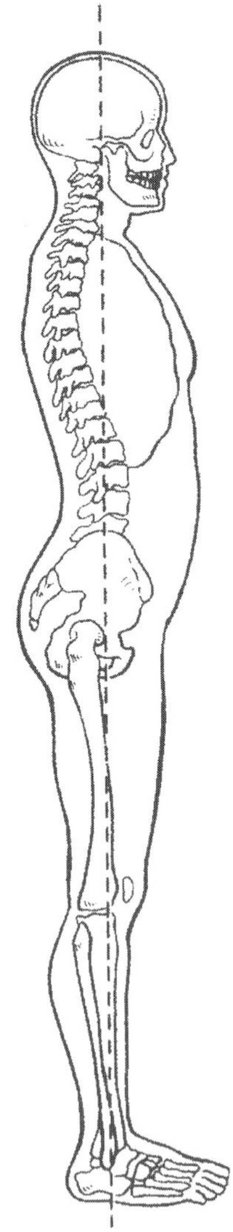

Figure 2-14
Neutral spine alignment with slight anterior (lordotic) curves at the neck and low back and a posterior (kyphotic) curve in the thoracic region

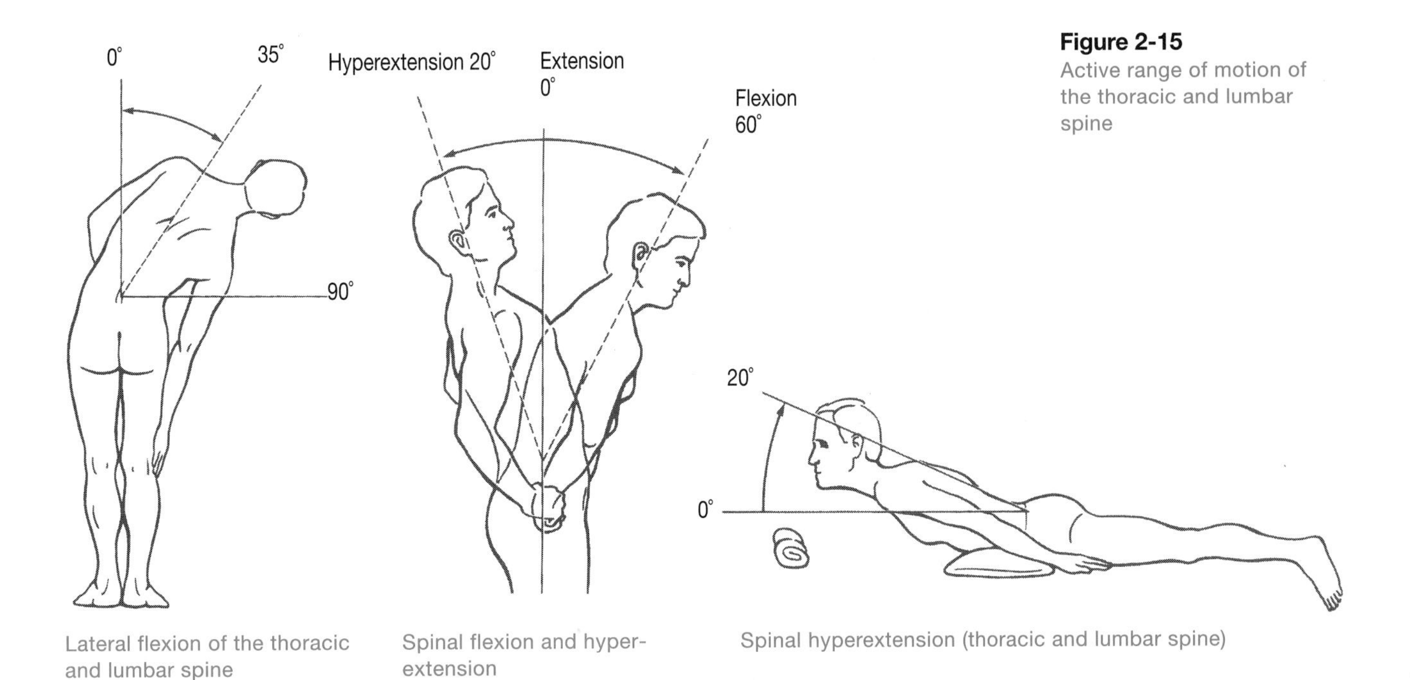

Lateral flexion of the thoracic and lumbar spine

Spinal flexion and hyperextension

Spinal hyperextension (thoracic and lumbar spine)

Figure 2-15
Active range of motion of the thoracic and lumbar spine

ity on both sides of the trunk—the trunk and hip flexors anteriorly and the trunk and spinal extensors posteriorly (Figure 2-16).

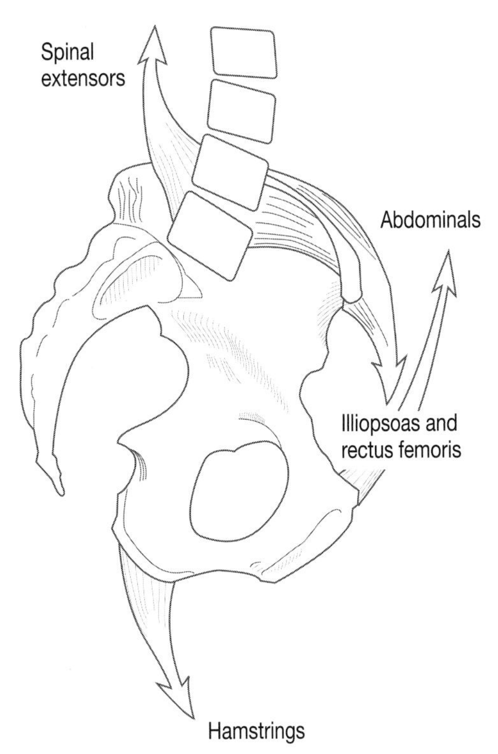

Figure 2-16
Muscular control of the pelvis by the abdominals and hip flexors (iliopsoas) anteriorly and the spinal extensors (erector spinae) and hamstrings posteriorly

Abnormal and Fatigue-related Postures

Deviations from neutral spine position can be temporary or permanent; muscle spasm and pain following a soft-tissue injury to the back, fatigue, or muscular imbalance may cause these deviations. When applied at the appropriate time with the correct dosage (frequency, intensity, and duration), exercise can help alleviate each of these conditions. Some postural deviations are structural (bony) in nature, and typically do not respond to corrective exercise. The three most common abnormal postures are lordosis, **kyphosis,** and **scoliosis.**

Lordosis is an excessive anterior curvature of the spine that typically occurs at the low back, but may also occur at the neck (Figure 2-17a). This lordotic posture has been associated with low-back pain, a condition commonly experienced by late-term pregnant women and individuals with large concentrations of abdominal fat. Lordotic posture will cause an anterior tilting of the pelvis, placing tension on the anterior longitudinal ligaments of the spine and compression on the posterior part of the intervertebral discs. If this posture is maintained over weeks and months, the back extensor and hip flexor muscles will adapt by losing their extensibility and adaptively shorten. In contrast, the hamstring and abdominal muscles will lengthen under these constant loads, becoming more lax and further decreasing their control of the pelvis. Unlike obesity, pregnancy has a finite beginning and end, and most back pain and changes in posture associated with pregnancy are resolved **postpartum.** The overweight or obese participant with lordosis presents a significant challenge to the LWMC. To correct the anterior pelvic tilt position associated with lumbar lordosis, the LWMC should focus on strengthening the client's abdominal and hip extensor (hamstring) muscles, while stretching the hip flexors (iliopsoas) and spine extensors (erector spinae).

Kyphosis is defined as an excessive posterior curvature of the spine, typically seen in the thoracic region (Figure 2-17b). The presence of kyphosis will give the individual a characteristic "humpback," with associated rounded shoulders, sunken chest, and head-forward posture with neck hyperextension. Kyphosis is a common postural abnormality among older adults with osteoporosis. In some instances, their rounded-shoulders posture is caused by weakness or disuse atrophy of the muscles that control scapular movement—the rhomboids and trapezius. Strengthening programs intended to correct this postural deformity have had varying levels of success.

Scoliosis is an excessive lateral curvature of the spine and is more prevalent among women than men (Figure 2-17c). With scoliosis, the pelvis and shoulders often appear uneven and the vertebrae may rotate, causing a posterior shift of the rib cage on one side.

If a participant has one of these three postural abnormalities and cannot actively assume a neutral spine posture, the LWMC should refer him or her to a physician.

Temporary lordotic (in standing position) or kyphotic (in sitting position) postures may occur every day when clients are tired—

Figure 2-17
Postural deviations

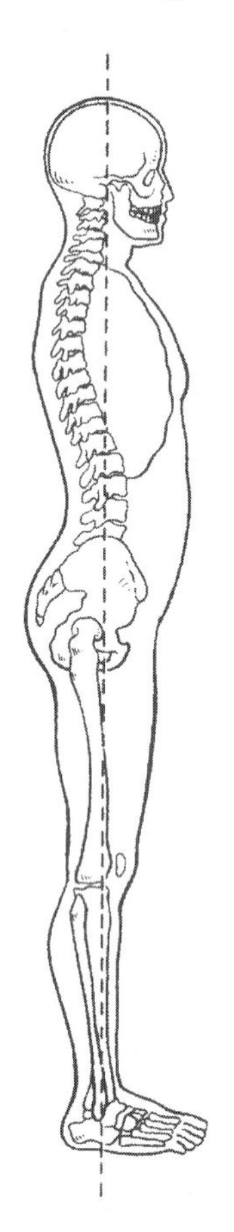

a. Lordosis: increased anterior lumbar curve from neutral

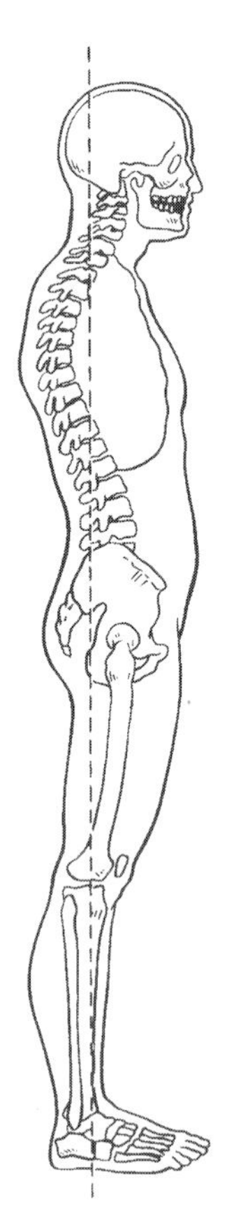

b. Kyphosis: increased posterior thoracic curve from neutral

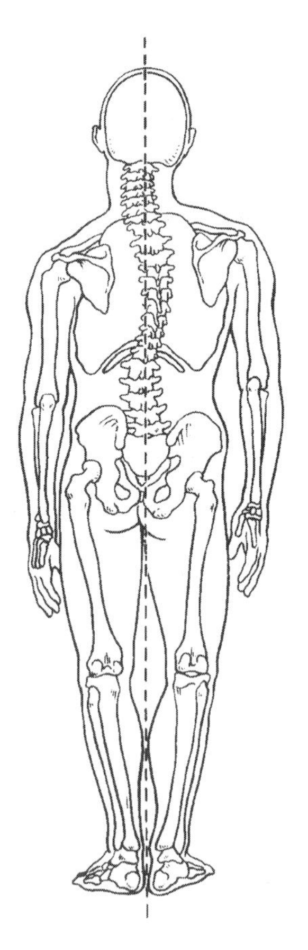

c. Scoliosis: lateral spinal curvature often accompanied by vertebral rotation

so-called fatigue postures. Fatigue postures may cause, or be the result of, physical stress, muscle imbalance, and/or pain. If these postures are continued for extended periods of time (e.g., months or years), the bones of the spine may adapt these postures, causing skeletal (rather than soft tissue) deviations that become irreversible.

Muscular Balance and Imbalance

When muscular balance is present on all sides of the cylindrical trunk, the neutral spine position can occur. However, a problem in one muscle group often creates problems in the opposing muscle group. If one muscle group is too tight (inflexible), it may pull the body out of the neutral position, causing increased stress and a tendency toward imbalance on the opposite side of the body. Conversely, if a particular muscle group is weakened from injury or fatigue, the body will fall out of alignment in the opposite direction.

The term muscular balance refers to the symmetry of the interconnected components of muscle and connective tissue. Specifically, muscular balance involves (a) equal strength and flexibility on the right and left sides of the body (bilateral symmetry); (b) proportional strength ratios in opposing (agonist/antagonist) muscle groups, although they may not be exactly equal; and (c) a balance in flexibility, in that normal ranges of motion are achieved but not exceeded.

One example of agonist/antagonist muscle imbalance is the relationship between the erector spinae and the abdominal muscles. Very commonly, the abdominals are overmatched by the muscles that extend the trunk, and neutral spine is lost. Persons with localized low-back pain from mechanical causes (no intervertebral disk or spinal nerve root involvement) are typically given abdominal-strengthening rehabilitation exercises to regain muscular control of the pelvis and balance with the erector spinae.

While not directly affecting the spine, a frequent muscular imbalance affects the function of the quadriceps and hamstrings. In untrained individuals, the naturally occurring size of the quadriceps is about twice that of the hamstrings, resulting in a significant imbalance in the agonist/antagonist relationship. With regular training, the ratio of hamstrings-to-quadriceps size and strength will improve, but hamstring strains unfortunately remain an all-too-frequent result of this muscular imbalance. Similarly, strength differences are often present between the dominant and nondominant limbs, particularly in the upper extremity. One method to counteract this is to have clients perform unilateral resistance exercises with dumbbells, isolating the right and left sides, rather than using a barbell to perform the same activity.

Core Stability

The axial skeleton (trunk) forms the "core" of the body, serving as the origin or insertion site for nearly 30 muscles in the abdomen, low back, pelvis, and hips. Biomechanically, the muscles that attach to the axial skeleton work to transfer forces to and from the upper and lower extremities. For example, a baseball pitch begins with generation of muscular force in the lower extremity (i.e., the forward stride toward home plate). These internal forces are transferred upward through a kinetic link system to the axial skeleton and into the throwing arm, concluding with the transfer of momentum to the ball via the fingers. While pitching coaches and athletic trainers go to great lengths to care for the shoulder muscles of professional pitchers, they, along with strength and conditioning specialists, also understand the need to develop trunk and lower-extremity muscular strength and endurance.

While not a particularly new concept, **core stability** is a popular topic of debate among fitness professionals, clinicians, coaches, and athletes. There is an increasing body of knowledge that suggests that core stability is a key component necessary for successful performance of most gross motor activities (Willson et al., 2005). Hip and trunk muscle strength, abdominal muscle endurance, the ability to maintain a particular spinal or pelvic alignment, and the absence of ligamentous laxity in the vertebral column have all been identified as "core stability."

The lumbo-pelvic-hip "core" is formed by the lumbar vertebrae, the pelvis, the hip joints, and the muscles, tendons, ligaments, and other connective tissues that either create or limit movement in any of these segments. **Static stabilizers** (the bony configuration of joints, fibrocartilages, and ligaments) and dynamic stabilizers (the muscles) contribute to the creation of core stability. When compared to the contributions to core stability made by the dynamic structures (muscles), the contributions of the static tissues are relatively small. There are three mechanisms by which the muscles that comprise the core contribute to the stability of the trunk: intra-abdominal pressure, spinal compressive forces, and hip and trunk **muscle stiffness,** which is the capacity of these tissues to resist internal and external loads (Willson et al., 2005).

Trunk Flexors: Abdominal Muscles

The abdominal muscles are found on the anterior and lateral surfaces of the trunk, and they flex, laterally flex, and rotate the trunk. Trunk flexion occurs in the sagittal plane, right and left lateral flexion occurs in the frontal plane, and right and left trunk rotation occurs in the **transverse plane.** The abdominal muscle group is composed of the rectus abdominis, the external oblique, the internal oblique, and the transverse abdominis (see Figure 1-29, page 37).

The fibers of the rectus abdominis are superficial and run longitudinally from the lower part of the chest to the pubic bone. Synergistic concentric actions of the right and left rectus abdominis muscles produce flexion of the trunk, as in the upward phase of an abdominal curl or crunch. While the anatomical movement during the return (downward) phase of the crunch is trunk extension, it is the eccentric muscle actions of the right and left rectus abdominis muscles (trunk flexors) that control the slow return to the mat. Unilateral concentric activation of the right or left rectus abdominis will result in lateral flexion of the trunk. Highly effective exercises to develop this muscle are posterior pelvic tilts, supine abdominal curls, straight reverse abdominal curls (eccentric action emphasized), and abdominal crunches (Figure 2-18a).

Also in the superficial layer of trunk muscles are the external obliques. These muscles originate on the ribs and attach to the iliac crest and the aponeurosis of the rectus abdominis; their fibers run diagonally downward and forward, as if into the front pockets of a pair of pants. When the right and left external obliques act together concentrically, they produce trunk flexion. The right and left sides can be activated independently to cause lateral flexion and, when combined with concentric action of the opposite internal oblique, produce trunk rotation to the opposite side. An example is the oblique (twisting) abdominal curl with the shoulder moved toward the opposite hip. Effective exercises to develop the external obliques are supine pelvic tilts, straight abdominal curls with the hips and knees partially extended to create more resistance, oblique abdominal curls, side-lying torso raises, and straight and oblique reverse abdominal curls (i.e., lifting the feet toward the ceiling until the buttocks leave the floor).

The internal oblique muscles are found deep to the external obliques, and their fibers run diagonally downward and posteriorly, as if into the back pockets of a pair of pants. Their functions include flexion, lateral flexion, and rotation of the trunk to the same side. Helpful exercises to develop and strengthen the internal obliques are supine pelvic tilts, straight and oblique reverse abdominal curls, and side-lying torso raises (Figure 2-18b).

Not too long ago, the transverse abdominis, which is found in the deepest layer of the abdominal wall, was thought to have no voluntary motor function; its only known anatomical contributions were to compress the viscera and support the spine. A series of studies have shown that the transverse abdominis, together with the multifidi muscles of

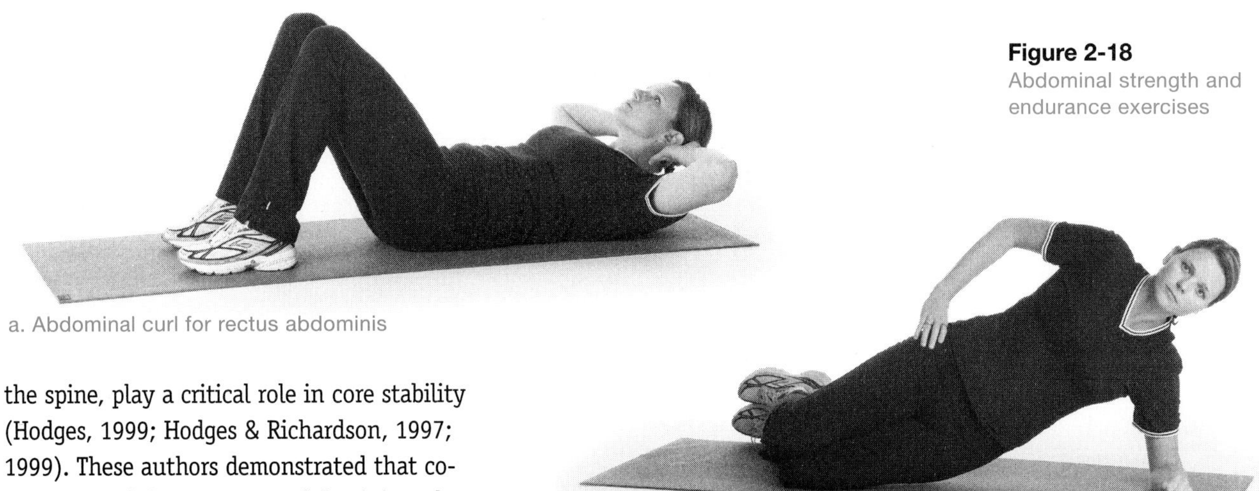

Figure 2-18
Abdominal strength and endurance exercises

a. Abdominal curl for rectus abdominis

b. Side-lying torso raise for internal and external obliques

the spine, play a critical role in core stability (Hodges, 1999; Hodges & Richardson, 1997; 1999). These authors demonstrated that co-activation of the transverse abdominis and multifidi muscles occurred before any movements of the limbs. Specifically, these two muscles were activated an average of 30 milliseconds before shoulder movement and 110 milliseconds before leg movement. What is the importance of this temporal pattern of trunk muscle recruitment? The transverse abdominis and multifidi muscles are thought to play a vital role in providing feedback about spinal joint position, and thus forewarn the central nervous system about impending dynamic forces to be created in the extremities that may destabilize the spine (Fredericson & Moore, 2005).

Knowing how to activate the transverse abdominis muscles is an important aspect of core stability. Have clients lie on their backs with their knees flexed and feet flat on the floor. While they are relaxed and breathing normally, have them visualize pulling their navel inward toward the spine. They should hold this position for several seconds, relax, and then repeat several times. There are several different floor and standing exercises that will help clients activate their transverse abdominis and multifidi muscles. If a participant has a history of low-back pain or injury, he or she may have difficulty recruiting the transverse abdominis and multifidi muscles early enough to stabilize the spine (Hides, Richardson, & Jull, 1996). An LWMC may need to refer these clients to a certified athletic trainer or physical therapist to assist them in learning these exercises. Figure 2-19 provides examples of static core stability exercises (prone plank, side plank) and dynamic core stability exercises (alternate leg bridges with shoulders on a stability ball, abdominal roll-out on a stability ball).

There are several effective methods of increasing the resistance and loading pattern during abdominal exercises; one such variation is to change body positions relative to gravity (e.g., partial abdominal curl on an incline bench with the head down rather than on a flat mat). Another variation is to change the end of the muscle that is stabilized and the one that is moved (e.g., perform abdominal curls with the shoulders lifted, and then change to a reverse curl with the hips elevated). Emphasize endurance training for the abdominals by having the participant hold an abdominal curl at various points in the arc of motion while performing exercises for the hip adductors or flexors.

Trunk Extensors: Erector Spinae Group

When acting bilaterally and concentrically, the erector spinae group of muscles, formed by the iliocostalis, longissimus, and spinalis, will produce trunk extension and hyperextension. These muscles also act eccentrically to control flexion of the spine from a standing position, as in bending over to pick up the morning newspaper. When the erector spinae muscles are stimulated unilaterally, they cause lateral flexion to that same side. In

Figure 2-19
Core stability exercises

Adapted from Fredericson & Moore, 2005

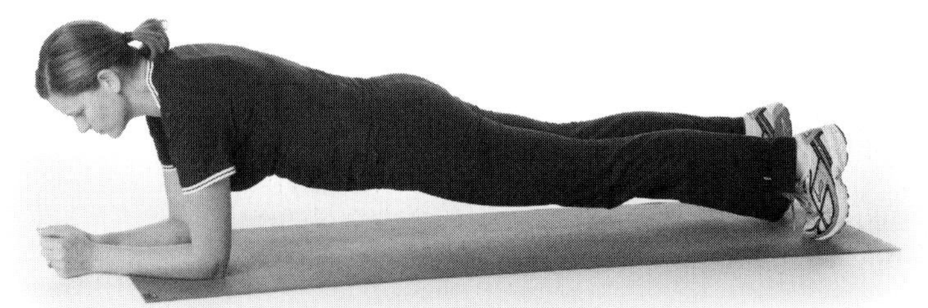

Prone plank with forearms on mat, elbows at 90 degrees

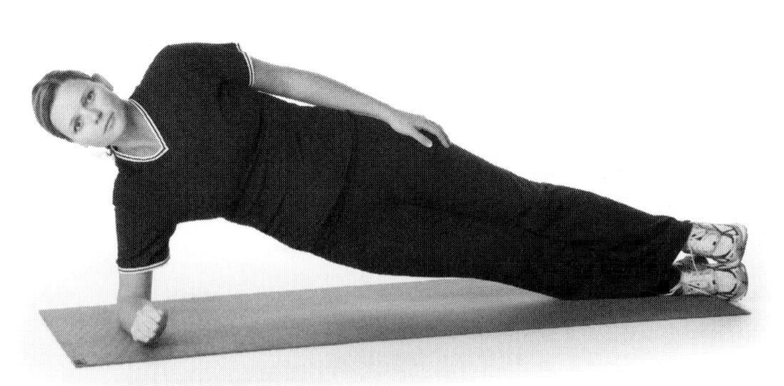

Side plank for abdominals and quadratus lumborum

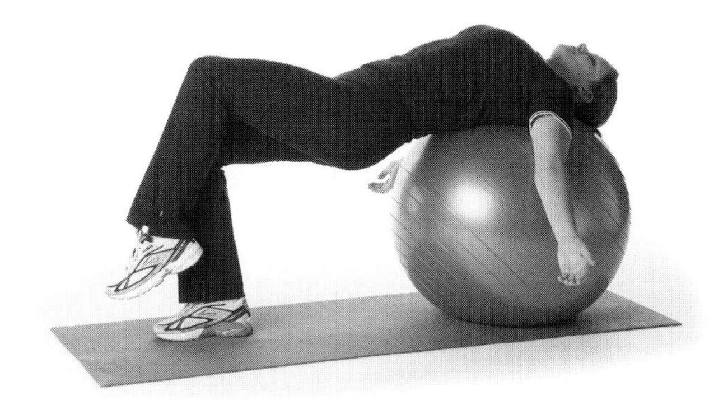

Alternate leg bridge with shoulders and head fully supported on a stability ball (extend the raised leg for a greater challenge)

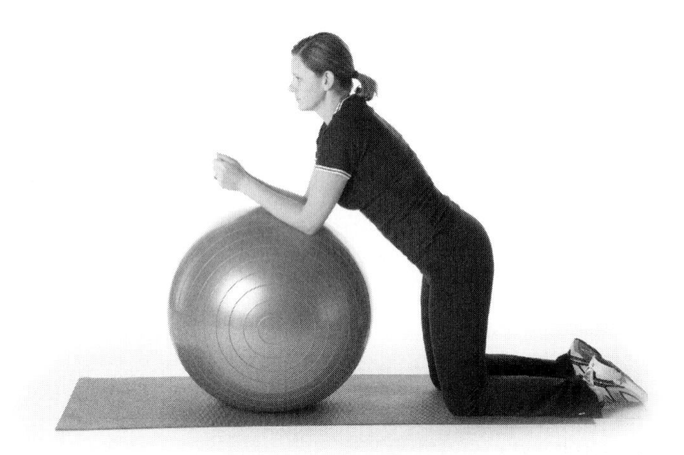

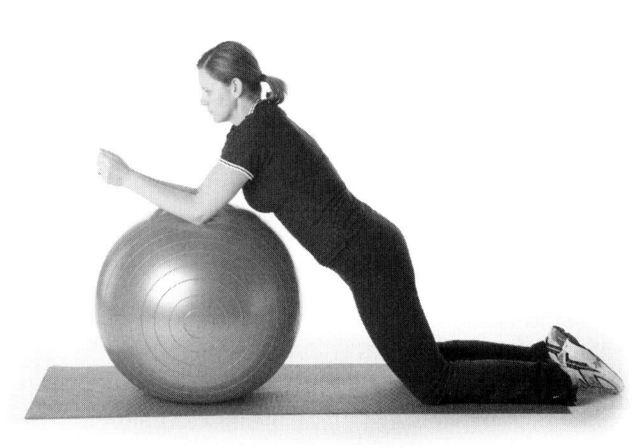

Abdominal rollout with stability ball; the farther the rollout, the more this exercise targets the latissimus dorsi

normal standing posture, the level of activity in these muscles is quite low.

Exercises that are effective for strengthening this muscle group include the prone trunk hyperextension lift (Figure 2-20a), and, from a kneeling (all-fours) position, simultaneous lifting of the opposite arm and leg (Figure 2-20b). The latter exercise causes the erector spinae muscles to function as stabilizers of the spine to maintain a neutral position. For clients seeking more advanced challenges, incorporate a BOSU™ into the exercise program to develop balance and proprioception along with trunk extensor strength (Figure 2-21).

To stretch the erector spinae group, have clients assume an all-fours position with the hands directly beneath the shoulders and the knees directly beneath the hips. Clients should arch their backs like a cat and then transition to the camel position (Figure 2-22). The posterior pelvic tilt position flattens the anterior (lordotic) curve in the lumbar region of the spine and places the erector spinae in a stretched position.

Figure 2-20
Basic and intermediate difficulty strength exercises for the trunk extensors

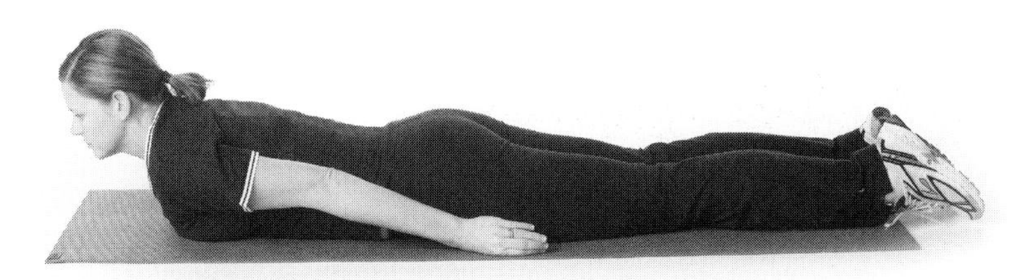

a. Prone hyperextension

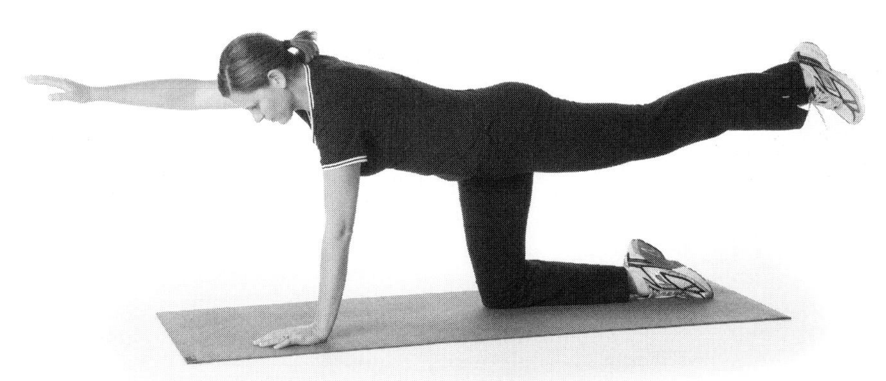

b. Birddog: lift the opposite arm and leg simultaneously while keeping the spine in neutral position

Figure 2-21
Advanced trunk extension exercise with a BOSU

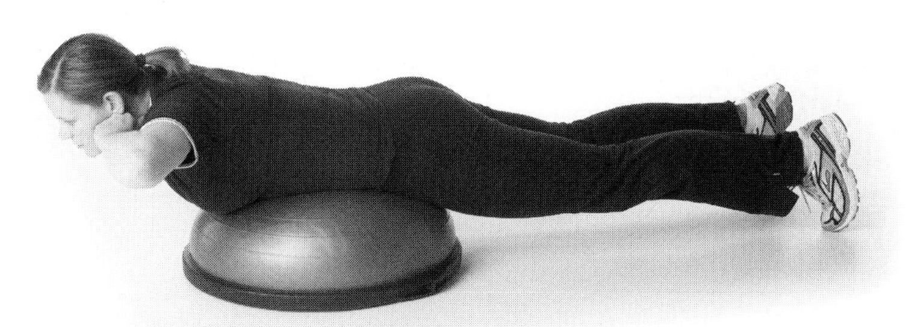

Starting position using both arms for balance

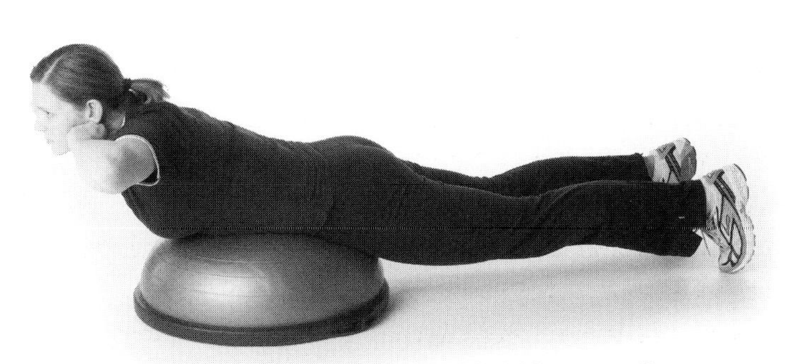

Trunk extension exercise (modified "Superman")

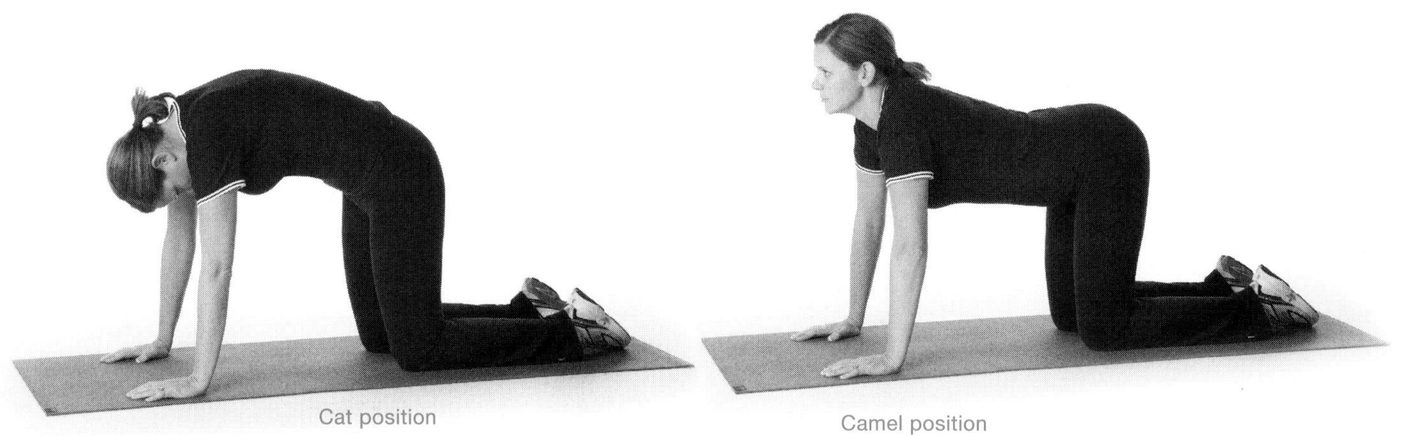

Figure 2-22
Cat-camel flexibility exercise for the erector spinae muscles

Kinesiology of the Upper Extremity

Upper-extremity segments include the head and neck, **shoulder girdle [scapulothoracic (S/T) articulation],** shoulders, elbows, wrists, and hands. Tables 1-7 through 1-10 summarize the muscles in each of these regions, their origins and insertions, primary function(s), and specific examples of exercises involving these muscles. Prior to discussion of the functional relationships of the muscles in the upper extremity, the terms **shoulder joint complex, glenohumeral (G/H) joint,** and shoulder girdle must be differentiated.

The term shoulder joint complex describes the coordinated functioning of four separate upper-extremity segments: the **sternoclavicular (S/C) joint,** the junction of the sternum and the proximal clavicle; the **acromioclavicular (A/C) joint,** the junction of the acromion process of the scapula with the distal clavicle; the G/H joint, the ball-and-socket joint composed of the glenoid fossa of the scapula and the humeral head; and the S/T articulation, the muscles and fascia connecting the scapulae to the thorax (Figure 2-23). The more general term, shoulder girdle, is synonymous with the formal anatomical term, scapulothoracic articulation.

The G/H joint is the most mobile joint in the body, the beneficiary of contributions to range of motion by the other components of the shoulder complex (S/C, A/C, and S/T). Voluntary movement at the G/H joint is possible in all three anatomical planes: flexion and extension in the sagittal plane, abduction and adduction in the frontal plane, circumduction in a combination of the sagittal and frontal planes, and internal and external rotation and horizontal flexion and extension in the transverse plane (Figure 2-24).

The glenohumeral joint and the scapulothoracic articulation work together to produce coordinated flexion and extension in the sagittal plane and abduction and adduction in the frontal plane. This relationship is referred

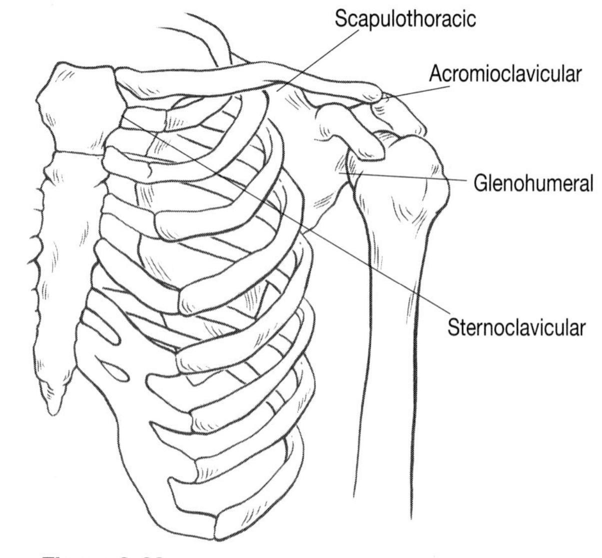

Figure 2-23
The four articulations of the shoulder joint complex

Figure 2-24
Shoulder joint range of motion

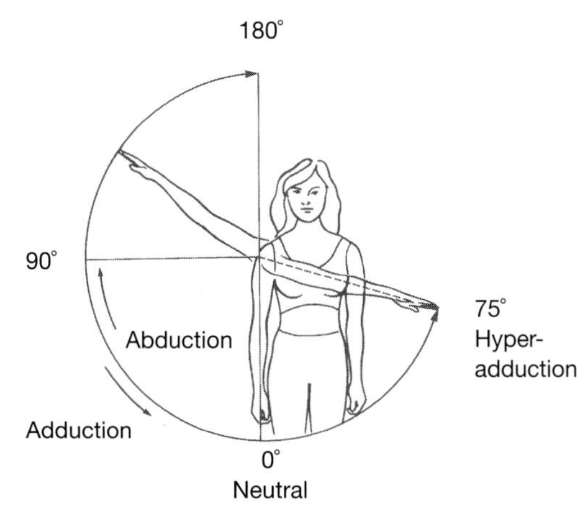

Shoulder range of motion in the frontal plane: abduction 180°, adduction to 0°, hyperadduction 75°

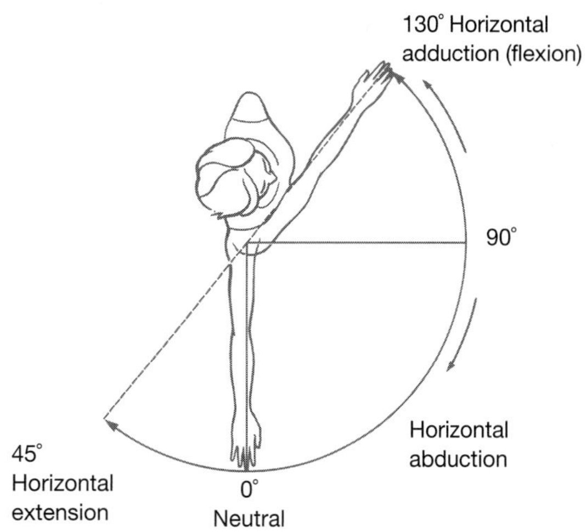

Shoulder range of motion in the transverse plane: horizontal adduction (flexion) 130°, horizontal abduction to 0°, horizontal extension 45° past neutral

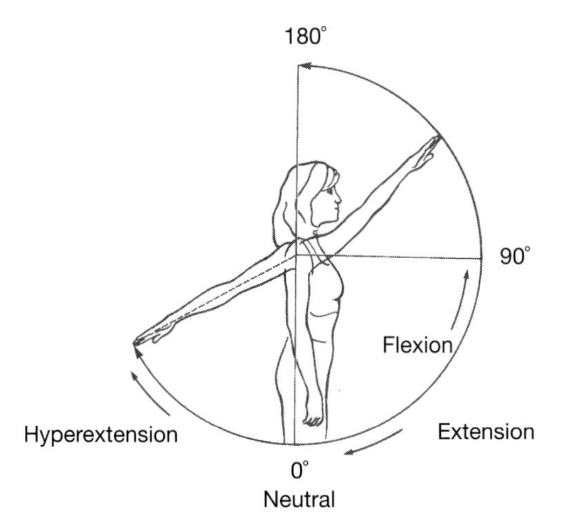

Shoulder range of motion in the sagittal plane: flexion 180°, extension to 0°, hyperextension 60°

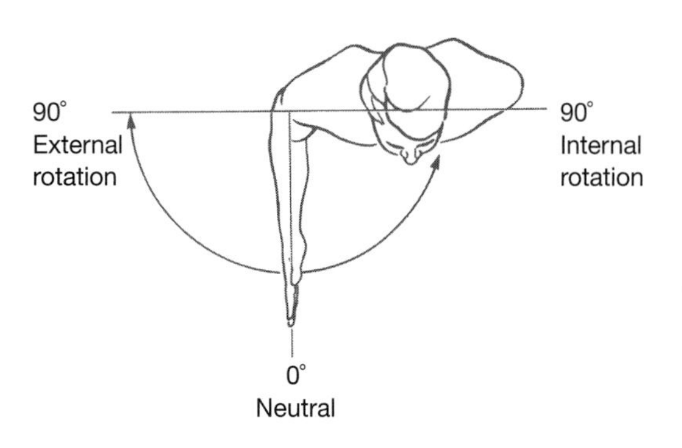

Shoulder rotation range of motion in the transverse plane (shoulder is adducted to 0°): external rotation 90°, internal rotation 90°

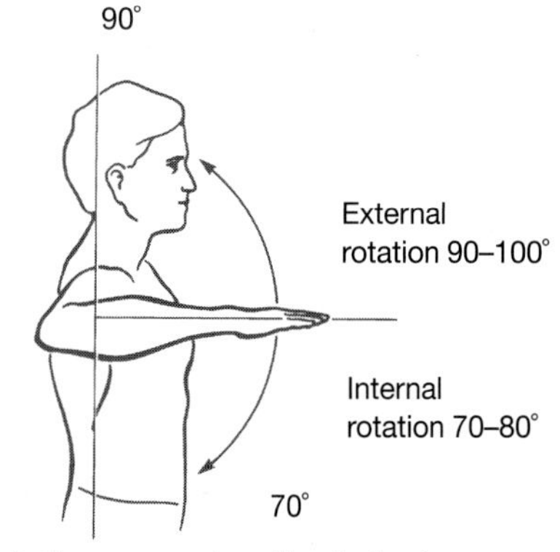

Shoulder rotation range of motion in the transverse plane, viewed from the sagittal plane: external rotation 90–100°, internal rotation 70–80°

to as **scapulohumeral rhythm** and, throughout the available range of motion for flexion/extension and abduction/adduction, approximately 2 degrees of humeral motion occurs for every 1 degree of scapular motion. Translated to absolute terms, to achieve 180 degrees of flexion or abduction, approximately 120 degrees of that motion occurs at the glenohumeral joint and 60 degrees of the motion occurs as the result of movement of the scapula on the thorax (Figure 2-25).

In common activities of daily living, the scapular muscles function primarily as stabilizers, but they also are powerful muscles involved in upper-extremity movements. Anatomical movements of the scapulae on the thorax include elevation and depression, abduction (also termed "**protraction**") and

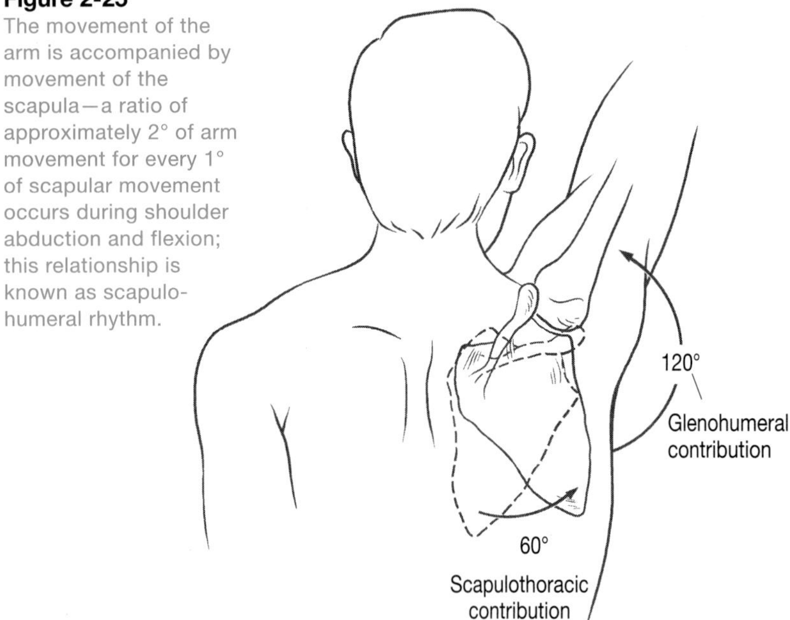

Figure 2-25
The movement of the arm is accompanied by movement of the scapula—a ratio of approximately 2° of arm movement for every 1° of scapular movement occurs during shoulder abduction and flexion; this relationship is known as scapulohumeral rhythm.

adduction (“**retraction**”), and upward and downward rotation (Figure 2-26). Scapular muscles are typically divided into two groups based on their location and function. Anterior shoulder girdle muscles connect the scapulae to the front of the trunk, while the posterior shoulder girdle muscles hold the scapulae to the back of the trunk.

There are many anatomical movements possible throughout the upper extremity. However, within the scope of this chapter, only the kinesiology of the scapulothoracic articulation and glenohumeral joint are addressed.

Anterior Shoulder Girdle Muscles

The major anterior shoulder girdle muscles—the pectoralis minor and serratus anterior—attach the scapula to the front of the thorax (Figure 2-27). Concentric and eccentric activity in these muscles results in scapular movement on the thorax; these muscles have no attachment to the humerus and thus do not directly cause glenohumeral motion. The pectoralis minor originates on the coracoid process of the scapula and inserts on the third, fourth, and fifth ribs. The pectoralis

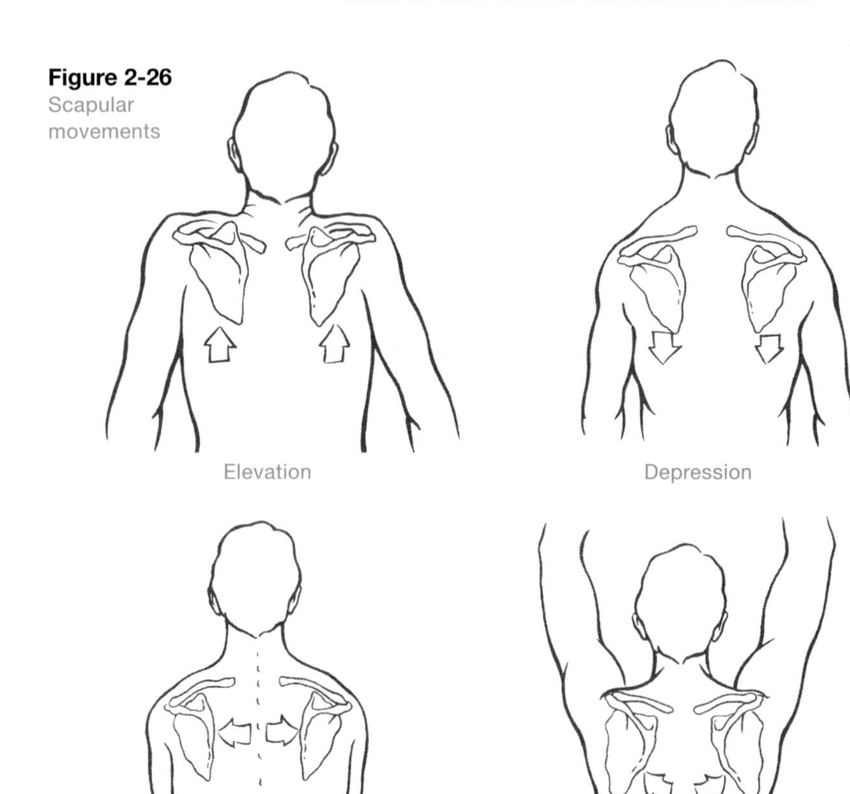

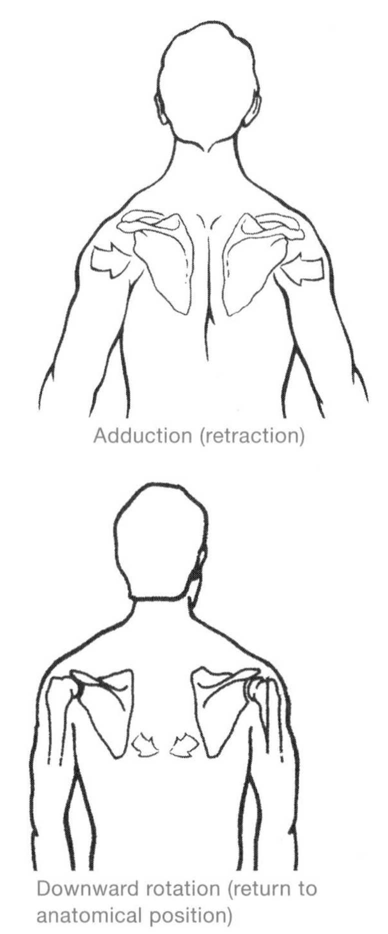

Figure 2-26
Scapular movements

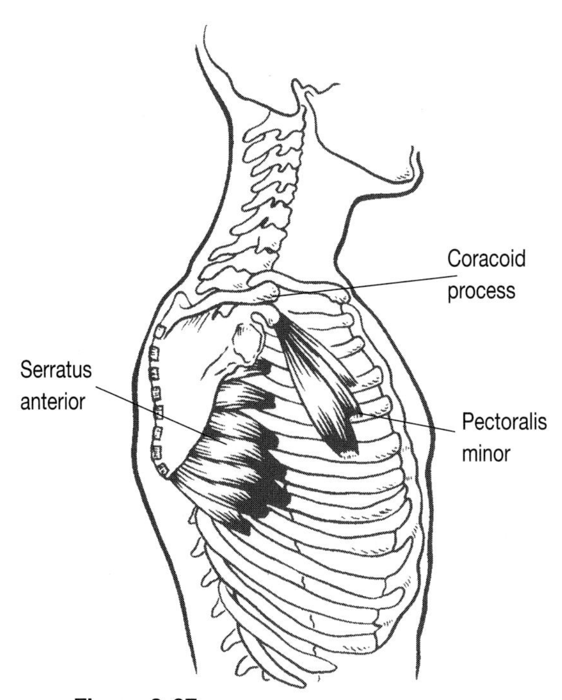

Figure 2-27
Anterior muscles of the shoulder girdle

minor can have a positive or negative effect on posture, depending on the amount of muscular tone in the scapular adductors, specifically the middle trapezius and rhomboids. Concentric activity of the pectoralis minor results in abduction, depression, and downward rotation of the scapula. However, if the scapular adductors are weak, fatigued, or injured, the muscular tension created by the pectoralis minor will tilt the scapulae forward and down, worsening a rounded-shoulders posture (kyphosis).

The serratus anterior is a broad, knife-edged muscle that originates along the underside of the entire length of the medial border of the scapula and inserts onto the front parts of the first through ninth ribs. The serratus anterior abducts the scapula and works as a synergist with the upper trapezius to produce upward rotation of the scapula. A key function of the serratus is to hold the medial border of the scapula firmly against the rib cage, preventing "winging" of the scapula posteriorly away from the thorax. Concentric action of the serratus anterior enables powerful forward motion of the arm, as in the overhead throwing motion. Strengthening of the serratus can be done from a supine position with the shoulder flexed to 90 degrees and the elbow extended, by pushing a dumbbell or medicine ball held in the hand toward the ceiling in a "punching" motion without bending the elbow. The shoulder blade(s) should lift off the floor slightly when performing this exercise (Figure 2-28). Another effective method of working the serratus anterior is to have clients perform push-ups with a "plus"—the addition of scapular abduction at the end of the upward phase of a regular push-up.

Figure 2-28
Exercise to strengthen the serratus anterior muscle

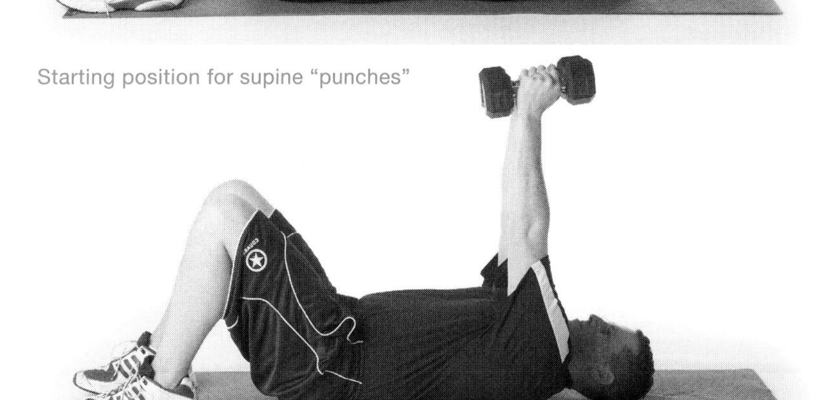

Starting position for supine "punches"

Shoulder blades lifted off the floor slightly; elbows fully extended

Posterior Shoulder Girdle Muscles

The posterior shoulder girdle muscles—the trapezius, rhomboids, and levator scapulae—attach the scapula to the back of the thorax. Since these muscles have no attachment to the humerus, their action does not directly result in glenohumeral motion.

The trapezius is the largest and most superficial of the posterior shoulder girdle muscles; it originates at the base of the skull and has attachments to all 19 vertebrae in the cervical and thoracic regions of the spine. Resembling the shape of a trapezoid, the muscle attaches laterally to the spine of the scapula and the lateral aspect of the clavicle. Recalling da Vinci's perspective of functional human anatomy as "cords attached to skeletons," it is easy to understand why the different sections of the trapezius have three different names. The trapezius is divided into three distinct units—upper, middle, and lower—because of the different directions and line of action of its fibers. The fibers of the upper trapezius are angled upward and obliquely, the muscle fibers of the middle trapezius are purely horizontal in their direction and pull, and the fibers of the lower trapezius are angled obliquely downward. Therefore, if the upper fibers are activated concentrically, they will produce elevation and adduction of the scapula. Stimulation of the fibers of the middle trapezius will cause pure adduction of the scapula, while concentric activity of the lower trapezius fibers will both depress and adduct the scapula.

The different fibers of the trapezius are alternately activated and relaxed to cause scapular rotation. If the arms are lifted in front (G/H flexion) or out to the side (G/H abduction), the shoulder blades rotate upward and away from the spine. This critical anatomical motion, upward rotation, occurs as the result of the upper and middle trapezius, rhomboids, and serratus anterior pulling on different aspects of the scapula. Concentric action of the lower trapezius, together with eccentric activity in the rhomboids and levator scapulae, will return the shoulder blades to their original (anatomical) position.

To design effective exercises to strengthen each of the sections of the trapezius, consider the stresses and loads that the muscle encounters regularly. In typical sitting and standing postures, the upper trapezius acts isometrically to support the arms and head. The upper trapezius is also active when a heavy weight or object is held at arm's length. This portion of the trapezius needs stretching and strengthening throughout the full range of motion and does not require long-duration, isometric-resistance activities. The upper trapezius and the levator scapulae are strengthened in an upright standing or a sitting position by performing shoulder shrugs with dumbbells or tubing with the arms extended behind (Figure 2-29).

The middle trapezius is commonly weak or fatigued in individuals who have rounded shoulders (kyphotic) in a standing or sitting posture. Typically, the middle trapezius does not need to be stretched, but rather strengthened in an "antigravity" position; that is, the muscle must be used to lift some resistance against gravity. Simply adducting the scapulae in a standing position does not overload the middle trapezius, because there is no resistance (other than gravity) to overcome. Examples of antigravity positions include a fully prone or a simulated-prone position (e.g., forward lunge, half-kneeling with the torso supported on the front thigh). Using dumbbells, the desired movement in the modified forward-lunge position is to "squeeze" the shoulder blades together, causing the arms to lift in the direction opposite the pull of gravity (Figure 2-30a). To isolate the middle trapezius in a standing position, use elastic bands or surgical tubing to provide resistance. Instruct clients to abduct their G/H joints to 90 degrees, maintain a neutral

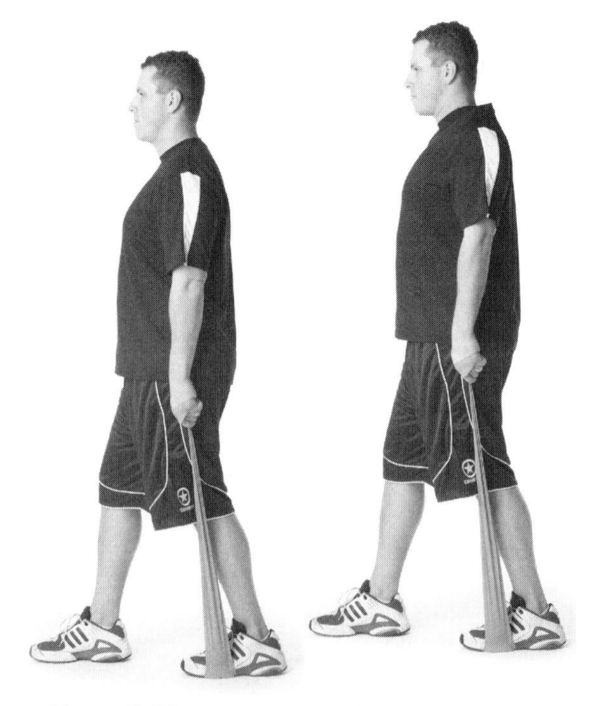

Figure 2-29
Exercise for the upper trapezius. The exerciser hyperextends the shoulders, then performs a full shoulder shrug.

spine, and then "pull" their scapulae together with no movement at the elbows or wrists (Figure 2-30b).

The rhomboid major and minor work together as one functional unit; the fibers of these muscles run upward and obliquely from the spine to the vertebral border of the scapulae. These muscles act primarily to adduct and elevate the scapulae and assist with downward rotation of the scapulae. When the rhomboids are weak or overstressed, the shoulder blades may tilt and pull away from the thorax due to the unopposed tension exerted by the serratus anterior and pectoralis minor. Bent-over rows with a weighted bar or pulley-machine weights or the use of a rowing ergometer are effective in strengthening the rhomboids (Figure 2-31).

Figure 2-30
Exercises for the middle trapezius

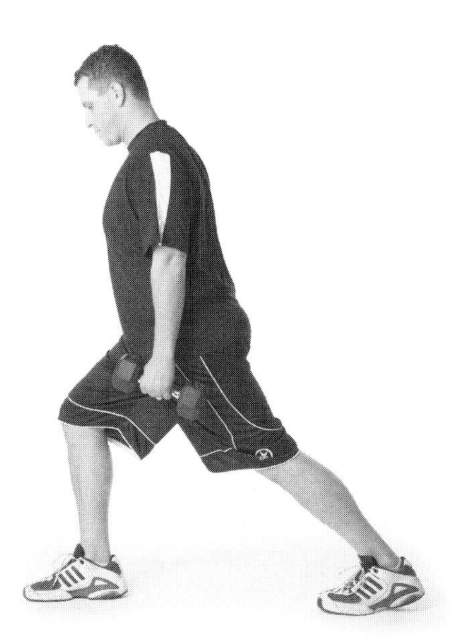

a. The exerciser should maintain neutral spine and pull the scapulae toward the spine, keeping the elbows straight and arms hanging down.

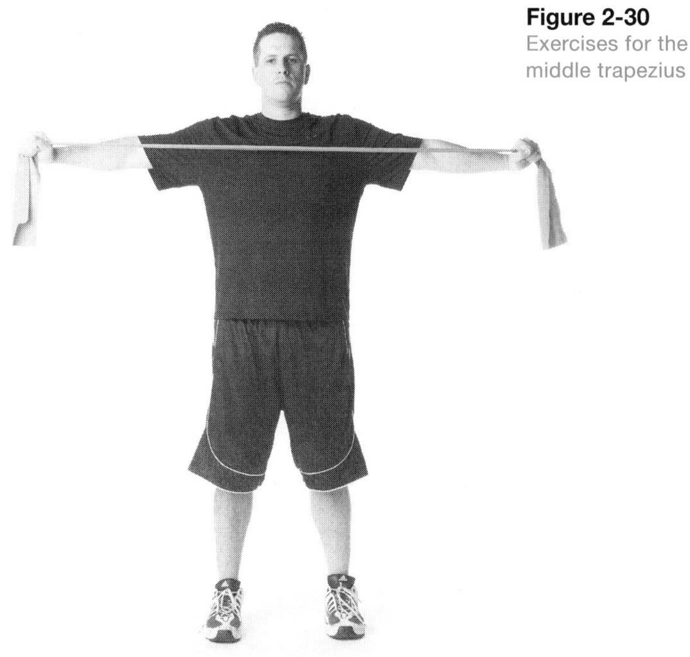

b. The exerciser should maintain neutral spine and pull the scapulae together with the elbows slightly bent and the wrists neutral.

Figure 2-31
Bent-over row to strengthen scapular retractors (rhomboids and middle trapezius muscles)

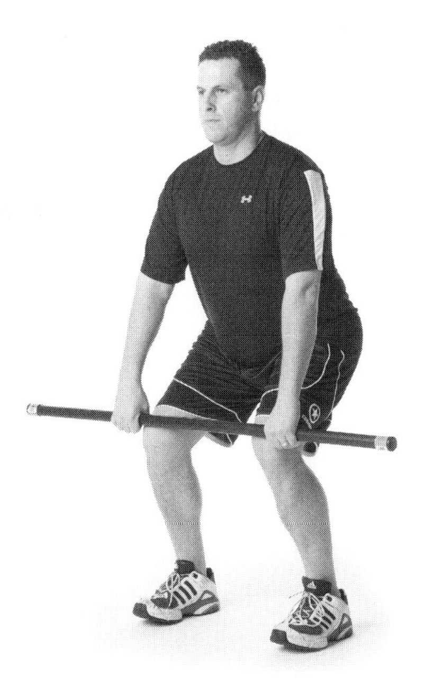

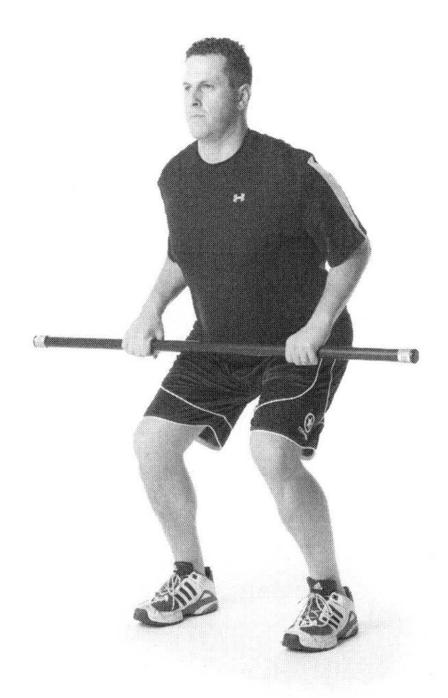

Glenohumeral Joint Muscles

The final muscles discussed in this section are those that directly produce movement at the glenohumeral joint. These prime movers include the pectoralis major, deltoid, rotator cuff, latissimus dorsi, and teres major (Figure 2-32). Due to the complexity of the anatomical functions of the major muscles acting at the G/H joint, they are not listed in groups as adductors, extensors, and so on.

The pectoralis major is a very large muscle that makes up the majority of the muscle mass on the anterior chest wall. The pectoralis major is divided into three sections, with each portion named for its attachment point to the axial skeleton: clavicular, sternal, and costal. The clavicular portion of the pectoralis major, originating on the anterior aspect of the clavicle, is located slightly superior to the G/H joint and acts concentrically as a flexor. The similar downward-oblique angles of the fibers of the sternal and costal portions of the pectoralis major allow them to be considered one functional unit. The inferior location of these muscles relative to the shoulder joint makes the sternal and costal portions powerful shoulder extensors. When considered as a whole unit, the pectoralis major is a prime mover in glenohumeral adduction, internal rotation, and horizontal flexion.

To strengthen the pectoralis major using hand-held weights, have clients lie supine on a mat or on top of a step bench. From this position, a pectoral fly exercise involving horizontal flexion will overload the pectoralis major. The push-up is also an effective exercise for the pectoral muscles. The pectoralis major, serratus anterior, and triceps brachii act eccentrically to slowly lower the body in the downward phase (same direction of movement as the force of gravity) of the push-up. These same muscles act concentrically during the upward phase of the push-up. As an added challenge for an advanced exerciser, utilize a step-bench as the starting position for the hands to increase the level of difficulty of the push-up, or have a client place two benches close together, positioning one hand on each and performing the push-up between the benches. The increased height off the ground will permit a larger range of motion during the eccentric and concentric phases of the push-up, creating a greater overload of these muscles. A study of 12 different types of push-up exercises reported that ballistic (plyometric) push-ups (e.g., those involving a hand-clap) elicited significantly higher levels of muscle activation in upper-extremity and core musculature than did push-ups performed with the hands on unstable surfaces

Figure 2-32
Superficial glenohumeral joint muscles

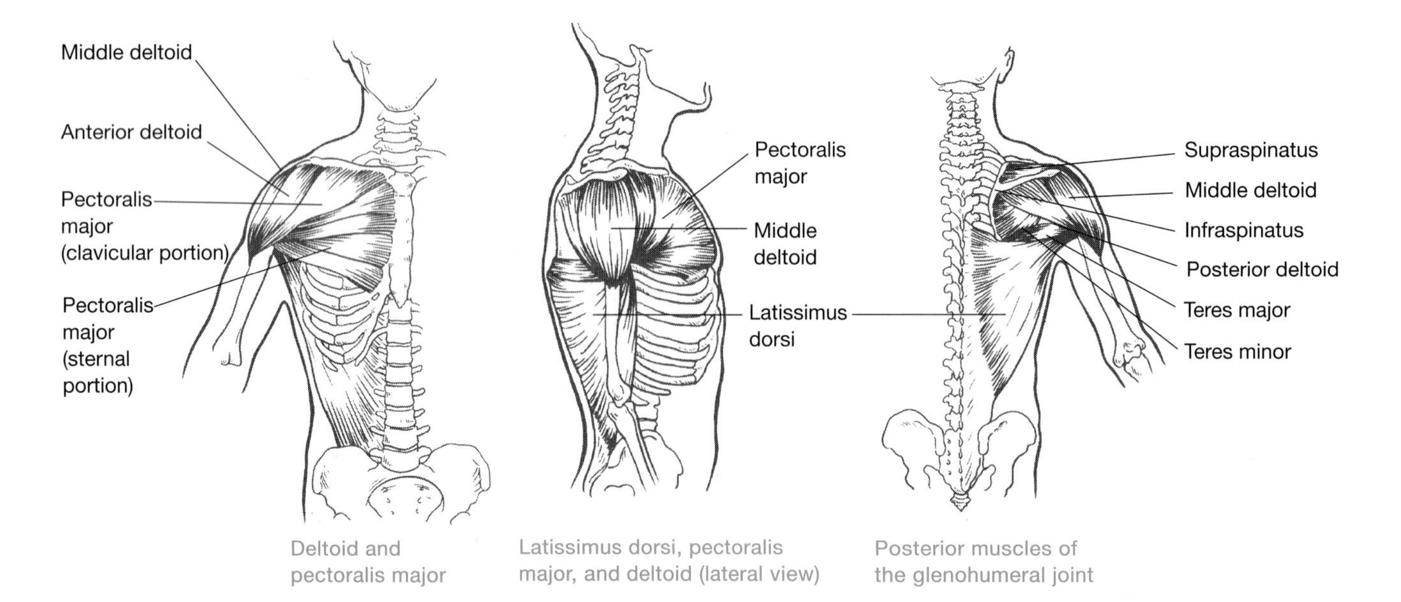

Deltoid and pectoralis major

Latissimus dorsi, pectoralis major, and deltoid (lateral view)

Posterior muscles of the glenohumeral joint

(e.g., using standard-size basketballs) (Freeman et al., 2006).

The deltoid has a configuration similar to the trapezius in that it has fibers running in three different directions and three names, according to location. As a whole, the deltoid muscle lies superior to the glenohumeral joint and collectively functions as the primary abductor of the shoulder joint. The anterior deltoid is easily palpated in the front of the shoulder, attaching to the lateral one-third of the clavicle. Since the anterior deltoid crosses the shoulder joint anteriorly, it flexes, internally rotates, and horizontally flexes the arm at the shoulder. The most effective positions to strengthen the anterior deltoid are sitting and standing. Using free weights or elastic tubing, clients can perform front shoulder raises in sets of eight to 12 repetitions.

The fibers of the middle deltoid are aligned perfectly with the frontal plane, and thus this muscle is the prime mover in concentric abduction of the shoulder joint (e.g., upward phase of a seated military press). During the downward phase of a seated military press, the middle deltoid acts eccentrically to control the lowering of the weight via adduction (Figure 2-33). When performing overhead resistance training, such as a shoulder press, it is important to maintain the glenohumeral joint in neutral or external rotation.

Shoulder abduction combined with internal rotation, particularly in clients over 40 years of age, will commonly irritate the rotator cuff muscles, impinging their tendons between the acromion process of the scapula, the subacromial bursa, and the head of the humerus. When clients who have existing shoulder pain or those who develop impingement symptoms, avoid recommending resistance exercises that combine shoulder abduction with internal rotation.

The posterior deltoid is located on the back side of the G/H joint and acts as an antagonist to the anterior deltoid. The posterior deltoid has the exact opposite functions as the anterior deltoid; it extends, externally rotates, and horizontally extends the arm at the shoulder. To strengthen the posterior deltoid, have clients stand in a forward lunge position with a neutral spine. Using hand weights, begin with the shoulder flexed, adducted, and internally rotated, and move into extension, abduction, and external rotation (Figure 2-34).

Figure 2-33
Seated military press for the deltoid muscle group

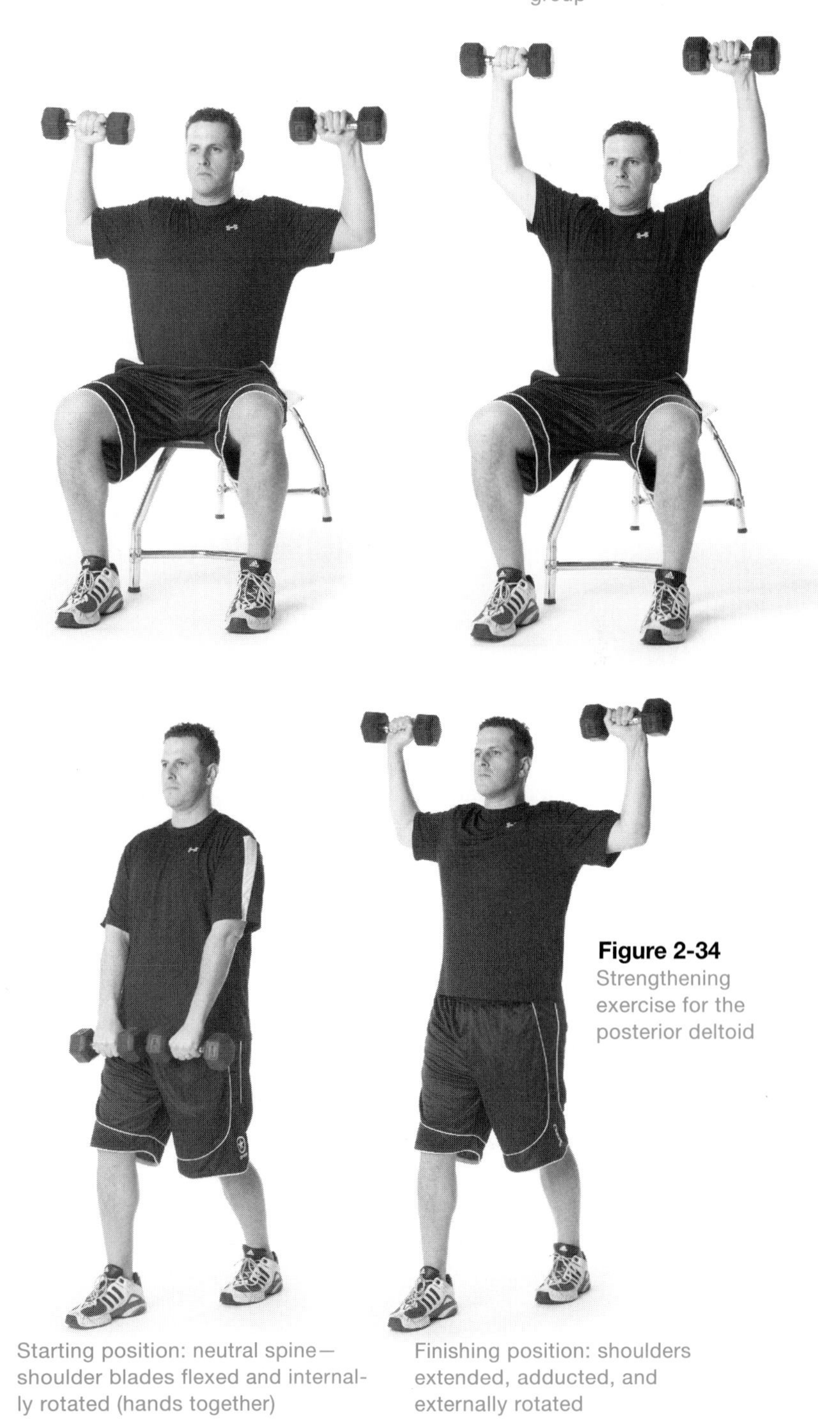

Figure 2-34
Strengthening exercise for the posterior deltoid

Starting position: neutral spine—shoulder blades flexed and internally rotated (hands together)

Finishing position: shoulders extended, adducted, and externally rotated

A group of four relatively small muscles comprise the rotator cuff (Figure 2-35). These muscles act synergistically to pull the head of the humerus down and into the glenoid fossa, thus helping to stabilize the G/H joint against the constant downward pull of gravity acting to dislocate the joint. The rotator cuff muscles are sometimes referred to as the "compressor cuff" because they stabilize the humeral head within the joint. The tendons of these muscles cover the head of humerus, while the muscles themselves are mostly named for their location in relation to the scapula. The acronym **SITS** is used as a memory device to recall the names of the muscles in this group. The supraspinatus, located superior to the spine of the scapula, initiates abduction and is a prime mover through the early abduction range of motion. The infraspinatus, found inferior to (below) the spine of the scapula, and the teres minor are synergists for external rotation of the G/H joint. The subscapularis, located on the anterior undersurface of the scapula, is not easily palpated and attaches to the anterior aspect of the joint. Since it is located anterior and medial, the subscapularis functions as an internal rotator of the humerus.

Caution must be used when working the rotator cuff in isolation; the four tendons (primarily the supraspinatus) can become inflamed as a result of performing many repetitions of movements that involve abduction, flexion, and rotation. For injury prevention, make sure that clients' shoulders are in neutral or external rotation any time the arms are abducted or flexed.

The latissimus dorsi and the teres major are similar muscles from a functional perspective (see Figure 1-24, page 33). Kinesiology instructors often nickname the teres major the "little lat" because its functions are identical to the much larger latissimus dorsi. The latissimus dorsi originates over a wide area in the lower thoracic and all of the lumbar regions of the spine, while the teres major arises from the inferior portion of the scapula. What makes these two muscles so functionally similar is the close proximity of their insertion sites on the medial aspect of the proximal humerus. Both muscles act concentrically to produce adduction, extension, and internal rotation of the glenohumeral joint. These muscles can be strengthened with elastic resistance or a cable pulley machine, starting with the arms overhead (elbows extended) and adducting and extending the G/H joint against the resistance provided by the tubing or machine. Performing this same exercise with dumbbells will not involve the latissimus and teres major in adduction, but rather recruit the abductors (deltoids) eccentrically to lower the weights. Regardless of the muscle targeted for strengthening, when working with hand-held weights, LWMCs must be sure that the initial effort is in a direction opposite the pull of gravity.

Figure 2-35
Rotator cuff muscles. Avoid resistance exercises that combine shoulder abduction and internal rotation to prevent irritation of the supraspinatus.

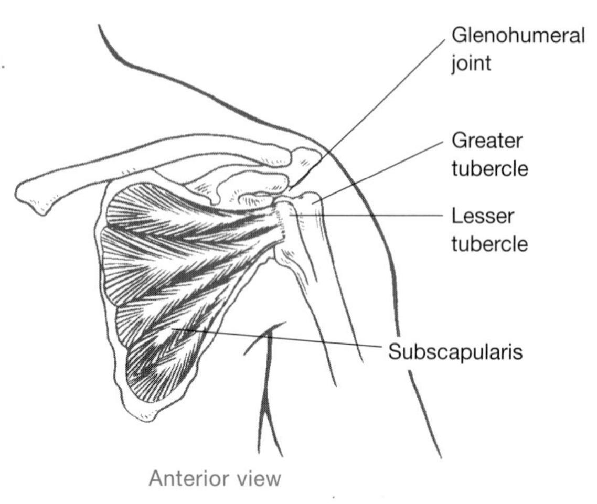

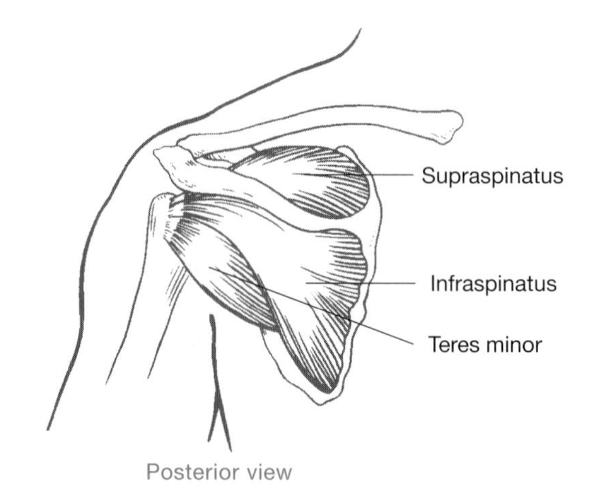

Obesity-related Biomechanics

Reports on the negative health effects of overweight and obesity, including an increased risk for **hypertension, dyslipidemia, type 2 diabetes, coronary heart disease, stroke,** and gallbladder disease, are seemingly ubiquitous. However, there has been less attention focused on the reporting of the posture and gait abnormalities associated with obesity that pose health risks for the joints and soft tissues of this population. LWMCs should recognize the functional limitations imposed by the additional loading of the locomotor system in obesity that results in abnormal mechanics and the potential for musculoskeletal injury.

Postural Balance

It has been proposed that body size and shape influence static postural stability by altering the location of the COG in overweight and obese individuals. It seems that an anterior displacement of the COG places obese individuals closer to their limits of stability and, as such, at greater risk of falling. Fortunately, regular physical activity has been shown to have a profound positive influence on balance performance in adults. Therefore, exercise programs that focus on weight reduction, balance training, and fall prevention in obese and overweight adults can help reduce the likelihood of falls occurring in this population.

Walking Gait

The calorie cost of walking in the overweight and obese population is greater than for the normal-weight population. Obese clients burn more calories during walking, in part because they are much less efficient at it than non-obese persons. In addition to weighing more and thereby expending more calories to perform physical activity, the greater energetic cost of the obese may be due to an altered step frequency (taking more steps to cover the same area), a greater vertical displacement of the COG, and extraneous movements resulting from greater limb dimensions. Additionally, research has shown that obese individuals shift their patterns of walking (i.e., use different muscles in a different order), which results in taking force off the knees and displacing it to the ankles (DeVita & Hortobagyi, 2003).

Individuals who are overweight or obese also increase their risk for the development of **osteoarthritis.** An increase in weight is significantly associated with increased pain in weightbearing joints. Small decreases in body weight (two BMI units) over a 10-year period has been associated with decreasing the odds for developing knee osteoarthritis by more than 50%, whereas weight gain is associated with a slight increase in risk (Wearing et al., 2006).

LWMCs should encourage physical activity among their obese clients that will not exacerbate their altered posture and gait biomechanics. Exercise intensities should be kept at a level that does not cause an increase in pain and soreness, since many overweight and obese individuals already have joint pain from simply performing their daily activities. **Cross-training** programs utilizing several exercise modalities within the same session are recommended. For example, cardio machines that impart less force and impact to the weightbearing joints, such as the elliptical trainer, stationary bike, and recumbent stepping machine, are popular with overweight and obese participants. Furthermore, a special effort should be made to steer clear of exercise equipment or positions that may be confining or uncomfortable for obese clients. Smaller seat surfaces, positions that allow the abdominal mass to restrict range of motion (e.g., seated leg press machine), and getting up and down from floor-lying positions should be avoided.

Summary

LWMCs are required to design exercise programs that are safe and effective, and that accomplish the desired fitness and/or personal goals of clients. Without a fundamental understanding of biomechanical principles and kinesiology, this task is nearly impossible. This chapter has provided a region-by-region summary of the functional relationships of skeletal muscles in the upper and lower extremities, as well as a review of the most current information available related to core stability. With this information, an LWMC has at his or her disposal sufficient tools to identify specific exercises and physical activities that will safely and efficiently accomplish the fitness goals of clients.

References

Clark, J.M. & Haynor, D. R. (1987). Anatomy of the abductor muscles of the hip as studied by computed tomography. *Journal of Bone and Joint Surgery,* 69A, 1021–1031.

DeVita, P. & Hortobagyi, T. (2003). Obesity is not associated with increased knee joint torque and power during level walking, *Journal of Biomechanics,* 36, 9, 1355–1362.

Fredericson, M. & Moore, T. (2005). Muscular balance, core stability, and injury prevention for middle- and long-distance runners. *Physical Medicine and Rehabilitation Clinics of North America,* 16, 3, 669–689.

Freeman, S. et al. (2006). Quantifying muscle patterns and spine load during various forms of the push-up. *Medicine & Science in Sports & Exercise,* 38, 570–577.

Hides, J.A., Richardson, C.A., & Jull, G.A. (1996). Multifidus muscle recovery is not automatic after resolution of acute, first-episode low-back pain. *Spine,* 21, 2763–2769.

Hodges, P.W. (1999). Is there a role for transverse abdominis in lumbo-pelvic stability? *Manual Therapy,* 4, 74–86.

Hodges, P.W. & Richardson, C.A. (1999). Altered trunk muscle recruitment in people with low back pain with upper limb movement at different speeds. *Archives of Physical Medicine and Rehabilitation,* 80, 1005–1012.

Hodges, P.W. & Richardson, C.A. (1997). Contraction of the abdominal muscles associated with movement of the lower limb. *Physical Therapy,* 77, 132–142.

Lindsay, D.M. et al. (1992). Comparison of isokinetic internal and external hip rotation torques using different testing positions. *Journal of Orthopedic and Sports Physical Therapy,* 16, 43–50.

Lundy, J. (2006). Gluteus medius stimulates lower extremity movement. *Biomechanics,* 13, 41–52.

Maybury, M.C. & Waterfield, J. (1997). An investigation into the relation between step height and ground reaction forces in step exercise: A pilot study. *British Journal of Sports Medicine*, 31, 109.

Neumann, D.A. (2002). *Kinesiology of the Musculoskeletal System.* St. Louis, Mo.: Mosby.

Wearing, S.C. et al. (2006). The biomechanics of restricted movement in adult obesity. *Obesity Reviews,* 7, 13–24.

Willson, J.D. et al. (2005). Core stability and its relationship to lower extremity function and injury. *Journal of the American Academy of Orthopaedic Surgeons,* 13, 316–325.

Suggested Reading

Golding, L.A. & Golding, S.M. (2003). *Musculoskeletal Anatomy and Human Movement.* Monterey, Calif.: Healthy Learning.

Hamilton, N. & Luttgens, K. (2002). *Kinesiology: Scientific Basis of Human Motion* (10th ed.). Boston, Mass.: McGraw-Hill.

Marieb, E.N., Mallatt, J., & Wilhelm, P.B. (2005). *Human Anatomy and Physiology* (4th ed.). Redwood City, Calif.: Benjamin-Cummings.

Mayo Clinic (2005). Core strengthening: Improve your balance and stability. *Mayo Clinic Women's HealthSource,* 9, 7.

Mow, V.C. & Huiskes, R. (Eds). (2005). *Basic Orthopaedic Biomechanics and Mechano-Biology* (3rd ed.). Philadelphia: Lippincott Williams & Wilkins.

Oates, C.A. (2004). *Kinesiology: The Mechanics and Pathomechanics of Human Movement.* Philadelphia: Lippincott Williams & Wilkins.

Watkins, J. (1999). *Structure and Function of the Musculoskeletal System.* Champaign, Ill.: Human Kinetics.

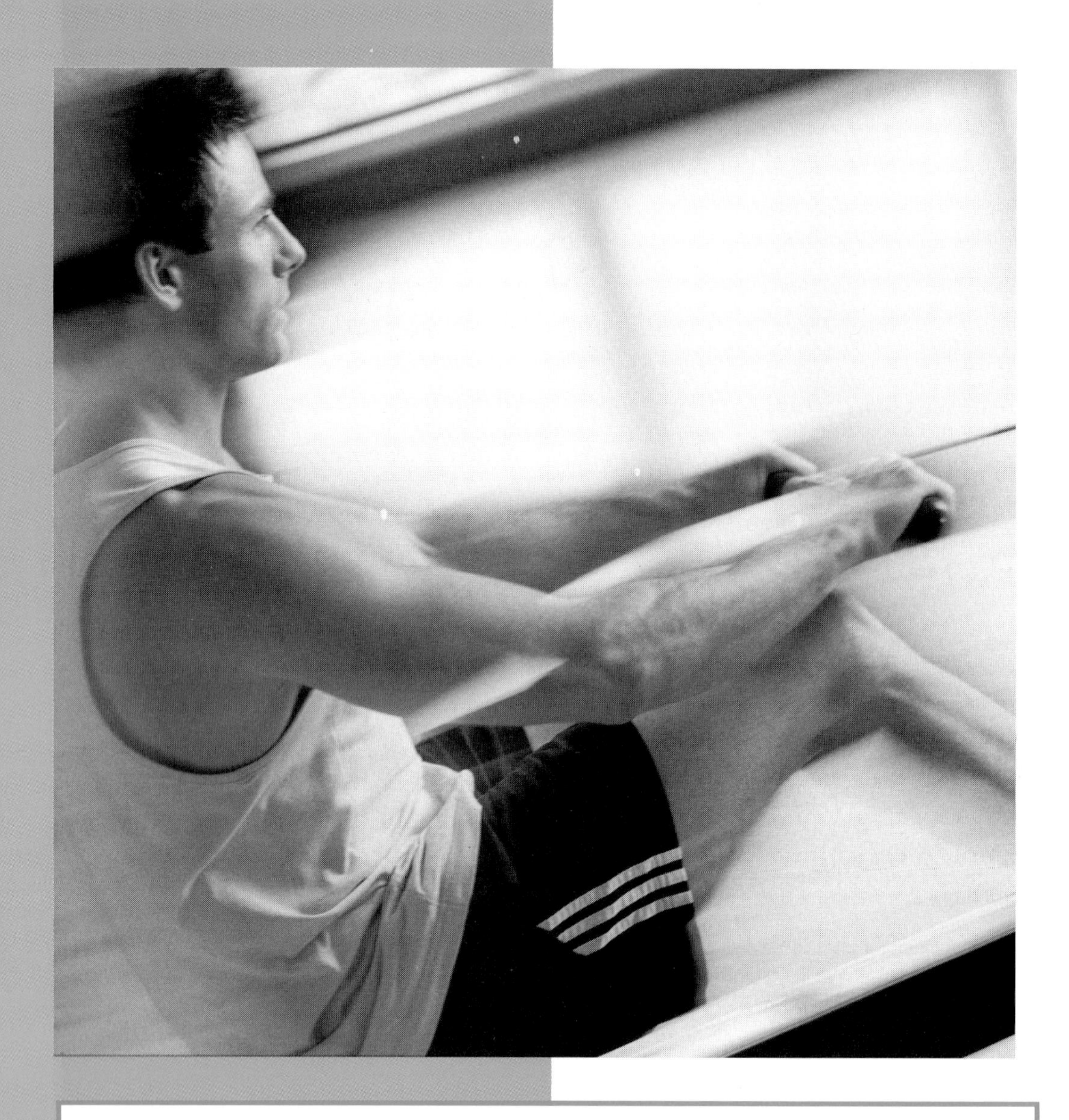

John P. Porcari

John P. Porcari, Ph.D., is a professor in the Department of Exercise and Sports Science and executive director of the La Crosse Exercise and Health Program at the University of Wisconsin – La Crosse. He is a fellow of the American College of Sports Medicine and of the American Association of Cardiovascular and Pulmonary Rehabilitation (AACVPR) and was the president of AACVPR in 2002–2003. Dr. Porcari's research interests have focused on the acute and training responses to exercising on a variety of exercise modalities, particularly new fitness products. He has authored more than 75 peer-reviewed publications and made more than 150 national presentations dealing with health and fitness.

Carl Foster

Carl Foster, Ph.D., is a professor in the Department of Exercise and Sports Science and director of the Human Performance Laboratory at the University of Wisconsin – La Crosse (UWL). He is a fellow of the American College of Sports Medicine (ACSM) and of the American Association of Cardiovascular and Pulmonary Rehabilitation. He was the 2005–2006 president of ACSM. Dr. Foster's research interests range from high-performance physiology (he is the head of sports science for U.S. Speedskating) to clinical exercise physiology (he is the research director for the Clinical Exercise Physiology graduate program at UWL). He has published more than 200 scientific papers and book chapters and 22 longer works (e.g., books, monographs, position stands, videos).

Chapter 3

Exercise Physiology

IN THIS CHAPTER:

Whenever the human body increases its activity, energy is required to fuel this movement, and the body has to make adaptations to provide this energy to the tissues. The study of exercise physiology provides an understanding of how the body responds to the acute and chronic demands placed upon on it by the increased energy demands of exercise. It is essential that Lifestyle & Weight Management Consultants (LWMCs) understand the basics of exercise physiology so that they can design safe and effective exercise programs for their clients.

Benefits of Physical Activity

There are many established benefits of being physically active, and new research is being published every day showing that exercise can aid in the prevention or treatment of most major diseases. It has often been said that if exercise could be packaged in a pill, it would be the most widely prescribed medication in the world. Some of the benefits of regular exercise include improved cardiovascular function, lower systolic and diastolic blood pressure, decreased body weight and fat mass, improved lipid profile, improved **glucose** control, decreased **anxiety** and **depression,** enhanced feelings of well-being, decreased incidence of several cancers (e.g., colon, breast, prostate), and decreased incidence of **osteoporosis.** Epidemiological studies have also found that regular exercisers live two to four years longer than sedentary individuals.

The benefits of exercise are most pronounced when sedentary individuals adopt even a minimal exercise program, but benefits continue to accrue whenever more exercise is performed.

The Concept of Physical Fitness

Before discussing the effects of exercise on the body, it is important to define what is meant by **physical fitness,** a commonly used term that has historically meant different things to different people. Much of the research on the benefits of exercise has focused on the role of physical activity in enhancing health status, as opposed to physical fitness. Physical activity can be defined as any bodily movement that comes about from the contraction of skeletal muscle and that increases energy expenditure. Many everyday activities are included under the umbrella of physical activity, including gardening, raking leaves, and performing household chores. Exercise is considered to be a more structured form of physical activity that has a specific purpose in mind. In many cases, that exercise is designed to improve specific aspects of physical fitness, which can be defined as a set of attributes that allow individuals to perform many types of physical activity with greater ease. A high level of physical fitness enables people to perform their required daily tasks without fatigue, thus enabling them to participate in additional pleasurable activities for personal enjoyment. Increased physical fitness is often reflected by physiological adaptations, such as a lowered heart rate during a standardized exercise test or an improved ability to mobilize and use body fuels. A high level of physical fitness implies optimal physical performance and good health.

Physical fitness is generally considered to have four major components, though many experts include **mind/body vitality** as a fifth component (see Chapter 13):

- **Muscular strength,** which is one component of muscular fitness, is the maximal force that a muscle or muscle group can exert during a contraction. Muscular strength is essential for normal everyday functioning, as individuals are required to lift and carry objects (e.g., groceries, suitcases) in their daily lives. Adequate muscular strength may even become more important as people age. Some elderly individuals, for instance, are not able to walk up stairs or even get up out of a chair due to inadequate lower-body strength.

  Muscular endurance, the second component of muscular fitness, is the ability of a muscle or muscle group to exert force against a resistance over a sustained period of time. Muscular endurance is assessed by measuring the length of time (duration) a muscle can exert force without fatigue, or by measuring the number of times (repetitions) that a given task can be performed without fatigue. Many everyday activities require a significant amount of muscular endurance (e.g., walking up stairs, shoveling snow).
- **Cardiovascular** or **cardiorespiratory endurance** (sometimes referred to as aerobic power or aerobic fitness) is the maximal capacity of the heart, blood vessels, and lungs to deliver oxygen and nutrients to the working muscles so that energy can be produced. The higher a person's cardiorespiratory endurance, the more physical work he or she can perform before becoming fatigued. Efficient functioning of the cardiorespiratory system is essential for physical activities such as walking, running, swimming, and cycling.
- **Flexibility** is the ability to move joints through their normal full **range of motion (ROM).** An adequate degree of flexibility is important to prevent musculoskeletal injuries, to maintain correct body posture, and to allow people to complete everyday bending and reaching tasks.
- **Body composition** refers to the makeup of the body in relation to proportions of **lean body mass** and body fat. Lean body mass consists of the muscles, bones, nervous tissue, skin, blood, and organs. These tissues have a relatively high metabolic rate and make a positive contribution to physical

performance. The primary role of body fat, or **adipose tissue,** the other component of body composition, is to store energy for later use. Body fat is further classified into **essential fat** and storage fat. Essential body fat is that amount of fat thought to be necessary for maintenance of life and reproductive function; 2 to 5% body fat is generally thought to be essential for men, while 10 to 13% is thought to be essential for women. The differences in these sex-specific essential-fat levels are due to hormonal differences related to childbearing, with the extra fat being located primarily in the breasts and pelvic regions. Excess body-fat storage is referred to as obesity and has been associated with a wide variety of health disorders, including **hypertension, type 2 diabetes,** and an increased incidence of **coronary artery disease.**

Physiology of the Cardiorespiratory System

Cardiorespiratory endurance is defined as the capacity of the heart and lungs to deliver blood and oxygen to the working muscles during sustained exercise. A person's capacity to perform aerobic exercise depends largely on the interaction of the cardiovascular and respiratory systems as they provide oxygen to the active cells so that carbohydrates and fatty acids can be converted to **adenosine triphosphate (ATP)** for muscular contraction. These two systems are also important for the removal of metabolic waste products, such as carbon dioxide and **lactate,** and for the dissipation of the internal heat produced by metabolic processes.

There are three basic processes that must interact to provide adequate blood and nutrients to the tissues:

- Getting oxygen into the blood—a function of pulmonary ventilation coupled with the oxygen-carrying capacity of the blood
- Delivering oxygen to the active tissues—a function of **cardiac output**
- Extracting oxygen from the blood to complete the metabolic production of ATP—a function of localizing the delivery of the cardiac output to the active muscles and the oxidative enzymes located within the active cells

Oxygen-carrying Capacity

The oxygen-carrying capacity of blood is determined primarily by two variables: the ability to ventilate the lungs adequately and the **hemoglobin (Hb)** content of the blood. **Pulmonary ventilation** is a function of both the rate and depth (**tidal volume**) of breathing. At the onset of exercise, both tidal volume and breathing rate increase. This increase in ventilation volume brings more oxygen into the lungs, where it can be absorbed into the blood. In normal individuals, respiration does not limit exercise performance. However, individuals with **emphysema** (degradation of the alveoli) or **asthma** (constriction of the breathing passages) cannot move enough air through their lungs to adequately oxygenate the blood. As a result, the blood leaving the lungs is not sufficiently loaded with oxygen, and exercise capacity is diminished.

Hemoglobin is a protein in red blood cells that is specifically adapted to bond with (i.e., carry) oxygen molecules. When oxygen enters the lungs, it diffuses through the pulmonary membranes into the bloodstream, where it binds to hemoglobin. The oxygen is then carried within the bloodstream throughout the body. Persons with low hemoglobin concentrations (i.e., **anemia**) cannot carry as much oxygen in their blood as persons with high hemoglobin concentrations. For example, in individuals with anemia (i.e., less than 12 g of Hb per 100 mL of blood), the blood's oxygen-carrying capacity is severely limited, and they fatigue very easily. In most healthy persons, the oxygen-carrying capacity of the blood is not a limiting factor in the performance of aerobic exercise.

Oxygen Delivery

Probably the most important factor in cardiorespiratory endurance is the delivery of blood to the active cells, which is a function of cardiac output. Cardiac output ($\dot{Q}$) is the product of **heart rate** (HR, in beats per minute) and **stroke volume** (SV, the quantity of blood pumped per heartbeat):

$$\dot{Q} = HR \times SV$$

At rest, cardiac output averages approximately 5 liters (1.3 gallons) per minute. During maximal exercise, this number can increase to up to 30 to 40 liters (8 to 10.5 gallons) per minute in highly trained individuals. The increase in cardiac output is brought about by increases in both HR and SV. HR generally increases in a linear fashion up to maximal levels, while SV increases up to approximately 40 to 50% of an individual's maximal capacity and then plateaus. The increase in SV is brought about by increases in both venous return and in the contractile force of the heart.

Oxygen Extraction

The third factor that is important in determining cardiorespiratory endurance is the extraction of oxygen from the blood at the cellular level for the aerobic production of ATP. The amount of oxygen extracted is largely a function of muscle-fiber type and the availability of specialized oxidative enzymes. For example, **slow-twitch muscle fibers** are specifically adapted for oxygen extraction and utilization due to their high levels of oxidative enzymes. Aerobic production of ATP takes place in the **mitochondria** of the cells. One of the most important adaptations to training is an increase in the number and size of the mitochondria, with a corresponding increase in the levels of oxidative enzymes used to aerobically produce ATP.

Bioenergetics of Exercise

The human body's cells require a continuous supply of energy to function. Ultimately, the food that people eat supplies this energy. However, the cells do not directly use the energy contained in food. Rather, they need ATP, which is the immediately usable form of chemical energy needed for all cellular function, including muscular contraction. While a small amount of ATP is actually stored within the muscles, the majority of the ATP used for muscular contraction is synthesized from foods consumed.

Foods are made up of **carbohydrates, fats,** and **proteins.** The process of digestion breaks these nutrients down to their simplest components (**glucose, fatty acids,** and **amino acids**), which are absorbed into the blood and transported to metabolically active cells, such as nerve or muscle cells. These components either immediately enter a metabolic pathway to produce ATP or are stored in body tissues for later use. For example, excess glucose will be stored as glycogen in muscle or liver cells. Fatty acids that are not immediately used for ATP production will be stored as adipose tissue (body fat). In contrast, relatively little of the protein (amino acids) a person eats is used for energy production. Instead, it is used for the growth or repair of cellular structures or is excreted as waste products. Figure 3-1 summarizes the fate of the carbohydrates, fats, and protein that people eat.

Stored ATP—The Immediate Energy Source

ATP is a complicated chemical structure made up of a substance called adenosine and three simpler groups of atoms called phosphate groups (P). Special high-energy bonds exist between the phosphate groups (Figure 3-2a). Breaking the phosphate bond releases energy (E) that the cell uses directly to perform its cellular function (Figure 3-2b). The specific cellular function performed depends on the type of cell. In a muscle cell, the breakdown of ATP allows the mechanical work known as muscular contraction. If ATP is not available, muscle contraction stops.

While ATP can be stored within the cells, the amount stored and immediately available for muscle contraction is extremely limited, and is sufficient for only a few seconds of muscular work. Therefore, ATP must be continuously resynthesized, which can be done

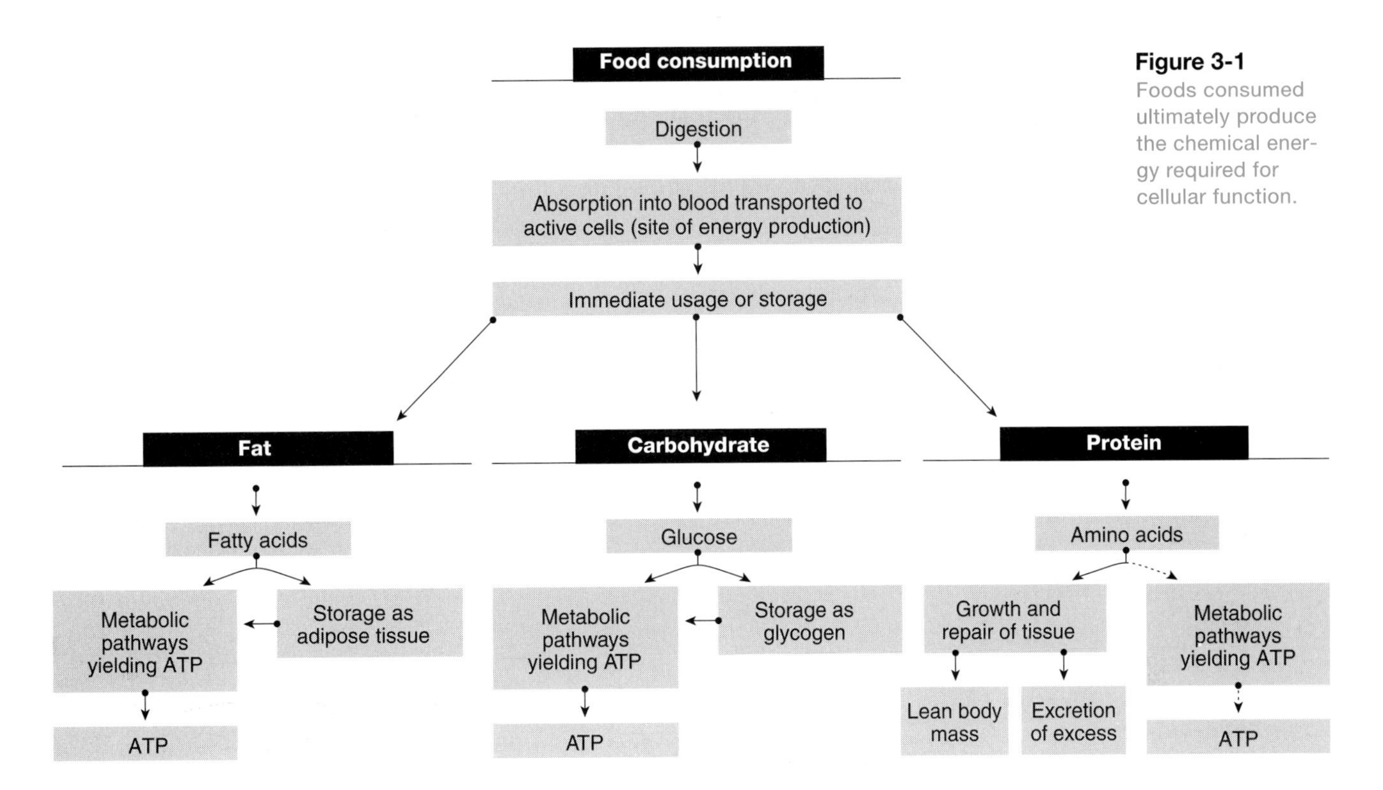

Figure 3-1
Foods consumed ultimately produce the chemical energy required for cellular function.

in several ways: immediately by the phosphagen system, somewhat more slowly with the **anaerobic** production of ATP from carbohydrate, or still more slowly with the **aerobic** production of ATP from either carbohydrate or fat. All three energy pathways are always active, but their relative activity varies from movement to movement, depending on the momentary level of muscular activity.

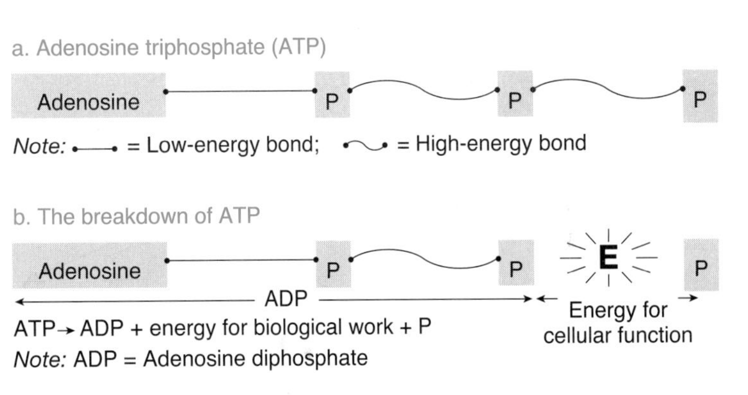

Figure 3-2
Breakdown of the ATP molecule

The Phosphagen System

Creatine phosphate (CP) is another high-energy phosphate compound found within muscle cells. Together, ATP and CP are referred to as the **phosphagens.** When ATP is broken down for muscular contraction, it is resynthesized very quickly from the breakdown of CP. The energy released from breaking the high-energy phosphate bond in CP is used to reconstitute ATP from **adenosine diphosphate (ADP)** and P (the phosphate group broken off from ATP), by-products of the initial reaction (Figure 3-3). The process is so efficient that the concentration of ATP only decreases during the most vigorous exercise (e.g., running 100 meters), and even then not by much. The concentration of CP, on the

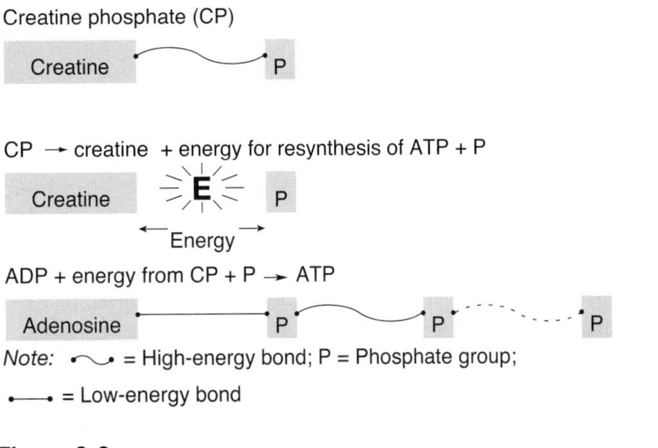

Figure 3-3
The immediate resynthesis of ATP by CP

other hand, can quickly drop to very low levels as CP is used up in reconstituting ATP.

The total amount of ATP and CP stored in muscle is very small, and thus the amount of energy available for muscular contraction is extremely limited. There is probably enough energy available from the phosphagens for only about 10 seconds of all-out exertion. However, this energy is instantaneously available for muscular contraction, and therefore is essential at the onset of physical activity and during short-term, high-intensity activities such as sprinting, performing a weight-lifting movement, or spiking a volleyball.

Anaerobic Production of ATP From Carbohydrate

The anaerobic production of ATP from carbohydrate is known as **anaerobic glycolysis.** Anaerobic literally means "without the presence of oxygen," and **glycolysis** refers to the breakdown of glucose or its storage form, glycogen. Thus, anaerobic glycolysis is a metabolic pathway that does not require oxygen, the purpose of which is to use the energy contained in glucose (or glycogen) for the formation of ATP.

Figure 3-4
Production of ATP via anaerobic and aerobic glycolysis and beta oxidation

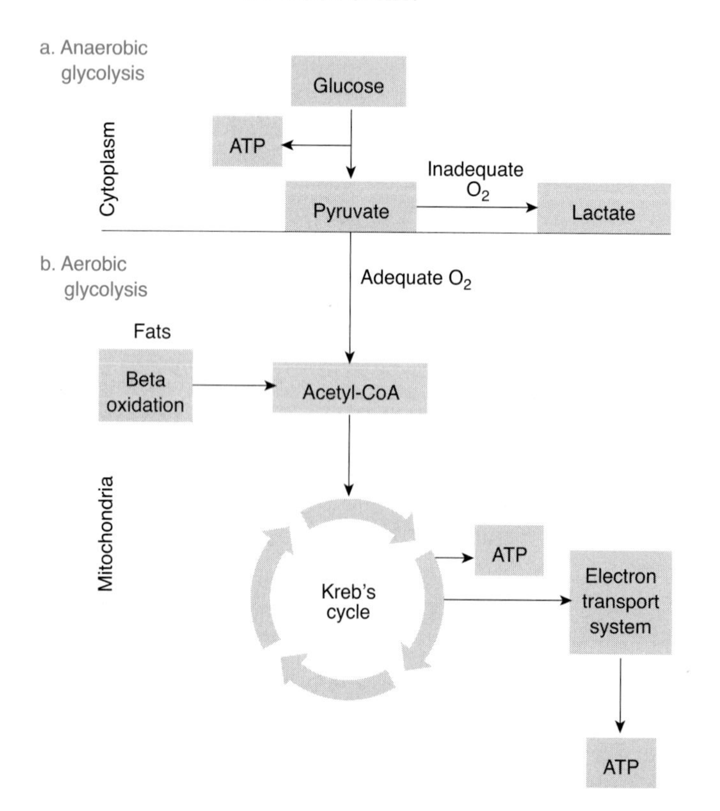

Anaerobic glycolysis is also capable of producing ATP quite rapidly, and thus is required when energy (ATP) is needed to perform activities requiring large bursts of energy over somewhat longer periods of time (typically one to three minutes) than the phosphagen system will allow. This metabolic pathway occurs within the cytoplasm of the cell and involves the incomplete breakdown of glucose (or glycogen) to a simpler substance called pyruvate, which may then be used in the mitochondria by the aerobic energy system. If exercise intensity is very high and adequate amounts of oxygen are not available, pyruvate is converted into lactate, as indicated in Figure 3-4a. Lactate may be transported out of the active cell and used for energy by other cells in the body.

The formation of lactate poses a significant problem because its accumulation is associated with changes in muscle pH (acidity) and eventual muscle fatigue. If the removal of lactate by the circulatory system cannot keep pace with its production in the active muscles, temporary muscle fatigue may occur, with painful symptoms usually referred to as "the burn." Thus, anaerobic glycolysis can only be used to a limited extent during sustained activity, but provides the main source of ATP for high-intensity exercise lasting up to a maximum of approximately three minutes.

Aerobic Production of ATP From Carbohydrate or Fat

The aerobic production of ATP is used for activities requiring sustained energy production. As aerobic literally means "in the presence of oxygen," aerobic metabolic pathways require a continuous supply of oxygen delivered by the circulatory system. Without oxygen, these pathways cannot produce ATP.

This metabolic pathway, called **aerobic glycolysis** or **oxidative glycolysis**, occurs within highly specialized cell structures called the mitochondria. Mitochondria, which are often called the powerhouses of the cell, contain specific enzymes (oxidative enzymes) needed by the cell to utilize oxygen. This highly efficient metabolic process is limited mainly by the capacity of the cardiorespiratory system to deliver oxygen to the active cells. When sufficient oxygen is available, pyruvate is converted into acetyl-CoA, which enters the Kreb's cycle and the electron-transport system, produces substantial amounts of ATP (Figure 3-4b), and produces CO_2 and H_2O, which are easily removed waste products.

Aerobic pathways are also available to break down fatty acids (the digested component of dietary fat) for the production of ATP. This metabolic pathway, called fatty acid oxidation, or **beta oxidation** (see Figure 3-4b), also occurs within the mitochondria and requires a continuous supply of oxygen (as does aerobic glycolysis). The aerobic metabolism of fat yields a very large amount of ATP. Therefore, fat is said to have a high caloric density. A calorie is a unit of energy. Fat yields nine kilocalories of energy per gram compared to the four kilocalories of energy yielded per gram of glucose. This difference is the reason why body fat is such an excellent source of stored energy (and is so hard to lose).

At rest, the body uses both glucose and fatty acids for energy production via aerobic pathways. The cardiorespiratory system can easily supply the oxygen necessary for this low rate of energy metabolism. During exercise, however, supplying the required amount of oxygen rapidly enough becomes more difficult. Because glucose metabolism requires less oxygen than fatty-acid metabolism, the body will use more glucose for energy production and less fat as exercise intensity increases. The **respiratory exchange ratio (RER)** can be used to determine the proportion of fat or carbohydrate that is being used for fuel at different exercise intensities. The RER is a ratio of the amount of carbon dioxide produced relative to the amount of oxygen consumed.

RER = carbon dioxide produced/oxygen consumed

Table 3-1 provides the RER values. When pure fat is being used as fuel, the RER value is 0.70. When pure carbohydrate (glucose) is being used for fuel, the RER is 1.00. At rest, RER values average approximately 0.75, indicating that the body is burning approximately 85% fat and 15% carbohydrate for fuel. As exercise intensity increases, the RER value also increases, reflecting a shift from primarily fat metabolism to primarily carbohydrate metabolism. For example, at a common submaximal intensity of approximately 60% of maximal heart rate, RER values might be in the range of 0.83, indicating that 58% of the energy is coming from fat and 42% is coming from carbohydrates. If the exercise intensity increases to 85% of maximal heart rate, the RER value would probably be in the range of 0.92, with 73% of the fuel coming from carbohydrates and only 27% coming from fat metabolism.

Table 3-1
Percentage of carbohydrate or fat burned as fuel based on the respiratory exchange ratio (RER)

RER	Carbohydrate	Fat
0.70	0	100
0.71	1	99
0.72	4	96
0.73	8	92
0.74	11	89
0.75	15	85
0.76	18	82
0.77	21	79
0.78	25	75
0.79	28	72
0.80	32	68
0.81	35	65
0.82	39	61
0.83	42	58
0.84	45	55
0.85	49	51
0.86	52	48
0.87	56	44
0.88	59	41
0.89	62	38
0.90	66	34
0.91	69	31
0.92	73	27
0.93	76	24
0.94	80	20
0.95	83	17
0.96	86	14
0.97	90	10
0.98	93	7
0.99	97	3
1.00	100	0

Fact or Fiction: Does Low-intensity Exercise Burn the Most Fat?

A very common misconception in the exercise literature is that low-intensity exercise is the best way to lose body weight and, more specifically, body fat. This misconception is based on the RER chart found in Table 3-1. Below an RER value of 0.86, a higher *percentage* of fat is being burned for fuel. Thus, it has been thought that by exercising at a low intensity (the lower the intensity of exercise, the lower the RER value), more fat would be burned for fuel and the fat stores would selectively decrease. This notion does not make sense mathematically and, more importantly, has never been proven in the laboratory.

To test this hypothesis, researchers at the University of Wisconsin, La Crosse, had subjects perform two 30-minute bouts of exercise: a relatively low-intensity bout (RER = 0.88) and a relatively high-intensity bout (RER = 0.93) (Porcari, 1994). The results, which are presented in Figure 3-5, show that for the low-intensity exercise, subjects burned a total of 240 calories, with 96 of those calories (41%) coming from fat. During the high-intensity bout, a total of 450 calories were burned, with 108 of those calories (24%) coming from fat. Therefore, during the low-intensity bout, there was a higher *percentage* of calories coming from fat, but the total number of fat calories was less than during the high-intensity trial.

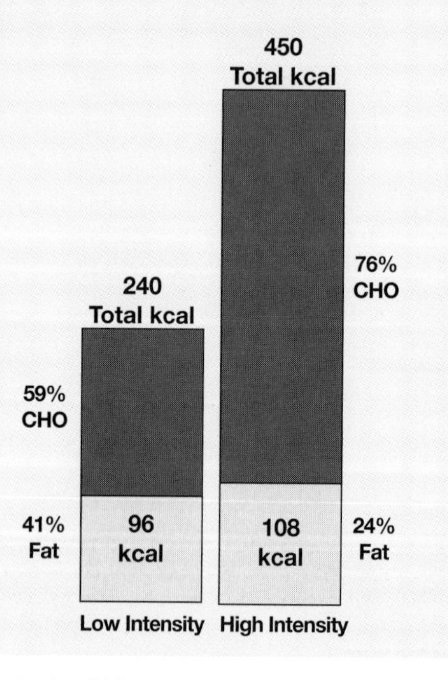

Figure 3-5
A breakdown of total calories, calories from fat, and calories from carbohydrates during 30 minutes of low-intensity (walking 3.8 mph) and high-intensity (running 6.5 mph) exercise.
Note: CHO = carbohydrate

Source: Reprinted with permission from Porcari, J.P. (1994). Fat-burning exercise: Fit or farce? *Fitness Management,* July, 40–42. Copyright *Fitness Management* magazine, www.fitnessmanagement.com.

It should be noted that no mention has been made of the use of protein as a fuel source, and that an RER value for protein is not included in Table 3-1. In a well-fed individual, only a negligible amount of protein is used to fuel muscular contraction. Exceptions to this rule are seen during the later stages of an exhausting exercise event (e.g., an ultramarathon) or in some clinical conditions, such as diabetes, where the body actually breaks down or catabolizes protein for fuel. Figure 3-6 provides an overview of the metabolic pathways of macronutrient utilization.

Aerobic Capacity and Oxygen Metabolism

Since the primary mechanism for creating energy is from the oxidation of glucose and fatty acids, quantifying an individual's **oxygen consumption** is an excellent measure of his or her ability to perform sustained endurance exercise. The more oxygen that an individual can take in, transport, and utilize, the more physical work he or she can perform. Oxygen consumption can be determined using specialized metabolic carts that determine the volume of air that an individual is breathing, as well as the concentrations of oxygen and carbon dioxide exhaled in comparison to room air (Figure 3-7).

When oxygen consumption is measured at maximal levels of exertion, it is referred to as **maximal aerobic capacity,** or **$\dot{V}O_2$max,** which is typically represented as milliliters of oxygen consumed per kilogram of body weight per minute (mL/kg/min). The dividing of oxygen consumption by body weight makes this a "relative" measurement. A larger person will invariably consume more oxygen to perform a given amount of work than a smaller person, just because he or she has a larger body to move. Dividing by body weight allows comparisons to be made between individuals of different body sizes.

Oxygen consumption can also be represented in absolute terms: liters of oxygen consumed per minute (L/min). This method is most commonly used to help in determining how many calories are being expended during a particular activity. On average, approximately 5 kilocalories (kcal) of energy are burned for every liter of oxygen consumed. For example, if someone were exercising at a level that requires 2 liters of oxygen per minute, he or she would be burning 10 kcal/min (2 L/min x 5 kcal/L = 10 kcal/min). Many books contain

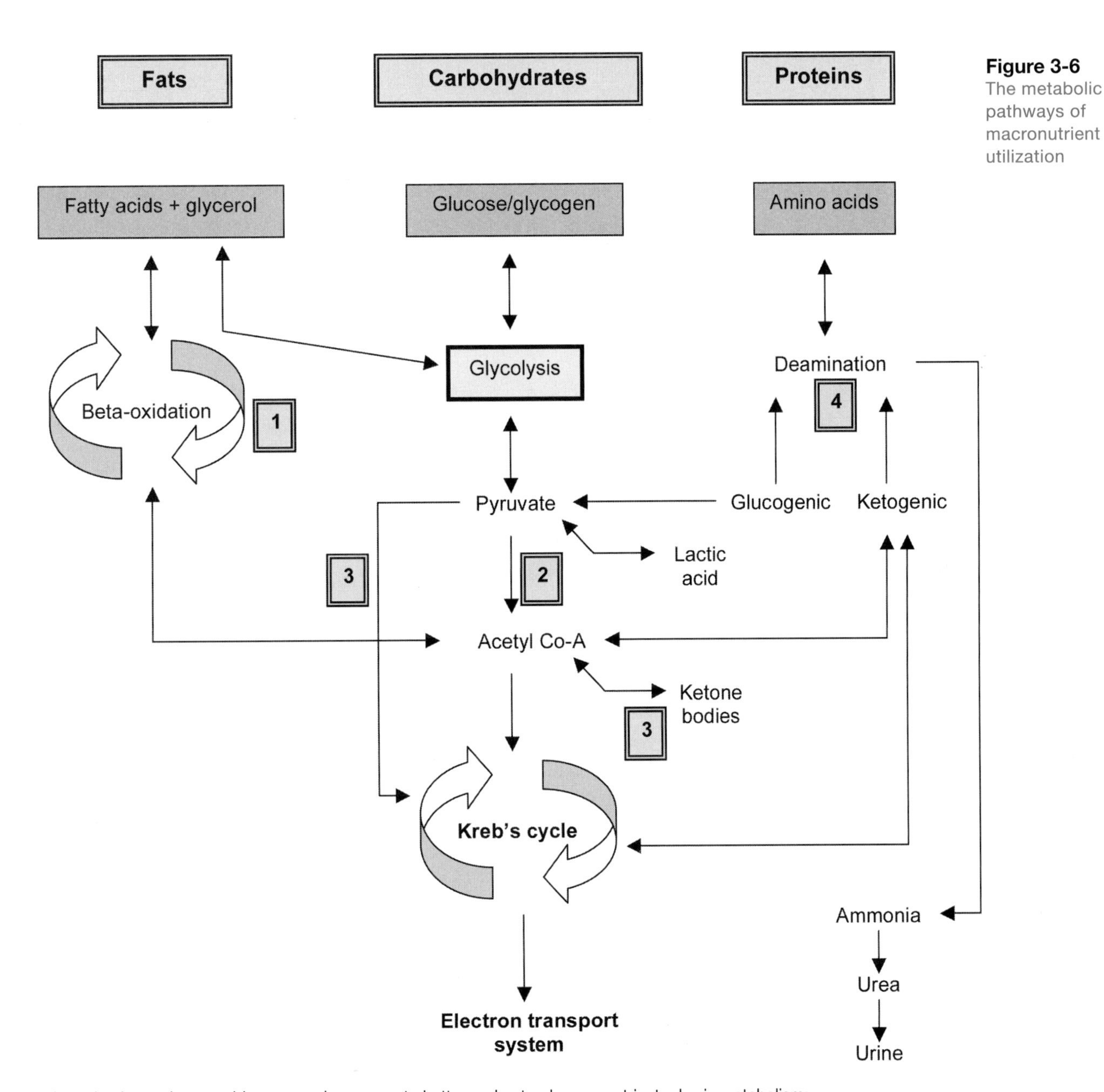

Figure 3-6 The metabolic pathways of macronutrient utilization

The following key points provide a general summary to better understand macronutrient roles in metabolism:

Number 1: Triglycerides are hydrolyzed to glycerol and free fatty acids. Because acetyl-CoA is a small carbon structure, the long-chain fatty acids must first be reduced to two-carbon structures via a fragmenting process called beta-oxidation. These two-carbon fragments are then converted to acetyl-CoA, where they have their point of entry into the Kreb's cycle.

Number 2: Note the multi- and unidirectional signs throughout all metabolic pathways, in particular the reaction where pyruvate forms acetyl-CoA. Once formed, it cannot be reconstituted back to pyruvate. The reaction of converting pyruvate to acetyl-CoA is irreversible, which explains why free fatty acids from fats cannot be utilized to form glucose. On the other hand, excess dietary carbohydrates that are not utilized for energy purposes can be converted to glycerol and enter the beta-oxidation process in reverse, manufacturing the two components needed to manufacture triglycerides. Consequently, excess carbohydrates can be converted to fat.

Number 3: Pyruvate additionally serves an important role as a precursor to the manufacture of an intermediate product of the Kreb's cycle that facilitates fat metabolism. Reductions in available pyruvate, as witnessed with carbohydrate-restricted diets or carbohydrate depletion, may impede the body's ability to properly metabolize fats. The accumulation of partially metabolized fats will result in the manufacture of ketone bodies as a means to rid the body of accumulated acetyl-CoA, a potential toxin. Likewise, the accumulation of ketone bodies can pose significant health risks to individuals. Carbohydrates (pyruvate), therefore, are essential to properly metabolize fats.

Number 4: Proteins must first undergo deamination to remove the amino group before they can be metabolized. They are defined as either glucogenic or ketogenic, based upon their point of entry into the pathways. Glucogenic amino acids can be converted to pyruvate, and therefore have the capacity to generate glucose via gluconeogenesis. Ketogenic amino acids, however, are converted to acetyl-CoA of Kreb's cycle intermediates, and therefore can only be used to generate energy.

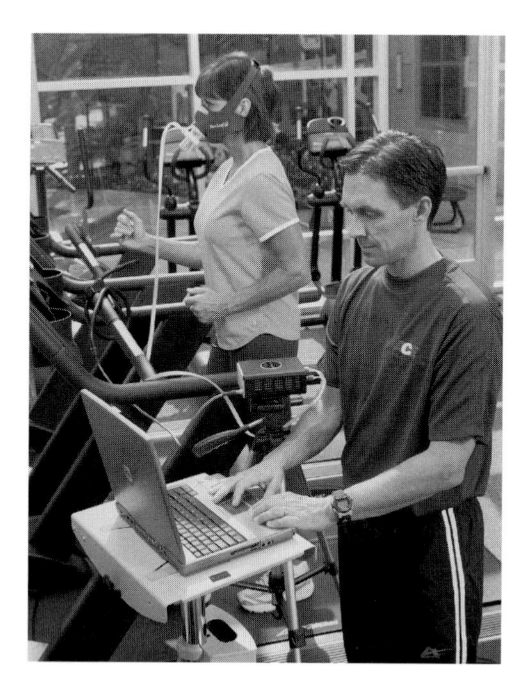

Figure 3-7
Example of a specialized metabolic cart system used to determine oxygen consumption

tables of the number of **calories** burned during various activities. To measure these values, researchers had subjects perform each activity and measured how much oxygen they were consuming, which was then converted to caloric-expenditure values. This was most likely done using a portable metabolic analyzer. It should also be noted that on most of those charts, the number of calories burned varies quite substantially based on body weight, because larger people consume more oxygen than smaller people when performing any amount of external work, thereby illustrating the concept just described.

Acute Responses to Aerobic Exercise

Aerobic exercise is best characterized as large-muscle, rhythmic activities (e.g., walking, jogging, aerobics, swimming, cross-country skiing) that can be sustained without undue fatigue for at least 20 minutes. Such movement patterns depend on the oxidative metabolic pathways to create ATP, and the goal of the body is to be in a **steady state**, where the energy needs are being met aerobically. The other metabolic pathways (i.e., the phosphagen system and anaerobic glycolysis) are used only to produce energy at the onset of these types of activity.

Figure 3-8 highlights the changes that take place with regards to oxygen consumption during aerobic exercise. When aerobic exercise begins, the body rapidly responds to increase the quantity of oxygen available to produce the ATP necessary to meet the molecular demands. At rest, the body is primarily under the control of the **parasympathetic nervous system,** which keeps heart rate, blood pressure, and metabolism low. With the onset of exercise, sympathetic stimulation (the "fight or flight" mechanism) increases and has many effects on the body. In addition to sending nervous signals to stimulate the cardiovascular system, signals are sent to the adrenal glands to release **epinephrine** and **norepinephrine** into the bloodstream. The purpose of these sympathetic hormones, which are also called **catecholamines,** is to stimulate the body to adjust to the increased metabolic demands of exercise. Cardiac output increases to deliver more blood to the active muscle cells. This increase is accomplished by an increase in both heart rate and stroke volume.

The heavy bold line in Figure 3-8 indicates the level of $\dot{V}O_2$ required at rest and the instantaneous increase that occurs with the commencement of exercise (at the upward arrow). The line returns to the resting level when exercise is abruptly stopped (at the downward arrow). The actual $\dot{V}O_2$ that results from the physiological responses to aerobic exercise is indicated by the sloping line in Figure 3-8. Notice that actual $\dot{V}O_2$ does not immediately meet the physiological requirement for oxygen. Instead, an oxygen deficit occurs.

The physiological responses that occur with the commencement of exercise take approximately two to four minutes to meet the increased metabolic demands for oxygen. During this time, the anaerobic metabolic systems—which are capable of producing energy more rapidly—produce the energy needed to carry out the exercise. During this period, the phosphagens are depleted and lactate accumulates. When the cardiorespira-

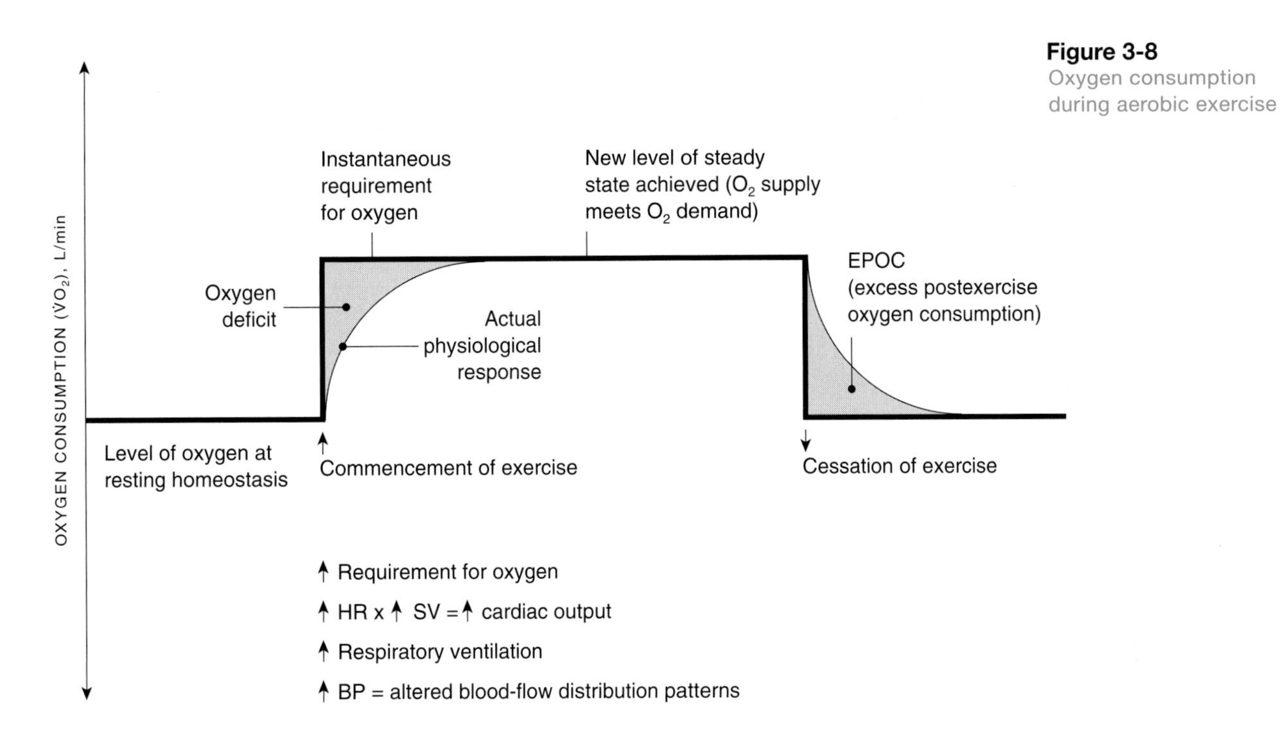

Figure 3-8
Oxygen consumption during aerobic exercise

tory systems have fully responded, a new level of oxygen consumption is achieved. If the exercise intensity is not too high relative to the body's ability to provide oxygen to the muscles, a steady state is achieved. The transition from rest to steady-state exercise is often uncomfortable for many people, as the body attempts to reach homeostasis. Once a steady state is reached, individuals usually feel more comfortable. Many people refer to this as having "caught their second wind." The $\dot{V}O_2$ during this period is usually referred to as steady state.

With cessation of exercise, the requirement for oxygen abruptly returns to the initial resting level. Again, however, the body responds more slowly. As cardiac output, blood pressure, and respiratory ventilation return to resting levels, oxygen consumption slowly declines as well, but is still elevated above resting levels. This is called **excess postexercise oxygen consumption (EPOC).** The energy produced during this time is used to replenish the depleted phosphagens, to eliminate accumulated lactate if it has not already been cleared from the blood, and to restore other homeostatic conditions (e.g., thermoregulation, tissue resynthesis).

If exercise intensity is so high that the body cannot meet all of the metabolic demands of the muscles via steady-state aerobic metabolism, the muscles have to supplement ATP production via anaerobic metabolism. When this occurs, the person is said to have exceeded the **anaerobic threshold (AT).** When someone exceeds the AT, lactate accumulates very rapidly in the blood, the oxygen deficit and corresponding EPOC are extremely high, and exercise cannot be performed for more than a few minutes. It is also at this point that hyperventilation begins to occur. As the body tries to buffer the lactate (i.e., remove it from the system), one of the by-products is carbon dioxide (CO_2). CO_2 provides a powerful stimulus to the respiratory system, and the body increases respiration in an attempt to "blow off" the excess CO_2. This increase in respiration is often called the **ventilatory threshold (VT)** and can be used as an indirect indicator of the AT.

During aerobic exercise, heart rate (HR) increases in a linear fashion and is proportional to the increase in oxygen consumption that occurs with increased amounts of physical work (Figure 3-9). Stroke volume also increases in up to about 40 to 50% of an individual's maximal aerobic capacity and then plateaus. **Systolic blood pressure** also increases as a result of the increase in contractile strength of the heart and is very important in blood-flow distribution because it provides the driving force that pushes blood through the circulatory system. Similar to HR, systolic blood pressure increases in a linear fashion throughout the range of exercise intensities. **Diastolic blood pressure,** which is a measure of the pressure in the arteries during the relaxation phase (**diastole**) of the heart, stays the same or decreases slightly because of the vasodilation of the blood vessels within the working muscles. More blood is allowed to enter the muscles with each heartbeat, so less blood is "trapped" in the arteries between heartbeats. Pulmonary ventilation also increases to provide more oxygen to the red blood cells in the lungs.

Much of the cardiovascular advantage in well-trained individuals and athletes is seen in the stroke volume due to a greater pumping capacity of the heart. This is analogous to a trained skeletal muscle being larger and stronger.

Blood-flow patterns also change during exercise according to metabolic need. Blood is shunted to the working muscles (to produce ATP for contraction) and to the skin (to dissipate the metabolic heat produced), while the amount of blood flowing to less-active organs such as the kidney and intestinal tract decreases (Table 3-2). Additionally, epinephrine causes the release of glucose from the liver, a process called **glycogenolysis,** which allows blood glucose levels to remain high to provide fuel for the exercising muscles.

Figure 3-9
Normal responses to blood pressure during exercise

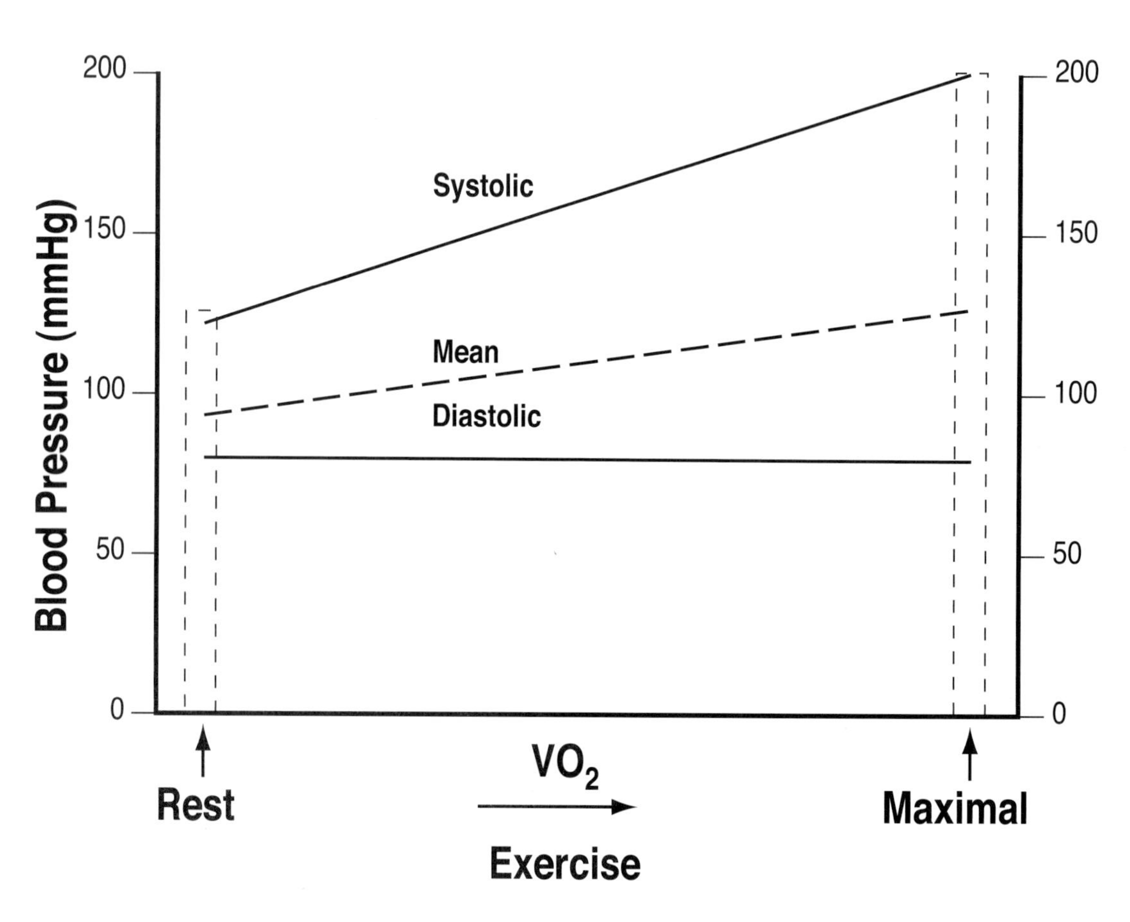

Table 3-2
Blood Flow Distribution at Rest and During Exercise

Organ	Rest	Exercise
Muscles	15–20%	84%
Liver	27%	2%
Heart	4%	4%
Skin	6%*	2%*
Brain	14%	4%
Kidneys	22%	1%
Other	7%	3%

*During light-intensity exercise in warm climates, skin blood flow might reach 12–14%. Reduced flow is seen during high-intensity exercise.

Chronic Training Adaptations to Aerobic Exercise

The benefits of any type of exercise-training program are said to follow the **SAID principle** (specific adaptation to imposed demands). The concept of the SAID principle is that the body will adapt to the specific challenges imposed upon it, as long as the program progressively overloads the system being trained. When performed appropriately, a regular program of aerobic exercise can have significant physiological benefits in as little as eight to 12 weeks. Changes to the cardiorespiratory system include improvements in cardiac efficiency (increased SV and a lower HR), increased respiratory capacity, and, ultimately, an increase in maximal oxygen consumption. These improvements provide individuals with a greater physiological reserve and allow them to perform everyday activities with less stress and strain. Regular exercise has also been shown to result in lowered blood pressure in moderately hypertensive individuals. This results in less work for the heart muscle and puts less stress on the blood vessels.

The benefits of aerobic exercise are not limited to the cardiovascular and respiratory systems. Studies have shown that weightbearing exercise promotes improved bone density, which is a key factor in the prevention of **osteoporosis,** particularly in women. Improvements in the control of blood glucose and blood lipids (e.g., **cholesterol, triglycerides**) are also associated with consistent physical activity. One of the primary reasons why many people exercise is to control body weight. Exercise burns calories, but, just as importantly, exercise serves to maintain or increase lean body mass, which is vital for maintaining resting metabolic rate. It is the decrease in muscle mass that contributes to the fall in metabolic rate as people age. And, finally, the psychological benefits of exercise cannot be overlooked. Exercise has long been associated with lower levels of anxiety and depression and a higher quality of life.

Neuromuscular Physiology

The basic anatomical unit of the nervous system is the **neuron,** or nerve cell. There are two kinds of neurons: sensory and motor. **Sensory neurons** convey electrochemical impulses from sensory organs in the periphery (such as the skin) to the spinal cord and the brain (called the **central nervous system,** or **CNS**). **Motor neurons** conduct impulses from the CNS to the periphery. Because the motor neurons carry electrical impulses from the CNS to the muscle cells, they signal the muscles to contract or relax and, therefore, regulate muscular movement. The endings of the motor neuron connect, or **synapse,** with muscle cells in the periphery of the body. This motor neuron–muscle cell synapse is called the **neuromuscular junction,** or **motor end plate** (Figure 3-10). The basic functional unit of the neuromuscular system is the **motor unit,** which consists of one motor neuron and the muscle cells that it innervates. The number of muscle cells that a motor neuron innervates can vary tremendously, depending upon the precision and accuracy required of that muscle. For example, the eye muscles, which require very fine adjustments, may have as few as one muscle fiber in a motor unit. In contrast, the quadriceps muscle, which generates high forces, may have more than a thousand muscle fibers per motor unit.

Figure 3-10
Basic anatomical structure of a motor neuron (or nerve cell) and motor end plate

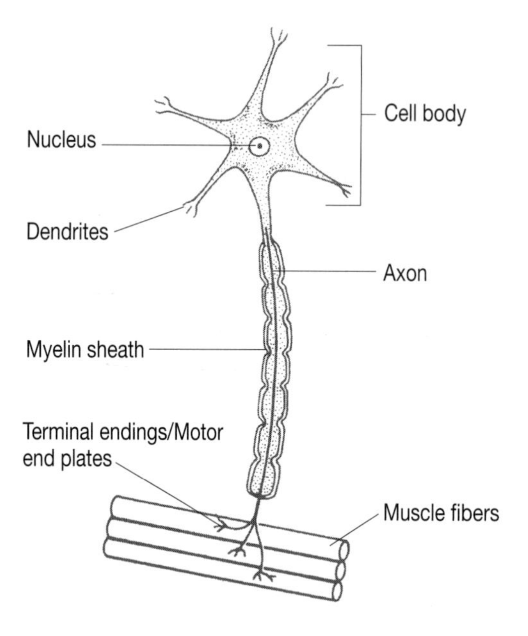

Muscles are composed of several kinds of fibers that differ in their ability to utilize the metabolic pathways previously described. **Fast-twitch (FT) muscle fibers** are rather poorly equipped in terms of the oxygen-delivery system, but have an outstanding capacity for the phosphagen system and a very high capacity for anaerobic glycolysis. Therefore, FT fibers are specialized for anaerobic metabolism. They are recruited by the nervous system predominantly for rapid, powerful movements such as jumping, throwing, and sprinting.

Slow-twitch (ST) muscle fibers, on the other hand, are exceptionally well equipped for oxygen delivery and have a high quantity of aerobic, or oxidative, enzymes. Although they do not have a highly developed mechanism for use of the phosphagens or anaerobic glycolysis, ST fibers have a large number of mitochondria and, consequently, are particularly well designed for use of aerobic glycolysis and fatty-acid oxidation. Thus, ST fibers are recruited primarily for low-intensity, longer-duration activities such as walking, jogging, and swimming.

Most people have roughly equal percentages of the two fiber types. Persons who excel in activities characterized by sudden bursts of energy, but who tire relatively rapidly, are probably born with a large percentage of FT fibers. Persons who are best at lower-intensity endurance activities are probably born with a large percentage of ST fibers. There are also a number of "intermediate" muscle fibers that have a fairly high capacity for both fast anaerobic and slow aerobic movements (see "Muscle-fiber Types," pages 26–27).

Muscle-fiber distribution (fast twitch, intermediate, or slow twitch) is determined to a large extent by genetic makeup. This is not to say, however, that muscle-fiber type is unresponsive to activity. All three types of muscle fiber are highly trainable. That is, they are capable of adapting to the specific metabolic demands placed on them. A person who regularly engages in low-intensity endurance activities improves his or her aerobic capacity. Although all three types of muscle fiber will show some improvement in aerobic ability, the ST fibers will be most responsive to this kind of training and will show the largest improvement in aerobic capacity. If, on the other hand, short-duration, high-intensity exercise such as interval training is performed regularly, other metabolic pathways will be emphasized, and the capabilities of the FT fibers to perform anaerobically will be enhanced. ST fibers are less responsive to this kind of training.

Muscular **hypertrophy** is often associated with a strength-development program. This hypertrophy is the result of an increase in the size of individual muscle cells. The increase in size is due to a proliferation of **actin** and **myosin** myofilaments within the myofibrils, especially within the FT muscle fibers. One common misconception is that women will develop "large" muscles if they strength train. Generally speaking, women do not experience muscular hypertrophy to the same extent as men, because the male hormone testosterone is important in synthesizing the contractile proteins. Nevertheless, women will increase substantially in strength in response to a progressive strength-training program.

Training for muscular endurance is specific to both ST and FT muscle fibers and motor units. Training increases the concentration of oxidative enzymes that extract oxygen from the blood in both types of fibers, thus making

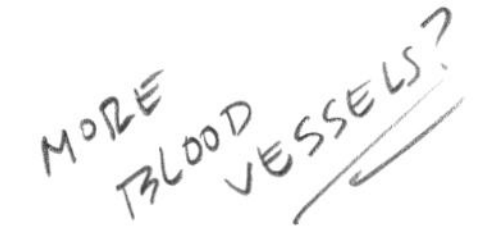

energy production more efficient. An increase in tissue **vascularity,** or an increase in the number and size of blood vessels, often accompanies this type of program. Increased vascularity enhances blood supply and, consequently, oxygen delivery to the myofibrils. It also aids in transporting metabolites, such as lactate, away from the contracting muscle.

Hormonal Responses to Exercise

The endocrine system plays a major role in regulating the body's response to exercise and training by releasing various **hormones** via glandular secretion. After binding to specific receptors on a target cell, these hormones perform a number of functions in the body, such as regulating cellular metabolism, facilitating the cardiovascular responses to exercise, and modulating protein synthesis. Even though the hormonal response to exercise is very complex, the integrated response of the various systems provides the changes necessary to help the body make the acute and chronic adaptations to exercise training.

- **Growth hormone (GH)** is secreted by the anterior pituitary gland and facilitates protein synthesis in the body. Many of growth hormone's effects are mediated by **insulin-like growth factors** (IGF-1 and IGF-2), which are synthesized in the liver as a result of GH release during exercise.
- **Antidiuretic hormone (ADH),** which is also called **vasopressin,** is released by the posterior pituitary gland during exercise. As its name implies, the primary function of ADH is to reduce urinary excretion of water. By conserving water during exercise, it helps to prevent dehydration.
- Epinephrine and norepinephrine are called catecholamines and are released by the adrenal medulla as part of the sympathetic response to exercise (the "fight or flight" mechanism). Epinephrine and norepinephrine play two major roles: to increase cardiac output by increasing heart rate and contractility during exercise and to cause **glycogenolysis** in the liver (i.e., glycogen breakdown), so that more glucose can be released into the bloodstream for use by the actively working muscles.
- **Aldosterone** and **cortisol** are two of the main hormones released by the adrenal cortex. Aldosterone acts to limit sodium excretion in the urine to maintain electrolyte balance during exercise. Cortisol is a **glucocorticoid** and plays a major role in maintaining blood glucose during prolonged exercise by promoting protein and triglyceride breakdown.
- **Insulin** and **glucagon** are both secreted by the cells of the **islets of Langerhans** in the pancreas, yet they have opposite effects. When blood glucose is high (e.g., after a meal), insulin is released from the **beta cells** in the islets of Langerhans to facilitate glucose removal from the blood and bring blood glucose back to within a normal range. When blood glucose levels are low (e.g., during prolonged endurance exercise), glucagon is released from the **alpha cells** in the islets of Langerhans to stimulate glucose release from the liver to increase blood glucose. Glucagon also causes the release of free fatty acids from adipose tissue so that they can be used as fuel.
- **Testosterone** (released by the testes) and **estrogen** (released by the ovaries) are the primary male and female sex hormones, respectively. Testosterone is responsible for the masculine characteristics associated with manhood (**androgenic** effects) and also has **anabolic** (muscle-building) effects. Because of potent anabolic effects, testosterone and its derivatives are often abused in attempts to enhance athletic performance. Estrogen is responsible for the feminine characteristics associated with being a woman and also plays a major role in bone formation and maintenance. High levels of chronic exercise training have been shown to decrease estrogen levels to the point where some female athletes no longer have their menstrual cycle, a condition called **amenorrhea,** which has been associated with osteoporosis and an increased risk of bone fractures.

Environmental Considerations When Exercising

Exercising under extreme environmental conditions can add significant stress to the cardiovascular system. Special precautions need to be taken when exercising in the heat or cold or at high altitude.

Exercising in the Heat

Exercising in the heat poses a significant threat to individuals if they do not take adequate precautions. The danger of heat overload is compounded if people are not adequately hydrated prior to starting exercise, wear excessive clothing, or are overweight or obese. For example, heat-induced problems are most common in football, where a number of issues combine to illustrate this point. The weight of the football padding adds to the external work that the person has to do. This added work increases the amount of heat build-up, as well as increases the amount of sweating and dehydration. The football padding also makes it difficult to dissipate the heat, as the heat effectively gets trapped beneath the padding. A similar phenomenon occurs when people are overweight or obese. The added body fat lies over the muscles and effectively traps the heat from escaping.

Considerable metabolic heat is produced during exercise. To reduce this internal heat load, venous blood is brought to the skin surface (i.e., peripheral vasodilation) to be cooled. When the sweat glands secrete water onto the skin, it is evaporated, which serves to cool the underlying blood. If environmental conditions are favorable, these mechanisms will adequately prevent the body temperature from rising by more than about 2 to 3 degrees Fahrenheit (° F), even during heavy exercise.

During exercise in the heat, however, dissipating internal body heat is difficult, and external heat from the environment may significantly add to the total heat load. This results in a higher heart rate than normal at any level of exercise. For example, if a man walks at three miles per hour and his heart rate is 125 beats per minute, walking at the same speed in the heat may result in a heart rate of 135 to 140 beats per minute. Thus, exercisers (regardless of the type of exercise performed) will have to decrease their absolute workload in the heat to stay within their target HR zones.

This elevated HR comes about primarily for two reasons. First, as the body tries to cool itself, the high degree of vasodilation in the vessels supplying the skin reduces venous return of blood to the heart, and SV declines. The heart attempts to maintain cardiac output by elevating HR. Second, sweating results in a considerable loss of body water. If lost fluids are not replenished, dehydration eventually results, and blood volume declines. This reduced blood volume also decreases venous return to the heart. Again, the body responds with a higher HR to maintain cardiac output.

The most stressful environment to exercise in is a hot, humid environment. When the air contains a large quantity of water vapor, sweat will not evaporate readily. Since it is the evaporative process that cools the body, adequate cooling may not occur in humid conditions. Under these conditions, heat exhaustion and heat stroke become dangerous possibilities. Heat exhaustion usually develops in nonacclimatized individuals and is typically a result of inadequate circulatory adjustments to exercise coupled with fluid loss. Heat stroke is a complete failure of the heat-regulating mechanisms, with the core temperature exceeding 104° F (40° C). Both conditions require immediate medical attention. Symptoms of heat exhaustion and heat stroke, as well as treatment options, are presented in Table 3-3.

Table 3-4 combines measures of heat and humidity into a simple-to-use **heat index** that provides guidelines regarding when exercise can be safely undertaken, and when it should be avoided.

Table 3-3
Heat Exhaustion and Heat Stroke

	Signs and Symptoms	Treatment
Heat Exhaustion	Weak, rapid pulse Low blood pressure Headache Nausea Dizziness General weakness Paleness Cold clammy skin Profuse sweating Elevated body core temp (≤104° F or 40° C)	Stop exercising Move to a cool, ventilated area Lay down and elevate feet 12–18 inches Give fluids Monitor temperature
Heat Stroke	Hot, dry skin Bright red skin color Rapid, strong pulse Labored breathing Elevated body core temp (≥105° F or 41° C)	Stop exercising Remove as much clothing as feasible Try to cool the body immediately in any way possible (wet towels, ice packs/baths, fan, alcohol rubs) Give fluids Transport to emergency room immediately

Table 3-4
Heat Index

TEMPERATURE (°F) (°C given in parentheses)

RELATIVE HUMIDITY %	70 (21)	75 (24)	80 (27)	85 (29)	90 (32)	95 (35)	100 (38)	105 (41)	110 (43)	115 (46)	120 (49)
	APPARENT TEMPERATURE* (°F) (°C given in parentheses)										
0	64 (18)	69 (21)	73 (23)	78 (26)	83 (28)	87 (31)	91 (33)	95 (35)	99 (37)	103 (39)	107 (42)
10	65 (18)	70 (21)	75 (24)	80 (27)	85 (29)	90 (32)	95 (35)	100 (38)	105 (41)	111 (44)	116 (47)
20	66 (19)	72 (22)	77 (25)	82 (28)	87 (31)	93 (34)	99 (37)	105 (41)	112 (44)	120 (49)	130 (54)
30	67 (19)	73 (23)	78 (26)	84 (29)	90 (32)	96 (36)	104 (40)	113 (45)	123 (51)	135 (57)	148 (64)
40	68 (20)	74 (23)	79 (26)	86 (30)	93 (34)	101 (38)	110 (43)	123 (51)	137 (58)	151 (66)	
50	69 (21)	75 (24)	81 (27)	88 (31)	96 (36)	107 (42)	120 (49)	135 (57)	150 (66)		
60	70 (21)	76 (24)	82 (28)	90 (32)	100 (38)	114 (46)	132 (56)	149 (65)			
70	70 (21)	77 (25)	85 (29)	93 (34)	106 (41)	124 (51)	144 (62)				
80	71 (22)	78 (26)	86 (30)	97 (36)	113 (45)	136 (58)					
90	71 (22)	79 (26)	88 (31)	102 (39)	122 (50)						
100	72 (22)	80 (27)	91 (33)	108 (42)							

How to Use Heat Index
1. Locate temperature across top
2. Locate relative humidity down left side
3. Follow across and down to find Apparent Temperature
4. Determine Heat Stress Risk on chart at right

Note: This Heat Index chart is designed to provide general guidelines for assessing the potential severity of heat stress. Individual reactions to heat will vary. In addition, studies indicate that susceptibility to heat disorders tends to increase among children and older adults. Exposure to full sunshine can increase Heat Index values by up to 15° F.

Apparent Temperature		Heat Stress Risk with Physical Activity and/or Prolonged Exposure
90–105	(32–41)	Heat cramps or heat exhaustion *possible*
105–130	(41–54)	Heat cramps or heat exhaustion *likely* Heat stroke *possible*
130–151	(54–66)	Heat stroke *highly likely*

*Combined index of heat and humidity and what it feels like to the body

LWMCs should share the following tips with clients before they consider exercising in the heat:

- Begin exercising in the heat gradually. Becoming acclimatized to exercising in the heat takes approximately seven to 10 days. Start by exercising for short periods of time each day.
- Always wear lightweight, well-ventilated clothing. Cotton materials are cooler; most synthetics retain heat. Wear light-colored clothing if exercising in the sun; white reflects heat better than other colors.
- Never wear impermeable or nonbreathable garments. The notion that wearing rubber suits or nonbreathable garments adds to weight loss is a myth, as the change in weight is due to fluid loss, not fat loss. Wearing impermeable clothing is a dangerous practice that could lead to significant heat stress and heat injury.
- Replace body fluids as they are lost. Drink fluids at regular intervals while exercising, but avoid overhydration, which can be as dangerous as dehydration. Frequent consumption of small amounts of fluid to minimize sweat-related weight loss is the best practice (see Table 7–6, page 170). While there are many commercially available sports drinks, rehydration with water is adequate except under extreme conditions where greater than 3% of a person's body weight is lost.
- Recording daily body weights is an excellent way to prevent accumulative dehydration. For example, if 5 pounds (2.27 kg) of body water is lost after aerobic exercise, this water should be replaced before exercising again the next day. If lost water has not been regained, exercise should be curtailed until the body is adequately rehydrated.

Exercising in the Cold

The major problems encountered when exercising in the cold are associated with an excessive loss of body heat, which can result in **hypothermia** or frostbite. Additionally, the cold can also cause a generalized **vasoconstriction** that can increase peripheral resistance and blood pressure. This may cause problems in people who are hypertensive or who have heart disease. Following exercise, chilling can occur quickly if the body surface is wet with sweat and heat loss continues.

Heat loss from the body becomes greatly accelerated when there is a strong wind. The wind chill factor can be quite significant. The wind chill index presented in Table 3-5 provides the various combinations of temperature and wind velocity that can be used as guidelines when deciding if it is safe to exercise in a cold environment.

LWMCs should share the following tips with clients before they consider exercising in a cold environment.

- Wear several layers of clothing, so that garments can be removed and replaced as needed. As exercise intensity increases, remove outer garments. Then, during periods of rest, warm-up, cool-down, or low-intensity exercise, put them back on. A head covering is also important, because considerable body heat radiates from the head.
- Allow for adequate ventilation of sweat. Sweating during heavy exercise can soak inner garments. If evaporation does not readily occur, the wet garments will continue to drain the body of heat during rest periods, when retention of body heat is important.
- Select garment materials that allow the body to give off body heat during exercise and retain body heat during inactive periods. Cotton is a good choice for exercising in the heat because it soaks up sweat readily and allows evaporation. For those same reasons, however, cotton is a poor choice for exercising in the cold. Wool is an excellent choice when exercising in the cold because it maintains body heat even when wet. Newer synthetic materials (e.g., polypropylene) are also excellent choices, as they wick sweat away from the body, thus preventing heat loss. When wind chill is a problem, nylon materials are good for outerwear. Synthetic materials like Gore-Tex®, although much more expensive than nylon, are probably the best choice for outerwear

Table 3-5
Windchill Factor Chart

Estimated wind speed (in mph) (km/h given in parentheses)	ACTUAL THERMOMETER READING (°F) (°C given in parentheses)											
	50 (10)	40 (4)	30 (-1)	20 (-7)	10 (-12)	0 (-18)	-10 (-23)	-20 (-29)	-30 (-34)	-40 (-40)	-50 (-46)	-60 (-51)
	EQUIVALENT TEMPERATURE (°F) (°C given in parentheses)											
calm	50 (10)	40 (4)	30 (-1)	20 (-7)	10 (-12)	0 (-18)	-10 (-23)	-20 (-29)	-30 (-34)	-40 (-40)	-50 (-46)	-60 (-51)
5 (8)	48 (9)	37 (3)	27 (-3)	16 (-9)	6 (-14)	-5 (-21)	-15 (-26)	-26 (-32)	-36 (-38)	-47 (-44)	-57 (-49)	-68 (-56)
10 (16)	40 (4)	28 (-2)	16 (-9)	4 (-16)	-9 (-23)	-24 (-31)	-33 (-36)	-46 (-43)	-58 (-50)	-70 (-57)	-83 (-64)	-95 (-71)
15 (24)	36 (2)	22 (-6)	9 (-13)	-5 (-21)	-18 (-28)	-32 (-36)	-45 (-43)	-58 (-50)	-72 (-58)	-85 (-65)	-99 (-78)	-112 (-80)
20 (32)	32 (0)	18 (-8)	4 (-16)	-10 (-23)	-25 (-32)	-39 (-39)	-53 (-47)	-67 (-55)	-82 (-63)	-96 (-71)	-110 (-79)	-124 (-87)
25 (40)	30 (-1)	16 (-9)	0 (-18)	-15 (-26)	-29 (-34)	-44 (-42)	-59 (-51)	-74 (-59)	-88 (-67)	-104 (-76)	-118 (-83)	-133 (-92)
30 (48)	28 (-2)	13 (-11)	-2 (-19)	-18 (-28)	-33 (-36)	-48 (-44)	-63 (-53)	-79 (-62)	-94 (-70)	-109 (-78)	-125 (-87)	-140 (-96)
35 (56)	27 (-3)	11 (-12)	-4 (-20)	-20 (-29)	-35 (-37)	-51 (-46)	-67 (-55)	-82 (-63)	-98 (-72)	-113 (-81)	-129 (-89)	-145 (-98)
40 (64)	26 (-3)	10 (-12)	-6 (-21)	-21 (-29)	-37 (-38)	-53 (-47)	-69 (-56)	-85 (-65)	-100 (-73)	-116 (-82)	-132 (-91)	-146 (-99)
[Wind speeds greater than 40 mph (64 km/h) have little additional effect.]	GREEN				YELLOW				RED			
	LITTLE DANGER (for properly clothed person). Maximum danger of false sense of security.				INCREASING DANGER Danger for freezing of exposed flesh.				GREAT DANGER			

because they can block the wind, are waterproof, and allow moisture to move away from the body.

- Replace body fluids in the cold, just as in the heat. Fluid replacement is also vitally important when exercising in cold air. Large amounts of water are lost from the body during even normal respiration, and this effect becomes magnified when exercising. Because sweat losses may not be as obvious as when exercising in the heat, monitoring of body weight over several days is recommended.

Exercising at Higher Altitudes

At moderate-to-high altitudes, the relative availability (i.e., **partial pressure**) of oxygen in the air is reduced. Because there is less pressure to drive the oxygen molecules into the blood in the lungs, the oxygen carried in the blood is reduced. Therefore, a person exercising at high altitude will not be able to deliver as much oxygen to the exercising muscles and exercise intensity will have to be reduced (e.g., the person will have to walk or run more slowly) to keep the HR in a target zone.

Signs and symptoms of altitude sickness include shortness of breath, headache, lightheadedness, and nausea. Generally, altitude sickness can be avoided by properly **acclimatizing** oneself by gradually increasing exercise and activity levels over the span of several days. A prolonged warm-up and cool-down and frequent exercise breaks at a lower intensity should help most people become accustomed to exercising at higher altitudes.

Exercising in Air Pollution

Some areas of the country have a high degree of airborne pollutants (i.e., smog) that can adversely affect exercise performance. These pollutants are the result of the combustion of fossil fuels and primarily include ozone, sulfur dioxide, and carbon monoxide. When these airborne particles are inhaled, they can have a number of deleterious effects on the body, such as irritating the airways and decreasing the oxygen-carrying capacity of the blood, both of which hamper performance. In individuals with cardiovascular disease, prolonged exposure to air pollution can even induce **ischemia** and **angina.** The overall physiological effects are determined by the degree of exposure (or dose) to pollutants that an individual is exposed to. This dose is related to the amount of pollutants in the air, the length of exposure, and the amount of air breathed. Practical suggestions to minimize the effects of air pollution include exercising early in the morning to avoid the build-up of pollutants associated with increased vehicular traffic, and avoiding high-traffic urban areas. Similar to exercising in the heat or at altitude, exercise pace may need to be reduced to keep HR in the desired training range. Under extreme conditions, exercising indoors is probably the best choice.

Summary

This chapter is designed to provide the LWMC with the basic principles of exercise physiology. Considerable content has been devoted to the presentation of aerobic and anaerobic metabolism, because the principle of **specificity** clearly dictates that physiological adaptations are specific to encountered stresses. The LWMC must understand the various methods of applying progressive overload and the physiological adaptations that result. Too often the exercising public falls victim to the poor advice of exercise leaders, coaches, and other "experts" who fail to apply the concept of exercise specificity because they simply do not understand basic principles.

Reference

Porcari, J.P. (1994). Fat-burning exercise: Fit or farce? *Fitness Management,* July, 40–42.

Suggested Reading

American College of Sports Medicine (2006). *ACSM's Guidelines for Exercise Testing and Prescription* (7th ed.). Philadelphia: Lippincott Williams & Wilkins.

American College of Sports Medicine (2005). *ACSM's Resource Manual for Guidelines for Exercise Testing and Prescription* (5th ed.). Philadelphia: Lippincott Williams & Wilkins.

Howley, E.T. & Franks, B.D. (2007). *Health Fitness Instructor's Handbook* (5th ed.). Champaign, Ill.: Human Kinetics.

McArdle, W., Katch, F., & Katch, V. (2006). *Exercise Physiology* (6th ed.). Philadelphia: Lippincott Williams & Wilkins.

Plowman, S.A. & Smith, D.L. (2007). *Exercise Physiology for Health, Fitness, and Performance.* Boston: Allyn and Bacon.

Wilmore, J.H., Costill, D.L., & Kenney, W.L. (2008). *Physiology of Sport and Exercise* (4th ed.). Champaign, Ill.: Human Kinetics.

Part II

Behavioral Science

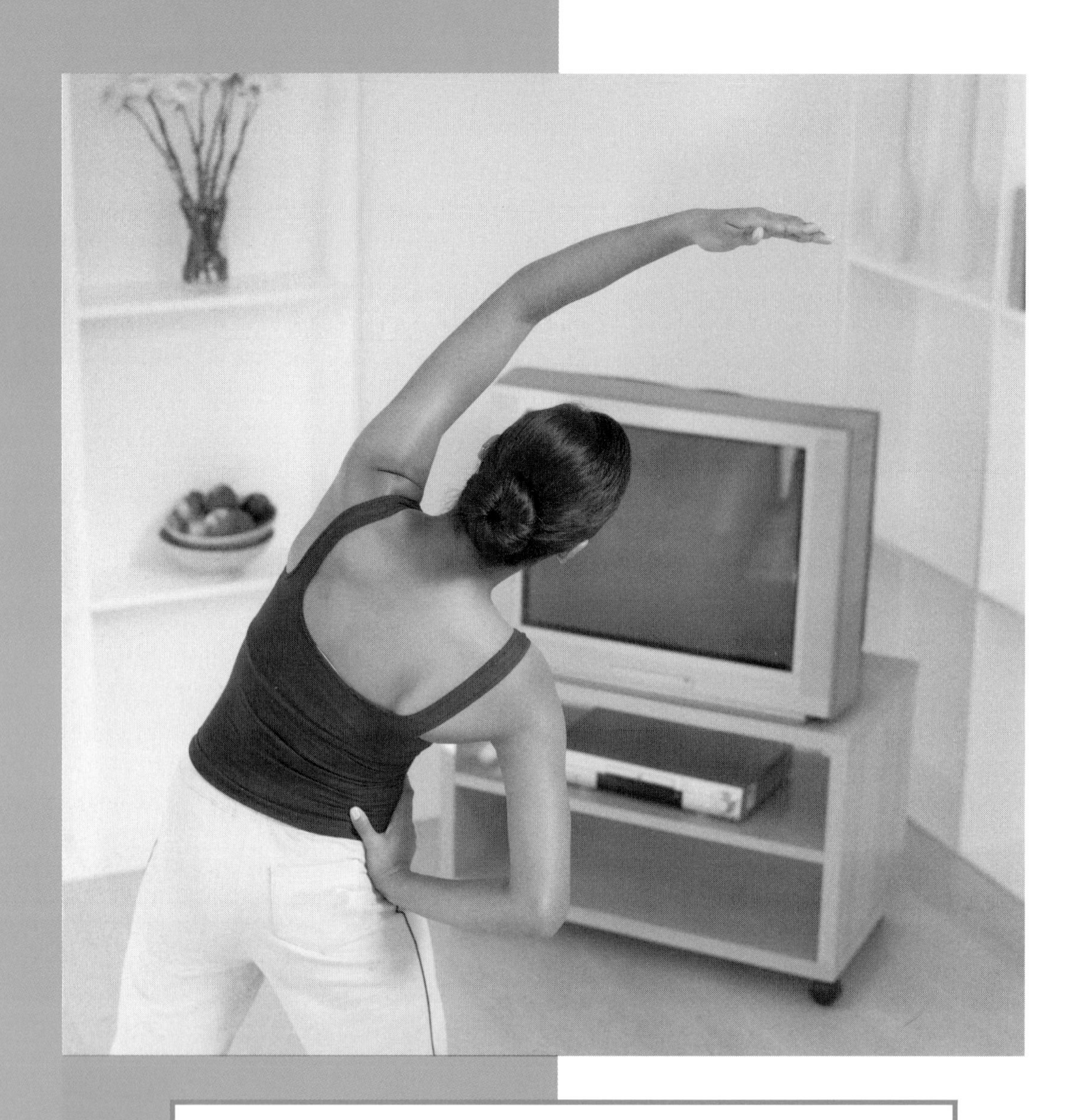

Tracie Rogers

Tracie Rogers, Ph.D., is a sport and exercise psychology specialist and owner of the BAR Fitness Studio located in Phoenix, Arizona. She teaches, speaks, and writes on psychological constructs related to physical-activity participation and adherence. She is also a faculty associate at Arizona State University in the department of kinesiology.

Chapter 4

Health Behavior Psychology

IN THIS CHAPTER:

Although the traditional biomedical model that explains diseases from a strictly physiological standpoint has led to great advances and understanding in the health and medical community, there are definitely flaws in this approach, as healthcare costs continue to rise along with the occurrence of lifestyle diseases. Therefore, **health psychology** emerged in the 1970s as a field of psychology that examines the causes of illnesses and studies ways to promote and maintain health, prevent and treat illnesses, and improve the healthcare system (Sarafino, 2006). Health psychology took the traditional biomedical model and added the individual to the equation. As a result, it has created a broader picture of the **correlates** of health and illness by examining not only the biological factors, but also the psychological and social factors that affect, and are affected by, a person's health (Engel, 1977). Under this new biopsychosocial model, behavioral risk factors, such as smoking, inactivity, alcohol abuse, and high dietary cholesterol, have been identified for each of the five leading causes of death.

As health and fitness professionals, LWMCs are in a position to greatly impact a client's overall health by decreasing behavioral risk factors of numerous diseases. Because LWMCs are working directly with clients on achieving long-term behavioral change, it is important that they understand the social and psychological factors that influence the adoption and maintenance of health behaviors.

Determinants of Behavior

Unfortunately, there is no simple answer to the question of why some people adopt healthy behaviors and others do not. In addition, the behavior of exercise is complicated, as it is perceived to take more time and effort than other health behaviors (Turk, Rudy, & Salovey, 1984). Also, different characteristics related to an exercise program can involve different determinants (Dishman, 1990), thereby further complicating the task of promoting activity adoption and maintenance. Nevertheless, researchers do have some understanding of factors that influence exercise behavior. The potential determinants for physical activity can be broken down into three categories: personal attributes, environmental factors, and the physical activity itself (Dishman & Sallis, 1994).

Personal Attributes

Demographic Variables

Demographic variables, including education, income, age, and gender, have been shown to be consistently linked with activity adherence (Morgan et al., 2003). Specifically, lower levels of activity are seen with increasing age, fewer years of education, and low income. Additionally, men demonstrate higher and more consistent activity adherence rates than women (Dishman & Buckworth, 1997). It is important to note that age is unrelated to activity adherence in supervised fitness settings (Oldridge, 1982). It is difficult to examine the specific influences of demographic variables, because they often occur concurrently, leaving researchers unable to separate the effects.

Biomedical Status

Biomedical status refers to health conditions, including **obesity** and **cardiovascular disease,** and is typically a weak predictor of exercise behavior. In general, research has shown that obese individuals are generally less active than normal-weight individuals and are less likely to adhere to supervised exercise programs. Unfortunately, these relationships have not remained consistent in more recent research, leaving experts a bit unsure about the exact relationship between obesity and activity-program adherence (Dishman & Buckworth, 1997). No consistent relationship between cardiovascular disease and activity adherence has been found.

Activity History

Activity history is arguably the most important and influential personal attribute variable. In supervised exercise programs, past program participation is the most reliable predictor of current participation. This relationship between past participation and current participation is consistent regardless of gender, obesity, and coronary heart disease status (Dishman & Buckworth, 1997).

Psychological Traits

Psychological traits refer to general tendencies that people have in their personality or psychological makeup. Psychological traits account for individual differences between people, and are often difficult to define and measure. However, the trait of self-motivation, which is reflective of one's ability to set goals, monitor progress, and self-reinforce, has been shown to have a relationship with physical-activity adherence (Dishman, 1982).

Knowledge, Attitudes, and Beliefs

Individuals have a wide variety of knowledge, attitudes, and beliefs about starting and sticking with an exercise program. Modifying the way an individual thinks and feels about exercise has been shown to influence his or her intentions for being active. Health perception, which is a knowledge, attitude, and belief variable, has been linked to adherence, such that those who perceive their health to be poor are unlikely to start or adhere to an activity program. Furthermore, if they do participate, it will likely be at an extremely low intensity and frequency (Dishman & Buckworth, 1997). **Locus of control** is another variable in this category, and, in healthy adults, a belief in personal control over health outcomes is a consistent predictor of unsupervised exercise activity. Finally, the variable of perceived barriers, such as lack of time, consistently demonstrates a negative relationship with activity-program adherence.

Environmental Factors

Access to Facilities

The notion of "access to facilities" most frequently refers to facility location. How convenient is it for clients to go to the gym? Is it close to their home or work, or are they driving out of the way to specifically see the LWMC? Access to facilities can be measured in two ways. First, it can be measured objectively, by assessing true access to, and availability of, fitness facilities. When measured in this way, access to facilities is a consistent predictor of physical-activity behavior, in that people with greater access are more likely to be physically active than people with less access. Access can also be measured subjectively by assessing perceived access to facilities. This has little to do with actual distance to, or availability of, a facility, but is instead a measure of an individual's perception of access. When measured this way, the research findings are much less consistent (Dishman, 1994).

Time

A perceived lack of time is the most common excuse for not exercising and for dropping out of an exercise program (Oldridge, 1982). The perception of not having enough time to exercise is likely a reflection of not being interested in or enjoying the activity, or not being committed to an activity program. The good news for LWMCs who are dealing with perceived lack of time with their clients is that this factor can be targeted and changed through thorough goal-setting, time-management, and prioritizing. If an individual makes health and activity a priority, he or she will make time to be active.

Social Support

Social support from family and friends is an important predictor of physical-activity behavior and has been consistently related to activity in both cross-sectional and prospective research designs (Duncan & McAuley, 1993). It is very difficult for an individual to maintain an exercise program if he or she does not have support at home. When support is broken down into specific types, support from a spouse is shown to be an important and reliable predictor of program adherence.

Physical-activity Factors

Intensity

Vigorous-intensity exercise programs have almost twice as much dropout as moderate-intensity activity programs. Additionally, when people are able to choose the type of activity they engage in, six times as many women and more than two times as many men choose to start moderate-activity programs than vigorous-activity programs. Intensity can be the actual exercise intensity as measured physiologically, such as by percent of **heart-rate reserve (HRR)**, or it can be measured psychologically, such as by a **rating of perceived exertion (RPE).** In either case, the same results are found with regards to exercise adherence (Sallis et al., 1986).

Injury

Injury is an important component of physical-activity behavior and adherence. There is a reliable relationship between physical activity and injury, and it is estimated that as many as half of all people who engage in high-intensity activities (such as running) are injured each year (Macera et al., 1989). The red flag with this statistic is that injuries that occur as a result of program participation are directly related to program dropout. Additionally, the relationship between injury and adherence is directly linked to exercise intensity, with high-intensity exercise being linked to greater injury risk. Research has also shown that injured exercisers are able to participate in modified exercise programs and often report engaging in significantly more walking than noninjured exercisers (Hofstetter et al., 1991).

Behavioral Theory Models

Each client will present new challenges and require the LWMC to develop unique techniques to achieve program adoption and maintenance. Because adopting a healthy lifestyle is complex, numerous explanations have been developed to explain the factors affecting health behaviors. One important factor in any lifestyle-modification program is the client's readiness to make a change. This individual readiness for change is the focus of a well-accepted theory examining health behaviors called the **transtheoretical model (TTM)** of behavioral change (Prochaska & DiClemente, 1984). For more information on the practical application of the TTM when designing exercise programs for clients, refer to Chapter 12. Chapter 16 also covers the TTM, but in the context of program adherence and maintenance. It is important that LWMCs understand this theory and are then able to apply it at various stages of a client's weight-management program.

Transtheoretical Model of Behavioral Change

Also called the stages-of-change model, the TTM is a critical construct to understand when promoting active lifestyles and healthy nutrition, because not all people are necessarily ready to make lifestyle changes. Both exercise and healthy eating need to be incorporated into a person's current lifestyle, making the TTM relevant and applicable to an LWMC.

Stages of Change

The first component of the TTM consists of five stages of behavior change:

- **Precontemplation:** People in this stage are sedentary, and are not even considering an activity program. These people do not see activity as relevant in their lives, and may even discount the importance or practicality of being physically active.
- **Contemplation:** People in this stage are still sedentary. However, they are starting to consider the importance of activity and have begun to identify the implications of being inactive. Nevertheless, they are still not ready to commit to making a change.
- **Preparation:** People in this stage perform some physical activity, as they are mentally and physically preparing to adopt an activity program. Activity during the preparation stage may be a sporadic walk, or even a visit to the gym, but it is still inconsistent. People in the preparation stage are ready to adopt and live an active lifestyle.
- **Action:** During this stage, people are engaging in regular physical activity, but have been doing so for less than six months.
- **Maintenance:** This stage is marked by regular physical-activity participation for longer than six months.

Processes of Change

The second component of the TTM consists of the processes of change that are used to pass from one stage to the next. Each transition has a unique set of processes and is based on specific individual decisions and mental states, such as individual readiness and motivation. The most effective change strategies are stage-specific interventions that target the natural processes people use as they move from one stage to the next (see Table 12-4, page 271). The first step is to identify the current stage of each client. If someone is in a fitness facility or has called a fitness facility, he or she is likely not a precontemplator. By listening to the types of questions being asked and to the types of hesitations an individual has, the LWMC will be able to identify the current stage of change and choose an appropriate intervention. The general goal of any interventions should be to advance the individual to the next stage of change.

Self-efficacy

The third component of the TTM is **self-efficacy,** which, in the lifestyle-modification context, is the belief in one's capabilities to be physically active and to maintain healthy nutrition (Bandura, 1986). Self-efficacy is an important component of lifestyle modification because it is strongly related to program adoption and maintenance. A circular relationship exists between self-efficacy and behavior change, so that a person's self-efficacy is related to whether he or she will participate in activity, and a person's participation in activity influences his or her self-efficacy level. Therefore, self-efficacy acts as both a determinant and an outcome of behavior change. Additionally, there is a reliable relationship between a person's self-efficacy for activity and his or her stage of behavior change, so that precontemplators and contemplators have significantly lower levels of self-efficacy than people in the action and maintenance stages. This relationship makes intuitive sense, as those in the precontemplation and contemplation stages are not exercising, which may be reflective of the belief that they do not have the ability to be active, and those in the action and maintenance stage are engaged in a regular activity program, and thus demonstrating a belief in the ability to be active. It is important to note that the most important and powerful predictor of self-efficacy is past performance experience. Therefore, an individual who has had past success in adopting and maintaining a physical-activity program will be more efficacious in his or her ability to be active in the future.

The documented relationship between stage of change and self-efficacy also implies that if self-efficacy is improved, the client may be helped in progressing through the stages. This is especially important for the people in the contemplation and preparation stages, as they are thinking about being active, or want to be active, and are working toward the point where they can be active regularly. By helping such individuals increase their self-efficacy, the LWMC may be able to move them through to the action stage more quickly.

Decisional Balance

The final of the four components of the TTM is **decisional balance,** which refers to the numbers of pros and cons an individual perceives regarding adopting and/or maintaining an activity program. Precontemplators and contemplators perceive more cons (e.g., sweating, sore muscles, time, finances, muscle hypertrophy, boredom) related to being regularly active than pros. The perceived cons do not have to be logical or realistic to prevent an individual from being active. As people progress through the stages of change, the balance of pros and cons shifts, so that people in the action and maintenance stages perceive more pros than cons. The active behavior of people in these later stages reflects this change in decisional balance.

The natural change in decisional balance that occurs as people progress through the stages of change implies that influencing their perceptions about being active may help in encouraging them to start an activity program. When working on shifting people's decisional balance, it is important to remember the processes of change related to moving from one stage to the next. For example, when working with a precontemplator or contemplator, an LWMC should emphasize the wide variety of benefits of being physically active and avoid arguing about the cons the client perceives about exercise. Often, the cons perceived by non-exercisers are a result of misinformation and a lack of experience. Additionally, it is important to discuss both short- and long-term benefits. An LWMC does not want to merely emphasize the long-term weight-loss benefits of an activity program, but also the more immediate benefits, including increased energy, improved mood, and enhanced mastery.

It is important to note that **relapse** can occur at any stage of the TTM, including the maintenance stage. Any change that may occur in an individual's life, such as moving, starting school, or suffering from an injury, can trigger a relapse into irregular activity or even no activity. The commitment of long-term exercisers should not be taken for granted, as this behavior can change and relapse can occur on any given day.

Additional Theories

In addition to examining how readiness to change influences health behavior, researchers have been interested in people's beliefs about their health and how these beliefs influence the adoption or non-adoption of health behaviors. The most accepted of these theories is called the **health belief model** (Becker, 1974).

Health Belief Model

The health belief model predicts that people will engage in a health behavior (i.e., exercise and/or healthy eating) based on the perceived threat they feel regarding a health problem, as well as the pros and cons of adopting that behavior. Perceived threat, which is defined as the degree to which a person feels threatened or worried by the prospect of a particular health problem, is influenced by several factors:

- The perceived seriousness of the health problem, or the feelings one has about the seriousness of contracting an illness or leaving it untreated. People take the severity of the potential consequences of the problem into consideration, and the more serious the consequences are perceived to be, the more likely people are to engage in a health behavior.
- The perceived susceptibility to the health problem is based on a person's subjective appraisal of the likelihood of developing the problem. People have a higher perceived threat and an increased likelihood to engage in a health behavior when they believe that they are vulnerable to a health problem.
- Cues to actions, or events, either bodily, such as physical symptoms, or environmental, such as health promotion information, motivate people to make a change. The more people are reminded about a potential health problem, the more likely they are to take action and engage in a health behavior.

The pros and cons of engaging in a health behavior are examined by the health belief model in terms of perceived benefits and perceived barriers of the health behavior. In other words, the client will assess the benefits, such a getting healthier and looking better, along with the barriers, such as financial cost and time, of making a lifestyle modification. According to the health belief model, if individuals perceive more barriers than benefits regarding a health behavior, they will be unlikely to make a behavior change.

However, if the perceived benefits outweigh the perceived barriers and the perceived threat of illness is high, people are likely to take preventative action, thus engaging in exercise and healthy nutrition behaviors. It is important for LWMCs to understand the perceptions their clients have regarding illness and a healthy lifestyle, including their perceived benefits and barriers to program participation. If individuals perceive little threat of developing an illness related to their lifestyle choices, the modification program is going to be difficult to implement without making the seriousness of the illness more apparent and making the individual feel more susceptible to developing the condition. It is important that LWMCs continuously use appropriate cues to action by introducing health information along with educating and focusing attention on physical symptoms.

Self-efficacy

Self efficacy is an important concept to understand when studying exercise and health behavior. As previously mentioned, self-efficacy is the belief in one's own capabilities to successfully complete a task. Self-efficacy beliefs are thought to influence thought patterns, affective responses, and action. Additionally, self-efficacy is positively related to motivation (Bandura, 1986). In the lifestyle-modification context, self-efficacy focuses on exercise behavior and healthy nutrition behaviors. What is the client's belief about his or her ability to be active, to be fit, to eat healthy, and to adhere to a program? This is important information to gather from all clients, as their self-efficacy levels will influence their program success. Furthermore, it is essential to understand how people develop self-efficacy. There are six sources of self-efficacy information:

- Past performance experience is the first and most influential source of self-efficacy information. What is the client's past experience with being physically active? This information is going to strongly influence his or her current self-efficacy level.
- Vicarious experience is the second source of self-efficacy. For a client who is starting a new lifestyle-modification program, observing someone else who is already successfully doing so, especially if the person is perceived to be similar to the client, can increase the client's self-efficacy.
- Verbal persuasion, the third source of self-efficacy, usually comes in the form of **feedback** (teaching) or motivational (encouraging) statements. These statements are most likely to influence self-efficacy if they come from a credible and knowledgeable source.
- A client's appraisal of his or her own physiological state as it relates to program participation is the fourth source of self-efficacy. From this appraisal, an individual may perceive arousal, pain, or fatigue. These appraisals lead people to make judgments about their ability to successfully participate.
- The appraisal of one's emotional state or mood related to program participation is the fifth source of self-efficacy information. Negative mood states, such as fear, anxiety, anger, and frustration, are related to lowered levels of both self-efficacy and participation.
- Imaginal experiences are the sixth source of self-efficacy information. A client's imagined experiences with program participation (positive or negative) will influence his or her actual self-efficacy levels.

It is always important to assess and understand clients' self-efficacy levels, because self-efficacy is related to ultimate success in a program. Self-efficacy influences three important participation variables:

- *Task choice:* Individuals with high self-efficacy are more likely to choose challenging tasks, as compared to individuals with low self-efficacy, who are more likely to choose very easy, non-challenging tasks.
- *Effort:* Individuals with high self-efficacy are more likely to display maximum effort when engaged in a lifestyle-modification program.
- *Persistence:* Individuals with high self-efficacy are more likely to overcome obstacles and challenges and stick with a program. Those with low self-efficacy are more likely to drop out as soon as a challenge arises.

Based on what researchers know about the construct of self-efficacy, it is important for LWMCs to always attempt to assess clients' efficacy levels for program participation and to understand why clients feel the way they do. This is best achieved through quality communication and continued interaction.

Principles of Behavior Change

The importance of understanding and applying theoretical constructs, such as the TTM and self-efficacy, is that they properly address exercise as a behavior. It is a mistake to think that starting and sticking with a lifestyle-modification program is simple, as it is a complicated process that requires replacing a lot of bad behaviors with new and healthy behaviors. The role of LWMCs is to influence the behaviors of clients by influencing attitudes, motives, emotions, and performances while simultaneously breaking old, destructive habits. This process does not happen in one day. Instead, individuals must develop into their new role of living a healthy lifestyle. To be successful, LWMCs must create a good learning environment and have an understanding of what controls peoples' behavior.

Operant Conditioning

An influential and effective approach to understanding human behavior is called **operant conditioning,** which considers how behaviors are influenced by their consequences and examines the relationships among **antecedents,** behaviors, and consequences (Martin & Pear, 1998).

Antecedents

Part of the learning experience is realizing which behaviors have consequences under certain conditions. Antecedents are stimuli that precede a behavior and often signal the likely consequences of the behavior. Antecedents help guide peoples' behavior so that it will most likely lead to positive or desirable consequences. Furthermore, antecedents can be manipulated in the environment to maximize the likelihood of desirable behaviors. This type of influence on behavior is called **stimulus control** and can be a valuable tool in behavior modification. For example, if a client frequently forgets his workout sessions, the LWMC may recommend that he leave his gym bag in the front seat of the car, serving as a visible reminder to go to the gym. Additionally, an LWMC can tell clients that keeping healthy snacks in their desks at work will increase their chances of choosing something healthy versus buying unhealthy snacks at the vending machine. Workout clothes and healthy snacks are examples of using stimulus control to modify behaviors.

Response Consequences

The most important component of operant conditioning is what happens after a behavior is executed. Different types of consequences lead to different behavioral outcomes, and consequences always involve the presentation, nonoccurrence, or removal of a positive or aversive stimulus. **Positive reinforcement,** or the presentation of a positive stimulus, increases the likelihood that a behavior will reoccur in the future. **Negative reinforcement,** which consists of the removal or avoidance of aversive stimuli following undesirable behavior, also increases the likelihood that the behavior will occur again. Extinction occurs when a positive stimulus that once followed a behavior is removed, which means that the likelihood of the behavior occurring again is decreased. **Punishment,** which consists of an aversive stimulus following an undesirable behavior, also decreases the likelihood of the behavior occurring again. Despite being effective in decreasing an unwanted behavior, punishment also increases fear and decreases enjoyment, so it must be used sparingly and only when appropriate (never for poor performance, only for lack of effort).

It is important that LWMCs provide appropriate feedback and consequences to client behaviors. LWMCs must positively reinforce the things that clients are doing well and must not ignore the things that need improvement. Clients need a clear understanding of the target behaviors, and providing consistent consequences will help decrease program ambiguity (Smith, 2005).

Shaping

Shaping occurs when reinforcements are used to gradually achieve a target behavior. This process begins with the performance of a basic skill that the client is currently capable of doing. The skill demands are then gradually raised and reinforcement is given as more is accomplished. This process of continually increasing the demands at an appropriate rate and providing positive reinforcement leads to the execution of the desired behavior and serves as a powerful behavioral control technique. Part of the reason that shaping is so effective is that it starts with having the client execute a task at an appropriate skill level (Smith, 2005). It is important to remember that each client is going to have his or her own starting point and that LWMCs will be most effective when they identify this level and design their programs from that starting point. Expecting too much from clients initially can lead to dropout, as they may feel overwhelmed and incapable.

Adherence and Motivation

Behavior Modification

To help enable clients to successfully stick with their lifestyle-modification programs, it is important to teach them behavior-modification strategies, which are tools that LWMCs will use to help their clients succeed in the adoption and maintenance of their activity programs. Regardless if clients are just beginning the program or if they have been participating for a long time, behavior-modification strategies are helpful and important. Just like turning on the television when getting home from work and talking on the telephone while driving can become habits in a person's life, being physically active and participating in activity throughout the day is also a habit, as is the avoidance of physical activity. When LWMCs help people find time in their schedule for regular activity, they often simultaneously help them identify undesirable behaviors or habits they can eventually replace with physical activity and healthy eating.

When tested in research, behavior-modification programs and tools have been shown to be consistently successful in helping people be regularly physically active. Behavior-modification methods change behavior by using the principles of operant and classical conditioning to help people learn to be more active (Dishman, 1991). There are numerous behavior-modification strategies, three of which are discussed in this section.

Written Agreements

Written agreements are useful tools for helping people stick with their activity programs. A written agreement can either be between the LWMC and the client or between the client and him- or herself. A written agreement should clearly specify what is expected of the client. One reason that agreements are successful is that they decrease any ambiguity and clarify all behaviors, commitments, and attitudes that the client expects of him- or herself and that the LWMC expects of the client. Written agreements are going to be less successful if the client does not take an active role in creating the contract. Telling people what to do and what is expected of them is never as helpful for behavior change as people setting their own expectations. Within a written agreement, the LWMC should also be specific in clarifying his or her own role in the activity program, along with the client's role. The LWMC and the client should both sign the agreement and hold each other accountable for the expected behaviors. Be flexible with the written agreement, and if circumstances or goals change, revise the agreement, so that it is always applicable to the activity program.

Behavioral Contracting

Behavioral contracting is another effective behavior-modification strategy. In behavior contracting for exercise adherence, the LWMC and the client will set up a system of rewards for sticking to the lifestyle-modification program. Behavioral contracting is most effective when the rewards are outlined by, and meaningful to, the client. If the rewards are not meaningful, the client may not find them to be worth working toward. Behavioral contracting works differently for each individual and LWMCs have to be careful not to push certain rewards on clients. Additionally, behavioral contracting is most effective when it is used consistently. Once certain goals are met, contracts need to be reconstructed throughout the duration of program participation.

Stimulus Control

A third effective behavior-modification strategy is stimulus control, which involves altering the environment to encourage healthy behaviors and to make following the modification program as easy as possible. Stimulus control is related to operant conditioning, as it refers to manipulating the stimuli in the environment to trigger the behavior of exercise or healthy eating. Stimulus-control strategies that LWMCs can recommend to their clients include the following:

- Having workout clothes, socks, and shoes ready for early-morning workouts
- Keeping a gym bag in the car with all necessary workout items
- Posting signs on pantry and refrigerator doors listing the foods they should be eating
- Making a grocery list and staying away from purchasing non-listed items
- Carrying or wearing comfortable shoes at work so that clients can take the stairs instead of the elevator

Another effective stimulus-control technique is to socialize with other people who live healthy lifestyles. By associating with people who have similar goals and interests, clients will create support systems for behavior change. Another effective strategy is to join a fitness facility located in the direct path between home and work, and scheduling workout times that concur with the times a person typically drives by the facility. If LWMCs start hearing a lot of excuses from their clients about why they are missing workouts or are unable to adhere, it may be a cue that a stimulus-control strategy is needed. LWMCs should always strive to make their clients' lifestyle-modification programs as convenient as possible in their everyday lives.

Cognitive Behavioral Techniques

In addition to behavior-modification strategies, cognitive behavioral techniques are also effective for changing behavior. Cognitive techniques alter behavior by changing how people feel and think. By using cognitive techniques, people are able to first identify and then change problematic beliefs that prevent them from making desired changes. Cognitive techniques can be used independently as intervention tools for behavior change, or in conjunction with other behavior-modification strategies (Dishman, 1991).

Goal-setting

Goal-setting is an effective and easy-to-use cognitive behavioral technique. However, for goal-setting to be optimally effective, it must be used systematically, meaning that it needs to be a regular part of the activity program. A common mistake made with goal-setting is sitting down at the start of program and creating program goals with a client—and then filing these goals away and not looking at them again. This type of goal-setting is not going to maximally benefit program adherence. Instead, clients need to be continually aware of their goals. Proper goals should be **SMART goals,** meaning that they should be specific, measurable, attainable, relevant, and time-bound (see Chapter 13). It is the LWMC's role to educate clients about these guidelines and help them create appropriate goals. It is important to avoid setting too many goals. Keeping the number of goals manageable and attainable prevents the LWMC from overwhelming the client. Also, LWMCs should avoid setting negative goals. If a client wants to set the goal to not miss any workouts, the LWMC can reword the goal to be positive: "Attend every scheduled workout session." When negative goals are set, it makes clients think about the behavior they want to avoid, when they should really be thinking about the behavior they want to achieve. Also, it is essential that the LWMC and client set both short- and long-term goals, as well as outcome goals and performance goals. LWMCs want their clients to achieve success in each workout. The most important thing that LWMCs can do to make goal-setting an effective behavior-change technique is to attend to the goals on a regular basis. LWMCs must adjust goals as needed and use them as tools to direct attention and effort, and to promote persistence.

Feedback

Feedback is an interesting technique that involves both the LWMC and the client. When most fitness professionals think of feedback, they think of providing reinforcement and encouragement to their clients. This is known as extrinsic or **external feedback,** and is critically important for initial program adoption. However, the type of feedback most important for long-term program adherence is **internal feedback,** which is provided by the clients themselves. To encourage the development of internal feedback for clients, LWMCs must taper off the amount of external feedback they provide. If LWMCs continue to reinforce every good behavior their clients engage in, the clients will never need to provide feedback for themselves. LWMCs must give clients the opportunity to provide their own reinforcement, encouragement, error correction, and, in some instances, punishment. By providing excessive amounts of external feedback, LWMCs cripple their clients' ability to achieve long-term adherence.

Decision-making

The utilization of decision-making entails encouraging clients to take control of the situation and choose between alternative courses of action. In using this technique, LWMCs enable their clients to make behavioral choices that impact program participation and success and increase the likelihood of program adherence. Encouraging clients to take this type of control over their program participation really empowers them with the knowledge that they have the ability to succeed and make changes in their lives that will influence that success.

Self-monitoring

Self-monitoring entails clients keeping track of information regarding their activity participation. This information should include their success and difficulties in adhering to their lifestyle-modification program. Self-monitoring provides clients with a lot of information about situations, people, and events that are barriers to adherence. This technique requires a great amount of client commitment and interest in becoming regularly active, but can be very effective in identifying barriers and developing strategies for long-term adherence.

Applying Theory to Practice

It is not only important that LWMCs understand the components and predictions of theoretical constructs, such as the TTM, but it is critical that they apply these concepts to their clients and their lifestyle-modification programs. Application of knowledge that stems from theoretical models will provide guidance in an LWMC's adherence-building strategies.

The most important skill that LWMCs can have in terms of the application of any theoretical concept is communication. Through effective communication techniques, LWMCs will be able to assess clients' self-efficacy and readiness to change. Based on initial information that LWMCs gather using effective communication techniques, they should then target the information in the program design to each client's stage of behavior change. This is an ongoing process and LWMCs should not expect changes in the stage of behavior based on one conversation or intervention. In conjunction with providing stage-specific information to a client or potential client, LWMCs want to start to manipulate decisional balance and self-efficacy. Provide information that logically disputes some of the perceived cons and give clients initial exercise or activity experiences that are positive. Additionally, create initial program experiences that are attainable and enjoyable. Give clients early success! Each client that LWMCs work with will have unique goals, needs, attitudes, and beliefs, and the programs are going to be most effective when they are customized to the individual, not just based on his or her physical abilities, but also on his or her psychological states.

Behavioral Interventions

To maximize behavior change and adherence, all behavior-modification programs should include a few specific things. First, LWMCs must always obtain information about clients' past activity experiences. When was the last time they were physically active, and did they have a positive or negative experience? Learn about their activity abilities and preferences, along with their activity hesitations. Also, it is extremely helpful when LWMCs start identifying potential and actual barriers to adopting and maintaining a regular activity program. The more LWMCs can learn about their clients at the start of a program, the more likely they will be able to customize the program and maximize adherence.

Second, LWMCs should always learn about each client's social support network. Does the rest of the family participate in activity? Do the family members and friends support the client in starting an activity program? Does the client have a work environment that supports and encourages an active lifestyle? This information will become clearer over time, but it is important to start gathering as much information as possible during initial client consultations.

Third, LWMCs should identify their clients' attitudes, opinions, and beliefs about physical activity. If LWMCs deal with individuals who have not engaged in regular activity in the recent past, they are going to be dealing with a lot of misconceptions about being active. Through education, experience, and rapport-building, LWMCs need to immediately start replacing illogical exercise perceptions with ones that represent a more realistic assessment of physical activity.

Finally, LWMCs need to provide education in effective goal-setting techniques and self-monitoring strategies. They must teach clients to take their activity experiences into their own hands and give them the power to succeed and the knowledge that they can do it.

If LWMCs keep these four guidelines in mind for all behavioral interventions, they will be off to a good start in creating programs for their clients. However, it is also important to remember that interventions do not end when program participation begins. For behavioral interventions to be effective, they need to continue through the duration of program participation. These interventions need to become part of the regular activity program and LWMCs need to continue to communicate, assess, and educate to maximize the likelihood of long-term adherence. Additionally, the best behavioral interventions are multifaceted, meaning that they include a variety of intervention techniques. LWMCs must not get overly focused on one intervention, but instead incorporate a variety of strategies for optimal success. Interventions must also be systematic and complete, meaning that LWMCs cannot neglect the behavioral-change aspect as they get caught up in the physical components of the program.

Relapse Prevention

Once an individual has reached the action stage of behavior change and has successfully adopted a regular activity program, the LWMC should start implementing strategies for relapse prevention. Relapse from regular physical-activity participation is extremely common, and LWMCs must educate their clients about potential relapse and prepare them with coping strategies to deal with adherence challenges. Because the vast majority of people face one or more barriers, such as time, finances, prioritizing, scheduling, support issues, or a dislike of, or dissatisfaction with, the program, it is important to develop strategies before adherence problems arise. Remember, ultimately the program has to be valued by the client for long-term adherence to occur.

Coping Strategies

An important coping strategy for relapse prevention is to increase and maintain social support for exercise. LWMCs must be creative in developing support systems at home. Get the family involved to some degree in the program so they can understand the commitment the client has made to lifestyle modification. Additionally, LWMCs can help create a support system within the exercise or activity environment by utilizing opportunities for group involvement and social interaction and making clients feel as though they belong in the program.

Assertiveness

Another strategy that can be used to help prevent program relapse is encouraging clients to be assertive. **Assertiveness** is an important characteristic for achieving success and is defined as the honest and straightforward expression of one's thoughts, feelings, and beliefs. Typically, when individuals are not assertive, it is because they lack self-confidence or they feel vulnerable. The more assertive clients are regarding their progress, concerns, accomplishments, and struggles, the more likely they are to achieve long-term success.

Self-regulation

The more effective that clients become at self-regulating their behaviors, schedules, time, and priorities, the more likely they will be to adhere to the program. LWMCs cannot try to regulate clients' behavior for them. Instead, LWMCs must teach clients to self-monitor and to make behavior changes that will optimize their success. Teaching self-regulation strategies will provide clients with control over their own lives. Once clients perceive control over their behavioral outcomes, they are more able to deal with barriers and challenges as they arise.

High-risk Situations

Identifying high-risk situations will make LWMCs more prepared to deal with program barriers and program relapse. Vacations, schedule changes, injuries, and holidays are some common situations in which many people relapse. LWMCs must be prepared for these events as they arrive and talk to their clients about the challenges of remaining physically active through these times. Also, identify clients who appear to be most at risk for program relapse. Those who have poor time-management skills, a lack of social support, or busy schedules are prime examples of people who will likely relapse. LWMCs should provide extra education, support, and guidance for these people as they adopt their programs and deal with barriers in sticking to the programs. Additionally, LWMCs must be observant of their clients' emotional states by watching for signs of being overwhelmed and worn out. LWMCS will be better able to help their clients maintain behavioral plans if they take the time to teach them additional coping skills, including time management and prioritizing, work with them on developing a plan for adherence, and remain supportive, understanding, and empathic.

Summary

Trying to predict health behavior is complex and requires the examination of numerous correlates. Understanding the theoretical models is important to create a foundation of knowledge about health behavior and behavior change. However, it is also critical that health professionals are aware of, and continuously evaluate, the numerous psychological and social factors that influence health. Furthermore, the success of a lifestyle-modification program will be related to the LWMC's ability to implement ongoing behavior-modification strategies and continual relapse-prevention techniques. Understanding how difficult making a lifestyle change can be will give the LWMC a better ability to create a program that inspires lasting behavior change.

References

Bandura, A. (1986). *Social Foundations of Thought and Action: A Social Cognitive Theory.* Englewood Cliffs, N.J.: Prentice-Hall.

Becker, M.H. (1974). The health belief model and personal health behavior. *Health Education Monographs,* 2, 324–473.

Dishman, R.K. (1994). *Advances in Exercise Adherence*. Champaign, Ill.: Human Kinetics.

Dishman, R.K. (1991). Increasing and maintaining exercise and physical activity. *Behavior Therapy,* 22, 345–378.

Dishman, R.K. (1990). Determinants of participation in physical activity. In: C. Bouchard et al. (Eds.). *Exercise, Fitness, and Health* (pp. 75–102). Champaign, Ill.: Human Kinetics.

Dishman, R.K. (1982). Compliance/adherence in health-related exercise. *Health Psychology,* 1, 237–267.

Dishman, R.K. & Buckworth, J. (1997). Adherence to physical activity. In: W.P. Morgan (Ed.). *Physical Activity & Mental Health* (pp. 63–80). Washington, D.C.: Taylor & Francis.

Dishman, R.K. & Sallis, J. (1994). Determinants and interventions for physical activity and exercise. In: C. Bouchard et al. (Eds.). *Exercise, Fitness, and Health*. Champaign, Ill.: Human Kinetics.

Duncan, T.E. & McAuley, E. (1993). Social support and efficacy cognitions in exercise adherence: A latent growth curve analysis. *Journal of Behavioral Medicine,* 16, 199–218.

Engel, G.L. (1977). The need for a new medical model: A challenge for biomedicine. *Science,* 196, 129–136.

Hofstetter, D.R. et al. (1991). Illness, injury, and correlates of aerobic exercise and walking: A community study. *Research Quarterly for Exercise and Sport*, 62, 1–9.

Macera, C. A. et al. (1989). Predicting lower-extremity injuries among habitual runners. *Archives of Internal Medicine*, 149, 2565–2568.

Martin, G. & Pear, J. (1998). *Behavior Modification: What It Is and How to Do It* (6th ed.). Englewood Cliffs, N.J.: Prentice-Hall.

Morgan, C.F. et al. (2003). Personal, social, and environmental correlates of physical activity in a bi-ethnic sample of adolescents. *Pediatric Exercise Science,* 15, 288–301.

Oldridge, N.G. (1982).Compliance and exercise in primary and secondary prevention of coronary heart disease: A review. *Preventive Medicine,* 11, 56–70.

Prochaska, J.O. & DiClemente, C.C. (1984). The *Transtheoretical Approach: Crossing Traditional Boundaries of Therapy.* Homewood, Ill.: Dow Jones/Irwin.

Sallis, J.F. et al. (1986). Predictors of adoption and maintenance of physical activity in a community sample. *Preventive Medicine,* 15, 331–341.

Sarafino, E.P. (2006). *Health Psychology: Biopsychosocial Interactions* (5th ed.). New York: John Wiley & Sons.

Smith, R.E. (2005). Positive reinforcement, performance feedback, and performance enhancement. In: J.M. Williams (Ed.). *Applied Sport Psychology: Personal Growth to Peak Performance.* Mountain View, Calif.: Mayfield Publishing Company.

Turk, D.C., Rudy, T.E., & Salovey, P. (1984). Health protection: Attitudes and behaviors of LPNs, teachers, and college students. *Health Psychology,* 3, 189–210.

Suggested Readings

Bandura, A. (2001). Social cognitive theory: An agentive perspective. *Annual Review of Psychology,* 52, 1–26.

Dishman, R.K. & Buckworth, J. (1996). Increasing physical activity: A quantitative synthesis. *Medicine and Science in Sports and Exercise,* 28, 706–719.

Dunn, A.L. & Blair, S.N. (1997). Exercise prescription. In: W.P. Morgan (Ed.). *Physical Activity & Mental Health* (pp. 49–62). Washington, D.C.: Taylor & Francis.

Kirschenbaum, D.S. (1997). Prevention of sedentary lifestyles: Rationale and methods. In: W.P. Morgan (Ed.). *Physical Activity & Mental Health* (pp. 33–48). Washington, D.C.: Taylor & Francis.

Masui, R. et al. (2002). The relationship between health beliefs and behaviors and dietary intake in early adolescence. *Journal of the American Dietetic Association,* 102, 421–424

McAuley, E., Pena, M.M., & Jerome, G.J. (2001). Self-efficacy as a determinant and an outcome of exercise. In: G.C. Roberts (Ed.). *Advances in Motivation in Sport and Exercise.* Champaign, Ill.: Human Kinetics.

Sallis, J.F. & Hovell, M.F. (1990). Determinants of exercise behavior. In: *Exercise and Sports Sciences Reviews*, 18. Baltimore: Williams and Wilkins, 307–330.

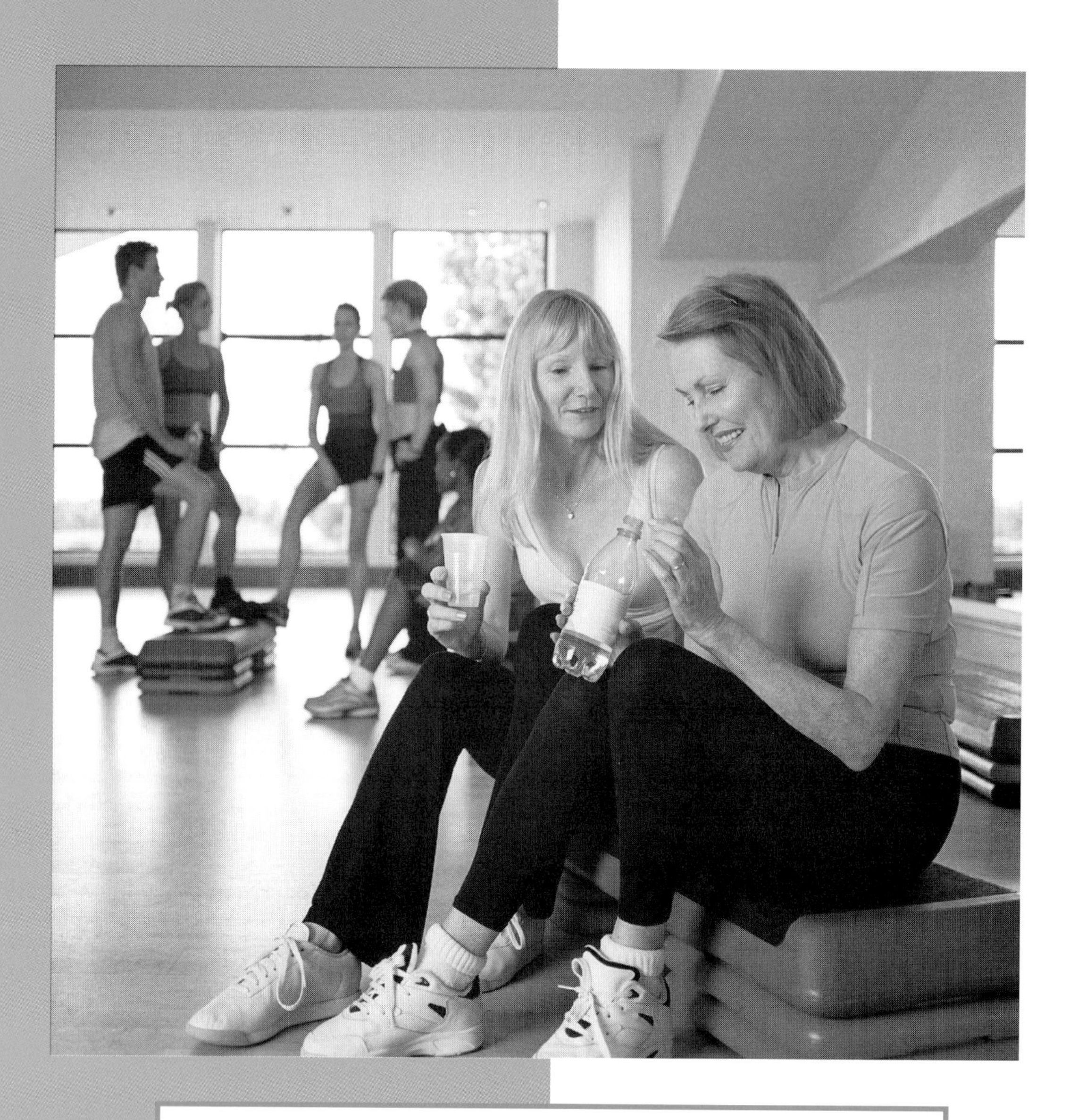

Tracie Rogers

Tracie Rogers, Ph.D., is a sport and exercise psychology specialist and owner of the BAR Fitness Studio located in Phoenix, Arizona. She teaches, speaks, and writes on psychological constructs related to physical-activity participation and adherence. She is also a faculty associate at Arizona State University in the department of kinesiology.

Chapter 5

Communication, Counseling, and Group Dynamics

IN THIS CHAPTER:

The ability to communicate effectively and efficiently is a crucial skill for achieving success in all personal and professional aspects of life, and the best relationships are those in which communication is clear and effective. This statement holds true for the relationships that Lifestyle & Weight Management Consultants (LWMCs) have with their clients. No matter how much LWMCs know about fitness testing, program design, and implementation, if they are not effective communicators, they will have great difficulty leading clients through successful modification programs, not to mention running a successful business. Most people have probably finished conversations and then thought, "I wish I would have said this or told them what I really thought." If an individual continually feels misunderstood and misrepresented, it is likely because he or she is not communicating effectively and efficiently with others. Effective communication does not always come naturally, and no one is always a perfect communicator. Communication, like all skills for success, must be learned, practiced, and perfected. In fact, some LWMCs may be very effective communicators in their personal lives, but struggle to communicate well in their professional lives. No matter how proficient a communicator a person thinks he or she is, everyone's communication skills can use some attention, and the development of effective communication requires continuous effort.

Rapport Building

LWMCs will be ineffective in their professional duties if they are unable to build quality relationships with their clients. A trusting relationship will serve as the solid foundation of all lifestyle-modification programs. Many clients are experiencing a new environment and new demands with the adoption of their programs, and they likely feel stressed, apprehensive, and insecure about their capabilities. Therefore, it is critical that the LWMC establishes **rapport** from the very beginning. Rapport is a relationship of trust and mutual understanding, and it is the LWMC's responsibility to establish this relationship from the outset. Without a foundation of trust, a working relationship cannot be effectively established.

Building rapport is critical in the client–consultant relationship, because the LWMC needs to know the expectations and needs of the client. When communicating with someone who is nervous, it is often a challenge to obtain all of this information. If the LWMC is unable to establish trust and open communication at the start of a program, working with the client will be a great challenge, and success will be limited. The process of opening communication starts with the LWMC. Because many fitness professionals, including LWMCs, are fit, it is important for them to realize that their physical appearance will affect their ability to establish trust and communication. If LWMCs want to be successful in creating and managing lifestyle-modification programs, they must be open-minded and compassionate with each client. The tendency to place blame on the client must be avoided and replaced with the teaching of responsibility and accountability for health behaviors. Additionally, LWMCs should always remember how difficult it is to maintain a healthy lifestyle and how challenging it is for people to make the decision to commit to changing their lifestyle. This compassion and understanding will give LWMCs a better chance of achieving success with all of their clients.

LWMCs must keep several things in mind as they work to establish rapport. First, it is important to be an active listener who is concerned about the content, intent, and feeling of the message (Yukelson, 2005). For initial consultations, it is always best to meet in person (not via email or telephone), and make eye contact throughout the conversation. **Active listening** is about being involved in the information being presented and asking questions to clarify points and express compassion. To display active listening, LWMCs should not take too many notes. Doing so will make it appear as though they are not paying attention or are uninterested in what is being said.

Second, LWMCs must be empathetic. **Empathy** is a learned skill that is marked by a display of concern and genuine interest. It is best described as an understanding of what the other person is experiencing. To be empathetic, it is important for LWMCs to restate what they have heard in their own words and to ask probing questions. Such statements and questions will demonstrate that they not only care about clients' feelings, but also that they understand their situations and needs.

Finally, to establish rapport, it is important to be aware of each client's goals and needs. What does the client hope to achieve by making lifestyle modifications and what does he or she expect the LWMC's role to be in the program? This information will help the LWMC understand how to be there for the client as a coach, cheerleader, and friend. Also, it will help identify unrealistic expectations and any issues with responsibility and accountability.

When building and maintaining rapport, it is useful to pay attention to the progress of the conversation and relationship. No two interactions will be the same, and LWMCs will be most effective if they are able to make adjustments based on the individual and the situation. If an LWMC perceives the conversation to be "slipping away" or notices that a client has lost interest and focus in the conversation, he or she should do a quick assessment of the environment, and his or her own body language, eye contact, and listening. For example, are there distracting noises preventing the conversation from moving forward? Is the client not making eye contact? Is the LWMC leaning back in the chair with arms crossed? All of these things can be indicators that the communication is less than ideal. Successful communicators have the ability to make the required adjustments to reestablish trust, understanding, and sharing.

Communication and Interviewing Techniques

It is difficult to come up with a universal definition of communication, as it is a dynamic and complex construct. However, high-quality communication can be described as effectively expressing one's thoughts, feelings, and needs, while understanding the thoughts, feelings, and needs of others. As reflected in this definition, communication not only encompasses expression, but also listening. Communication is truly a process of mutual sharing and understanding that is critical to success (Orlick, 1986).

Nonverbal Communication

Ideas, information, thoughts, and feelings are not only expressed verbally in communication, but nonverbally as well. Nonverbal communication, which can include body language, gestures, facial expressions, and body positioning, should not be overlooked as an important component of quality interaction. In fact, how LWMCs say things is just as important as the content of their message. In other words, if an LWMC is trying to be empathic and understanding, but has his or her arms crossed and is looking at his notes, then the nonverbal cues are sending a different message than the words. As a result, the message is unclear, and the LWMC may have missed an opportunity to establish trust and credibility with a new client. Nonverbal communication should be used to strengthen the verbal message, and to confirm active listening. In fact, an LWMC can show support, understanding, respect, and emotion, all of which are important for establishing rapport and building professional relationships, by using only nonverbal cues. Key points for good nonverbal communication include the following:

- *Eye contact*: Maintaining eye contact will be difficult for clients who feel anxious about the meeting or the beginning of a program. LWMCs must be receptive to their clients' nonverbal cues, so they do not become intimidated or uncomfortable, yet strive to maintain a relaxed focus on the client when talking. This can be done by glancing away momentarily as needed, but then returning focus on the client's face and eyes. When LWMCs are listening, they should look at the client to show interest in, and understanding of, what he or she is saying.
- *Body posture:* The way LWMCs hold their bodies can portray confidence, credibility, compassion, and empathy. LWMCs should be relaxed, but strong in their posture—shoulders back, head up, and directly facing the client. LWMCs should keep their arms and legs uncrossed and lean forward as they listen to display interest. This type of posture will make an LWMC feel like a leader, and look like one as well.
- *Body movement:* All body movements should be natural and relaxed. LWMCs should make their movements meaningful and avoid fidgeting or rocking, as these nervous movements will portray an image of insecurity and self-doubt.

Verbal Communication

The ability to effectively interview and communicate with clients and prospective clients relies on the LWMC's ability to display active listening and understanding. Through listening, an LWMC must be able to demonstrate that he or she is hearing clients' viewpoints, experiences, and emotions. Additionally, the LWMC must be psychologically and physically attentive to the client to be aware of what he or she is trying to say (Yukelson, 2005). It is important for the LWMC to question, encourage, paraphrase, reflect on, and summarize ideas as the client speaks. Doing so demonstrates that the LWMC is listening (Egan, 1994). To become a better listener, an LWMC must learn to put the client's needs, feelings, and thoughts ahead of his or her own. The LWMC must make a conscious effort to be concerned about the content, intent, and feeling of what is being heard by asking questions, expressing empathy, and providing insight. Additionally, LWMCs must make a real effort to avoid turning the focus of a conversation to themselves. The key to being an effective listener is to truly listen, not talk.

Good communication skills will help LWMCs get the information they need to start a program, make a client feel comfortable and safe, express empathy, and bring clarity and purpose to the program design and implementation. Finally, LWMCs must make the conversation a top priority during consultations. Minimizing outside distractions, such as the telephone or other interruptions, ensures that the client remains the focus.

Communication Problems

One of the biggest problems in any relationship is that people make assumptions. When people stop making an effort to communicate, they start assuming that other people know what they think and feel, and assume that they know the thoughts and feelings of others. As a result, they are less clear with their expressions and expectations than they should be. Because of their leadership position, it is critical that LWMCs learn to express expectations clearly and take the time to listen to others as they express their challenges, concerns, and insights. Stress, ambiguity, and lack of motivation can all be alleviated by clear and consistent expression of program goals, expectations, and progress.

When communication breaks down, it is easy to place the blame on the other party. However, it is the LWMC's responsibility to continually make the effort to establish and maintain communication.

Communication Factors

Many factors influence the way messages are expressed, conveyed, received, and interpreted, making it very easy for miscommunications to occur. Because miscommunication happens so frequently, health professionals should tailor their conversation to the specific client based on his or her needs, interests, and concerns (Kreuter & Wray, 2003). Specifically, two important components of any communication are the individuals involved and the environment in which the communication is taking place.

Psychological and Personal Factors

Because communication is a dynamic process, it is ever-changing based on the people involved. A person's personality traits and communication styles can significantly alter the quality of communication. Personality traits, such as shyness, extroversion, and **assertiveness,** in addition to the need to belong, be recognized, feel powerful, and feel secure, will not only alter how a message is transmitted, but also how it is received by the other party. It is important for an LWMC to be aware of the personalities of clients and to understand how his or her own personality influences personal communication skills. Furthermore, the individual's motivation for making a lifestyle change should be assessed, as his or her reasons for starting a program should influence the focus of the information the LWMC presents.

Assertiveness

A person's ability to tell others what he or she feels, thinks, and believes will influence the quality of one's communication, confidence, perceived control, and ultimately, achievements. These critical skills are encompassed in the trait of assertiveness, which is one of the most important psychological skills related to success. For some people, being assertive may come very naturally, while others continually struggle with expressing themselves to others. Like all communication skills, assertive behavior can be learned, practiced, and perfected.

Assertive behavior is defined as the ability to honestly and straightforwardly express thoughts, feelings, and beliefs (Yukelson, 2005). This does not mean that people should go around telling everyone exactly how they feel and what they think in an effort to be assertive. The vital part of being assertive is learning to express oneself in a socially appropriate manner, meaning that an individual must understand and take into consideration the situation, environment, and people involved in all interactions (Lazarus, 1973). Individuals must learn to become aware of the potential consequences of their behavior. Additionally, by reflecting on their own behavior, people become more aware of the consequences of either not expressing themselves or of being disruptive with their self-expression. Whatever people's natural behavioral tendencies may be, taking the time to work on assertiveness will increase the quality and satisfaction of their interactions.

Assertiveness can be broken down into four specific behaviors that can be targeted and practiced individually. The first of these behaviors is being able to say no. This is an important skill to develop, as it reflects an understanding of one's own needs and limitations. When people are unable to say no to other people, they end up losing focus on their priorities and possibly their professional responsibilities. Being assertive is about maintaining control of one's time, resources, and beliefs. Learning to say no is the first step in this direction.

The second component of assertive behavior is being able to start, continue, and end conversations. If people are going to be able to express themselves, they obviously have to be able to talk to people. New clients are often going to perceive the situation as stressful, so it is the LWMC's responsibility to initiate and carry on conversations. This skill helps develop confidence in expressing how one feels and what one thinks.

The third component of assertive behavior is being able to express both positive and negative feelings. A person should be able to easily express pride, excitement, and happiness. Additionally, a person should be able to express negative feelings, including disappointment, sadness, and discouragement. The quality of a person's relationships will improve when people understand how he or she feels.

The final component of assertive behavior is being able to ask for help. An LWMC must be aware of his or her limitations. When overwhelmed, overworked, or underqualified, LWMCs must ask others to help out. If LWMCs ignore these feelings and attempt to take on too many roles, they will be ineffective.

Environmental, Ethnic, and Cultural Factors

In addition to individual differences such as personality, situational differences also influence the quality of client–consultant interactions. First, the relationship the LWMC has with the other person will change the dynamic of the conversation. Specifically, the length of time the consultant and client have known each other, the history they share, the amount of trust and respect perceived, and the structure of power all affect communication. Second, the environment in which the communication takes place is important. Communication will be different if it takes place in a private, quiet office, as compared to a public space with a lot of foot traffic and commotion. The stress of the situation also influences the quality of communication. When the situation is emotionally charged in any way, the structure of the communication will change. If LWMCs are feeling stressed or pressured in a situation, it is important to remember that the effectiveness of communication will be diminished and that they need to focus on successfully transmitting their message.

Cultural differences influence the effectiveness of both verbal and nonverbal communication and, if misinterpreted, such differences can jeopardize trust and the ability to share thoughts, feelings, and beliefs. As a result, LWMCs should be aware of cultural differences in communicative behaviors. Cultural differences may influence facial expressions, eye-contact patterns, gestures, expectations, family background, diet, language, and values. It is also important for LWMCs to understand how cultural differences may influence a client's level of support and encouragement for lifestyle modification. It is not the norm in all cultures to exercise and eat healthy. This may provide unique challenges in program development and adherence. If an LWMC is working with clients from different cultural and racial backgrounds, it would be beneficial for the LWMC to seek out more specific information as needed. Many local and state health agencies will be able to provide specific information as it relates to race and health conditions, including obesity and diabetes.

It is an LWMC's responsibility to be sensitive and accommodating to all clients' cultural differences and needs. Therefore, the LWMC needs to be receptive to potential cultural differences by not making immediate assumptions regarding differences in communication styles. Once rapport has been established, the LWMC can talk to the client about cultural factors that are related to program participation. LWMCs should work with their clients to develop a lifestyle-modification program that is not only effective, but culturally sensitive as well.

Group Consulting

Much of the work of an LWMC will likely be done with clients on an individual basis. However, an LWMC may develop a business model that focuses on a group approach, which, if implemented properly, can maximize program adherence and enjoyment, as well as increase the number of clients with whom the LWMC is able to work.

The key to successfully implementing group programming is to be organized and efficient in communication and leadership. When working with a small group, there is no room to "fake it." If the LWMC does not have a plan before a group session begins, the clients will see the lack of preparedness and possibly doubt the LWMC's capability and credibility. Therefore, the first step in group consulting is preparation.

In creating group programming, it is important to remember that a group environment may not be the best option for all clients. Some people will need constant one-on-one supervision that is not available in a group setting. For example, if a new client has no previous experience with exercise or healthy eating or has low **self-efficacy,** he or she may do better by starting in a one-on-one situation. The LWMC should make this decision by gathering information in the initial consultation. Additionally, if a client is obviously not succeeding in a group environment, the LWMC should never hesitate to make a change to a one-on-one setting for that individual. On the other hand, some clients will benefit from the social interaction, support, and peer accountability that exists in group consulting. Clients will likely be apprehensive about working in a group, so the LWMC needs to be able to clearly explain the potential benefits of such participation, and then allow clients to decide if it is right for them.

Once an LWMC has created a group for a lifestyle-modification program, the group members must build rapport with one another and with the LWMC. It is important to provide time for the group members to get to know each other, as this will enable them to work together in a supportive environment. Additionally, the LWMC must clarify the expectations of the individual members and of the group as a whole. The group must take time to set effective goals and discuss strategies for goal attainment. The group, including the LWMC, must make a commitment to work together and hold each other accountable to the program. The LWMC should encourage group members to call each other for support and motivation. Additionally, it is a good idea to provide time for the group members to discuss their perceived challenges and barriers to program adherence and encourage them to support one another and help each other develop strategies for success. Each group should also have a set of norms for acceptable behaviors. These norms should be specified at the beginning of the program, and the expected behavior—along with the consequences for unacceptable behavior—should be clear to all members.

As the facilitator of the group programming, it is important for the LWMC to realize that the dynamic of each group will be unique, and that each group will have unique needs. The size of a group should be kept between four and eight people, allowing for optimal communication, cohesion, and trust (Widmeyer, Brawley, & Carron, 1990). It is the responsibility of the LWMC to be aware of problems that may emerge in groups. It is essential that the LWMC watches for breakdowns in communication, clashes of personalities, or a lack of support. Anytime LWMCs see accusations or assumptions being made about group members, they need to step in and attempt to rectify the situation. The most important thing that LWMCs can do when conflict arises is to communicate. As the leader, an LWMC must communicate with the group and create the environment and opportunity for the group members to communicate with one another. With clear communication, problems will work themselves out, either when the individuals come to an understanding of each other or agree that they will not be able to work together. In the latter instance, the LWMC must be flexible in making group changes as required. The entire group should not fall apart as a result of changing members.

If implemented properly, group consulting can be a rewarding and successful experience for all involved, including the LWMC. It creates an opportunity for people to share their challenges—and more importantly, their triumphs—in making behavioral changes.

Professional Responsibilities

LWMCs are in a position of trust and responsibility, not only with their clients, but also with their entire network of healthcare professionals. LWMCs' effectiveness will often be based on their ability to communicate and understand when a client's needs require attention that is beyond an LWMC's capabilities.

Scope of Practice

It is an LWMC's primary responsibility to clients and to the profession to act only within the defined **scope of practice** of an LWMC (see Chapter 19). Despite how clear scope-of-practice issues may seem in theory, they can quickly become somewhat blurred in practice. As a result of the rapport and trust an LWMC builds with his or her clients, clients will often come to the LWMC with medical, psychological, social, and nutritional concerns. In their minds, the LWMC seems qualified to answer all of their questions. However, it is critical that the LWMC maintain the proper scope of practice and not diagnose injuries or illnesses, prescribe injury treatments or diets, or attempt to deal with psychological disorders. LWMCs must be very careful with the advice they give and must not be afraid to say that they are not qualified to answer a question. LWMCs must never hesitate to ask for help, and if they have even the slightest doubt about their actions being within the scope of practice, they should ask for advice from other consultants or refer the client to a qualified professional. Additionally, it is an LWMC's responsibility to understand the legal issues in the state where he or she works (see Chapter 19). An LWMC must also understand and adhere to the ACE Code of Ethics (Appendix A).

Referral Networks

One way for LWMCs to ensure that they work within their scope of practice is to establish a network of qualified professionals in the community with whom they have regular contact (see Chapter 11). It is important to build relationships with physicians, registered dietitians, and mental-health practitioners. LWMCs should talk to these professionals about the lifestyle-modification programs they create for clients and discuss the need for these other healthcare professionals to be part of the team. If LWMCs establish professional relationships of trust and respect, they will feel more comfortable when referring clients to outside services.

Documentation Procedures

LWMCs will often work with a client's network of health professionals, which may include a physician and dietitian, among others. Therefore, it is critical, not only for the LWMC's records, but also in terms of communication with the team, that the LWMC consistently document all aspects of the client's participation. From the client's complaints of pain to the results of fitness testing, the client file should be kept updated and complete. **SOAP notes** provide an organized and professional way to record, store, and share this information with the healthcare team.

SOAP Notes

When an LWMC is working with a team of healthcare professionals, SOAP notes should be used to establish and maintain communication among everyone involved in caring for a client. SOAP notes are a systematic way to record progress, issues, and ailments related to program participation. SOAP notes are divided into four sections: subjective, objective, assessment, and plan.

Under the subjective section of the notes, LWMCs record any information that the client verbally provides regarding complaints, participation, symptoms, and feelings. This portion of the SOAP notes contains information about the client's perceptions and descriptions.

The next part of the SOAP notes is reserved for information gathered from objective observation techniques. In other words, anything that the LWMC can measure or see should be documented under the objective category. For example, the results of fitness testing and the client's weight are objective measures. In addition to the results of the objective measures, the date, time, and location of measurement should be documented.

The assessment portion of SOAP notes is an interpretation of both the subjective and objective observations. In other words, what do the tests show with regard to fitness, posture, strength, flexibility, weight, and blood pressure? LWMCs must be as clear and concise as possible in their assessment of clients, and if more than one interpretation exists, it is essential that LWMCs document each possible meaning. LWMCs must be careful not to make any medical diagnoses in the assessment section, as that is outside the scope of practice. Furthermore, when reviewing the subjective and objective measurement information, LWMCs should refer to appropriate healthcare professionals as necessary. The final component of SOAP notes is the client plan. Based on the information contained in the other sections of the notes, the best course of action should be documented in the plan section. From an exercise perspective, this should contain exercise type, frequency, duration, and intensity information. Refer to Chapter 11 for comprehensive coverage of the proper use of SOAP notes.

Records and Confidentiality

Effective LWMCs will keep a detailed file on each of their clients. In addition to their SOAP notes, which contain detailed program and personal information, several other documents should be kept in a client file, including a complete health history, release of liability, client goals, and possible payment or financial information. It is the LWMC's responsibility to be organized and professional with this information, which means that the LWMC is accountable for keeping it confidential. Clients should never be concerned about other people finding out anything about them, from their weight and the medications they take to their credit card numbers. Everything that takes place as part of the lifestyle-modification program must be kept private and confidential. Client files need to be kept in locked area (either an office or cabinet), and should never be left on a desk or in a public cabinet. If client information is stored in a personal computer, the LWMC should restrict access by using a protected password.

Also, information about client progress must be kept confidential. LWMCs must not discuss clients' program participation with other fitness professionals, friends, or family members. If someone is requesting information on a client, the LWMC must get written permission from the client before releasing anything to anyone, including their own family. If and when a client gives permission to release his or her information to an authorized individual or party, LWMCs must use secure methods of communication such as certified mail, a dedicated private fax line, or email with encryption.

Summary

The ultimate success of an LWMC is based on the ability to build and maintain trusting relationships. This is best done through consistent communication that is marked by active listening and honest self-expression. These skills should always be practiced and never assumed to be perfect. The more an LWMC is able to understand the needs and feelings of the client, the better he or she will be at creating supportive programs that maximize lifestyle-modification adherence and success.

References

Egan, B. (1994). *The Skilled Helper: A Problem Management Approach to Helping* (5th ed.). Pacific Grove, Calif.: Brooks/Cole.

Kreuter, M.W. & Wray, R.J. (2003). Tailored and targeted health communication: Strategies for enhancing information relevance. *American Journal of Health Behavior,* 27, S227–S232.

Lazarus, A.A. (1973). On assertive behavior: A brief note. *Behavior Therapy,* 4, 697–699.

Orlick, T. (1986). *Psyching for Sport.* Champaign, Ill.: Human Kinetics.

Widmeyer, W.N., Brawley, L.R., & Carron, A.V. (1990). The effects of group size in sport. *Journal of Exercise and Sport Psychology,* 12, 177–190.

Yukelson, D.P. (2005). Communicating effectively. In: J.M. Williams (Ed.). *Applied Sport Psychology: Personal Growth to Peak Performance.* Mountain View, Calif.: Mayfield Publishing Company.

Suggested Reading

Carron, A.V. & Hausenblas, H.A. (2005). *Group Dynamics in Sport* (3rd ed.). Morgantown, W.V.: Fitness Information Technology.

Malouf, D. (2000). *Power Up Your People Skills: Communication in the New Millennium.* Australia: Australian Print Group.

Okun, B.F. (2007). *Effective Helping: Interviewing and Counseling Techniques* (7th ed.). Belmont, Calif.: Wadsworth Publishing Company.

Part III

Nutritional Science

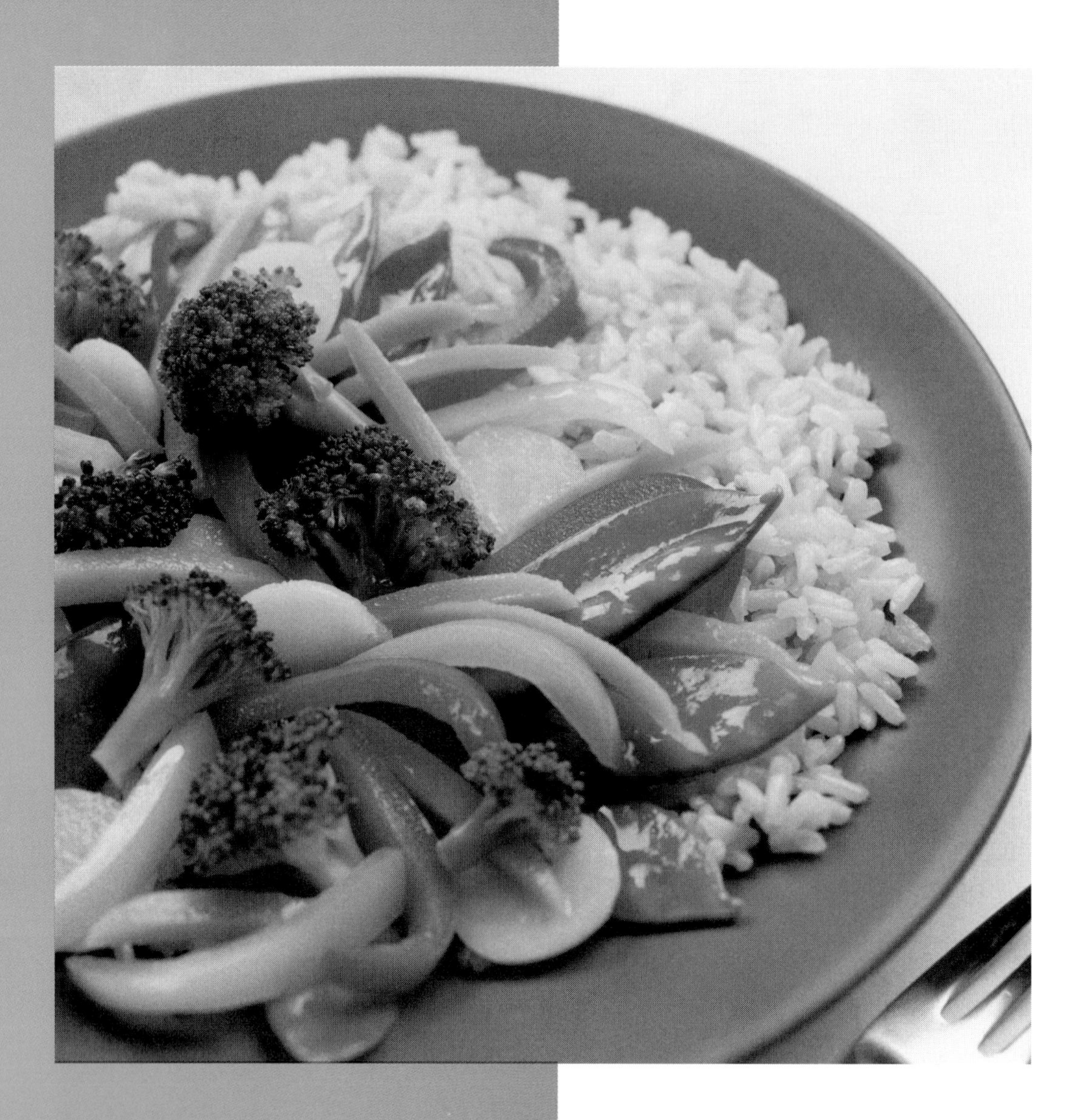

Natalie Digate Muth

Natalie Digate Muth, M.P.H., R.D., is currently pursuing a medical doctor degree at the University of North Carolina at Chapel Hill. In addition to being a registered dietitian, she is an ACE-certified Personal Trainer and Group Fitness Instructor, an American College of Sports Medicine Health and Fitness Instructor, and a National Strength and Conditioning Association Certified Strength and Conditioning Specialist. She is also an ACE Master Trainer and a freelance nutrition and fitness author.

Karen Friedman-Kester

Karen Friedman-Kester, M.S., R.D., L.D.N., is an instructor of nutrition at Harrisburg Area Community College. She is the author of several books and magazine articles on food, food safety, and nutrition. She has appeared on regional and national radio and television. She also lectures on various nutrition topics across the country.

Chapter 6

Basic Nutrition and Digestion

IN THIS CHAPTER:

Most clients will know that eating a healthful diet is good for their bodies. What they may not understand is why certain foods are considered healthier than others, such as why **protein** helps build muscle or why **carbohydrate** is the best energy source for endurance training. While Lifestyle & Weight Management Consultants (LWMCs) should focus on practical recommendations and suggestions when counseling and educating their clients, they should understand basic nutrition, **digestion,** and **absorption.** After acquiring this knowledge, LWMCs can better explain recommendations; provide clear answers to clients' questions; and have a knowledge base when they attend continuing-education classes, read about scientific findings in relevant articles, and communicate with their colleagues. From a discussion of macro- and **micronutrient** structure and function to the processes of **nutrient** digestion and absorption, this chapter provides a foundation of knowledge in nutritional sciences, an exciting scientific field that encompasses biology, chemistry, biochemistry, physiology, and psychology.

A few concepts and definitions will serve LWMCs well as they guide their clients in making healthful nutritional choices. It is important to know the role of various nutrients that are essential for optimal functioning. While everyone needs these nutrients, people require varying amounts depending on gender, age, activity level, health status, and other factors. The federal government has taken these issues into consideration when developing recommended intakes. The 2005 Dietary Guidelines (www.health.gov/dietaryguidelines) and MyPyramid Food Guidance System (www.mypyramid.gov) provide individualized nutrition recommendations for a healthy diet (see Chapter 7).

The description of reference values for optimal intake of various nutrients has been revamped over the years. In the past, **Recommended Dietary Allowances (RDAs)** were published for the different nutrients based on age and gender. The RDAs were defined as "the levels of intake of essential nutrients that, on the basis of scientific knowledge, are judged by the Food and Nutrition Board to be adequate to meet the known needs of practically all healthy persons." Current reference values, known as **Dietary Reference Intakes (DRIs)** are more descriptive. DRI is a generic term used to refer to three types of reference values: RDA; **Estimated Average Requirement (EAR),** an adequate intake in 50% of an age- and gender-specific group; and **Tolerable Upper Intake Level (UL),** which is the maximum intake that is unlikely to pose risk of adverse health effects to almost all individuals in an age- and gender-specific group. **Adequate Intake,** which is used when an RDA cannot be based on an EAR, is a recommended nutrient intake level that, based on research, appears to be sufficient for good health.

DRIs have been established for calcium, vitamin D, phosphorus, magnesium, and fluoride; folate and other B vitamins; **antioxidants** (vitamins C and E and selenium); **macronutrients** (protein, carbohydrate, and **fat**); trace elements (vitamins A and K, iron, and zinc); and **electrolytes** and water. The complete set of DRIs is available through the Institutes of Medicine (www.iom.edu).

Macronutrient Structure and Function

Food is composed of some combination of three macronutrients: carbohydrate, protein, and fat. The term macronutrient simply means that the nutrient is needed in large quantities for normal growth and development. Macronutrients are the body's source of **calories,** or energy to fuel life. The sun is the initial energy supply for all living organisms, though only green plants are able to directly take the energy from the sun and convert it into chemical energy through a process known as **photosynthesis.** This chemical energy is stored by linking carbon dioxide to hydrogen and other carbons. Carbohydrates are the first macronutrient formed through this process. The carbohydrates are then used as an energy source for the plant, and also as a precursor to make protein and fat.

Carbohydrates

Carbohydrates contain approximately four calories per gram and are the body's preferred energy source. Plants produce a variety of types of carbohydrates, which vary in sweetness, texture, rate and ease of digestion, and degree of absorption. These varying properties are partially determined by the type of carbohydrate—**monosaccharide, disaccharide, oligosaccharide,** or **polysaccharide.** A monosaccharide is the simplest form of sugar and cannot be broken down any further. Monosaccharides are rarely found free in nature. Instead, they are usually found joined together as di-, oligo-, or polysaccharides. Three monosaccharides found in nature can be absorbed and utilized by humans—**glucose, fructose,** and **galactose.** Glucose is the predominant sugar in nature and the basic building block of most other carbohydrates (Figure 6-1). Fructose, or fruit sugar, is the sweetest of the monosaccharides and is found in varying levels in different types of fruits. Galactose joins with glucose to form the disaccharide **lactose,** the principal sugar found in milk. (**Lactose intolerance** results from a deficiency in the **enzyme** lactase, which is necessary to break the bond between the glucose and galactose molecules so that they can be digested.) Other disaccharides include **maltose,** which is two glucose molecules bound together, and **sucrose** (table sugar), which is formed by glucose and fructose.

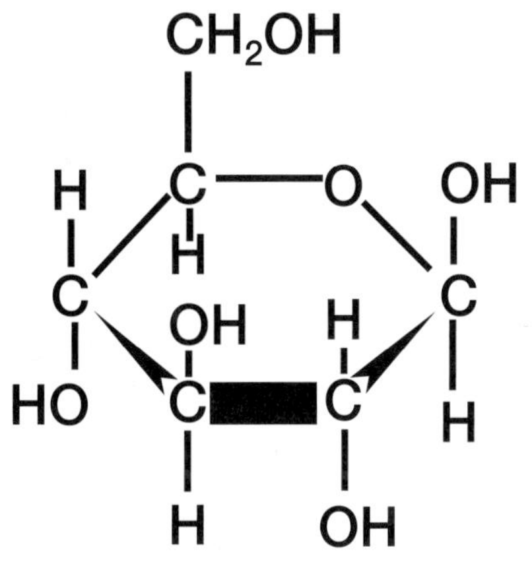

Figure 6-1
Glucose structure

Most caloric sweeteners are disaccharides. Raw sugar, granulated sugar, brown sugar, powdered sugar, and turbinado sugar (Sugar in the Raw®) all are sucrose. Honey is a natural form of sucrose that is made from plant nectar and harvested by honeybees, which secrete an enzyme that hydrolyzes sucrose to glucose and fructose. Corn sweeteners, such as the corn syrup commonly found in sodas, baked goods, and some canned products, are a liquid combination of maltose, glucose, and dextrose. Sorbitol, which is used in many diet products, is produced from glucose and found naturally in some berries and fruits. It is absorbed by the body at a slower rate than sugar. Noncaloric sweeteners—which are calorie-free because the body cannot metabolize them—also are used to add sweet taste to foods and beverages. Aspartame, also known as Equal® in packaged sweetener and NutraSweet® in foods and beverages; Acesulfame K, which is called Sunett® in cooking products and Sweet One® as a tabletop sweetener; saccharin; sucralose (Splenda®); and neotame all are approved for use in the United States. While early studies found that certain sweeteners may cause bladder cancer in laboratory rats, subsequent studies have found no association in humans.

An oligosaccharide is a chain of approximately three to 10 simple sugars. **Fructooligosaccharides,** a category of oligosaccharides that are mostly indigestible, may help relieve constipation, improve triglyceride levels, and decrease production of foul-smelling digestive by-products.

A long chain of sugar molecules is referred to as a polysaccharide. **Glycogen,** an animal carbohydrate found in meat products and seafood, and **starch,** a plant carbohydrate found in grains and vegetables, are the only polysaccharides that humans can fully digest. Both are long chains of glucose and are referred to as **complex carbohydrates** (vs. **simple carbohydrates,** which are short chains of sugar). Animals store excess carbohydrates as glycogen. Although glycogen can be found in animal products, most glycogen stores are depleted before meat enters the food supply. Therefore, while humans do not consume large amounts of glycogen, excess carbohydrates from starch or other sugars are stored in the human liver and muscles as glycogen. Because glycogen contains many water molecules, it is large and bulky, and therefore unsuitable for long-term energy storage. Approximately 90 grams of glycogen is stored in the liver. About 150 grams of glycogen is stored in muscle, though this amount can be increased five-fold with physical training (Mahan & Escott-Stump, 2007). Carbohydrate loading also increases glycogen stores.

Historically, much debate has centered on whether consumption of simple or complex carbohydrates is better for athletic performance. It seems as though the role of a particular carbohydrate in athletic performance may be better determined by its **glycemic index,** a measure of the rise in blood glucose following consumption, rather than its structure. Research suggests that a diet based on consumption of high-glycemic carbohydrates promotes greater glycogen storage following strenuous exercise (Jentjens & Jeukendrup, 2003). For a more complete discussion of the glycemic index, refer to Chapter 8.

Plants store carbohydrates as starch granules. Edible plants make two types of starch: amylase (a small, linear molecule) and the more prevalent amylopectin (a larger, highly branched molecule). Because starches are longer than disaccharides and oligosaccharides, they take longer to digest. Still, humans are able to easily break down and digest starches with specific self-produced enzymes. However, the rest of the plant, which is formed largely of the carbohydrate **cellulose** and other fibers such as **hemicellulose, lignin**, gums, and **pectin,** is indigestible. These fibers pass through the human body undigested, as humans do not produce the necessary enzymes to break the sugar bonds. Because no chemical bonds are broken, no energy is released, and therefore **fiber** does not contain calories.

Fiber is classified as either soluble or insoluble. **Soluble fiber** forms gels in water. It helps prevent heart disease and stroke by binding bile and cholesterol; diabetes by slowing glucose absorption; and constipation by holding moisture in stools and softening them [American Dietetic Association (ADA), 2002]. Soluble fibers include gums found in foods such as oats, legumes, guar, and barley, as well as pectin found in foods like apples, citrus fruits, strawberries, and carrots. **Insoluble fiber** comprises the structural part of the plant. It reduces constipation and lowers the risk of hemorrhoids and diverticulosis by adding bulk to the feces and reducing transit time in the colon (ADA, 2002). Other insoluble fibers include cellulose found in whole-wheat flour, bran, and vegetables; hemicellulose found in whole grains and bran; and lignin found in mature vegetables, wheat, and fruits with edible seeds (like strawberries). Increased consumption of insoluble fiber helps to increase **satiety,** and the feeling of fullness may lead to decreased caloric intake (ADA, 2002). As a result, a diet high in insoluble fiber may promote weight loss.

Fats and Lipids

The most energy-dense of the macronutrients, fat provides nine calories per gram, which is 225% more calories than both carbohydrate and protein (four calories per gram). Because of this high caloric value, foods that are high in fat should be consumed in moderation if weight control is the goal, but they should not be avoided altogether. Research suggests that certain types of fat, namely mono- and polyunsaturated fats, are heart-healthy (though still calorie-dense) (Hu & Willett, 2002; Zarraga & Schwarz, 2006). In addition, fats serve many critical functions in the human body, including insulation, cell structure, nerve transmission, vitamin absorption, and hormone production. But some fats—notably saturated fats and **trans fats**—also lead to clogging of the arteries, increased risk for heart disease, and myriad other problems. Consumption of these fats should be avoided or strictly limited.

To understand how various fats function in the human body, first consider their structure. All fats are made up of hydrogen, carbon, and oxygen, and all fats are insoluble in water. Beyond that, they are a very heterogeneous group of molecules. Figure 6-2 presents a pictorial representation of various physiologically important fats and lipids.

Fatty acids, which are usually found linked to other molecules in nature, are long hydrocarbon chains with an even number of carbons and varying degrees of saturation with hydrogen. **Saturated fatty acids** contain no double bonds between carbon atoms, are typically solid at room temperature, and are very stable. Foods high in saturated fat include red meat, full-fat dairy products, and tropical oils such as coconut and palm oil. Saturated fat increases levels of **low-density lipoprotein (LDL),** which is sometimes called the "bad" cholesterol.

Unsaturated fatty acids contain one or more double bonds between carbon atoms, are typically liquid at room temperature, and are fairly unstable, which makes them susceptible to oxidative damage and a shortened shelf life. Monounsaturated fats contain one double

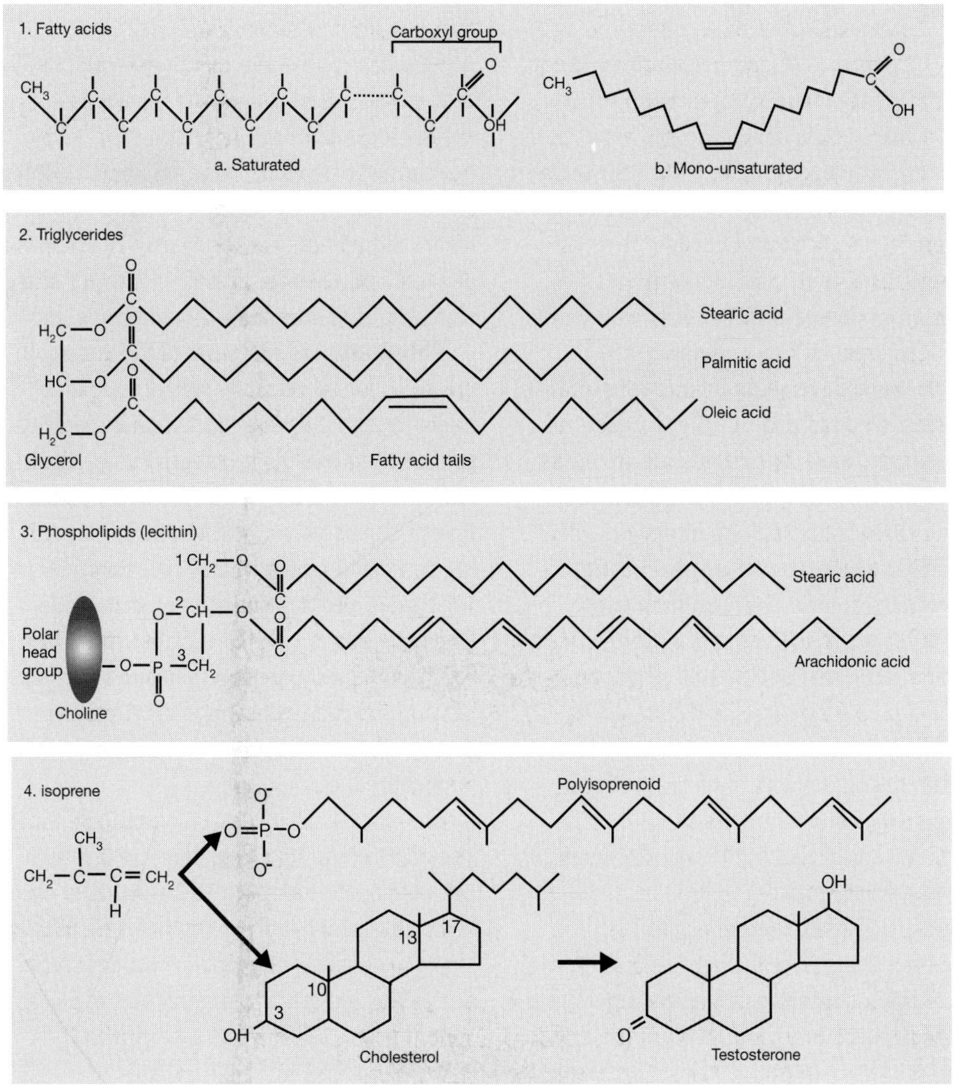

Figure 6-2
Structures of physiologically important fats and lipids

Source: Reprinted with permission from Mahan, L.K. & Escott-Stump, S. (2007). *Krause's Food Nutrition and Diet Therapy* (12th ed.). Philadelphia: W.B. Saunders Company.

bond between two carbons and increased levels of **high-density lipoprotein (HDL),** which is sometimes called the "good cholesterol." Common sources include olive, canola, and peanut oils. Polyunsaturated fat contains a double bond between two or more sets of carbons. Sources include corn, safflower, and soybean oils, and cold-water fish. **Essential fatty acids** are polyunsaturated fats that must be obtained from the diet. Unlike other fats, the body cannot produce **omega-3 fatty acids** or **omega-6 fatty acids,** which are also called **linolenic acid** and **linoleic acid,** respectively. Omega-3 is an essential fatty acid found in egg yolk and cold-water fish, including tuna, salmon, mackerel, and cod, as well as in crabs, shrimp, and oysters. These fatty acids promote a healthy immune system and help protect against heart disease and other diseases. Americans tend not to get enough omega-3 fatty acids. On the other hand, omega-6 fatty acids, which are found in flax seed, canola, and soybean oils and green leaves, are generally consumed in abundance. Polyunsaturated fats decrease total cholesterol, LDL cholesterol, and HDL cholesterol.

Both types of essential fatty acids are used to make **eicosanoids,** which are oxygenated fatty acids that the body uses to signal cellular responses. Eicosanoids made from omega-6 fatty acids tend to cause inflammation and increase blood pressure and blood clotting.

Eicosanoids made from omega-3 fatty acids have the opposite effect: They reduce blood clotting, dilate blood vessels, and reduce inflammation. This balancing act between omega-6 and omega-3 is essential for maintaining normal circulation and other important processes. Reducing consumption of omega-6 fatty acids and increasing consumption of omega-3 fatty acids may lower chronic disease risk (Simopoulos, 1999), though research remains inconclusive. Table 6-1 offers a comparison of dietary fats.

In nature, most fatty acids are found as part of triglycerides, which are formed by joining three fatty acids to a glycerol (carbon and hydrogen structure) backbone. Triglycerides are the chemical form in which most fat exists in food as well as in the body.

Trans fat, listed as "partially hydrogenated" oil on a food ingredient list, results from a manufacturing process that makes unsaturated fat solid at room temperature with a goal of prolonging its shelf life. The process involves breaking the double bond of the unsaturated fat. The product is a heart-damaging fat that increases LDL cholesterol even more than saturated fat. Legislation requiring food manufacturers to include the amount of trans fat on the nutrition label if it is more than 0.5 grams per serving has resulted in many processed foods that were once high in trans fat, such as chips, crackers, cakes, peanut butter, and margarine to be made "trans-fat free." LWMCs should advise their clients to look on the label's ingredients list for "partially hydrogenated" oil to determine if a food contains trans fat. If so, the food should be avoided.

Phospholipids such as lecithin and sphingomyelin are structurally similar to triglycerides, but the glycerol backbone is modified, so that the molecule is water-soluble at one end and water-insoluble at the other end. Phospholipids play a critical role in maintaining cell-membrane structure and function. Lecithin is also a major component of HDL, which functions to remove cholesterol from cell membranes. Common food sources of lecithin include liver, egg yolks, soybeans, peanuts, legumes, spinach, wheat germ, and animal products.

Cholesterol, a fat-like, waxy, rigid four-ring steroid structure, plays an important role in cell-membrane function. It also helps to make bile acids (which are important for fat absorption), metabolize fat-soluble vitamins (A, D, E, and K), and make vitamin D and some steroid hormones, such as estrogen and

Table 6-1
A Comparison of Dietary Fats

	Type	Dietary Fat	Dietary Cholesterol (mg/Tbsp)	% Saturated Fat	% Polyunsaturated Fat	% Monounsaturated Fat
Vegetable Fats	M	Canola oil	0	6	32	62
	P	Safflower oil	0	10	77	13
	P	Sunflower oil	0	11	69	20
	P	Corn oil	0	13	62	25
	M	Olive oil	0	14	9	77
	P	Soybean oil	0	15	61	24
	M	Peanut oil	0	18	33	49
Animal Fats	S	Chicken fat	11	31	22	47
	S	Lard	12	41	12	47
	S	Beef fat	14	52	4	44
	S	Butter	33	66	4	30

Note: M = Monounsaturated fat P = Polyunsaturated fat S = Saturated fat

Source: U.S Department of Agriculture

testosterone. Saturated fat, once it is converted to cholesterol in the liver, is the main dietary cause of **hypercholesterolemia** (i.e., high blood levels of cholesterol), though high levels of cholesterol are also found in animal products such as egg yolks, meat, poultry, fish, and dairy products.

Too much cholesterol in the bloodstream causes problems. For cholesterol to get from the liver to the body's cells (in the case of endogenously produced cholesterol), or from the **small intestine** to the liver and adipose tissue (in the case of exogenously consumed cholesterol) it must be transported through the bloodstream. Because it is fat-soluble, it needs a water-soluble carrier protein to transport it. When the cholesterol combines with this protein en route to the body's cells, it is an LDL and therefore susceptible to attaching to inner linings or walls of arteries, where it forms a plaque and ultimately causes **atherosclerosis.** HDLs remove excess cholesterol from the arteries and carry it back to the liver, where it is excreted.

Proteins

Proteins contain four calories per gram and are the building blocks of human and animal structure. Proteins serve innumerable functions in the human body, including the following:

- Formation of the brain, nervous system, blood, muscle, skin, and hair
- Transportation of iron, **vitamins, minerals,** fats, and oxygen
- Maintenance of acid–base and fluid balance

Proteins form enzymes, which can speed up chemical reactions to milliseconds that might otherwise take years. Antibodies that the body makes to fight infection are made from proteins. Finally, during periods of energy deprivation, the body can break down proteins for energy.

Proteins are built from **amino acids,** which are carbohydrates with an attached nitrogen-containing amino group and, in some cases, sulfur. Proteins form when amino acids are joined together through peptide bonds. The completed protein is a linear chain of amino acids. Attractions between different amino acids then create what are known as helices and pleated structures. These structures fold, creating a unique three-dimensional **polypeptide.** Individual polypeptides may remain free-standing or may bind together to form a larger complex. Figure 6-3 illustrates the peptide bond and folding protein.

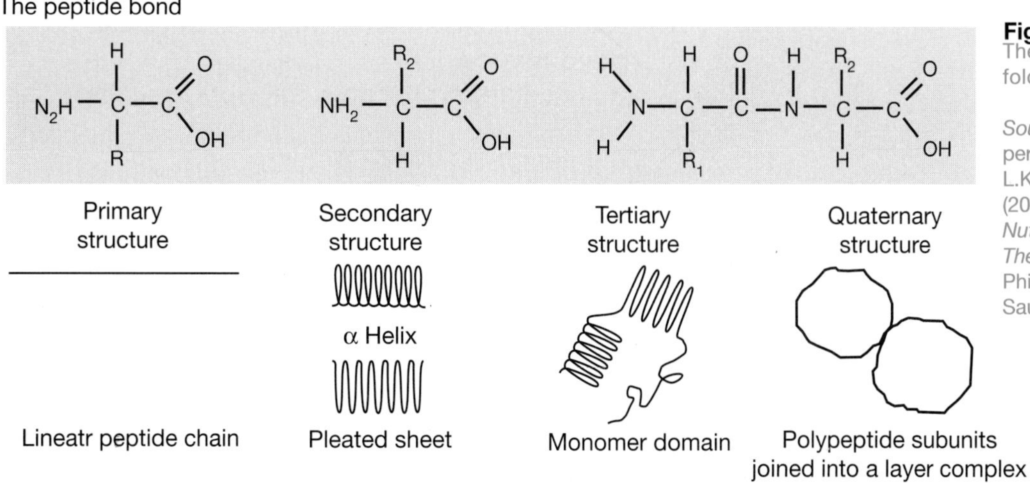

Figure 6-3
The peptide bond and folding protein

Source: Reprinted with permission from Mahan, L.K. & Escott-Stump, S. (2007). *Krause's Food Nutrition and Diet Therapy* (12th ed.). Philadelphia: W.B. Saunders Company.

Many of the 20 amino acids that bind together to form proteins can be made in the body, and therefore are called nonessential amino acids. Of the 20 amino acids, all but eight to 10 can be manufactured by the body. Those the body cannot make are called **essential amino acids** and must be consumed in the diet. Because humans have carbon skeletons, they cannot manufacture the essential amino acids. Generally, protein-containing animal products contain all of the essential amino acids, which is why they are called **complete proteins.** Proteins in plant foods usually do not contain all of the essential amino acids, making them **incomplete proteins.** One notable exception is soy, a plant-based complete protein. When combined, incomplete plant proteins (such as rice and beans) can together provide all of the essential amino acids through a process called **protein complementarity** (see Figure 7-3, page 177).

Micronutrient Structure and Function

Micronutrients, by definition, are only needed in small amounts. The World Health Organization (WHO) refers to these nutrients as the "'magic wands' that enable the body to produce enzymes, hormones, and other substances that are essential for proper growth and development" (WHO, 2007). When the body is deprived of micronutrients, the consequences are severe. But when the micronutrients are consumed in just the right amounts, they lead to optimal health and function.

Water

When people think of nutrition, they often forget to think about water. Although it provides no calories and is **inorganic** in nature, it is as important as oxygen. Loss of only 20% of total body water could cause death. A 10% loss causes severe disorders (Figure 6-4). In

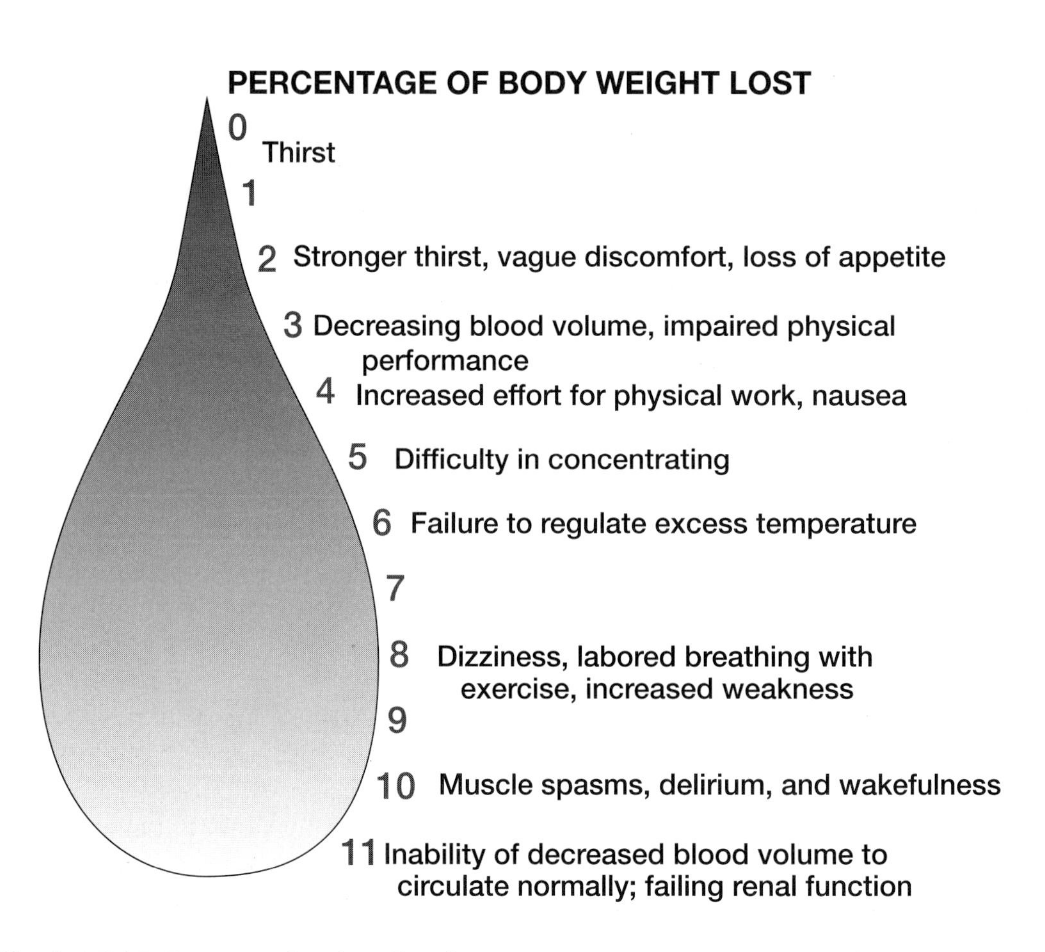

Figure 6-4
Adverse effects of dehydration

Source: Reprinted with permission from Mahan, L.K. & Escott-Stump, S. (2007). *Krause's Food Nutrition and Diet Therapy* (12th ed.). Philadelphia: W.B. Saunders Company.

general, adults can survive up to 10 days without water, while children can survive for up to five days (Mahan & Escott-Stump, 2007). But why is water so necessary?

Water is the single largest component of the human body, making up approximately 50 to 70% of body weight. In other words, about 85 to 119 pounds (39 to 54 kg) of a 170-pound (77-kg) man is water weight. Physiologically, water has many important functions, including regulating body temperature, protecting vital organs, providing a driving force for nutrient absorption, serving as a medium for all biochemical reactions, and maintaining a high blood volume for optimal athletic performance. In fact, total body weight is higher in athletes compared to nonathletes, and tends to decrease with age due to diminishing muscle mass.

Water volume can be influenced by a variety of factors, such as food and drink intake; sweat, urine, and feces excretion; metabolic production of small amounts of water; and losses of water that occur with breathing. These factors play an especially important role during exercise, as metabolism is increased. The generated body heat is released through sweat, which is a solution of water, sodium, and other electrolytes.

If fluid intake is not increased to replenish the lost fluid, the body attempts to compensate by retaining more water and excreting more concentrated urine. Under these conditions, the person is said to be dehydrated. Severe **dehydration** can lead to heat stroke. On the other hand, if people ingest excessive amounts of fluid to compensate for minimal amounts of water lost in sweat, they may become overloaded with fluid, a condition called **hyponatremia.** When the blood's water-to-sodium ratio is severely elevated, excess water can leak into brain tissue, leading to **encephalopathy,** or brain swelling.

Fortunately, the human body is well-equipped to withstand dramatic variations in fluid intake during exercise and at rest with little or no detrimental health effects. Most recreational exercisers will never suffer from serious hyponatremia or dehydration.

Common wisdom calls for drinking approximately 64 ounces (eight glasses) of water per day, and to "stay ahead of thirst" while exercising. The latest recommendations are to follow individualized hydration regimens and let thirst be the guide—if thirsty, drink water [Von Duvillard et al., 2004; American College of Sports Medicine (ACSM), 2007]. Exceptions include infants, vigorously exercising athletes, hospitalized patients, and the sick and elderly, who may have diminished thirst sensation. Because these individuals have higher water needs, they should be closely monitored and encouraged to drink more.

Do not follow

Vitamins

Vitamins are **organic,** noncaloric micronutrients that are essential for normal physiological function. Vitamins must be consumed through foods, with only three exceptions: vitamin K and biotin, which can be produced by normal intestinal flora (bacteria that live in the intestines and are critical for normal gastrointestinal function), and vitamin D, which can be self-produced with sun exposure. No "perfect" food contains all the vitamins in just the right amount. Instead, a variety of nutrient-dense foods must be consumed to ensure adequate vitamin intakes. Many foods (such as breads and cereals) have been fortified with some nutrients to cut the risk of vitamin deficiency. And some foods contain inactive vitamins, which are called **provitamins.** Fortunately, the human body contains enzymes to convert these inactive vitamins into active vitamins.

Humans need 13 different vitamins, which are divided into two categories: water-soluble vitamins (the B vitamins and vitamin C) and fat-soluble vitamins (vitamins A, D, E, and K). Choline—called a "quasi-vitamin" because it can be produced in the body, but also provides additional benefits through consumption of foods—plays a crucial role in neurotransmitter and platelet functions, and may help prevent Alzheimer's disease (McDaniel, Maier, & Einstein, 2003). Table 6-2 presents the vitamin DRIs.

Table 6-2
Vitamin Facts

Vitamin	RDA/AI* Men[†]	RDA/AI* Women[†]	Best Sources	Functions
A (carotene)	**900 µg**	**700 µg**	Yellow or orange fruits and vegetables, green leafy vegetables, fortified oatmeal, liver, dairy products	Formation and maintenance of skin, hair, and mucous membranes; helps people see in dim light; bone and tooth growth
B1 (thiamine)	**1.2 mg**	**1.1 mg**	Fortified cereals and oatmeals, meats, rice and pasta, whole grains, liver	Helps the body release energy from carbohydrates during metabolism; growth and muscle tone
B2 (riboflavin)	**1.3 mg**	**1.1 mg**	Whole grains, green leafy vegetables, organ meats, milk, eggs	Helps the body release energy from protein, fat, and carbohydrates during metabolism
B6 (pyridoxine)	**1.3 mg**	**1.3 mg**	Fish, poultry, lean meats, bananas, prunes, dried beans, whole grains, avocados	Helps build body tissue and aids in metabolism of protein
B12 (cobalamin)	**2.4 µg**	**2.4 µg**	Meats, milk products, seafood	Aids cell development, functioning of the nervous system, and the metabolism of protein and fat
Biotin	30 µg	30 µg	Cereal/grain products, yeast, legumes, liver	Involved in metabolism of protein, fats, and carbohydrates
Choline	550 mg	425 mg	Milk, liver, eggs, peanuts	A precursor of acetylcholine; essential for liver function
Folate (folacin, folic acid)	**400 µg**	**400 µg**[‡]	Green leafy vegetables, organ meats, dried peas, beans, lentils	Aids in genetic material development; involved in red blood cell production
Niacin	**16 mg**	**14 mg**	Meat, poultry, fish, enriched cereals, peanuts, potatoes, dairy products, eggs	Involved in carbohydrate, protein, and fat metabolism
Pantothenic Acid	5 mg	5 mg	Lean meats, whole grains, legumes	Helps release energy from fats and vegetables
C (ascorbic acid)	**90 mg**	**75 mg**	Citrus fruits, berries, and vegetables—especially peppers	Essential for structure of bones, cartilage, muscle, and blood vessels; helps maintain capillaries and gums and aids in absorption of iron
D	5 µg	5 µg	Fortified milk, sunlight, fish, eggs, butter, fortified margarine	Aids in bone and tooth formation; helps maintain heart action and nervous system function
E	**15 mg**	**15 mg**	Fortified and multigrain cereals, nuts, wheat germ, vegetable oils, green leafy vegetables	Protects blood cells, body tissue, and essential fatty acids from harmful destruction in the body
K	120 µg	90 µg	Green leafy vegetables, fruit, dairy, grain products	Essential for blood-clotting functions

* Recommended Dietary Allowances are presented in bold type; Adequate Intakes are presented in non-bolded type.

[†] RDAs and AIs given are for men aged 31–50 and nonpregnant, nonbreastfeeding women aged 31–50; mg = milligrams; µg = micrograms

[‡] This is the amount women of childbearing age should obtain from supplements or fortified foods.

Water-soluble Vitamins

Thiamin, riboflavin, niacin, pantothenic acid, folate, vitamin B6, vitamin B12, biotin, and vitamin C are referred to as the water-soluble vitamins. Their solubility in water (which gives them similar absorption and distribution in the body) and their role as **cofactors** of enzymes involved in metabolism (i.e., without them, the enzyme will not work) are common traits. With the exception of vitamins B6 and B12, water-soluble vitamins cannot be stored in the body and are readily excreted in urine. This decreases the risk of toxicity from overconsumption and makes their regular intake a necessity.

Certain B vitamins—thiamin (vitamin B1), riboflavin (vitamin B2), niacin (vitamin B3), and pantothenic acid (vitamin B5)—are cofactors in energy metabolism. In other words, these vitamins are necessary to unlock the energy in food.

Thiamin

Thiamin is essential for carbohydrate metabolism. It also is thought to play a nonmetabolic role in nerve function. Thiamine deficiency is characterized by **anorexia,** weight loss, and cardiac and neurologic manifestations that progress to beriberi—a constellation of symptoms that includes mental confusion, muscular wasting, swelling, decreased sensation in the feet and hands, a fast heart rate, and an enlarged heart. Thiamin deficiency is rare in the U.S. because of supplementation in rice and cereal products. Deficiency occasionally manifests in alcoholics, who are often malnourished and have impaired absorption of the nutrient.

Riboflavin

Riboflavin assists in carbohydrate, amino-acid, and lipid metabolism. It also helps with antioxidant protection through its role in reduction-oxidation (redox) reactions. Consumption of meat, dairy products, and green leafy vegetables helps prevent riboflavin deficiency, which causes eye problems, including photophobia, excessive tearing, burning and itching, and loss of vision, as well as soreness and burning of the mouth, tongue, and lips.

Niacin

Niacin acts as a cofactor for more than 200 enzymes involved in carbohydrate, amino-acid, and fatty-acid metabolism. Lean meats, poultry, fish, peanuts, and yeast contain ample amounts of niacin. Muscular weakness, anorexia, indigestion, and skin abnormalities are early signs of niacin deficiency and can cause the disease pellagra, which is characterized by the "three Ds": dermatitis (eczema), dementia, and diarrhea.

Pantothenic Acid

Panthothenic acid, which is present in all plant and animal tissues, forms an integral component of coenzyme A and acyl-carrier protein. These proteins are essential for metabolism of fatty acids, amino acids, and carbohydrates, as well as for normal protein function. Because this vitamin is ubiquitous, deficiency is rare.

Vitamin B6

Vitamin B6 (pyridoxine) plays an important role in many bodily functions, including protein metabolism, red blood cell production, glycogenolysis (in which glycogen is broken down to glucose), conversion of the protein tryptophan to niacin, neurotransmitter formation, and immune-system function. Meats, whole-grain products, vegetables, and nuts contain high concentrations of vitamin B6, though **bioavailability** of the nutrient is highest in animal products. Deficiency leads to decreased neurologic and dermatologic function and weakened immunity.

Folate

Folate (vitamin B9; also known as folic acid in its supplement form) is named for its abundance in plant foliage (like green leafy vegetables). Folate plays a crucial role in the production of **deoxyribonucleic acid (DNA),** formation of red and white blood cells, formation of neurotransmitters, and metabolism of amino acids. Deficiency is relatively common, as folate is easily lost during cooking and food preparation, and also because most people do not eat enough green leafy vegetables. Folate deficiency early in pregnancy can be devastating for a developing fetus and can lead to neural tube defects such as spina bifida. For this reason, all women of childbearing age are advised to take a daily folate supplement. Deficiency also causes megaloblastic anemia, skins lesions, and poor growth. Notably, excessive consumption of folate can mask a vitamin B12 deficiency.

Vitamin B12

Vitamin B12 (cobalamin) is important for the normal function of cells of the **gastrointestinal tract,** bone marrow, and nervous tissue. The richest sources of vitamin B12 include clams and oysters, milk, eggs, cheese, muscle meats, fish, liver, and kidney. Long-time **vegans** are at risk for deficiency, as are the elderly, who tend to have a decreased ability to absorb the nutrient. Deficiency leads to megaloblastic anemia and neurologic dysfunction, in which neurons become demyelinated. This causes numbness, tingling, and burning of the feet, as well as stiffness and generalized weakness of the legs.

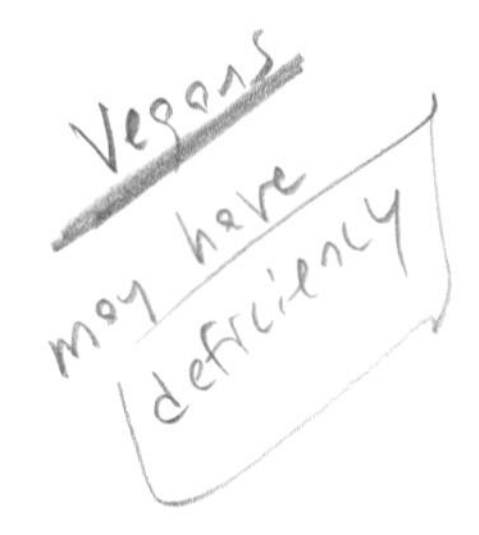

Biotin

Biotin (vitamin B7) is the ultimate "helper vitamin." Typically bound to protein, it carries around a carboxyl (-COOH) group. It then lends this carboxyl group to any of four different enzymes that are important in various metabolic functions. Ultimately, biotin plays an important role in the metabolic functions of pantothenic acid, folic acid, and vitamin B12. The most important sources of biotin include milk, liver, egg yolk, and a few vegetables. Deficiency is uncommon.

Vitamin C

Vitamin C plays an important role as an antioxidant. Deficiency can result in scurvy (a deficiency disease that can cause dark purplish spots on the skin and spongy or bleeding gums). Vitamin C is also necessary to make collagen, a fibrous protein that is part of skin, bone, teeth, ligaments, and other connective structures. Vitamin C improves iron absorption, promotes resistance to infection, and helps with steroid, neurotransmitter, and hormone production. Citrus fruits and green leafy vegetables are excellent sources of vitamin C. Signs of deficiency include impaired wound healing, swelling, bleeding, and weakness in bones, cartilage, teeth, and connective tissues.

Fat-soluble Vitamins

Vitamins A, D, E, and K are the fat-soluble vitamins and are often found in fat-containing foods. They are stored in the liver or adipose tissue until needed, and therefore are closely associated with fat. If fat absorption is impaired, so is fat-soluble-vitamin absorption. Unlike water-soluble vitamins, fat-soluble vitamins can be stored in the body for extended periods of time and eventually are excreted in feces. This storage capacity increases the risk of toxicity from overconsumption, but also decreases the risk of deficiency.

Vitamin A

Vitamin A and its provitamin beta-carotene are important for vision, growth, and development; the development and maintenance of epithelial tissue, including bones and teeth; immune function; and reproduction. Animal products, including liver, milk, and eggs, are rich in preformed vitamin A. Dark green leafy vegetables, and yellow-orange vegetables and fruit contain lots of provitamin A carotenoids. (A good rule of thumb: The deeper the color, the higher the level of carotenoids.) Deficiency of vitamin A is the most common cause of blindness in the developing world. It begins with night blindness and progresses to poor growth and increased susceptibility to infection. Excess consumption, which overwhelms the capacity of the liver to store the vitamin (generally resulting from supplement misuse), leads to dryness and cracking of the skin and mucous membranes, headache, nausea and vomiting, and liver disease. Intake of more than 20,000 IU of vitamin A in pregnant women is associated with fetal malformations; pregnant women are advised to limit intake to less than 10,000 IU per day.

Vitamin D

Vitamin D is essential for calcium and phosphorus absorption and homeostasis, though a mild deficiency is present in many Americans (Looker et al., 2003). Vitamin D is referred to as the "sunshine vitamin," because small amounts of sunlight exposure (about 10 to 15 minutes twice a week) induce the body to make sufficient vitamin D from cholesterol. Fish liver oils provide an abundance of vitamin D. Smaller amounts are found in butter cream, egg yolk, and liver. Typically, Americans get the majority of their vitamin D intake from fortified milk. Regardless of the source, adequate vitamin D intake is critical. Without it, adults can develop **osteomalacia,** a condition in which the bones become weak and susceptible to pseudo-fractures, leading to muscular weakness and bone tenderness. This increases the risk of fracture, in particular of the wrist and pelvis. Low vitamin D intake may also play a role in the development of **osteoporosis** in **postmenopausal** women. Without Vitamin D, children whose bones have not yet fully developed will experience impaired mineralization, leading to rickets and bowing of the legs. Too much vitamin D causes elevated calcium and phosphorus levels and may lead to headache, nausea, and eventually calcification of the kidney, heart, lungs, and the tympanic membrane of the ear, leading to deafness.

Vitamin E

Vitamin E, which is also known as alpha-tocopherol, plays a fundamental role in the metabolism of all cells. It may help protect against conditions related to oxidative stress, including aging, air pollution, **arthritis,** cancer, **cardiovascular disease,** cataracts, **diabetes,** and infection, though research remains contradictory and inconclusive. (A more detailed discussion of the role of antioxidants is presented later in this chapter.) Vitamin E is only synthesized by plants. The richest sources of vitamin E are polyunsaturated plant oils, wheat germ, whole grains, green leafy vegetables, nuts, and seeds. Vitamin E is easily destroyed by heat and oxygen. Therefore, its richest source, oils, should be stored in a cool, dark location. Vitamin E deficiency is rare in humans and tends to only occur in cases of fat malabsorption and transport problems. Toxicity is uncommon, though when present may decrease the absorption of other fat-soluble vitamins, impair bone mineralization, and lead to prolonged clotting times. This is especially relevant for individuals on anticlotting medication, such as coumadin.

Vitamin K

Vitamin K, which is produced by bacteria in the colon and present in large amounts in green, leafy vegetables (especially broccoli, cabbage, turnip greens, and dark lettuce), is important for blood clotting and maintaining strong bones. Due to vitamin K's critical role in blood clotting, individuals on blood-thinning medications that interfere with vitamin K absorption need to carefully titrate their vitamin K intake through diet under the supervision of a physician. Insufficient vitamin K intake can lead to hemorrhage, and potentially fatal **anemia.** Fortunately, vitamin K deficiency is rare, and usually only found in association with lipid malabsorption, destruction of intestinal flora (often due to chronic antibiotic therapy), and liver disease. Newborns are at risk for vitamin K deficiency, as the vitamin does not cross the placenta and is negligible in breast milk. For this reason, newborn infants routinely receive a vitamin K shot after birth to prevent (or slow) a rare problem of bleeding into the brain weeks after birth. Vitamin K also promotes blood clotting. Toxicity of vitamin K only occurs with excessive intake of the synthetic form, which is called menadione. At doses of about 1000 times the RDA, vitamin K can cause severe jaundice in infants and hemolytic anemia.

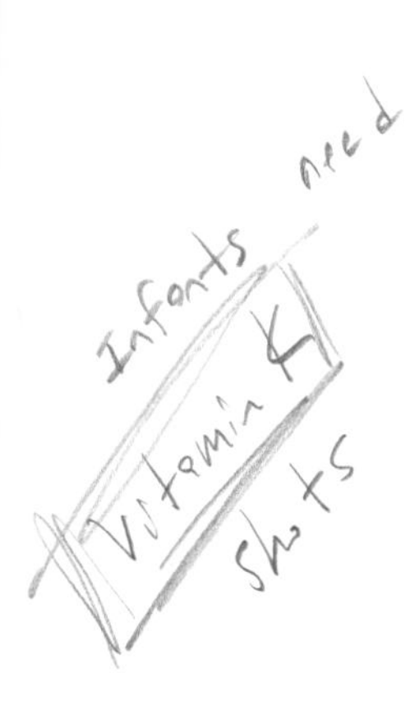

Minerals

Minerals are an important group of micronutrients. With roles ranging from regulating enzyme activity and maintaining acid–base balance to assisting with strength and growth, minerals are critical for human life. Unlike vitamins, many minerals are found in the body as well as in food. The body's ability to use the minerals is dependent upon their bioavailability, or the degree to which the mineral can be absorbed by the body. Nearly all minerals, with the exception of iron, are absorbed in their free form—that is, in their ionic state unbound to organic molecules and complexes. When bound to a complex, the mineral is not bioavailable, and will be excreted in feces. Typically, minerals with high bioavailability include sodium, potassium, chloride, iodide, and fluoride. Minerals with low bioavailability include iron, chromium, and manganese. All other minerals, including calcium and magnesium, are of medium bioavailability.

An important consideration when consuming minerals, and particularly when taking mineral supplements, is the possibility of mineral–mineral interactions. Minerals can interfere with the absorption of other minerals. For example, zinc absorption may be decreased through iron supplementation. Similarly, zinc excesses can decrease copper absorption. Too much calcium limits the absorption of manganese, zinc, and iron. When a mineral is not absorbed properly, a deficiency may develop.

Minerals are typically categorized as macrominerals (bulk elements) and microminerals (trace elements). Macrominerals include calcium, phosphorus, magnesium, sulfur, sodium, chloride, and potassium. Microminerals include iron, iodine, selenium, zinc, and various other minerals that do not have an established DRI, and will not be discussed in this chapter. Table 6-3 presents the DRIs for many minerals.

Macrominerals (Bulk Elements)

By definition, macrominerals are essential for adults in amounts of 100 mg/day or more.

Calcium

Calcium is the most abundant mineral in the human body and serves various functions, including mineralization of the bones and teeth, muscle contraction, blood clotting, blood-pressure control, immunity, and possibly colon-cancer prevention (Mahan & Escott-Stump, 2007). Significant sources of calcium include milk products, small fish with bones, green leafy vegetables, and legumes. Most people in the U.S. do not consume the recommended amounts of calcium from food sources. To help counter this problem, calcium supplements are often used to increase intake. Calcium deficiency in childhood and adolescence can contribute to decreased peak bone mass and suboptimal bone strength. Calcium deficiency in adulthood, particularly in postmenopausal women, can lead to osteomalacia, **osteopenia,** and/or osteoporosis. Calcium toxicity, particularly when combined with vitamin D toxicity, can lead to hypercalcemia and calcification of soft tissues, particularly of the kidneys. High calcium intake also interferes with the absorption of other minerals, including iron, zinc, and manganese. Constipation and renal stone formation are possible.

Phosphorus

Phosphorus is the second most abundant mineral in the body (Mahan & Escott-Stump, 2007). Like calcium, phosphorus plays a role in mineralization of bones and teeth. Phosphorous also helps filter out waste in the kidneys and contributes to energy production in the body by participating in the breakdown of carbohydrates,

Table 6-3
Mineral Facts

Mineral	RDA/AI*		Best Sources	Functions
	Men†	Women†		
Calcium	1,000 mg	1,000 mg	Milk and milk products	Strong bones, teeth, muscle tissue; regulates heart beat, muscle action, and nerve function; blood clotting
Chromium	35 µg	25 µg	Corn oil, clams, whole-grain cereals, brewer's yeast	Glucose metabolism (energy); increases effectiveness of insulin
Copper	**900 µg**	**900 µg**	Oysters, nuts, organ meats, legumes	Formation of red blood cells; bone growth and health; works with vitamin C to form elastin
Fluoride	4 mg	3 mg	Fluorinated water, teas, marine fish	Stimulates bone formation; inhibits or even reverses dental caries
Iodine	**150 µg**	**150 µg**	Seafood, iodized salt	Component of hormone thyroxine, which controls metabolism
Iron	**8 mg**	**18 mg**	Meats, especially organ meats, legumes	Hemoglobin formation; improves blood quality; increases resistance to stress and disease
Magnesium	**420 mg**	**320 mg**	Nuts, green vegetables, whole grains	Acid/alkaline balance; important in metabolism of carbohydrates, minerals, and sugar (glucose)
Manganese	2.3 mg	1.8 mg	Nuts, whole grains, vegetables, fruits	Enzyme activation; carbohydrate and fat production; sex hormone production; skeletal development
Molybdenum	**45 µg**	**45 µg**	Legumes, grain products, nuts	Functions as a cofactor for a limited number of enzymes in humans
Phosphorus	**700 mg**	**700 mg**	Fish, meat, poultry, eggs, grains	Bone development; important in protein, fat, and carbohydrate utilization
Potassium	4700 mg	4700 mg	Lean meat, vegetables, fruits	Fluid balance; controls activity of heart muscle, nervous system, and kidneys
Selenium	**55 µg**	**55 µg**	Seafood, organ meats, lean meats, grains	Protects body tissues against oxidative damage from radiation, pollution, and normal metabolic processing
Zinc	**11 mg**	**8 mg**	Lean meats, liver, eggs, seafood, whole grains	Involved in digestion and metabolism; important in development of reproductive system; aids in healing

* Recommended Dietary Allowances are presented in bold type; Adequate Intakes are presented in non-bolded type.

† RDAs and AIs given are for men aged 31–50 and nonpregnant, nonbreastfeeding women aged 31–50; mg = milligrams; µg = micrograms

protein, and fats. It also may help reduce muscle pain after a strenuous workout. Phosphorus is needed for the growth, maintenance, and repair of all tissues and cells, and for the production of the genetic building blocks, DNA and RNA. Phosphorus is also needed to balance and metabolize other vitamins and minerals, including vitamin D, calcium, iodine, magnesium, and zinc. Animal products such as meat, fish, poultry, eggs, and milk are excellent sources of phosphorus. As a general rule, any food high in protein is also high in phosphorus. The outer coating of many grains contains phosphorus, but in the form of phytic acid, a bound form of phosphorus that is not bioavailable. The leavening process unbinds the phosphorus, making leavened breads a good source of the mineral. Phosphorus is also present in sodas. Deficiency of phosphorus is practically unheard of in the United States. In fact, most individuals consume much more than the DRIs. People taking phosphate-binding medications may be at risk of deficiency, which can present with neuromuscular, skeletal, hematologic, and renal abnormalities and may be deadly. Too much phosphorus intake interferes with calcium absorption and may lead to decreased bone mass and density.

Magnesium

Magnesium, which is present primarily in bone, muscle, soft tissue, and body fluids, is important for bone mineralization, protein production, muscle contraction, nerve conduction, enzyme function, and healthy teeth. Excellent food sources include nuts, legumes, whole grains, dark green leafy vegetables, and milk. In general, a diet high in vegetables and unrefined grains will include more than adequate amounts of magnesium. Unfortunately, most Americans eat a diet high in refined foods and meat and do not meet recommended magnesium intakes. High intakes of calcium, protein, vitamin D, and alcohol increase the body's magnesium requirements. Magnesium deficiency is very rare, but moderate depletion is fairly common, especially in the elderly. Magnesium depletion may contribute to many chronic illnesses and is associated with heart arrhythmias and myocardial infarction. Magnesium toxicity may prevent bone calcification, but toxicity is also very rare, even in cases of supplement overuse.

Sodium, Potassium, and Chloride

Known as electrolytes, these minerals exist as ions in the body and are extremely important for normal cellular function. Sodium is an **extracellular cation,** choloride is an **extracellular anion**, and potassium is an **intracellular cation.** All three electrolytes play at least four essential roles in the body: water balance and distribution, osmotic equilibrium [i.e., assuring that the negative ions (anions) balance with positive ions (cations) when electrolytes move in and out of cells], acid–base balance, and intracellular/extracellular differentials (i.e., assuring that the sodium and chloride stay mostly outside of the cell while potassium stays mostly inside the cell).

When electrolytes are out of balance, such as in a state of dehydration (high concentration of electrolytes) or hyponatremia (low concentration of electrolytes), serious consequences may occur. Symptoms of dehydration include nausea, vomiting, dizziness, disorientation, weakness, irritability, headache, cramps, chills, and decreased performance. Symptoms of hyponatremia include nausea, vomiting, extreme fatigue, respiratory distress, dizziness, confusion, disorientation, coma, and seizures. In severe cases, both conditions can result in death. Electrolytes are excreted in urine, feces, and sweat.

Generally, electrolyte deficiencies do not occur. In fact, sodium excess (and consequently, **hypertension**) is increasingly common given the typical American diet of highly processed and salty foods. Sodium excess may also contribute to osteoporosis, as high sodium increases calcium excretion. Potassium tends to be underconsumed, because most people don't consume enough fruits and vegetables. Insufficient potassium intake is linked to hypertension and osteoporosis.

Sulfur

Sulfur is an important component of many important bodily constituents, including the following: two amino acids (cystine and methionine); three vitamins (thiamin, biotin, and pantothenic acid); and heparin, an anticoagulant found in the liver and other tissues. Meat, poultry, fish, eggs, dried beans, broccoli, and cauliflower are good food sources of the mineral. Sulfur deficiency is relatively uncommon and does not appear to cause any symptoms. Excess sulfur intake may lead to decreased bone mineralization, though sulfur toxicity is very rare.

Microminerals (Trace Elements)

Trace elements are found in minute amounts (less than 1 teaspoon) in the human body. Despite the need for minimal doses of these minerals, they are critical for optimal growth, health, and development. RDAs have been established for only four trace elements: iron, iodine, selenium, and zinc.

Iron

Iron plays a very important role in normal human function. It is essential for the production of **hemoglobin,** the protein that carries inhaled oxygen from the lungs to the tissues, and **myoglobin,** the protein responsible for making oxygen available for muscle contraction. It also regulates cell growth and differentiation. Iron can be stored in the human body for future use as the protein complex **ferritin.** Liver, oysters, seafood, kidney, heart, lean meat, poultry, and fish are excellent food sources, though many people use iron supplements to meet recommended intake amounts. Regardless of the source of iron intake, it is important to meet recommended intakes, as iron deficiency leads to fatigue, poor work performance, and decreased immunity. It is equally important to not exceed recommended intakes, as excess amounts can lead to accumulation of iron in the liver, causing toxicity, and sometimes even death.

Iodine

Iodine, a mineral stored in the thyroid gland and essential for normal growth and metabolism, is found naturally in seafood, though the most common source of iodine in the U.S. is iodized salt. Thanks to this fortification, iodine deficiency is rare in developed countries. However, in some developing countries, deficiency can cause goiter (enlargement of the thyroid gland) and mental retardation in children of mothers who were iodine-deficient during pregnancy. Excessive iodine intake also causes goiter and, potentially, thyroid disease.

Selenium

Selenium, an important antioxidant found mostly in plant foods grown in selenium-rich soil, is needed only in small amounts for optimal function. A lack of this mineral may lead to heart disease, hypothyroidism, and a weakened immune system. Low selenium intake may also have implications in some cancers, for the **human immunodeficiency virus (HIV),** and arthritis, though the research is inconclusive [National Institutes of Health (NIH), 2004a]. Too much selenium can lead to a condition called selonosis, which is manifested as gastrointestinal distress, hair loss, white blotchy nails, garlic breath odor, fatigue, irritability, and nerve damage.

Zinc

Zinc is found in almost every cell and is second only to iron among the trace elements in terms of abundance. It stimulates the activity of enzymes, supports a healthy immune system, assists with wound healing, strengthens the senses (especially taste and smell), supports normal growth and development, and helps with DNA synthesis. Foods rich in zinc include meat, fish, poultry, milk products, and seafood such as oysters and other shellfish. Zinc deficiency causes delayed wound healing and immune-system dysfunction. Toxicity is rare in otherwise healthy individuals, although too much zinc as a result of overzealous supplementation can decrease healthy HDL cholesterol, interfere with copper absorption, and alter iron function (NIH, 2002).

Antioxidants and Phytochemicals

Many of the vitamins and minerals already discussed, including vitamin C, beta-carotene, vitamin E, and selenium, function as antioxidants. Just as metal rusts over time when exposed to water and oxygen, cells are damaged from chronic oxygen exposure. This damage-causing process is called **oxidation,** and can set in motion various chemical reactions that at best cause aging and at worst cause cancer. Antioxidants function to prevent or repair oxidative damage. In the past, antioxidants were considered potent disease fighters. Subsequent research suggests that the agents not only fail to protect against disease, but also that some of them may act to increase the risk of cancer, heart disease, and mortality in some individuals (Bejelakovic et al., 2007; Halliwell, 2007). Their true role in disease pathology has yet to be determined. What remains undisputed is that a diet high in fruits and vegetables is associated with a lower risk of developing chronic disease, such as heart disease, cancer, and possibly Alzheimer's disease. The source of this health-promoting benefit is uncertain. Foods and beverages derived from plants are chemically complex. Their beneficial effects could be due to antioxidants, fiber, agents that stimulate the immune system, monounsaturated fatty acids, B vitamins, folic acid, or various other potential **phytochemicals**—substances in plants that are not necessarily required for normal functioning, but improve health and reduce the risk of disease.

Engineered Foods, Alcohol, Drugs, and Stimulants

While nature has produced an abundance of nutrient-rich foods for human consumption, man has developed an ability to alter the natural form to create engineered foods, various alcoholic beverages, drugs, stimulants, and other compounds. Scientists have learned to process foods to make them taste better (though in general, the greater the processing, the lesser the nutritional value). Humans genetically modify foods to make a more perfect and abundant plant, and they manufacture products to help people lose weight or gain muscle. The processed-food industry is huge, with people spending billions of dollars each year to reap the promised benefits.

Some of these food products are considered **functional foods.** While various definitions exist, the ADA considers a functional food to be any whole food or fortified, enriched, or enhanced food that has a potentially beneficial effect on human health beyond basic nutrition (ADA, 2004). Whole foods such as phytochemical-containing fruits and vegetables are functional foods, as are modified foods that have been fortified with nutrients or phytochemicals. Because functional foods may play a role in decreasing signs of aging, altering disease prevalence and progression, and providing various other benefits, the public is willing to pay more for these products. As a result, many manufacturers and various other companies and individuals are interested in profiting from these products. At times, promises are made that are not backed by quality research or Food and Drug Administration (FDA) approval. LWMCs play an important role in helping clients sift through quality products and hyped junk.

Clients also may be interested in learning how alcohol intake affects their weight-loss plans. Alcohol is a non-nutritive calorie-containing beverage (seven calories per gram). Moderate alcohol consumption provides many health benefits, such as increased HDL cholesterol and reduced risk for cardiovascular disease. However, too much alcohol may contribute to weight gain, regretful behavior, and serious accidents. In addition, alcohol use during pregnancy is linked to birth defects, and alcohol in excess can cause cirrhosis of the liver. Therefore, alcohol is best avoided altogether for those who are pregnant, cannot control intake, or take certain medications.

Herbal supplements, as well as legal and illicit drugs, have been used and abused in weight-loss efforts. While some herbs and other supplements may in fact have beneficial effects, consumers should purchase and use these products cautiously, as they are not regulated by the FDA. The **Dietary Supplement and Health Education Act (DSHEA)** of 1994 dictates supplement production, marketing, and safety guidelines. The following are the highlights of the legislation. LWMCs and their clients must be aware that savvy product manufacturers and marketing experts have found ingenious ways to get around some of the rules.

- A **dietary supplement** is defined as a product (other than tobacco) that functions to supplement the diet and contains one or more of the following ingredients: a vitamin, mineral, herb or other botanical, amino acid, a nutritional substance that increases total dietary intake, metabolite, constituent, or extract, or some combination of these ingredients.
- Safety standards provide that the Secretary of the Department of Health and Human Services may declare that a supplement poses imminent risk or hazard to public safety. A supplement is considered adulterated if it, or one of its ingredients, presents a "significant or unreasonable risk of illness or injury" when used as directed, or under normal conditions. It may also be considered adulterated if too little information is known about the risk of an unstudied ingredient.
- Retailers are allowed to display "third-party" materials that provide information about the health-related benefits of dietary supplements. The Act stipulates the guidelines that this literature must follow, including the fact that it must not be false or misleading, and cannot promote a specific supplement brand.
- Supplement labels cannot include claims that the product diagnoses, prevents, mitigates, treats, or cures a specific disease. Instead, they may describe the supplement's effects on the "structure or function" of the body or the "well-being" achieved by consuming the substance. Unlike other health claims, these nutritional support statements are not approved by the FDA prior to marketing the supplement.
- Supplements must contain an ingredient label, including the name and quantity of each dietary ingredient. The label must also identify the product as a "dietary supplement" (FDA, 1995).

Many clients experiment with various herbs and supplements. Only a few of the most commonly used herbs and supplements are discussed in this chapter. However, the websites of the FDA (www.fda.gov) and the National Institutes of Health Office of Dietary Supplements (www.dietary-supplements.info.nih.gov) provide reputable, up-to-date information about numerous supplements and herbs.

The Chinese botanical **ma huang,** also known as **ephedra,** reduces appetite, but also is associated with significant life-threatening side effects, including dangerously increased blood pressure, heart attack, seizure, stroke, and serious psychiatric illness. The drug works as a **stimulant** to the **central nervous system. Ephedrine,** a synthetic derivative of ephedra, causes the release of **norepinephrine** and stimulates the heart rate, leading to increased cardiac output. It also causes peripheral constriction, and thus, elevated blood pressure. Ephedrine relaxes bronchial smooth muscle and works as a decongestant for temporary relief of shortness of breath caused by asthma. Stimulants also function like adrenaline and release glucose from glycogen, so that blood glucose levels increase. The elevated glucose may suppress appetite. Ephedrine also may work in the hypothalamus, causing a decrease in hunger. However, the drug is not approved by the FDA for weight loss (NIH, 2004b). Another product on the market is Hoodia. Claims that Hoodia promotes weight loss have not yet been thoroughly evaluated by research. The safety of this product has yet to be determined.

Caffeine, which is found in coffee, tea, soft drinks, chocolate, and various other foods and drinks, also acts as a stimulant by increasing alertness, mood, and physical performance. However, too much caffeine causes restlessness, irritability, and anxiety. It can also interfere with sleep and cause headaches, abnormal heart rhythms, and other problems. As a diuretic, caffeine promotes increased urination and may lead to dehydration. If a person has developed a dependence on caffeine, discontinuation could cause withdrawal symptoms such as headache.

Physiology of Digestion

To fully understand the basics of nutrition, LWMCs not only need to know what the macronutrients, micronutrients, and other substances do in the body, but also how they are converted from a molecule contained within a piece of food or pill into a usable form.

Digestive Pathway

The gastrointestinal tract, which is where digestion and absorption occur, forms a long hollow tube from mouth to **anus** (Figure 6-5). Digestion takes two forms. Mechanical digestion is the process of chewing, swallowing, and propelling food through the gastrointestinal tract, while chemical digestion entails the addition of enzymes that break down nutrients. To visualize how this process works, consider the following scenario.

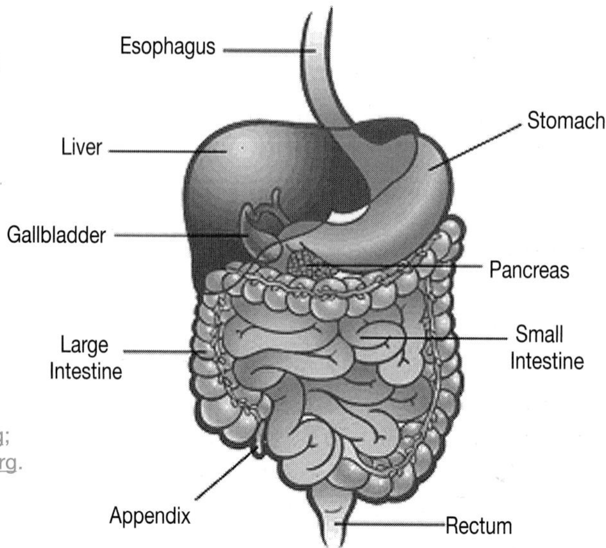

Figure 6-5
The gastrointestinal tract

Source: This information was provided by KidsHealth, one of the largest resources online for medically reviewed health information written for parents, kids, and teens. www.KidsHealth.org; www.TeensHealth.org.

Imagine a person just woke up to the aroma of homemade pancakes and turkey bacon cooking on the stove. Before the person even gets out of bed, his digestive system is preparing to break down the food into nutrients and usable energy by forming enzyme-rich **saliva.** When he finally takes the first bite, the saliva begins to digest and moisten the food, forming a **bolus.** As he swallows, the food passes through the **pharynx** to enter the **esophagus** (the epiglottis prevents food from entering the trachea). Muscles in the esophagus push food to the stomach through a wave-like motion called **peristalsis.** The stomach mixes up the food, liquids, and its homemade digestive juices to break down the pancakes and turkey bacon into absorbable nutrients and energy. Finally, the stomach empties its contents into the small intestine. (The **esophageal sphincter,** also known as the **cardiac sphincter,** prevents food and stomach acid from splashing back into the esophagus from the stomach, while the **pyloric sphincter** separates the stomach from the small intestine.) The amount of time it takes for the **gastric emptying** depends on the type of food (carbohydrates are emptied the fastest, followed by protein and then fat), and the amount of muscle action of the stomach and the receiving small intestine.

The gallbladder and pancreas play key roles in digestion, but are not part of the long gastrointestinal tube. With some help from pancreatic digestive juices and bile produced in the liver and stored in the gallbladder, the 22-foot (7-meter) small intestine spends approximately one to four hours further digesting the food, now called **chyme,** and finally absorbing the nutrients and energy into the blood. This blood gets fast-tracked directly to the liver for the processing and distribution of nutrients to the rest of the body. All of the waste and indigestibles left over in the small intestine (such as fiber)
are passed through the ileocecal valve to the 5-foot (1.5-meter) large intestine, where a few minerals and lots of water are reabsorbed into the blood. As more water gets reabsorbed, the waste passing through the colon

portion of the large intestine gets harder until it is finally excreted as solid waste from the rectum and anus. Food can stay in the large intestine from hours to days. Total transit time from mouth to anus usually takes anywhere from 18 to 72 hours. Therefore, what's considered to be a "normal" frequency of bowel movements can range from three times daily to once every three days or more.

Digestive Enzymes

Numerous enzymes play important roles in digestion. The salivary enzymes α-amylase and lingual lipase initiate carbohydrate and triglyceride digestion, respectively. Protein digestion begins in the stomach, where **endopeptidases, exopeptidases,** and pepsin are secreted. The enzymes break the long chain of amino acids into smaller chains called peptides. Mixing or churning of the bolus of food in the stomach helps to break lipids into droplets to increase their surface area for digestion by pancreatic enzymes.

The final steps of digestion for each of the macronutrients occur in the small intestines. Carbohydrates—now oligosaccharides or disaccharides after initial digestion in the saliva—are digested into monosaccharides. Maltase, α-dextrinase, and sucrase in the intestinal **brush border** hydrolyze the oligosaccharides, while **lactase, trehalase,** and sucrase degrade their respective disaccharides. Ultimately, carbohydrates must be degraded into monosaccharides—glucose, galactose, or fructose—for absorption.

Various pancreatic proteases are activated in the small intestines. Their job is to further digest peptides into amino acids, dipeptides, and tripeptides. Lipid droplets from the stomach pass into the small intestine, where bile acids **emulsify** the lipids, further increasing surface area so that pancreatic lipases can hydrolyze the lipids into fatty acids, monoglycerides, cholesterol, and lysolecithin.

Gastrointestinal Hormones and Gastrointestinal Control

Both neural pathways and hormones facilitate digestion and absorption of food. The neural control of gastrointestinal contractile and secretory activity consists of a local system—the enteric nervous system, which is located in the gut wall—and the systemic **autonomic nervous system.** Receptors sensitive to acidity and stretch send messages to the muscular and secretory cells of the intestinal tract via various neurotransmitters and hormones.

The hormone **gastrin** maintains the pH of the stomach by signaling the cells that produce hydrochloric acid whenever food enters the stomach. When the correct pH is reached, the gastrin-producing cells are turned off via a feedback mechanism similar to the furnace turning off when the correct temperature is reached. **Secretin** is a hormone that tells the pancreas when to produce and secrete bicarbonate to neutralize the stomach acid. It is released when the pH of the small intestine is too low and is turned off when the pH is neutral. **Cholecystokinin** is also released in the small intestine when fat is present. The hormone causes the gallbladder to contract and release bile. When all of the fat is emulsified, the hormone release is halted. Both cholecystokinin and **gastric-inhibitor peptide** slow motility of the intestine to allow the absorption of foods that require more time for digestion and absorption.

Physiology of Absorption

Carbohydrates, proteins, lipids, vitamins, and minerals are absorbed through the walls of the small intestines. The cells are uniquely formed to maximize absorptive capability and help transfer nutrients into the circulation so that they can be used by the body.

Absorptive Cells

To maximize surface area, and thus absorptive capacity, the walls of the small intestine contain many folds and hairlike projections, called **villi** and **microvilli.** These villous structures form a brush border where nutrient absorption occurs.

Types of Absorption

Once digested, individual nutrients must be absorbed across the brush border. Nutrients are absorbed by different mechanisms depending on their solubility, size, and relative concentration. Some nutrients, such as water, can readily diffuse across the membrane in a process called simple diffusion. Other nutrients, such as water-soluble vitamins, require a carrier; this process is called **facilitated diffusion.** Amino acids and glucose require **active transport,** in which energy is needed to move nutrients across a concentration gradient. Products of lipid digestion and fat-soluble vitamins are carried by **micelles** to the absorptive surface of the intestinal cells, where they diffuse across the luminal membrane, are converted back into triglycerides, cholesterol, and phospholipids, and join an apoprotein to form a **chylomicron.** Other substances, such as vitamin B12, calcium, and iron, have special requirements for absorption. Vitamin B12 requires intrinsic factor, a glycoprotein produced in the stomach. Calcium relies on adequate amounts of active vitamin D, or 1,25-dihydroxycholecalciferol . Iron is absorbed in its free form or bound to hemoglobin or myoglobin. In the intestinal cells, all of the iron is converted into its free form and bound to transferrin in the blood.

Portal and Lymphatic Roles in Absorption

Once across the mucosal membrane, sugar, amino acids, water-soluble vitamins, and minerals enter **portal circulation.** This system takes nutrients through the bloodstream to the liver, which acts to detoxify any harmful substances prior to sending them to the brain or heart. Because chylomicrons are too large to enter the capillaries, fats and fat-soluble vitamins are transferred into the **lymphatic system** and added to the bloodstream through the thoracic duct, a large lymphatic vein that drains into the heart. Ultimately, the nutrients are distributed to muscles, organs, and other tissues.

Summary

An individual's health is at least partially determined by the nutrients he or she chooses to consume. While each nutrient plays a specific role in the body's well-being, it is the balance among these different nutrients that allows the body to function optimally. As such, a balanced and varied diet is the foundation for good health. LWMCs should arm their clients with an understanding and appreciation of basic nutrition, digestion, and absorption to help them make proper choices and follow the path toward optimal health and well-being.

References

American College of Sports Medicine (2007). American College of Sports Medicine Position Stand: Exercise and fluid replacements. *Medicine & Science in Sports & Exercise,* 39, 2, 377–390.

American Dietetic Association (2004). Position of the American Dietetic Association: Functional foods. *Journal of the American Dietetic Association,* 104, 814–826.

American Dietetic Association (2002). Position of the American Dietetic Association: Health implications of dietary fiber. *Journal of the American Dietetic Association,* 102, 7, 993–1000.

Bjelakovic, G. et al. (2007). Mortality in randomized trials of antioxidant supplements for primary and secondary prevention. *Journal of the American Medical Association,* 297, 842–857.

Food and Drug Administration (1995). Dietary Supplement Health and Education Act of 1994. http://www.cfsan.fda.gov/~dms/dietsupp.html

Halliwell, B. (2007). Dietary polyphenols: Good, bad, or indifferent for your health? *Cardiovascular Research,* 73, 341–347.

Hu, F.B. & Willett, W.C (2002). Optimal diets for prevention of coronary heart disease. *Journal of the American Medical Association,* 288, 2569–2578.

Jentjens, R. & Jeukendrup, A.E. (2003). Determinants of post-exercise glycogen synthesis during short-term recovery. *Sports Medicine,* 33, 2, 117–144.

Looker, A.C. et al. (2003). Serum 25-hydroxy vitamin D status of adolescents and adults in two seasonal subpopulations from NHANES III. *Bone,* 30, 771–777.

Mahan, L.K. & Escott-Stump, S. (2007). *Krause's Food Nutrition and Diet Therapy* (12th ed.). Philadelphia: W.B. Saunders Company.

McDaniel, M.A., Maier, S.F., & Einstein, G.O. (2003). "Brain-specific" nutrients: A memory cure? *Nutrition*, 19, 957–975.

National Institutes of Health Office of Dietary Supplements (2004a). Dietary supplement fact sheet: Selenium. http://dietary-supplements.info.nih.gov/factsheets/selenium.asp

National Institutes of Health Office of Dietary Supplements (2004b). Dietary supplement fact sheet: Ephedra and ephedrine alkaloids for weight loss and athletic performance. http://ods.od.nih.gov/factsheets/ephedraandephedrine.asp

National Institutes of Health Office of Dietary Supplements (2002). Dietary supplement fact sheet: Zinc. http://ods.od.nih.gov/factsheets/cc/zinc.html

Simopoulos, A.P. (1999). Essential fatty acids in health and chronic disease. *American Journal of Clinical Nutrition*, 70, 560S–569S.

Von Duvillard, S.P. et al. (2004). Fluid and hydration in prolonged endurance performance. *Nutrition,* 20, 651–656.

World Health Organization (2007). Micronutrients. http://www.who.int/nutrition/topics/micronutrients/en/index.html

Zarraga, I.G.E. & Schwarz, E.R. (2006). Impact of dietary patterns and interventions on cardiovascular health. *Circulation,* 114, 961–973.

Recommended Reading

Dunford, M. (Ed.) (2006). *Sports Nutrition: A Practice Manual for Professionals* (4th ed.). Washington, D.C.: SCAN Dietetic Practice Group: The American Dietetic Association.

Duyoff, R.L. & American Dietetic Association (2006). *Complete Food and Nutrition Guide* (3rd ed.). Hoboken, N.J.: John Wiley and Sons.

Institutes of Medicine (2005). Dietary reference intakes. http://www.iom.edu/CMS/3788/4574.aspx

Kleiner, S.M. (2007). *Power Eating: Build Muscle, Gain Energy, Lose Weight* (3rd ed.). Champaign, Ill: Human Kinetics.

National Institutes of Health, Office of Dietary Supplements: Vitamin and Mineral Supplement Fact Sheets. http://ods.od.nih.gov/Health_Information/Vitamin_and_Mineral_Supplement_Fact_Sheets.aspx

United States Department of Health and Human Services (2005). Dietary Guidelines for Americans 2005. www.health.gov/dietaryguidelines

Willett, W. (2006). *Eat, Drink, and Be Healthy: The Harvard Medical School Guide to Healthy Eating* (2nd ed.). New York: Free Press.

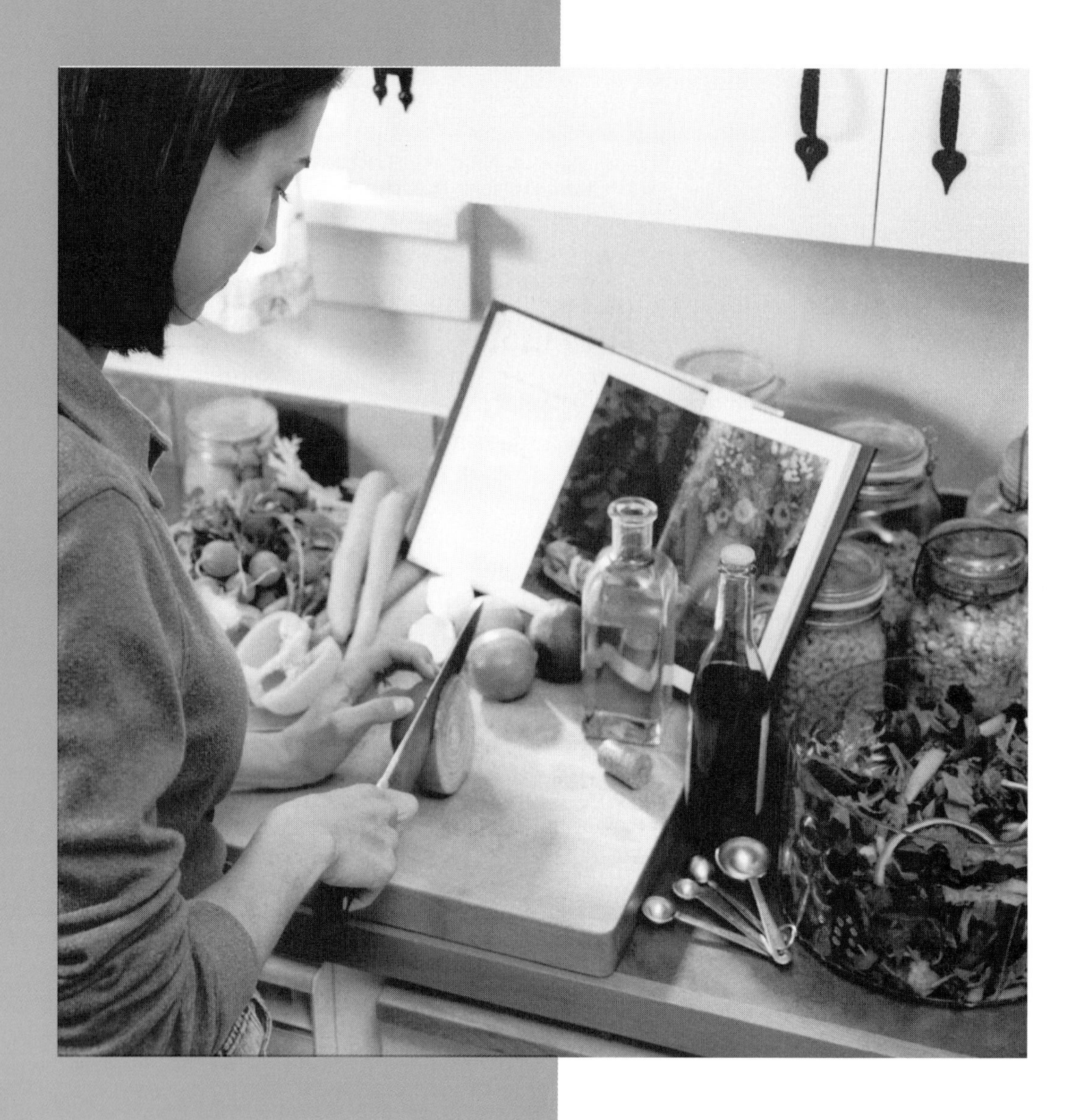

Natalie Digate Muth

Natalie Digate Muth, M.P.H., R.D., is currently pursuing a medical doctor degree at the University of North Carolina at Chapel Hill. In addition to being a registered dietitian, she is an ACE-certified Personal Trainer and Group Fitness Instructor, an American College of Sports Medicine Health and Fitness Instructor, and a National Strength and Conditioning Association Certified Strength and Conditioning Specialist. She is also an ACE Master Trainer and a freelance nutrition and fitness author.

Chapter 7

Application of Nutrition

IN THIS CHAPTER:

Lifestyle & Weight Management Consultants (LWMCs) provide nutrition guidance and recommendations to clients who have struggled with myriad challenges, health conditions, and weight-management successes and failures. To provide clients with the highest quality of care and help them to achieve their goals, LWMCs must have knowledge of the latest nutrition recommendations and guidelines for optimal health. But, more importantly, to empower clients to adopt healthful lifestyle changes, an LWMC must be adept at translating nutrition knowledge into action. While diets come and go with the pounds lost and regained, healthful habits that are adopted, reinforced, and encouraged are the keys to a client's weight-management success.

Dietary Guidelines and Recommended Dietary Allowances

Credible resources are essential to effectively apply nutrition principles and make appropriate nutrition recommendations. While only a registered dietitian (R.D.) is trained to provide specific and individualized nutrition eating plans, LWMCs can use well-established guidelines to help clients adopt healthful and appropriate nutrition habits. The government-issued Dietary Guidelines for Americans, **Dietary Reference Intakes,** and the **MyPyramid Food Guidance System** are ready sources of nutrition recommendations and advice that apply to most Americans.

Dietary Guidelines and the DASH Eating Plan

Every five years, the United States Department of Agriculture (USDA) publishes updated Dietary Guidelines, the government's best advice to Americans on how to eat to promote health and prevent **chronic diseases** such as **cardiovascular disease, stroke, hypertension, diabetes, osteoporosis,** and some cancers. In response to the rise in **obesity** among Americans, the 2005 guidelines also emphasize engaging in ample physical activity and decreasing caloric consumption for weight control. The 2005 guidelines are the most comprehensive recommendations to date, with 84 pages devoted to describing 41 key recommendations in nine topic areas. The major points in each of the key topic areas for the general population are presented in this section (USDA, 2005). Nutrition recommendations for special populations are discussed later in this chapter.

- *Adequate nutrients within calorie needs:* The guidelines encourage Americans to choose a variety of nutrient-dense foods, such as fruits, vegetables, and whole grains, and limit foods high in saturated and **trans fats, cholesterol,** added sugars, salt, and alcohol. The food choices should be distributed within a balanced eating plan such as the MyPyramid Food Guidance System or the **DASH (Dietary Approach to Stop Hypertension) eating plan.** This strategy allows individuals to get all of the **nutrients** the body needs without exceeding caloric requirements.
- *Weight management:* The key to weight control is to balance caloric intake from food and beverages with caloric expenditure. Most adults tend to gradually gain weight with age. For adults to prevent weight gain, the guidelines suggest a 50- to 100-calorie decrease in intake each day, combined with up to 60 minutes of physical activity per day. Those trying to lose weight should aim for a 500-calorie deficit per day achieved through decreased caloric intake and/or increased physical activity. For optimal long-term success and overall health, gradual weight loss is best. And to keep the weight off, clients may need to engage in physical activity for 60 to 90 minutes per day.
- *Physical activity:* All Americans are encouraged to be active and reduce **sedentary** activity. To prevent disease, individuals should engage in at least 30 minutes of moderate activity most days of the week. More or higher-intensity activity will lead to even greater health benefits, as well as help prevent weight gain. A balanced physical-activity program includes cardiovascular training, muscular strength and endurance training, and flexibility training.
- *Food groups to encourage:* Fiber-dense fruits, vegetables, and whole grains are the staples of a healthy diet. Americans should aim to consume nine total servings of fruits (2 cups, or four servings) and vegetables (2.5 cups, or five servings) each day for a standard 2,000-calorie diet. A variety of colorful fruits and vegetables, including dark green and orange vegetables, legumes, and starchy vegetables, will optimize **vitamin, mineral,** and **phytochemical** intake. The guidelines also encourage Americans to consume three or more servings of whole grains daily to meet fiber requirements and three or more cups per day of low-fat milk (or equivalent) products to assure adequate calcium intake.
- *Fats:* The guidelines advise individuals to eat less than 10% of calories from artery-clogging **saturated fat** and less than 300 mg per day of cholesterol. Trans fat, now included on nutrition labels, should be avoided because, like saturated fat, it causes **atherosclerosis.** Ideally, fat intake should contribute 20 to 35% of daily caloric intake, with the majority of fat coming from polyunsaturated or **monounsaturated fat** (e.g., fish, nuts, vegetable oils). To minimize unhealthy fat intake, individuals should

choose lean or low-fat meat, poultry, dry beans, and milk products.

- *Carbohydrates:* Fiber-rich fruits, vegetables, and whole grains are optimal sources of carbohydrate. The guidelines encourage all Americans to limit added sugars and caloric sweeteners, which contain little nutritional value, to practice good oral hygiene, and to eat sugar-laden foods less often to prevent dental caries.
- *Sodium and potassium:* To prevent hypertension, the guidelines recommend that people consume less than 2,300 mg of sodium per day (i.e., one teaspoon of salt). In general, fast food, canned food, and frozen dinners contain an abundance of salt and should be avoided in favor of foods with little salt, such as fresh fruits, vegetables, and unprocessed whole grains.
- *Alcoholic beverages:* Drink in moderation (i.e., <1 drink per day for women; <2 drinks per day for men). While a moderate intake of alcohol has been shown to help prevent cardiovascular disease, individuals who abstain from alcohol are not encouraged to begin drinking to realize these benefits. The guidelines emphasize that people who cannot control intake, pregnant women, children, and those on medications that interact with alcohol should avoid alcoholic beverages.
- *Food safety:* Food safety is discussed in more detail later in this chapter.

The DASH Eating Plan

One in four, or 50 million, American adults between the ages of 20 and 74 years have hypertension, which is defined as a blood pressure higher than 140/90 mmHg. Millions more are **prehypertensive,** with a blood pressure greater than 120/80 mmHg [Centers for Disease Control and Prevention (CDC), 2004]. Hypertension is the leading cause of stroke in the United States, and thus blood pressure should be carefully controlled. While prescription medications are highly effective in reducing blood pressure, nutrition and physical activity are also important in the treatment and prevention of hypertension. In fact, multiple studies have shown that the DASH eating plan, combined with decreased salt intake, can substantially reduce blood pressure levels, and potentially make blood pressure medications unnecessary (Champagne, 2006).

Although it was developed to reduce blood pressure, the DASH eating plan is an overall healthy approach to eating that can be adopted by anyone, regardless of whether he or she has elevated blood pressure. In fact, some studies suggest that the DASH eating plan may also reduce **coronary heart disease** risk by lowering total cholesterol and **low-density lipoproteins (LDL)** in addition to lowering blood pressure (Champagne, 2006). The eating plan is low in saturated fat, cholesterol, and total fat, and consists primarily of fruits, vegetables, and low-fat dairy products. Fish, poultry, nuts, and other unsaturated fats, as well as whole grains, are also encouraged. Red meat, sweets, and sugar-containing beverages are very limited. Table 7-1 describes the DASH eating plan in more detail.

The MyPyramid Food Guidance System

The MyPyramid Food Guidance System is an interactive online tool (www.MyPyramid.gov) designed to replace the well-known but poorly adopted 1992 Food Guide Pyramid. The significance of each component of the MyPyramid symbol is described in Figure 7-1. The goal of the new pyramid is to provide updated guidelines based on the latest scientific research and to offer consumers an online feature to personalize dietary guidelines in accordance with their individual needs and lifestyle.

A major criticism of the 1992 Food Guide Pyramid was that it did not differentiate between healthy and unhealthy choices in a given food group. For example, ice cream and skim milk were lumped together in the dairy group, as were french fries and spinach under the category of vegetables. MyPyramid describes

Table 7-1
The DASH Eating Plan

Food Group	Daily Servings (except as noted)	Serving Sizes	Examples and Notes	Significance of Each Food Group to the DASH Eating Plan
Grains and grain products	7–8	1 slice bread 1 oz dry cereal* ½ cup cooked rice, pasta, or cereal	Whole-wheat bread, English muffin, pita bread, bagel, cereals, grits, oatmeal, crackers, unsalted pretzels, popcorn	Major sources of energy and fiber
Vegetables	4–5	1 cup raw leafy vegetable ½ cup cooked vegetable 6 oz vegetable juice	Tomatoes, potatoes, carrots, green peas, squash, broccoli, turnip greens, collards, kale, spinach, artichokes, green beans, lima beans, sweet potatoes	Rich sources of potassium, magnesium, and fiber
Fruits	4–5	6 oz fruit juice 1 medium fruit ¼ cup dried fruit ½ cup fresh, frozen, or canned fruit	Apricots, bananas, dates, grapes, orange juice, grapefruit, grapefruit juice, mangoes, melons, peaches, pineapples, prunes, raisins, strawberries, tangerines	Important sources of potassium, magnesium, and fiber
Low-fat or fat-free dairy foods	2–3	8 oz milk 1 cup yogurt 1½ oz cheese	Fat-free (skim) or low-fat (1%) milk, fat-free or low-fat buttermilk, fat-free or low-fat regular or frozen yogurt, low-fat and fat-free cheese	Major sources of calcium and protein
Meats, poultry, and fish	2 or less	3 oz cooked meats, poultry, or fish	Select only lean; trim away visible fats; broil, roast, or boil, instead of frying; remove skin from poultry	Rich sources of protein and magnesium
Nuts, seeds, and dry beans	4–5 per week	⅓ cup or 1½ oz nuts 2 Tbsp or ½ oz seeds ½ cup cooked dry beans	Almonds, filberts, mixed nuts, peanuts, walnuts, sunflower seeds, kidney beans, lentils, peas	Rich sources of energy, magnesium, potassium, protein, and fiber
Fats and oils†	2–3	1 tsp soft margarine 1 Tbsp low-fat mayonnaise 2 Tbsp light salad dressing 1 tsp vegetable oil	Soft margarine, low-fat mayonnaise, light salad dressing, vegetable oil (such as olive, corn, canola, or safflower)	DASH has 27% of calories as fat, including fat in or added to foods
Sweets	5 per week	1 Tbsp sugar 1 Tbsp jelly or jam ½ oz jelly beans 8 oz lemonade	Maple syrup, sugar, jelly, jam, fruit-flavored gelatin, jelly beans, hard candy, fruit punch, sorbet, ices	Sweets should be low in fat

* Equals ½–1¼ cups, depending on cereal type. Check the product's Nutrition Facts label.

† Fat content changes serving counts for fats and oils. For example, 1 Tbsp of regular salad dressing equals one serving; 1 Tbsp of a low-fat dressing equals ½ a serving; 1 Tbsp of a fat-free dressing equals 0 servings.

Source: National Heart Lung and Blood Institute of the National Institutes of Health

the best choices in each food group. For example, people are encouraged to consume:

- Mostly whole grains, as opposed to refined sugars
- Ample nutrient-dense dark green and orange vegetables, such as broccoli and carrots, rather than disproportionate amounts of starchy vegetables such as white potatoes and corn, which contain fewer vitamins and minerals
- A variety of fruits, preferably from whole-food sources, as opposed to fruit juices
- Oils in moderation with an emphasis on mono- or **polyunsaturated fats** instead of trans or saturated fats
- Low- or nonfat milk products rather than whole-milk products
- Lean meats and bean products instead of higher-fat meats such as regular (75 to 80% lean) ground beef or chicken with the skin

The MyPyramid Food Guidance System tailors nutrition advice to individual caloric needs. For example, a consumer can go to www.MyPyramid.gov to calculate his or her estimated energy expenditure based on age, gender, and typical amount of physical activity. Within seconds, he or she will be categorized into one of 12 different energy levels (from 1,000 to 3,200 calories) and will be given the recommended number of servings—measured in cups and ounces—to eat from each of the seven food groups. A set number of discretionary calories (i.e., the leftover calories available for sugar or additional fats or an extra serving from any of the food

Figure 7-1
Anatomy of MyPyramid

Anatomy of MyPyramid

One size doesn't fit all

USDA's new MyPyramid symbolizes a personalized approach to healthy eating and physical activity. The symbol has been designed to be simple. It has been developed to remind consumers to make healthy food choices and to be active every day. The different parts of the symbol are described below.

Activity
Activity is represented by the steps and the person climbing them, as a reminder of the importance of daily physical activity.

Moderation
Moderation is represented by the narrowing of each food group from bottom to top. The wider base stands for foods with little or no solid fats or added sugars. These should be selected more often. The narrower top area stands for foods containing more added sugars and solid fats. The more active you are, the more of these foods can fit into your diet.

Personalization
Personalization is shown by the person on the steps, the slogan, and the URL. Find the kinds and amounts of food to eat each day at MyPyramid.gov.

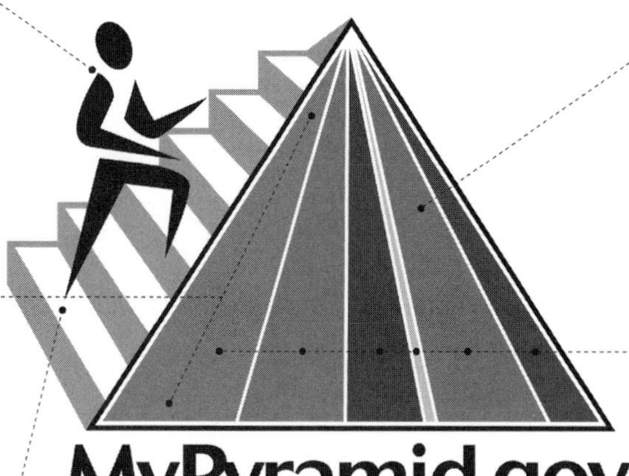

MyPyramid.gov
STEPS TO A HEALTHIER YOU

Proportionality
Proportionality is shown by the different widths of the food group bands. The widths suggest how much food a person should choose from each group. The widths are just a general guide, not exact proportions. Check the Web site for how much is right for you.

Variety
Variety is symbolized by the 6 color bands representing the 5 food groups of the Pyramid and oils. This illustrates that foods from all groups are needed each day for good health.

Gradual Improvement
Gradual improvement is encouraged by the slogan. It suggests that individuals can benefit from taking small steps to improve their diet and lifestyle each day.

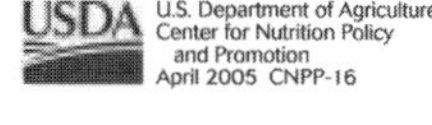

U.S. Department of Agriculture
Center for Nutrition Policy and Promotion
April 2005 CNPP-16

USDA is an equal opportunity provider and employer.

GRAINS | VEGETABLES | FRUITS | OILS | MILK | MEAT & BEANS

groups) will also be allocated. By following these recommendations, that individual will have the optimal diet for disease prevention and weight maintenance based on his or her personalized needs. The website also has a variety of online tools, including:

- *MyPyramid Plan:* Provides an estimate of what and how much food to eat based on the user's age, gender, and activity level
- *MyPyramid Tracker:* Cites detailed information on the quality of an individual's diet and his or her physical-activity status
- *Inside MyPyramid:* Provides in-depth data for every food group, including recommended daily amounts
- *Tips and Resources:* Offers a variety of suggestions to eat healthier and be more active (e.g., a tip sheet that describes how to eat healthy when eating out) (Table 7-2)

Table 7-2
Eating Healthy When Eating Out

- As a beverage choice, ask for water or order fat-free or low-fat milk, unsweetened tea, or other drinks without added sugars.
- Ask for whole-wheat bread for sandwiches.
- In a restaurant, start your meal with a salad packed with veggies, to help control hunger and feel satisfied sooner.
- Ask for salad dressing to be served on the side. Then use only as much as you want.
- Choose main dishes that include vegetables, such as stir fries, kebobs, or pasta with a tomato sauce.
- Order steamed, grilled, or broiled dishes instead of those that are fried or sautéed.
- Choose a "small" or "medium" portion. This includes main dishes, side dishes, and beverages.
- Order an item from the menu instead of heading for the "all-you-can-eat" buffet.
- If main portions at a restaurant are larger than you want, try one of these strategies to keep from overeating:
    - Order an appetizer or side dish instead of an entrée.
    - Share a main dish with a friend.
    - If you can chill the extra food right away, take leftovers home in a "doggy bag."
    - When your food is delivered, set aside or pack half of it to go immediately.
    - Resign from the "clean your plate club"—when you've eaten enough, leave the rest.
- To keep your meal moderate in calories, fat, and sugars:
    - Ask for salad dressing to be served "on the side" so you can add only as much as you want.
    - Order foods that do not have creamy sauces or gravies.
    - Add little or no butter to your food.
    - Choose fruits for dessert most often.
- On long commutes or shopping trips, pack some fresh fruit, cut-up vegetables, low-fat string cheese sticks, or a handful of unsalted nuts to help you avoid stopping for sweet or fatty snacks.

Source: www.MyPyramid.gov

The MyPyramid Food Guidance System also emphasizes the importance of staying active and provides a resource page filled with tips on how to move more frequently. Despite its improvements from the 1992 Food Guide Pyramid, MyPyramid is not without flaws. After all, transferring the 85 pages of nutrition information contained in the 2005 Dietary Guidelines into a simple symbol is no easy task. The committee formed to create the MyPyramid Food Guidance System also faced immense pressures from food-industry lobbyists. And, because it is a Web-based program, MyPyramid is less accessible to seniors and low-income individuals who are less likely to have access to a computer. Nonetheless, the MyPyramid Food Guidance System is a valuable tool that can be used to help improve clients' nutrition and activity habits.

Food Labels

To make healthy nutrition decisions, individuals must understand what nutrients contribute to a healthy diet and know which foods contain those nutrients. LWMCs play an important role in providing clients with accurate nutrition information. The food label, a required component of nearly all packaged foods, can help individuals turn knowledge into action (Figure 7-2).

Encourage clients to dissect the food label by starting from the top—the serving size and the number of servings per container. In general, serving sizes are standardized so that consumers can compare similar products. All of the nutrient amounts listed on the food label are for one serving, so it is important to determine how many servings an individual

Serving Size
Is your serving the same size as the one on the label? If you eat double the serving size listed, you need to double the nutrient and calorie values. If you eat one-half the serving size shown here, cut the nutrient and calorie values in half.

Calories
Are you overweight? Cut back a little on calories! Look here to see how a serving of the food adds to your daily total. A 5' 4", 138-lb active woman needs about 2,200 calories each day. A 5' 10", 174-lb active man needs about 2,900. How about you?

Total Carbohydrate
Carbohydrates are in foods like bread, potatoes, fruits and vegetables. Choose these often! They give you more nutrients than sugars like soda pop and candy.

Dietary Fiber
Grandmother called it "roughage," but her advice to eat more is still up-to-date! That goes for both soluble and insoluble kinds of dietary fiber. Fruits, vegetables, whole-grain foods, beans and peas are all good sources and can help reduce the risk of heart disease and cancer.

Protein
Most Americans get more than they need. Where there is animal protein, there is also fat and cholesterol. Eat small servings of lean meat, fish, and poultry. Use skim or low-fat milk, yogurt, and cheese. Try vegetable proteins like beans, grains, and cereals.

Vitamins and Minerals
Your goal here is 100% of each for the day. Don't count on one food to do it all. Let a combination of foods add up to a winning score.

Nutrition Facts

Serving Size ½ cup (114g)
Servings Per Container 4

Amount Per Serving	
Calories 90	Calories from Fat 30
	% Daily Value*
Total Fat 3g	**5%**
Saturated Fat 0g	0%
Trans Fat 0g	0%
Cholesterol 0mg	0%
Sodium 300mg	13%
Total Carbohydrate 13g	4%
Dietary Fiber 3g	12%
Sugars 3g	
Protein 3g	

Vitamin A	80%	•	Vitamin C	60%
Calcium	4%	•	Iron	4%

*Percent Daily Values are based on a 2,000 calorie diet. Your daily values may be higher or lower depending on your calorie needs:

	Calories	2,000	2,500
Total Fat	Less than	65g	80g
Sat Fat	Less than	20g	25g
Cholesterol	Less than	300mg	300mg
Sodium	Less than	2,400mg	2,400mg
Total Carbohydrate		300g	375g
Fiber		25g	30g

Calories per gram:
Fat 9 • Carbohydrate 4 • Protein 4

(More nutrients may be listed on some labels)

mg = milligrams (1,000 mg = 1 g)
g = grams (about 28 g = 1 ounce)

Total Fat
Aim low: Most people need to cut back on fat! Too much fat may contribute to heart disease and cancer. Try to limit your calories from fat. For a healthy heart, choose foods with a big difference between the total number of calories and the number of calories from fat.

Saturated Fat
Saturated fat is part of the total fat in food. It is listed separately because it's the key player in raising blood cholesterol and your risk of heart disease. Eat less!

Trans Fat
Trans fat works a lot like saturated fat, except it is worse. This fat starts out as a liquid unsaturated fat, but then food manufacturers add some hydrogen to it, turning it into a solid saturated fat (that's what "partially hydrogenated" means when you see it in the food ingredients). They do this to increase the shelf-life of the product, but in the body the trans fat damages the blood vessels and contributes to increasing blood cholesterol and the risk of heart disease.

Cholesterol
Too much cholesterol—a second cousin to fat—can lead to heart disease. Challenge yourself to eat less than 300 mg each day.

Sodium
You call it "salt," the label calls it "sodium." Either way, it may add up to high blood pressure in some people. So, keep your sodium intake low—2,400 to 3,000 mg or less each day. (The American Heart Association recommends no more than 3,000 mg sodium per day for healthy adults.)

Daily Value
Feel like you're drowning in numbers? Let the Daily Value be your guide. Daily Values are listed for people who eat 2,000 or 2,500 calories each day. If you eat more, your personal daily value may be higher than what's listed on the label. If you eat less, your personal daily value may be lower. For fat, saturated fat, cholesterol and sodium, choose foods with a low % Daily Value. For total carbohydrates, dietary fiber, vitamins, and minerals, your daily value goal is to reach 100% of each.

Figure 7-2
How to Read the New Food Label

actually consumes to accurately assess nutrient intake.

Next, clients should look at the total number of calories and the number of calories from fat. The total number of calories indicates how much energy a person gets from a particular food. Americans tend to consume too many calories without meeting daily nutrient requirements. This part of the nutrition label is the most important factor for weight control. In general, 40 calories per serving is considered low, 100 calories is moderate, and 400 or more calories is considered high. The Dietary Guidelines encourage consuming less than 20 to 35% of calories from fat. To determine the percentage of calories from fat, divide the number of calories from fat by the total number of calories per serving.

The next two sections of the label note the nutrient content of the food product. Clients should try to minimize intake of the first three nutrients listed: fat (especially saturated and trans fat), cholesterol, and sodium. They should aim to consume adequate amounts of fiber, vitamin A, vitamin C, calcium, and iron.

The **percent daily values (PDV)** are listed for key nutrients to facilitate the comparing of products (clients must make sure that the serving sizes are similar), nutrient content claims (e.g., does a cereal with a reduced sugar content really contain less carbohydrate than a similar cereal of a different brand?), and dietary trade-offs (e.g., balance consumption of a high-fat product for lunch with lower-fat products throughout the rest of the day). In general, 5% daily value or less is considered low, while 20% daily value or more is considered high.

The footnote at the bottom of the label reminds consumers that all percent daily values are based on a 2,000-calorie diet. Individuals who need more or less calories should adjust the recommendations accordingly. For example, 3 grams of fat provides 5% of the recommended amount for someone on a 2,000-calorie diet and 7% for someone on a 1,500-calorie diet. The footnote also includes daily values for nutrients that should be limited (i.e., total fat, saturated fat, trans fat, cholesterol, sodium), recommended carbohydrate intake for a 2,000-calorie diet (i.e., 60% of calories), and minimal fiber recommendations for 2,000- and 2,500-calorie diets [U.S. Food and Drug Administration (FDA), 2004].

Legislation passed in 2006 also requires food manufacturers to list all potential food allergens on food packaging. The most common food allergens are fish, shellfish, soybean, wheat, egg, milk, peanuts, and tree nuts. This information usually is included near the list of ingredients on the package. Note that the ingredient list is in decreasing order of substance weight in the product. That is, the ingredients listed first are the most abundant ingredients in the product. Clients should try to avoid foods that contain low-nutrient-density foods such as sugar, high-fructose corn syrup (and other common sweeteners), bleached flour, or partially hydrogenated oils at the top of the list.

While the food label is found on the side or the back of products, myriad health and nutrition claims are visibly displayed on the front of the box. The FDA closely regulates these claims, which must meet strict criteria (Table 7-3).

Food Safety and Selection

Another key to healthy eating is to avoid foods contaminated with harmful bacteria, viruses, parasites, and other microorganisms. Nearly 76 million people in the United States become ill each year from foodborne illnesses (USDA, 2005). Special populations most at-risk include pregnant women, infants and young children, older adults, and people who are immunocompromised. The majority of foodborne illnesses are preventable with a few simple precautions (Table 7-4). Refer to www.fightbac.org or www.foodsafety.gov for more information.

Clients should follow these tips while grocery shopping to reduce the risk of foodborne illnesses:

- Check produce for bruises, and feel and smell for ripeness.

Table 7-3
Nutrient Content Claims

Requirements for Health Claims

According to government requirements, foods must meet three criteria to carry a health claim:

- Not exceed specific levels for total fat, saturated fat, cholesterol, and sodium. These are the main nutrients that health professionals suggest consumers limit in their daily diets.
- Contain at least 10% of the daily value, before supplementation, for any one or all of the following: protein, dietary fiber, vitamin A, vitamin C, calcium, and iron. These are the nutrients that health professionals suggest consumers get adequate amounts of in their daily diets.
- Meet nutrient levels that are specific for each approved health claim.

Allowable Health Claims

Calcium and osteoporosis
The food or supplement must be "high" in calcium and must not contain more phosphorus than calcium. Claims must cite other risk factors; state the need for regular exercise and a healthful diet; explain that adequate calcium early in life helps reduce fracture risk later by increasing as much as genetically possible a person's peak bone mass; and indicate that those at greatest risk of developing osteoporosis later in life are white and Asian teenage and young adult women, who are in their bone-forming years. Claims for products with more than 400 mg of calcium per day must state that a daily intake over 2,000 mg offers no added known benefit to bone health.

Sodium and hypertension (high blood pressure)
Foods must meet criteria for "low sodium." Claims must use "sodium" and "high blood pressure" in discussing the nutrient-disease link.

Dietary fat and cancer
Foods must meet criteria for "low fat." Fish and game meats must meet criteria for "extra lean." Claims may not mention specific types of fats and must use "total fat" or "fat" and "some types of cancer" or "some cancers" in discussing the nutrient-disease link.

Dietary saturated fat and cholesterol and risk of coronary heart disease
Foods must meet criteria for "low saturated fat," "low cholesterol," and "low fat." Fish and game meats must meet criteria for "extra lean." Claims must use "saturated fat and cholesterol" and "coronary heart disease" or "heart disease" in discussing the nutrient-disease link.

Fiber-containing grain products, fruits, and vegetables and cancer
Foods must meet criteria for "low fat" and, without fortification, be a "good source" of dietary fiber. Claims must not specify types of fiber and must use "fiber," "dietary fiber," or "total dietary fiber" and "some types of cancer" or "some cancers" in discussing the nutrient-disease link.

Fruits, vegetables, and grain products that contain fiber, particularly soluble fiber, and risk of coronary heart disease
Foods must meet criteria for "low saturated fat," "low fat," and "low cholesterol." They must contain, without fortification, at least 0.6 g of soluble fiber per reference amount, and the soluble fiber content must be listed. Claims must use "fiber," "dietary fiber," "some types of dietary fiber," "some dietary fibers," or "some fibers" and "coronary heart disease" or "heart disease" in discussing the nutrient-disease link. The term "soluble fiber" may be added.

Fruits and vegetables and cancer
Foods must meet criteria for "low fat" and, without fortification, be a "good source" of fiber, vitamin A , or vitamin C. Claims must characterize fruits and vegetables as foods that are low in fat and may contain dietary fiber, vitamin A, or vitamin C; characterize the food itself as a "good source" of one or more of these nutrients, which must be listed; refrain from specifying types of fatty acids; and use "total fat" or "fat," "some types of cancer" or "some cancers," and "fiber," "dietary fiber," or "total dietary fiber" in discussing the nutrient-disease link.

Folate and neural tube birth defects
Foods must meet or exceed criteria for "good source" of folate—that is, at least 40µg of folic acid per serving (at least 10% of the Daily Value). A serving of food cannot contain more than 100% of the Daily Value for vitamin A and vitamin D because of their potential risk to fetuses. Claims must use "folate," "folic acid," or "folacin" and "neural tube defects," "birth defects spina bifida or anencephaly," "birth defects of the brain or spinal cord anencephaly or spina bifida," "spina bifida and anencephaly, birth defects of the brain or spinal cord," "birth defects of the brain and spinal cord," or "brain or spinal cord birth defects" in discussing the nutrient-disease link. Folic acid content must be listed on the Nutrition Facts panel.

Dietary sugar alcohol and dental caries (cavities)
Foods must meet the criteria for "sugar free." The sugar alcohol must be xylitol, sorbitol, mannitol, maltitol, isomalt, lactitol, hydrogenated starch hydrolysates, hydrogenated glucose syrups, erythritol, or a combination of these. When the food contains a fermentable carbohydrate, such as sugar or flour, the food must not lower plaque pH in the mouth below 5.7 while it is being eaten or up to 30 minutes afterwards. Claims must use "sugar alcohol," "sugar alcohols," or the name(s) of the sugar alcohol present and "dental caries" or "tooth decay" in discussing the nutrient-disease link. Claims must state that the sugar alcohol present "does not promote," "may reduce the risk of," "is useful in not promoting," or "is expressly for not promoting" dental caries.

Dietary soluble fiber, such as that found in whole oats and psyllium seed husk, and coronary heart disease
Foods must meet criteria for "low saturated fat," "low cholesterol," and "low fat." Foods that contain whole oats must contain at least 0.75 g of soluble fiber per serving. Foods that contain psyllium seed husk must contain at least 1.7 g of soluble fiber per serving. The claim must specify the daily dietary intake of the soluble fiber source necessary to reduce the risk of heart disease and the contribution one serving of the product makes toward that intake level. Soluble fiber content must be stated in the nutrition label. Claims must use "soluble fiber" qualified by the name of the eligible source of soluble fiber and "heart disease" or "coronary heart disease" in discussing the nutrient-disease link. Because of the potential hazard of choking, foods containing dry or incompletely hydrated psyllium seed husk must carry a label statement telling consumers to drink adequate amounts of fluid, unless the manufacturer shows that a viscous adhesive mass is not formed when the food is exposed to fluid.

Source: Food and Drug Administration

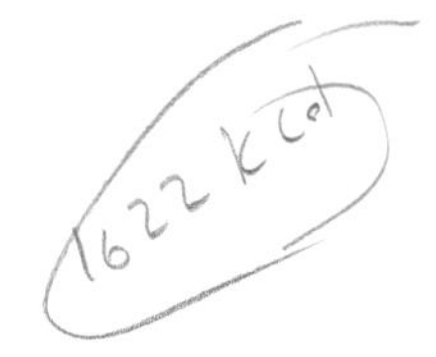

Table 7-4
Steps to Safe Food Handling

To avoid microbial foodborne illness:

- Clean hands, food contact surfaces, and fruits and vegetables. Meat and poultry should not be washed or rinsed.
- Separate raw, cooked, and ready-to-eat foods while shopping, preparing, or storing foods.
- Cook foods to a safe temperature to kill microorganisms [bacteria grow most rapidly between the temperatures of 40 and 140° F (4 and 60° C)]. Pregnant women should only eat certain deli meats and frankfurters that have been reheated to steaming hot.
- Refrigerate perishable food promptly (within two hours) and defrost foods properly. Eat refrigerated leftovers within three or four days.
- Avoid raw (unpasteurized) milk or any products made from unpasteurized milk, raw or partially cooked eggs, or foods containing raw eggs, raw or undercooked meat and poultry, unpasteurized juice, and raw sprouts. This is especially important for infants and young children, pregnant women, older adults, and those who are immunocompromised.

Source: U.S. Department of Agriculture (2005). Dietary Guidelines for America. www.health.gov/dietaryguidelines.

- Look for a sell-by date for breads and baked goods, a use-by date on some packaged foods, an expiration date on yeast and baking powder, and a packaged date on canned and some packaged foods.
- Make sure packaged goods are not torn and cans are not dented, cracked, or bulging.
- Separate fish and poultry from other purchases by wrapping them separately in plastic bags.
- Pick up refrigerated and frozen foods last. Try to make sure all perishable items are refrigerated within one hour of purchase (Clemson University Cooperative Extension, 1999).

Nutritional Needs for Active Adults

Active adults require conscientious fueling and refueling to maintain optimal performance and overall health. Nutrition recommendations can be tailored to individual clients by determining their daily energy needs. For healthy adults, the most accurate estimation of **resting metabolic rate (RMR),** an approximation of the energy expended at rest each day, is the Mifflin-St Jeor equation (Frankenfield, Routh-Yousey, & Compher, 2005):

For men: RMR = 9.99 x wt (kg) + 6.25 x ht (cm) – 4.92 x age (yrs) + 5
For women: RMR = 9.99 x wt (kg) + 6.25 x ht (cm) – 4.92 x age (yrs) – 161

Moderately active people are generally advised to consume about 1.5 to 1.7 times the calculated RMR (ADA, 2000). For example, a 30-year-old female who is 5'6" (1.7 m), weighs 145 pounds (66 kg), and engages in 40 to 60 minutes of vigorous physical activity most days of the week would need approximately 2,200 calories per day for weight maintenance.

The Institute of Medicine's (IOM) 2005 Dietary Reference Intakes (DRI) recommend that approximately 45 to 65% of calories come from carbohydrate, 10 to 35% from protein, and 20 to 35% from fat (IOM, 2005). Although active individuals require ample carbohydrates to maintain blood **glucose** and replace muscle **glycogen** expended during exercise, as well as increased protein for muscle repair, research suggests that active individuals do not need a greater percentage of calories from carbohydrate or protein than the average population. However, they are able to meet the increased demands created by a greater overall caloric intake (ADA, 2000).

The ADA suggests that active individuals consume 6 to 10 grams of carbohydrates per kilogram of body weight per day, depending on total daily energy expenditure, type of exercise done, gender, and environmental conditions. Endurance athletes are advised to eat 1.2 to 1.4 grams of protein per kilogram of body weight per day, while strength and conditioning athletes may need up to 1.6 to 1.7 grams of protein per kilogram of body weight. These recommendations can usually be met through diet alone without protein supplementation (ADA, 2000).

Active individuals who eat a well-balanced diet are not at increased risk of micronutrient deficiencies compared to their sedentary counterparts. Thus, no vitamin and mineral supplements are necessary beyond those recommended for reasons unrelated to exercise, such as folic acid in women of childbearing age (ADA, 2000).

Nutritional Requirements for Fitness and Sport

Optimal nutrition and athletic performance go hand in hand. Advise clients to eat a small snack before exercising to maximize the training session. The food should be something that is relatively high in carbohydrate to maximize blood glucose availability, relatively low in fat and fiber to minimize gastrointestinal distress and facilitate gastric emptying, moderate in protein, and well-tolerated by the individual. Many people prefer a bagel or a granola bar, for example.

During extended training sessions, clients should aim to replace fluid losses and consume 30 to 60 grams of carbohydrate per hour of training to maintain blood glucose levels. This is especially important for extended training sessions lasting longer than one hour; exercise in extreme heat, cold, or high altitude; and when adequate amounts of food or drink have not been consumed prior to a training session (ADA, 2000).

After the exercise session, clients should focus on carbohydrates and protein. Studies show that the best meals for post-workout refueling include an abundance of carbohydrates accompanied by some protein. The carbohydrates replenish the used-up energy that is normally stored as glycogen in muscle and in the liver. The protein helps to rebuild the muscles that were fatigued with exercise. About 75 to 90 grams of carbohydrate (approximately five to six servings of whole grains, fruit, or vegetables) per hour over the course of five hours after training are recommended for optimal refueling (Jentjens & Juekendrup, 2003). The ADA recommends a carbohydrate intake of 1.5 g/kg of body weight in the first 30 minutes after exercise and then every two hours for four to six hours thereafter (ADA, 2000). Certainly, the amount of refueling necessary depends on the intensity and duration of the training session.

As far as refueling goes, not all carbohydrates are created equal. Carbohydrates with a high **glycemic index,** such as instant white rice and dried fruit, are more rapidly absorbed and more quickly release sugar into the bloodstream (Table 7-5). Thus, they are more effective at replenishing energy stores than low-glycemic foods, which are broken down more slowly and take longer to release sugar into the bloodstream. And glucose, found in non-fruit carbohydrates, is better absorbed than fructose, the sugar in fruit (Jentjens & Jeukendrup, 2003). However, although high-glycemic, glucose-rich foods are good for refueling and athletic performance, lower-glycemic foods and fruits may be a better choice for overall heart health (Thomas, Elliott, & Baur, 2007). The goal is to find a balance.

Remind clients to eat as soon after exercising as possible, preferably within 30 minutes. This is the time when the muscles are best able to replenish energy stores, enabling the body to prepare for the next big workout.

Table 7-5
Glycemic Index of Various Foods

High GI ≥70	Medium GI 56–69	Low GI ≤55
White bread	Rye bread	Pumpernickel bread
Corn Flakes®	Shredded Wheat®	All Bran®
Graham crackers	Ice cream	Plain yogurt
Dried fruit	Blueberries	Strawberries
Instant white rice	Refined pasta	Oatmeal

Fluid and Hydration

Acutely aware of the detrimental health and performance effects of **dehydration,** health and fitness experts have long urged recreational exercise enthusiasts and athletes alike to hydrate continuously. In fact, a 1996 American College of Sports Medicine (ACSM) position stand encouraged exercisers to drink "the maximal amount that can be tolerated" (Convertino et al., 1996). But the latest research reveals that **hyponatremia**—or severely reduced blood sodium concentration resulting from overhydration—may be of equal or greater concern. In response, ACSM updated its guidelines and the United States Track and Field Association (USATF) developed guidelines for optimal hydration during exercise (Table 7-6) (Casa, Clarkson, & Roberts, 2005):

- *Use thirst to determine fluid needs:* Advise clients to drink when they are thirsty and stop drinking when they feel hydrated.
- *Aim for a 1:1 ratio of fluid replacement to fluid lost via sweat:* Ideally, people should consume the same amount of fluid as is lost in sweat. Clients can check their hydration status by comparing pre- and post-exercise weight. Perfect hydration occurs when no weight is lost or gained during exercise. Another simple way to determine adequate hydration status is to check urine color. Individuals will know that they are adequately hydrated when their urine is clear or pale yellow. Because people sweat at varying rates, the typical recommendation to consume 3 to 6 ounces of water for every 20 minutes of exercise may not be appropriate for everyone. However, when individual assessment is not possible, this recommendation works for most people. Experts advise small athletes exercising in mild environmental conditions to consume slightly smaller amounts of fluids, and competitive athletes working at higher intensities in warmer environments to consume slightly more (Noakes, 2003).

Table 7-6
Fluid-intake Recommendations During Exercise

2 hours prior to exercise, drink 500–600 mL (17–20 oz)
Every 10–20 minutes during exercise, drink 200–300 mL (7–10 oz) or, preferably, drink based on sweat losses
Following exercise, drink 450–675 mL for every 0.5 kg body weight lost (or 16–24 oz for every pound)

Adapted with permission from Casa, D.J. et al. (2000). National Athletic Trainers' Association: Position statement: Fluid replacement for athletes. *Journal of Athletic Training,* 35, 212–224.

- *Measure fluid amounts:* When exercisers know how much they are actually drinking, they may be able to better assess if they are consuming appropriate amounts.
- *Drink fluids with sodium during prolonged exercise sessions:* If an exercise session lasts longer than two hours, experts recommend that the athlete consume a sports drink that contains elevated levels of sodium (Coyle, 2004). Note that researchers did not find a benefit from sports drinks that contained only 18 mmol/L (100 mg/8 oz) of sodium, which is the level typical of most sports drinks, and thus concluded that higher levels would be needed to prevent hyponatremia during prolonged exercise (Almond et al., 2005). Alternatively, exercisers can consume extra sodium with meals and snacks prior to a lengthy exercise session or a day of intensive physical activity (Casa, 2003).
- *Drink carbohydrate-containing sports drinks to reduce fatigue:* With prolonged exercise, muscle glycogen stores become depleted and blood glucose becomes a primary fuel source. To maintain performance levels and prevent fatigue, urge clients to consume drinks and snacks that provide 30 to 60 grams of rapidly absorbed carbohydrate for every hour of training (Coyle, 2004). As long as the carbohydrate concentration is less than about 6 to 8%, it will have little effect on gastric emptying (Coombes & Hamilton, 2000).
- *Hydrate appropriately pre- and post-event:* To maximize pre-event hydration, USATF recommends consuming 17 to 20 ounces of water or sports drink two to three hours before exercise, and 10 to 12 ounces of water or sports drink within 10 minutes of beginning exercise. Following exercise, the athlete should aim to correct any fluid imbalances that occurred during the exercise session. This includes con-

suming water to restore hydration, carbohydrates to replenish glycogen stores, and electrolytes to speed rehydration (Casa, 2003). Those at greatest risk of hyponatremia should be careful not to consume too much water following exercise and should focus instead on replenishing sodium.

- *Pay attention to environmental conditions:* Athletes who are well-acclimatized to heat will have reduced sodium losses in sweat, which lowers their risk of hyponatremia (Casa, 2003). Risk of heat stroke is elevated in conditions of elevated temperature and humidity and little or no wind due to the body's diminished ability to dissipate heat into the environment (Noakes, 2003).

The human body is well-equipped to withstand dramatic variations in fluid intake during exercise and at rest with little or no detrimental health effects. For this reason, most recreational exercisers will never suffer from serious hyponatremia or dehydration and should not be alarmed. It is under extreme situations of prolonged or very high-intensity exercise in excessive heat and humidity that risk is elevated. And even then, if athletes replenish sweat loss with equal amounts of fluid, hydration problems can be avoided.

Nutrition Applications in the Lifecycle

A well-balanced eating plan often extends beyond a one-size-fits-all dietary recommendation. At certain times, some individuals need slightly modified dietary recommendations to best meet their lifestyle, nutritional, and cultural needs.

While the USDA Dietary Guidelines are intended for all Americans ages two and older, some stages of the human lifecycle require special nutritional needs. LWMCs can best serve their clients who are in the midst of these stages by tailoring recommendations to address their specific needs.

Nutrition in Childhood and Adolescence

The American Academy of Pediatrics (AAP) and the American Heart Association (AHA) recommend a diet rich in fruits, vegetables, whole grains, low-fat and nonfat dairy products, beans, fish, and lean meat for children and adolescents, as well as for adults (AHA et al., 2006). Strategies to implement these recommendations are listed in Table 7-7.

A wide gap exists between nutrition recommendations for children and what children actually eat. Compared to the recent past, children and adolescents eat breakfast less often, eat meals away from home more often, and consume a greater proportion of calories from snacks and fried and nutrient-poor foods, larger portion sizes, fewer fruits and vegetables, excessive amounts of sodium, more sweetened beverages, and fewer dairy products (French, Story, & Jeffrey, 2001). In fact, on average children consume approximately 12 ounces of soft drinks per day, compared to just 5 ounces in 1978 (French, Lin, & Guthrie, 2003). And nearly 25% of adolescents drink more than 26 ounces of soda per day. Research suggests that high soda consumption displaces milk intake; that is, those who drink the most soda drink the least amount of milk (Harnack, Stang, & Story, 1999). As a result, children and especially

Table 7-7
Dietary Strategies for Individuals >2 Years

- Balance dietary calories with physical activity to maintain normal growth.
- Perform 60 minutes of moderate to vigorous play or physical activity daily.
- Eat vegetables and fruits daily, and limit juice intake.
- Use vegetable oils and soft margarines low in saturated fat and trans fatty acids instead of butter or most other animal fats in the diet.
- Eat whole-grain breads and cereals rather than refined-grain products.
- Reduce the intake of sugar-sweetened beverages and foods.
- Use nonfat (skim) or low-fat milk and dairy products daily.
- Eat more fish, especially oily fish, broiled or baked.
- Reduce salt intake, including salt from processed foods.

Source: American Heart Association et al. (2006). Dietary recommendations for children and adolescents: A guide for practitioners. *Pediatrics*, 117, 544–559.

adolescents consume less than the recommended values of many nutrients, including calcium and potassium (IOM, 2004).

The AAP and AHA recommend that the family and cultural background of the child be considered when making nutrition recommendations. Media messages, cultural beliefs that a chubby child is a healthy child, immediate access to inexpensive fast food, and motivation to change are all important determinants of a child's nutrition status. LWMCs are encouraged to adjust the recommendations presented in Table 7-8 based on each family's individual situation and circumstances.

Adolescents face unique nutritional challenges due to rapid bone growth and other maturational changes associated with the onset of puberty. While caloric and some micronutrient needs increase to support growth, adolescence is also a time of decreasing physical activity for many teens and increased independence when making food choices. Ready access to soda machines in schools, the prevalence of fast food restaurants, and peer and media pressure to eat fat- and sugar-laden foods make it easy for many teens to eat more calories than they expend, which puts them at greater risk for obesity. While the Dietary Guidelines and the MyPyramid Food Guidance System provide scientifically sound nutrition guidelines for teens, any nutrition advice offered must be individualized and consistent with the teen's readiness to change if it is to be successful (AHA et al., 2006).

Table 7-8
Improving Nutrition in Young Children

- Parents choose meal times, not children.
- Provide a wide variety of nutrient-dense foods such as fruits and vegetables instead of high-energy-density/nutrient-poor foods such as salty snacks, ice cream, fried foods, cookies, and sweetened beverages.
- Pay attention to portion size; serve portions appropriate for the child's size and age.
- Use nonfat or low-fat dairy products as sources of calcium and protein.
- Limit snacking during sedentary behavior or in response to boredom and particularly restrict the use of sweet/sweetened beverages as snacks (e.g., juice, soda, sports drinks).
- Limit sedentary behaviors, with no more than one to two hours per day of video screen/television and no televisions sets in children's bedrooms.
- Allow self-regulation of total caloric intake in the presence of normal BMI or weight for height.
- Have regular family meals to promote social interaction and role model food-related behavior.

Source: American Heart Association et al. (2006). Dietary recommendations for children and adolescents: A guide for practitioners. *Pediatrics*, 117, 544–559.

Nutrition in Aging

Optimal nutrition choices are important for successful aging, which is defined as the ability to maintain a low risk of disease, high mental and physical function, and active engagement in life (Rowe & Kahn, 1998). In fact, research suggests that eating a nutritious diet, engaging in regular physical activity, and not smoking are more important than genetics in helping people to avoid the deteriorating effects of aging (CDC, 2007).

While the U.S. suffers from an epidemic of obesity at least partly due to excessive caloric intake, many older adults are at risk of inadequate caloric intake to supply needed nutrients. Appetite often decreases with age and, as a result, many older adults do not consume enough of certain nutrients such as calcium, zinc, iron, and B vitamins. The decreased appetite likely is due to a combination of decreased taste and smell and altered appetite and **satiety** regulation. Older adults are also at risk of age-related nutrient malabsorption and dehydration resulting from a blunted thirst sensation, decreased functioning of the kidneys, medication side-effects, and other factors.

Though caloric intake may decrease, many older adults are overweight or obese because the age-related decrease in physical activity and metabolic rate is often more pronounced than reduced caloric intake. This scenario leads to a **positive energy balance** and weight gain.

The ADA recommends that older adults consume a variety of healthful foods to assure adequate nutrient intake and also adopt a healthful eating plan such as DASH to control chronic disease (ADA, 2005a). Furthermore, because up to 20% of people over age 65 suffer from constipation, the Dietary Guidelines recommend that older adults pay particular attention to consuming foods high in fiber (USDA, 2005). Nutrient supplementation may be necessary for some older adults with poor dietary intake. In these situations, referral to a registered dietitian is prudent.

Nutrition and Special Considerations

Many clients will have medical diagnoses such as cardiovascular disease or diabetes that require special nutrition recommendations beyond those articulated in the Dietary Guidelines. In these cases, it is advisable that the client work closely with his or her physician and a registered dietitian to develop an individualized eating plan. The LWMC's role is to provide support and encouragement for the client to follow the recommended plan. To be effective, it is important to understand the basic disease processes, as well as the general nutrition recommendations for these conditions.

Obesity

Nearly one-third of American adults are obese (Ogden et al., 2006). Obesity is defined as excess body fat and is often described as a body mass index greater than 30. Obese individuals face increased risk of myriad health problems, including many of the diseases discussed in this section (see Chapter 17 for more information about the causes and consequences of obesity). The key to successful nutritional management of obesity is to decrease caloric intake and increase caloric expenditure to create a **caloric deficit.** For these changes to be sustainable, the client must enjoy the overall eating plan and the recommended physical activities and be committed to maintaining a lifelong lifestyle change (ADA, 2005b).

Cardiovascular Disease

Cardiovascular disease is a leading killer of both men and women in the United States. It often results from atherosclerosis, which is a buildup of fatty plaques in the lining of arteries. The buildup causes the arteries to lose their elasticity and reduces the flow of blood to the rest of the body. When the atherosclerosis is particularly bad in the coronary arteries, which are the arteries that supply oxygen and nutrients to the heart, it can prevent oxygenation of the heart, leading to a **myocardial infarction,** or heart attack.

The AHA advises the following specific dietary strategies for optimal cardiovascular risk reduction (Lichenstein et al., 2006):

- Balance caloric intake and physical activity to achieve and maintain a healthy weight.
- Consume a diet rich in fruits and vegetables.
- Choose whole-grain, high-fiber foods.
- Consume fish, especially oil fish such as salmon and tuna, at least two times per week.
- Limit intake of saturated fat to less than 7% of energy, trans fat to less than 1% of energy, and cholesterol to less than 300 mg per day by choosing lean meats, vegetable alternatives, and low- and nonfat dairy products, and minimizing intake of partially hydrogenated fats.
- Minimize intake of beverages and foods with sugars.
- Choose and prepare foods with little or no salt.
- Consume alcohol in moderation, or not at all.
- Follow these recommendations when eating food prepared outside the home.

Hypertension

Hypertension is often called the "silent killer" because it is asymptomatic in most individuals, and often causes substantial damage in the heart, kidneys, and nervous system without the individual ever knowing that something is wrong. The best nutritional management for the prevention and treatment of hypertension is the DASH eating plan, along with sodium restriction in salt-sensitive individuals.

Diabetes

Diabetes is a condition that results from abnormal regulation of blood glucose. **Type 1 diabetes** results from the inability of the pancreas to secrete **insulin,** the hormone that allows the cells to take up glucose from the bloodstream. Type 2 diabetes results from the cells' decreased ability to respond to insulin. In most cases, the nutrition recommendations for individuals with diabetes closely resemble the Dietary Guidelines. However, it is especially important for people with diabetes to balance food intake with exercise and insulin or other medications to maintain a regular blood sugar level throughout the day.

A low-glycemic eating plan may be beneficial for people with diabetes (Brand-Miller et al., 2003). Remember, the glycemic index (GI) ranks carbohydrates based on their blood glucose response. High-GI foods break down rapidly, causing a large glucose spike; low-GI foods are digested more slowly and cause a smaller glucose increase. Thus, blood glucose levels are lower after eating a low-GI food versus a high-GI food. In general, foods high in soluble fiber, such as whole-grain barley, rye, oats, pasta, and less-starchy vegetables have low GI. The **glycemic load (GL)** accounts for GI as well as portion size.

GL = [GI x grams of carbohydrate]/100

A low-GL diet can create a more favorable glucose and insulin profile than a high-GL diet. Thus, without having to make drastic dietary changes, individuals with diabetes may benefit from reducing the consumption of soft drinks and from replacing high-GI grains with low-GI grains, and starchy vegetables with less-starchy vegetables (Liu, 2006).

Cancer

Nutrition plays an important role both in the treatment, and possibly the prevention, of cancer, a disease in which abnormal cells grow uncontrollably. For cancer prevention, the American Cancer Society (ACS) recommends a diet high in fruits, vegetables, and whole grains, and limited in red meat and alcohol, along with regular physical activity and maintenance of a healthy weight (ACS, 2002). The National Cancer Institute (NCI) also emphasizes the important role of nutrition in the treatment of cancer. A nutrient-dense diet can help a person enduring chemotherapy treatment to maintain strength and positive mood, and also improve prognosis. However, treatment often causes symptoms, such as nausea, vomiting, diarrhea, constipation, and decreased appetite, that interfere with optimal intake (NCI, 2005). Assuring adequate protein and calorie intake are the primary goals of a meal plan for an individual with cancer.

Osteoporosis

Osteoporosis is defined as a weakening of the bones due to excessive bone mineral loss that can lead to fractures of the hip, spine, and other skeletal sites. The disease most often affects elderly women, although it can occur in men and younger women as well. Nutrition therapy for the prevention and treatment of osteoporosis includes adequate calcium intake, which is modestly correlated with bone mineral density, and adequate vitamin D intake. Vitamin D deficiency is associated with higher bone turnover, reduced calcium absorption, and decreased bone mass. To protect against bone weakening and osteoporosis, the IOM recommends that most adults consume 1000 mg of calcium, which is the equivalent of three glasses of milk (far more than most Americans consume), and 400 to 600 IU of vitamin D each day (Ma et al., 2007; IOM, 2004). Smoking and a sedentary lifestyle also increase the risk of osteoporosis, while engaging in weightbearing physical activity may decrease risk (Mahan & Escott-Stump, 2007).

Iron-deficiency Anemia

Up to 20% of women age 18 to 44 have **iron-deficiency anemia** (ADA, 2004). Iron is an important component of hemoglobin, the protein complex responsible for delivering oxygen to muscles and the body's other cells. With iron deficiency, less oxygen is available for cells to use to make energy. As a result, iron deficiency decreases energy levels and endurance capacity. It also can induce preterm labor and result in low birth weight. Infants, adolescent girls, pregnant women, endurance athletes, and elderly women are at highest risk of iron-deficiency anemia (ADA, 2004). To prevent iron-deficiency anemia, advise clients to consume adequate amounts of iron-rich foods; consume a source of vitamin C at each meal to increase iron absorption; include a serving of meat, fish, or poultry at each meal; and avoid drinking large amounts of coffee or tea, which contain tannins that interfere with iron absorption (Mahan & Escott-Stump, 2007).

Pregnancy and Breastfeeding

During pregnancy, an expectant mother requires adequate nutrients not only to fuel her own body, but also to provide for the growth and development of the fetus. The most important nutritional consideration for pregnant women begins before conception. All women of childbearing age should take a 400-microgram folic acid supplement for at least four months prior to conception and during pregnancy to prevent neural tube defects in the developing fetus. Because the brain and spinal cord develop early in the first trimester—often before a woman even knows that she is pregnant—folic acid is vital for all women of reproductive age, regardless of when they intend to become pregnant. **Vegans** and strict **vegetarians** should also take a vitamin B12 supplement, because the vitamin is present only in meat products and, like folic acid, helps to ensure healthy **central nervous system (CNS)** development. The Dietary Guidelines also suggest that women of childbearing age consume foods high in iron, such as lean red meats and dark green vegetables; fruits and other foods with high levels of vitamin C will help to increase iron absorption (USDA, 2005).

During pregnancy, caloric needs increase by approximately 300 calories per day. Pregnant women are encouraged to meet increased energy demands by following the 2005 Dietary Guidelines and consuming a healthful diet containing a wide variety of wholesome foods for optimal nutrition and growth of the fetus. Women should consume the appropriate number of calories to gain a healthy amount of weight during the pregnancy. Table 7-9 provides recommendations for weight gain during pregnancy based on pre-pregnancy **body mass index (BMI)** (ADA, 2002a). Research suggests that women of normal weight who adhere to weight-gain guidelines have a lower risk of poor pregnancy outcomes (DeVader et al., 2007), while obese women who gain little or no weight during pregnancy fare best (Kiel et al., 2007). Some women may require other nutritional guidance and supplementation during pregnancy. A woman's obstetrician and/or a registered dietitian are most qualified to make supplementation and specific dietary recommendations, as this is beyond the **scope of practice** of an LWMC.

Prior to the child's birth, most women will decide whether or not to breastfeed. An LWMC can play an important role in encouraging breastfeeding, although the woman's healthcare providers are formally charged with the responsibility. Ultimately, however, the decision of whether or not to breastfeed is up to the woman and should be respected.

Table 7-9
Recommended Weight Gain During Pregnancy

	Recommended Weight Gain	Weight Gain per Week After 12 Weeks
BMI <19.8	28–40 lb (12.7–18.2 kg)	1 lb (0.5 kg)
BMI of 19.8–26.0	25–35 lb (11.4–15.9 kg)	0.4 kg
BMI of 26.0–29.0	15–25 lb (6.8–11.4 kg)	0.3 kg
BMI >29.0	at least 15 lb (6.8 kg)	—
Twin pregnancy	34–45 lb (15.4–20.4 kg)	0.7 kg
Triplet pregnancy	overall gain of 50 lb (22.7 kg)	—

Note: BMI = Body mass index

Source: Reprinted from *Journal of the American Dietetic Association,* Vol. 102: Position of the American Dietetic Association: Nutrition and lifestyle for a healthy pregnancy outcome. 1479–1490, 2002a, with permission from Elsevier.

Breastfeeding, as opposed to formula, is thought to provide optimal nutrition and health protection for the first six months of life, according to a position statement of the ADA. Six to 12 months of breastfeeding combined with the introduction of complementary foods is optimal (ADA, 2005b). Table 7-10 outlines the benefits of breastfeeding for both mother and child. Women who breastfeed require approximately 500 additional calories per day for weight maintenance. Thus, breastfeeding generally facilitates postpartum weight loss.

LWMCs can also assist with postpartum weight loss by reinforcing the positive lifestyle changes that were likely made during pregnancy. For example, LWMCs should encourage the client to maintain behaviors such as quitting smoking and eating more fruits, vegetables, and whole grains. Also, LWMCs should facilitate entry or re-entry into a regular physical-activity program.

Vegetarian Diets

A growing number of Americans are vegetarians, which means they do not eat meat, fish, poultry, or products containing these foods. Vegetarian diets come in several forms, all of which are healthful, nutritionally adequate, and effective for disease prevention if carefully planned. A **lacto-ovo-vegetarian** does not eat meat, fish, or poultry, but does eat dairy products and eggs. A **lacto-vegetarian** does not eat eggs, meat, fish, or poultry, but does eat dairy products. A vegan does not consume any animal products, including dairy products such as milk and cheese.

Vegetarian diets provide several health advantages. These diets are generally low in saturated fat, cholesterol, and animal protein, and high in fiber, folate, vitamins C and E, carotenoids, and some phytochemicals. Compared to nonvegetarians, vegetarians have lower rates of obesity, death from cardiovascular disease, hypertension, **type 2 diabetes,** and prostate and colon cancer. However, if poorly planned, vegetarian diets (especially vegan diets) may include insufficient amounts of protein, iron, vitamins B12 and D, calcium, and other nutrients (ADA, 2003).

Quality protein intake is crucial for vegetarians. A main determinant of protein quality is whether a food contains all of the **essential amino acids** in amounts proportional to need. **Amino acids** are the basic building blocks of protein. There are eight to 10 essential amino acids, which are amino acids that the body cannot produce itself and therefore must be consumed in the diet. Most meat-based products are higher-quality proteins, because they have varying amounts of the essential amino acids, while plant proteins (other than soy) are incomplete proteins, because they do not contain all of the

Table 7-10
The Benefits of Breastfeeding

Benefits for Infant	Benefits for Mother
• Provides optimal nutrition for infant	• Promotes faster shrinking of the uterus
• Guarantees safe, fresh milk	• Reduces postpartum bleeding
• Enhances immune system	• Decreases risk of breast and ovarian cancer
• Protects against infectious and non-infectious diseases	• Delays resumption of the menstrual cycle
• Protects against allergies and intolerances	• Improves bone density
• Decreases risk of diarrhea and respiratory infections	• Decreases risk for hip fracture
• Promotes correct development of jaws, teeth, and speech patterns	• Improves glucose profile in gestational diabetics
• Decreases risk of childhood obesity	• Strengthens bond with the infant
• Increases cognitive function	• Enhances self-esteem in the maternal role
• Reduces risk for heart disease	• Eliminates the need for preparing and mixing formula
• Increases bonding with mother	• Saves money not spent on formula

Source: Reprinted from *Journal of the American Dietetic Association,* Vol. 105: Position of the American Dietetic Association: Nutrition and lifestyle for a healthy pregnancy outcome. 1479–1490, 2005a, with permission from Elsevier.

essential amino acids in the amount proportional to individual need. However, complementary plant products such as rice and beans (or other grains and legumes) consumed during the course of the day combine to provide all the essential amino acids in appropriate amounts (Figure 7-3). Research suggests that most vegetarians consume adequate amounts of complementary plant proteins throughout the day to meet their protein needs. It is important to note that the complementary proteins do not need to be consumed in the same meal (ADA, 2003).

Vegetarians must carefully plan their diets to ensure adequate nutrient intake of a variety of micronutrients. The vegetarian food guide pyramid (Figure 7-4) provides minimum recommendations for each of the food groups to assure adequate nutrient intake. The minimum recommendations provide approximately 1,400 to 1,500 calories per day; vegetarians are encouraged to consume additional servings to meet caloric needs (Messina, Melina, & Mangels, 2003).

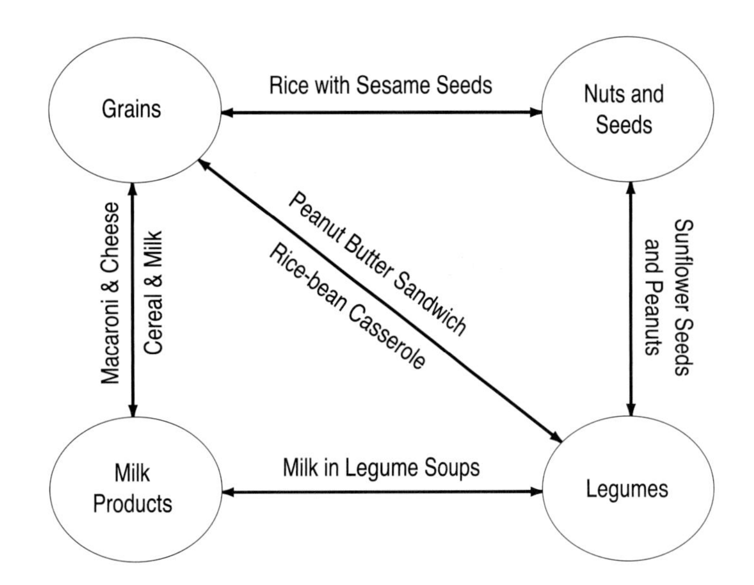

Figure 7-3
Protein complementarity chart

Adapted with permission from Lappé, F.M. (1992). *Diet for a Small Planet.* New York: Ballantine Books.

Cultural Considerations

Flavor, price, tradition, and emotional and social meaning of food are critical factors to consider when providing dietary recommendations. It is important to recommend healthful food choices that are compatible with the client's typical eating patterns, cultural beliefs about food, and overall lifestyle. In most situations, retaining pieces of the

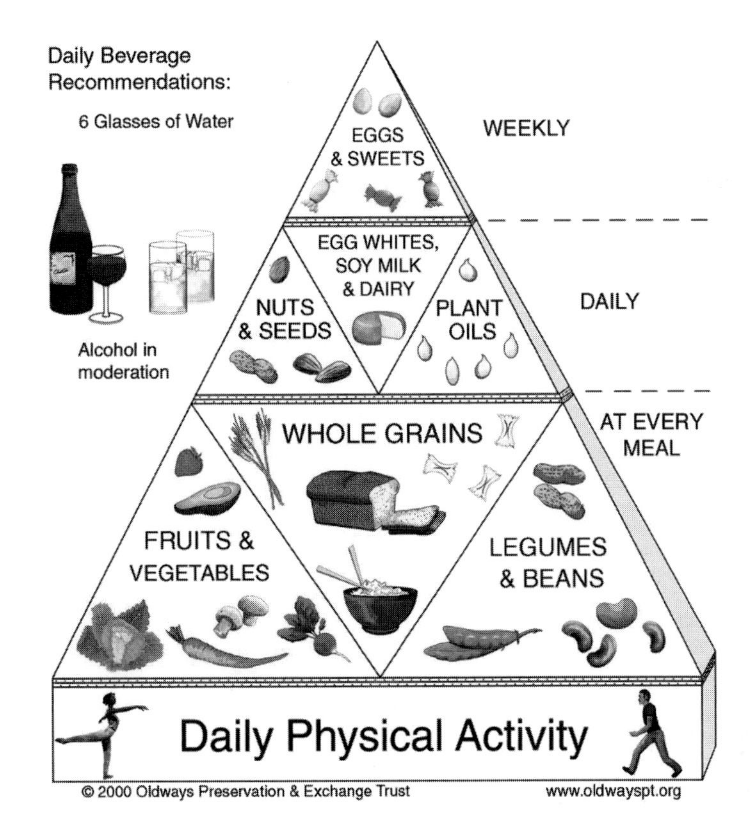

Figure 7-4
Vegetarian Food Guide Pyramid

Source: Reprinted with permission from www.oldwayspt.org

individual's customary eating habits is advisable. After all, adopting a more Westernized diet often leads to increased intake of calories, refined carbohydrates, fat, processed foods, and sodium, and reduced consumption of complex carbohydrates, fruits, and vegetables. Together, these changes lead to dramatic increases in obesity. However, some traditional eating patterns, such as the typical diet in the Southeastern United States, are less healthy than the standard American fare. In those cases, it may be advisable to help individuals adopt more mainstream eating habits, or better yet, make healthy substitutions for high-fat and low-nutrient-density foods in their traditional diets (Kumanyika, 2006).

Summary

Clients rely on LWMCs to provide them with credible nutrition recommendations and advice to develop a healthy eating plan and lifestyle. Utilize sources such as the Dietary Guidelines and MyPyramid when making recommendations to clients and refer to a registered dietitian when clients need individualized nutrition plans. And remember that the primary objective of an LWMC is to help clients transform nutrition information and recommendations into action.

References

Almond, C.S.D. et al. (2005). Hyponatremia among runners in the Boston Marathon. *New England Journal of Medicine,* 352, 15, 1550–1556.

American Cancer Society (2002). The complete guide—nutrition and physical activity. http://www.cancer.org/docroot/PED/content/PED_3_2X_Diet_and_Activity_Factors_That_Affect_Risks.asp?sitearea=PED.

American Dietetic Association (2005a). Position paper of the American Dietetic Association: Nutrition across the spectrum of aging. *Journal of the American Dietetic Association,* 105, 4, 616–633.

American Dietetic Association (2005b). Position of the American Dietetic Association: Promoting and supporting breastfeeding. *Journal of the American Dietetic Association,* 105, 5, 810–818.

American Dietetic Association (2004). Position of the American Dietetic Association and Dietitians of Canada: Nutrition and women's health. *Journal of the American Dietetic Association,* 104, 6, 984–1001.

American Dietetic Association (2003). Position of the American Dietetic Association and Dietitians of Canada: Vegetarian diets. *Journal of the American Dietetic Association,* 103, 6, 748–765.

American Dietetic Association (2002a). Position of the American Dietetic Association: Nutrition and lifestyle for a healthy pregnancy outcome. *Journal of the American Dietetic Association,* 102, 10, 1479–1490.

American Dietetic Association (2002b). Position of the American Dietetic Association: Weight management. *Journal of the American Dietetic Association,* 102, 8, 1145–1155.

American Dietetic Association (2000). Position of the American Dietetic Association, Dietitians of Canada, and the American College of Sports Medicine: Nutrition and athletic performance. *Journal of the American Dietetic Association,* 100, 12, 1543–1556.

American Heart Association et al. (2006). Dietary recommendations for children and adolescents: A guide for practitioners. *Pediatrics,* 117, 544–559.

Brand-Miller, J., et al. (2003). Low-glycemic index diets in the management of diabetes: A meta-analysis of randomized controlled trials. *Diabetes Care,* 26, 8, 2261–2267.

Casa, D.J. (2003). Proper hydration for distance running—identifying individual fluid needs: A USA Track & Field advisory. www.usatf.org/groups/Coaches/library/hydration/ProperHydrationForDistanceRunning.pdf.

Casa, D.J., Clarkson, P.M., & Roberts, W.O. (2005). American College of Sports Medicine roundtable on hydration and physical activity: Consensus statements. *Current Sports Medicine Reports,* 4, 115–127.

Casa, D.J. et al. (2000). National Athletic Trainers' Association Position Statement: Fluid replacement for athletes. *Journal of Athletic Training,* 35, 212–224

Centers for Disease Control and Prevention (2007). Healthy aging: Preserving function and improving quality of life among older Americans. www.cdc.gov/nccdphp/aag/aag_aging.htm.

Centers for Disease Control and Prevention (2004). Health, 2004 with chartbook on trends in the health of Americans. www.cdc.gov/nchs/data/hus/hus04trend.pdf#067.

Champagne, C.M. (2006). Dietary interventions on blood pressure: The Dietary Approaches to Stop Hypertension (DASH) trials. *Nutrition Reviews,* 64, 2, (II), S53–S56.

Clemson University Cooperative Extension (1999). Food selection and storage. http://hgic.clemson.edu/factsheets/HGIC3480.htm.

Convertino, V.A. et al. (1996). American College of Sports Medicine position stand: Exercise and fluid replacement. *Medicine & Science in Sports & Exercise.* 28, 1, i–vii.

Coombes, J.S. & Hamilton, K.L. (2000). The effectiveness of commercially available sports drinks. *Sports Medicine,* 29, 3, 181–209.

Coyle, E.F. (2004). Fluid and fuel intake during exercise. *Journal of Sports Sciences,* 22, 1, 39–55.

DeVader, S.R. et al. (2007). Evaluation of gestational weight gain guidelines for women with normal pre-pregnancy body mass index. *Obstetrics & Gynecology,* 110, 4, 745–751.

Frankenfield, D., Routh-Yousey, L., & Compher, C. (2005). Comparison of predictive equations of resting metabolic rates in healthy non-obese and obese adults: A systematic review. *Journal of the American Dietetic Association,* 105, 5, 775–789.

French, S.A., Lin, B., & Guthrie, J.F. (2003). National trends in soft drink consumption among children and adolescents age 6 to 17 years; prevalence, amounts, and sources, 1977–1978 to 1994–1999. *Journal of the American Dietetic Association,* 103, 1326–1331.

French, S.A., Story, M., & Jeffrey, R.W. (2001). Environmental influences on eating and physical activity. *Annual Reviews of Public Health,* 22, 309–335.

Harnack, L., Stang, J., & Story, M. (1999). Soft drink consumption among U.S. children and adolescents: Nutritional consequences. *Journal of the American Dietetic Association,* 99, 436–441.

Institute of Medicine (2005). Dietary Reference Intakes for energy, carbohydrate, fiber, fat, fatty acids, cholesterol, protein, and amino acids. Washington, D.C.: National Academy Press.

Institute of Medicine (2004). Dietary Reference Intakes for calcium, magnesium, phosphorus, vitamin D, and fluoride. Washington, D.C.: National Academy Press.

Jentjens, R. & Jeukendrup, A.E. (2003). Determinants of post-exercise glycogen synthesis during short-term recovery. *Sports Medicine,* 33, 2, 117–144.

Kiel, D.W. et al. (2007). Gestational weight gain and pregnancy outcomes in obese women: How much is enough? *Obstetrics & Gynecology,* 110, 4, 752–758.

Kumanyika, S. (2006). Nutrition and chronic disease prevention: Priorities for U.S. minority groups. *Nutrition Reviews,* 64, 2, (II), S9–S14.

Lichenstein, A.H. et al. (2006). Diet and lifestyle recommendations revision 2006: A scientific statement from the American Heart Association Nutrition Committee. *Circulation,* 114, 82–96.

Liu, S. (2006). Lowering dietary glycemic load for weight control and cardiovascular health: A matter of quality. *Annals of Internal Medicine,* 166, 1428–1439.

Ma, J. et al. (2007). Americans are not meeting current calcium recommendations. *American Journal of Clinical Nutrition,* 85, 5, 1361–1366.

Mahan L.K. & Escott-Stump, S. (2007). *Krause's Food Nutrition and Diet Therapy* (12th ed.). Philadelphia, Pa.: W.B. Saunders Company.

Messina, V., Melina, V., & Mangels, A.R. (2003). A new food guide for North American vegetarians. *Canadian Journal of Dietetic Practice and Research,* 64, 2, 82–86.

National Cancer Institute (2005). Overview of nutrition in cancer care. http://www.cancer.gov/cancertopics/pdq/supportivecare/nutrition/Patient/page1.

Noakes, T. (2003). Fluid replacement during marathon running. *Clinical Journal of Sport Medicine,* 13, 309–318.

Ogden, C.L. et al. (2006). Prevalence of overweight and obesity in the United States, 1999–2004. *Journal of the American Medical Association,* 295, 13, 1549–1555.

Rowe, J.W. & Kahn R.L. (1998). *Successful Aging.* New York: Pantheon Books.

Thomas, D.E., Elliott, E., & Baur, L. (2007). Low glycemic index or low glycemic load diets for overweight and obesity. *Cochrane Database of Systematic Reviews,* 18, 3, CD005105.

U.S. Department of Agriculture (2005). Dietary Guidelines for Americans 2005. www.health.gov/dietaryguidelines.

U.S. Food and Drug Administration, Center for Food Safety and Applied Nutrition (2004). How to understand and use the nutrition facts label. http://www.cfsan.fda.gov/~dms/foodlab.html#twoparts.

Suggested Reading

Clark, N. (2003). *Nancy Clark's Sports Nutrition Guidebook* (3rd ed.). Champaign, Ill.: Human Kinetics.

Dunford, M. (2005). *Sports Nutrition: A Practice Manual for Professionals* (4th ed.). Washington, D.C.: American Dietetic Association.

Institute of Medicine (1990). *Nutrition During Pregnancy, Weight Gain and Nutrient Supplements: Report of the Subcommittee on Nutritional Status and Weight Gain During Pregnancy*. Washington, D.C.: National Academy Press.

National Heart Lung and Blood Institute. The DASH eating plan. http://www.nhlbi.nih.gov/health/public/heart/hbp/dash.

Willett, W. (2006). *Eat, Drink, and Be Healthy: The Harvard Medical School Guide to Healthy Eating* (2nd ed.). New York: Free Press.

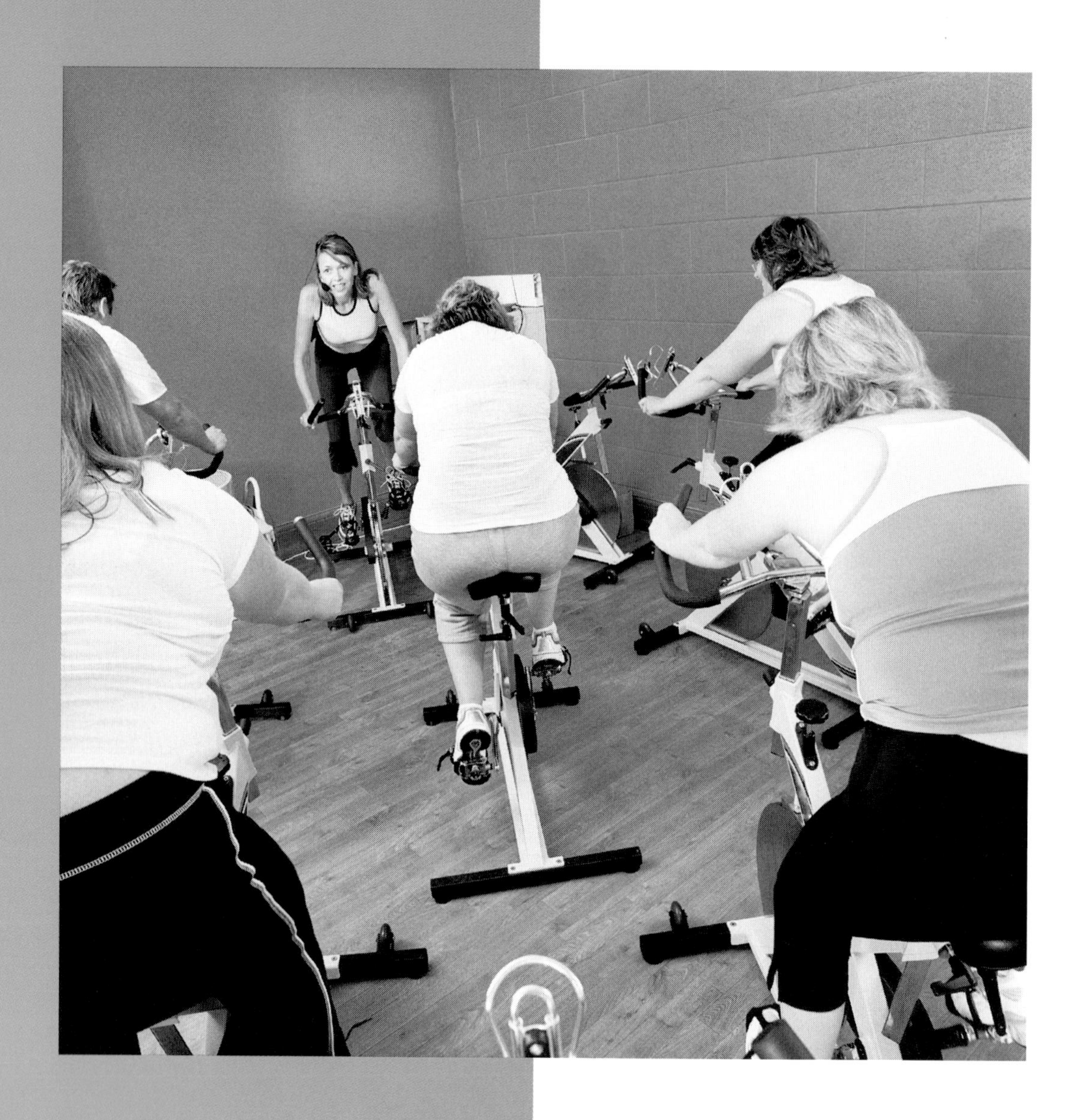

Jenna A. Bell-Wilson

Jenna A. Bell-Wilson, Ph.D., R.D., C.S.S.D., is a board-certified specialist in sports dietetics and a nutrition consultant. Dr. Bell-Wilson's areas of focus include sports nutrition, weight loss, healthy living, metabolism, and exercise physiology. Dr. Bell-Wilson earned her doctorate in exercise science at the University of New Mexico (UNM), master's degree in nutrition and dietetic internship at UNM, and bachelor's degree in nutritional sciences from the University of New Hampshire.

Chapter 8

Current Concepts in Weight Management

IN THIS CHAPTER:

The number of **overweight** and obese individuals in the United States frequently makes headlines in both consumer magazines and scientific journals. The growth in **obesity** numbers is rivaled only by the increase in weight-loss fads, from Internet programs to best-selling books. Health professionals are concerned and consumers are eager to find quick-fix solutions and remedies. This chapter reviews some popular diets and their associated health risks, details the slippery slope to eating disorders, and explains the health consequences of each eating disorder. To begin the discussion, a review of energy balance—the calories taken in compared to those expended—is provided. Chapter 17 offers a more detailed look at the development of obesity and the way in which the body regulates energy balance through hormones, genetics, and intake.

Energy Balance and Weight Control

It is sometimes said that "life is a balancing act." Each day, financial statements are balanced, work is balanced against play, and individuals pursue a balance between their home lives and careers. Unbeknownst to many, the body is busy balancing energy as well. The balance between energy intake and energy output influences energy stores, such as body fat and **lean body mass.** This balance can be mathematically described with the following equations:

Energy intake – Energy output = Energy balance
Calories consumed – Calories expended = Energy balance

When an individual finds himself in a state of **positive energy balance,** the storage of energy exceeds the amount expended. This state may be achieved by either consuming too many calories or by not using enough. Times of positive energy balance, during which an increase in calories is required, include phases of growth—infancy, childhood, and pregnancy. Otherwise, a positive energy balance results in weight gain.

On the other hand, a **negative energy balance** reflects a state in which the number of calories expended is greater than what is taken in, thereby contributing to weight loss. For example, if an individual eats fewer calories than she works off through her exercise program and burns via basic metabolism and food digestion, she will find herself in a calorie deficit and weight loss will result.

Finding a balance between intake and output throughout life is the cornerstone of maintaining a healthy weight and has been linked to numerous longevity-related benefits (Stubbs & Tolkamp, 2006). Achieving this balance, although seemingly straightforward, is very challenging over time, as evidenced by the growing number of overweight and obese Americans and the continual struggle to find the perfect diet.

Energy Requirements

The components of an individual's energy requirements must be considered in the pursuit of weight loss and the balance between intake and output. An understanding of the factors that contribute to a person's overall energy (or calorie) requirements allows for an assessment of the efficacy of popular diets and answers questions regarding how an energy deficit can be created for weight loss.

Energy Intake

The amount of food eaten in a day is dictated by a variety of factors. Availability, personal preferences, traditions, culture, social influences, psychological factors, and nutrition goals are on the long list of reasons why people eat what they do. The primary reason for taking in food, however, is to support the demands put on the body, from normal metabolism to physical work. This process has evolved over the centuries as the environment has changed. Food ingestion is imperative to survival and ecologists have studied the alterations that have occurred as eating has transitioned from being strictly survival-related to a behavioral response. Food establishments riddle major and minor roadways, eliminating the need for hunting and gathering meals. Therefore, the need to salvage and store intake has lessened. The environment may be overly dictating people's intake, thereby ameliorating the focus on food as a means of survival (see Chapter 17).

Energy Output

The determinants of calorie needs are influenced by energy output. This output includes calories "burned," or used, for normal metabolic functions, during physical activity, and as a result of the **thermic effect of food (TEF).** Add these factors together, and an estimate of **total energy expenditure (TEE)** can be determined.

Basal Metabolism

For all systems to work properly, a minimum amount of energy is required. This is referred to as basal metabolism, or **basal energy expenditure (BEE).** BEE allows the body to rest, maintain core temperature in ambient conditions, and survive. BEE, the calorie expenditure in a fasting state (12 to 14 hours after a meal), is influenced by several factors (Table 8-1), and makes up approximately 60 to 70% of the TEE (Shetty, 2005).

Physical Activity

Energy is needed to sustain the work of physical activity. The calories expended above and beyond BMR via physical activity make up approximately 25 to 40% of TEE. The amount of physical activity varies from per-

Table 8-1
Factors Affecting Basal Energy Expenditure (BEE)

Factor	Affect on BEE	Comments
Age	↓	Metabolism declines with age; age-related loss of lean body mass likely contributes to this decline
Body Temperature	↑	Seen with temperature extremes; fever and hypothermia (shivering)
Caffeine and Nicotine	↑	Act as stimulants to increase BEE
Gender	↑ ↓	Males tend to have higher BEEs due to increases in lean body mass
Sympathetic Nervous System Activity	↑ ↓	Norepinephrine is associated with an increase in BEE
Nutritional Status	↓	Reduced calorie intake can depress BEE
Pregnancy	↑	BEE increases gradually throughout pregnancy
Thyroid Hormones	↑ ↓	People with too much thyroid hormone (hyperthyroidism) have increased RMR, and those (hypothryroidism) have decreased BEE

Note: ↑ = increase; ↓ = decrease; ↑ ↓ = variable

Sources: Shetty, P. (2005). Energy requirements of adults. *Public Health Nutrition*, 8, 7A, 994–1009; Wardlaw, G.M. & Hampl, J.S. (2006). *Perspectives in Nutrition* (7th ed.). New York: McGraw-Hill.

son to person, with many unfortunately choosing a sedentary lifestyle.

Physical activity is the most easily manipulated component of TEE, and therefore plays a key role in creating an energy deficit when weight loss is desired. An individual can expend hundreds of calories on a daily basis by consistently performing exercise. Chapter 12 reviews the process of designing a weight-loss program and covers the importance of exercise.

Thermic Effect of Food

To digest and absorb **nutrients** from food, energy must be used. The total cost of this process makes up approximately 5 to 10% of TEE. Interestingly, the **macronutrient** composition of a meal can affect the thermic effect, or the number of calories required to digest and absorb it. The thermic effect of food (TEF) associated with the consumption of a high-protein meal is significantly higher than it is following a high-carbohydrate or high-fat meal. (Wardlaw & Hampl, 2006). The significance of this difference is still unclear in the long-term view of diet programs and weight-loss success.

Popular Diets and Associated Health Risks

If there is any question about whether diets are popular, simply typing the term "weight loss" into any online search engine will provide answers. It is likely that more than one million sites will pop up, many of which make grandiose claims and promises, and offer twists on similar themes. The search for weight-loss solutions hasn't relented in the recent past in either pop culture or the world of research. Investigations have continued, as individuals diligently pursue the easiest way to balance energy and lose weight. The following sections review popular diets and describe the health-related risks associated with them. Also, see Appendix C for additional information regarding the evaluation of popular diets.

Carbohydrate-restricted Diets

A number of popular diets with a variety of names and catchphrases fall under the umbrella of carbohydrate-restricted diets. Because of the plethora of diets touting themselves as carbohydrate-restricted plans, and with science testing a variety of carb levels, consumers are often confused by what carb restriction entails. There are carbohydrate-modified diets, such as The Zone®, Carbohydrate Addict's Diet®, and the South Beach diet®, but a low-carb diet is defined by Last and Wilson (2006) as a diet plan consisting of less than 20% of a day's calories from carbohydrate, or 20 to 60 grams per day. Arguably the most popular of its kind, the Atkins Diet® epitomizes this blend of low-carb eating with generous protein and fat.

Proponents of low-carbohydrate diets claim that by eliminating or restricting sugars and carbohydrates, weight loss will ensue. Health professionals, including those in the American Dietetic Association and the American Heart Association, express concerns about the long-term safety of such diets and encourage individuals to tread lightly (Stein, 2000; St. Jeor et al., 2001). Reservations exist regarding the influence that carb restriction could have on chronic disease development, especially cardiovascular disease risk factors, **type 2 diabetes,** and **osteoporosis,** as well as nutrient deficiencies (Bravata et al., 2003). Low-carbohydrate diets have been associated with deficiencies of vitamin A, B6, C, and E; thiamine; folate; calcium; magnesium; iron, potassium; and fiber (Freedman, King, & Kennedy, 2001). Headaches and constipation are common complaints among people following a carbohydrate-restrictive diet (Astrup, Larsen, & Harper, 2004).

Several controlled trials have attempted to find answers to the following questions: Do carbohydrate-restricted diets promote weight loss? And more importantly, are they safe?

A randomized, controlled trial published in the *New England Journal of Medicine* sought to compare the traditional, higher-carbohydrate, energy-restricted diet to the Atkins low-carbohydrate plan. At six months, participants abiding by the Atkins principles showed a significantly greater weight loss (7.0%, SD 6.5) than those following the traditional plan (3.2%, SD 5.6) However, at 12 months, no difference between the groups could be detected (Foster et al., 2003).

Identified as diets of less than 20% of total calories from carbohydrates, modified carbohydrate diets have also become popular. These versions of "low-carb" diets typically are below the **Acceptable Macronutrient Distribution Range** of 45 to 65% of total calories from carbohydrates (Krieger et al., 2006). A meta-regression was performed by Krieger and colleagues (2006) to see how these low-carb diets performed during calorie restriction and to observe the effect that varying levels of protein have on body mass and composition. After sorting through the research, 87 studies were included in their analysis in an effort to delineate the predictors of weight and body composition. After researchers divided the data into quartiles of lower and higher intakes of protein and carbohydrate, protein was found to be a significant predictor of fat-free mass maintenance during a calorie reduction (an average level of 1.05 g/kg/day as opposed to the 0.8 g/kg/day prescribed by the RDA). The *lowest* levels of carbohydrate intake (less than 35 to 41.5% of total calories) were associated with a greater amount of body-weight loss and body-fat reduction. However, low-carbohydrate diets were also linked to a loss of fat-free mass that was greater than those seen with the low-fat diets. The authors concluded that a more generous amount of protein (>1.05 g/kg/day) may be beneficial during calorie restriction. It is important to note that the level of carbohydrate is above that suggested by the more restrictive carb diets, such as the Atkins Diet.

In an attempt to address the safety and efficacy concerns, Bravata and colleagues (2003) extensively reviewed the low-carb-related literature. Studies were evaluated for changes in weight, serum lipids, blood glucose, serum insulin, and blood pressure in outpatient settings. The researchers concluded that the data were insufficient to support the claim that low-carb diets promote weight loss better than traditional diets. As may be expected, diets that restricted calories and had a longer duration yielded improved weight-loss outcomes. Carbohydrate restriction alone was not associated with alterations in serum lipid, fasting glucose, or blood pressure.

Experts appear to agree that an insufficient amount of evidence is available to support the claim that carbohydrate restriction alone promotes weight loss. Despite the lack of certainty that such diets are the ideal approach to losing extra pounds, they appear to be safe in the short term. However, long-term studies are lacking.

High-fat Diets

Dietary fat has long been synonymous with "unhealthy" and "disease-promoting." It is often considered the root of obesity and assumed to be the greatest culprit in its development. As discussed in Chapter 6, dietary fat has specific and important purposes in the human body. Despite its necessity, fat can be prohibitive in terms of an individual's efforts to lose weight. Remembering that energy balance is achieved through equalizing energy intake and output, fat, which has nine calories per gram, compared to the four calories per gram found in carbohydrates and protein, can substantially influence the ability to create the negative caloric balance needed for weight reduction. In considering the role that fat plays, experts review its affect on **satiety, thermogenesis,** and fat storage (Wenk, 2004; Westerterp-Plantenga, 2004).

Simply put, satiety is the feeling of fullness after eating. If a person is satiated, it will be reflected in how much he or she chooses to eat after the meal. When assessed for its affect on satiety, as well as thermogenesis, a high-fat diet shows a lesser influence on satiety during the meal and throughout the day, and a lower thermogenic effect compared to a protein/carbohydrate diet (Westerterp-Plantenga, 2004). With less of an effect on how full a person feels, as well as a lower thermogenic effect, a high-fat diet could be an obstacle to weight loss.

In addition to its relatively limited effect on fullness and thermogenesis, dietary fat is easily stored as fat (Wenk, 2004). Forming body fat from dietary fat is easy compared to doing so from carbohydrates and protein because of fat's high digestibility and metabolic efficiency. As a result of the aforementioned effects, a high-fat diet is generally incompatible with the quest to lose weight.

High-protein Diets

As discussed earlier in this chapter, de-emphasizing carbs, while pushing protein, has become a popular weight-loss technique. The promotion of protein dates back to the 1860s, when William Banting attributed his 21-kg (46.2-pound) weight loss to his ample protein intake, exclaiming that he did this without feeling hungry (Astrup, Larsen, & Harper, 2004). High-protein diets (above the 0.8 g/kg RDA) have received attention in the public, media, and among researchers. Protein's role in weight maintenance stems from its potential for increasing satiety and thermogenesis, and its role in maintaining fat-free mass. During a calorie restriction, fat-free mass is lost and could potentially decrease calorie needs, thereby challenging even the most dedicated dieter.

Studies have supported the positive effects of protein on both satiety and thermogenesis (Westerterp-Plantenga & Lejeune, 2005). Individuals ingesting a greater amount of protein—approximately 30% of total calories—report less hunger and consume fewer calories. The thermogenic effect of protein is greater than that of carbohydrates and fat, which also shows its potential for weight-loss promotion. Noakes and colleagues (2005) challenged this potential to see if improvements could be detected in weight loss, body composition, nutritional status, and markers for cardiovascular health in obese women. Subjects were assigned to one of two groups that were given the same number of calories. Their diets differed only by whether they were high in protein or carbohydrate. While both groups showed relatively similar reductions in body weight, individuals in the high-protein group with high **triacylglycerol** levels (a marker for cardiovascular disease) exhibited more fat loss and noticeable reductions in triacylglycerol levels. In their evaluation of nutritional status and renal function, researchers found that the high-protein diet did not negatively affect measurements, leading them to state that a high-protein diet is a safe and viable option for weight loss.

Having already discussed carbohydrate-restrictive diets at levels below 20% of total calories, it is imperative to note that this particular study provided 34% of its energy from protein, 20% from fat, and 46% from carbohydrate in the high-protein group. The high-carbohydrate diet provided 17% protein, 20% fat, and 64% carbohydrate. While the aforementioned high-protein dietary protocol does not represent a ketogenic-inducing increase in protein intake, it is double that of the recommended level for protein intake and was found to be safe in this investigation (Noakes et al., 2005).

The ability to keep the weight off following a weight-loss program is an essential component of a successful program. Because of its role in satiety and thermogenesis, protein was assessed for its ability to moderate the reduction in energy expenditure associated with weight loss (Westerterp-Plantenga, 2004). After a four-week weight-loss program, subjects participated in a three-month follow-up for weight maintenance, with half the group receiving an additional 48.2 grams of protein per day (an approximate increase of 20% per day, or 18% vs. 15% of total calories from protein). Those who had a modest bump in their protein intake showed a 50% lower regain of body weight and reported feeling fuller. Interestingly, the weight gain was predominantly fat-free mass, not fat mass, in the protein group, leading to a lower percent of body fat. This data suggests that even moderate increases in protein intake can help keep the weight off after a short-term weight-loss program.

To date, ill health consequences have not been documented with the higher-protein diets described in this section. As discussed, a severe carbohydrate restriction cannot be safely recommended for weight loss, but a modest increase in protein may be beneficial in helping to maintain weight loss.

Pharmacological Agents for Weight Loss

In an effort to decrease the health impact of obesity and provide individuals with pharmacological options for weight loss, medications have been developed to block fat absorption, increase energy expenditure, and suppress appetite. Pharmacological agents have not shown themselves to be "magic pills," and do not promote weight loss independently. Drugs are constantly hitting the market—often as others disappear—and it is the responsibility of the fitness professional to be aware of what is happening on the pharmacological side of the weight-loss industry. The following sections provide a brief review of several weight-loss medications that have received a fair amount of attention in the marketplace.

Lipase Inhibition: Fat Malabsorption Agents

Orlistat (Xenical®)

Dietary fat provides more calories per gram than carbohydrates and protein, and can impede weight loss when consumed in excess. Because of fat's predominance in the diet and its affect on obesity development as a high calorie contributor, inhibiting its digestion and absorption may help reduce intake and calorie contribution. Orlistat (Xenical) is a drug developed to block the digestion and absorption of **triglycerides** so that they are excreted in the stool undigested. A review of orlistat trials in humans reveals that weight loss was modestly greater in the groups receiving the recommended dosages of the drug as compared to a placebo (Halford, 2004).

Despite its success in promoting weight loss, orlistat's side effects cannot be overlooked. Patients taking orlistat report flatulence, oily stool, fecal urgency, incontinence, and abdominal pain prior to modifying their dietary fat intake. The absorption of fat-soluble vitamins is also decreased, thereby putting an individual at risk for deficiency if he or she does not take a vitamin supplement. However, few such cases have been reported (Halford, 2006).

The gastrointestinal distress experienced with orlistat use may also modify dietary intake. To avoid gastrointestinal distress, people taking the drug can reduce their fat intake. Unfortunately, human trials have revealed a compensatory increase in carbohydrate consumption—a response that could weaken this drug's weight-loss benefits (Halford, 2004).

In June 2007, Alli™ became the first over-the-counter diet pill approved by the Food and Drug Administration (FDA). It is a half-strength version of the prescription weight-loss drug Xenical (orlistat). For best results, Alli should be taken before every meal that contains fat. It works by decreasing the amount of fat absorbed by the gastrointestinal tract during the digestive process. Research has shown that when individuals use Alli in combination with diet and exercise, they lose up to 50% more weight on average compared to dieting and exercising alone. As with any drug, Alli has several documented side effects, including excessive flatulence and oily, difficult-to-control bowel movements. Those individuals hailing Alli as the next "magic bullet" for weight loss should bear in mind that most weight-loss experts contend that without the contributory effects of diet and exercise, Alli's beneficial weight-loss effects will be very limited.

Appetite Suppressants and Energy Expenditure–increasing Agents

Fen-Phen

In 1959, the FDA approved a drug called phentermine (Phen) for weight loss (Wellman & Maher, 1999). It acted like an amphetamine and reduced appetite. A drug with a different mechanism, but similar results, called fenfluramine (Fen) was introduced and approved in 1973. Acting alone, these drugs suppressed appetite modestly and produced few safety issues. Researchers began investigating the combination of the two drugs to see if coupling enhanced results. They found that the combination caused further appetite suppression and weight loss. Although the combination was not approved by the FDA, their safety and effectiveness was assumed.

Following the prescription and use of "fen-phen," investigations and reports surfaced of a negative and dangerous synergistic effect. Reports of primary pulmonary hypertension and valvular heart disease began to emerge in people taking the fen-phen combination. Once a rare disorder, primary pulmonary hypertension increased in appearance following the fen-phen therapy. In addition, a thickening of the heart valves leading to valvular heart disease was discovered, with a greater incidence among users of the drug combination (Wellman & Maher, 1999). In July 1997, the FDA issued a warning regarding the safety of fen-phen, and two months later, removed it from the market.

Sibutramine

Efforts to find a way to decrease people's appetite for food are ongoing. Sibutramine (trade name is Meridia® in the United States and Reductal® in Europe) has been investigated as a tool to help reduce intake and hunger, as well as increase energy expenditure (Halford, 2004). Sibutramine acts to increase **norepinephrine** and **serotonin** activity in the brain by decreasing reuptake, thereby reducing feelings of hunger. The evidence supporting its role in enhancing energy expenditure is mixed. It has produced a stimulatory effect in rodent studies, but shows less of an impact when taken by humans (Halford, 2006).

As with most medications, side effects are par for the course. Patients report dry mouth, constipation, and insomnia, with some reporting mild increases in blood pressure and heart rate. In addition to its mild negative side effects, sibutramine appears to beneficially affect triglyceride, **high-density lipoprotein (HDL),** and blood glucose levels, therefore making it a viable option for obese individuals to use in combination with a diet and exercise program.

Glycemic Index

The use of the **glycemic index (GI)** as a weight-loss tool has been accepted in consumer publications and debated by the scientific community. GI is a value used to rate or categorize the impact that a carbohydrate-containing food has on blood glucose levels. Foods have been categorized as low, moderate, or high, compared to the reference food, which is glucose or white bread (Table 8-2).

The challenge lies in the fact that determining a food's GI is difficult without testing. GI is affected by cooking, ripeness, protein and fat content, and handling, and therefore cannot be easily determined by consumers. The GI of a food also does not reflect its overall nutritional value. A high-glycemic food is not necessarily "unhealthier" or less nutritious, nor is a low-glycemic food necessarily "healthier" or more nutritious.

It should also be noted that when these carbohydrates are combined with other nutrients, such as protein or fat, it changes the glycemic effect. For this reason, some experts consider the **glycemic load** to be a more realistic approach.

Glycemic load is a measure of the glycemic index, multiplied by the number of carbohydrates (CHO) consumed, divided by 100:

Glycemic load = Glycemic index x CHO (g)/100

The glycemic load is useful in that it represents how much a given amount of a food will affect blood sugar levels. The thinking behind glycemic index and glycemic load is that if blood sugar is rapidly increased, **insulin** levels will rise quickly and lead to increased fat deposition.

A link between the GI and weight loss may stem from epidemiological studies that show an inverse relationship between the intake of sugary, carbohydrate-containing foods and obesity (Saris, 2003). This relationship leads to speculation that even though carbohydrates, as a whole, promote a feeling of fullness, high-glycemic foods that cause a spike in blood glucose may instead lead to overeating and subsequent weight gain (Anderson & Woodend, 2003).

When the glycemic index is investigated for its effect on weight loss, the research is inconclusive at best. Sloth et al. (2004) evaluated the influence of GI on appetite and body weight, as well as risk factors for type 2 diabetes over a 10-week intervention. After dividing groups into high-glycemic and low-glycemic diet programs, researchers assessed diet intake, body weight, and blood samples for lipids, glucose, and insulin. Upon completion, no differences in energy intake, body weight, or fat mass were detected. The low-glycemic group showed a significantly greater decrease in **low-density lipoproteins (LDL)** as the only change in blood levels. The results fail to support the assumption that a low-glycemic diet will be more satiating or that high-glycemic diets promote an increase in intake (Sloth et al., 2004). The lack of difference in body weight and fat mass implies that the glycemic index alone is an ineffective tool for weight maintenance. In fact, experts agree that the evidence is insufficient to support the use of GI as an agent for weight loss (Saris, 2003).

A controlled clinical trial was initiated to determine if diets with a low GI and high level of protein had a beneficial effect on weight loss in 129 overweight or obese young adults (McMillan-Price et al., 2006). The subjects were randomly assigned to one of three diet regimens:

- A reduced-fat, high-fiber diet

Table 8-2
Glycemic Index of Various Foods

High GI ≥70	Medium GI 56–69	Low GI ≤55
White bread	Rye bread	Pumpernickel bread
Corn Flakes®	Shredded Wheat®	All Bran®
Graham crackers	Ice cream	Plain yogurt
Dried fruit	Blueberries	Strawberries
Instant white rice	Refined pasta	Oatmeal

- A high-carbohydrate diet with either high- or low-GI carbohydrates
- A high-protein diet with either high- or low-GI carbohydrates

The results showed that although all participants lost similar amounts of weight (on average), there was a higher proportion of individuals that lost 5% or more of their body weight in the high-carbohydrate, low-GI (40 GI, 75 glycemic load) and the high-protein (25% of total calories), high-GI (57 GI, 87 glycemic load) diets. These same two groups showed a greater loss of fat mass than those on the high-carbohydrate, high-GI diet. In review of the biomarkers for cardiovascular disease risk, the high-carbohydrate, low-GI diet group showed a decrease in LDL-cholesterol, although no differences were seen in lipid profiles between the other diet groups. The results of this study should be considered when encouraging people to consume more quality whole grains, thus moving toward a lower-GI diet composition (Liu, 2006). Researchers in both studies agree that further investigations are warranted.

Fasting

Many frustrated individuals turn to fasting as a means of kicking off a weight-loss plan. Fasting, or inadequate food intake to produce a negative energy balance, appears enticing, as weight can be lost rapidly. Unfortunately, the consequences of fasting may make weight-loss efforts difficult and include unfavorable changes to the body.

Short-term calorie deficiencies lead to initial weight reductions, and can lead to changes in energy expenditure as they progress. As inadequate calorie intake continues, the body will make modifications to survive on the insufficient calories being supplied. This achievement of a new **steady state** can wreak havoc on a weight-loss plan. In the initial stages of a short-term calorie restriction, the body will rapidly lose weight. Glycogen reserves will decline, protein will be used to make glucose, and water will be lost (Kurpad, Muthayya, & Vaz, 2005). Fat loss occurs, but there will also be a decline in lean body tissue (i.e., muscle). During this time, the person can experience a drop in **basal metabolic rate (BMR),** thereby decreasing the number of calories needed to survive. Over time, if the energy deficiency persists, metabolic rate and total energy expenditure can plummet. Lean-body-mass loss continues and nutrient deficiencies can ensue.

Therefore, fasting is not recommended to create the negative energy balance required for weight loss. Increasing activity, with a modest restriction in calories, is still the most advisable way to tip the scale.

Eating Disorders and Associated Health Risks

Eating disorders are defined as disturbances in eating behavior or methods to control weight that contribute to impairments in physical and mental health, and are not related to another medical or psychiatric disturbance (Klein & Walsh, 2004). The American Dietetic Association (ADA) estimates that more than five million Americans suffer from **anorexia nervosa (AN), bulimia nervosa (BN),** or **binge eating disorder (BED)** (ADA, 2001). Regardless of the specific disorder, medical complications can occur and, in extreme cases, result in death. The following sections review the clinical features and health complications associated with eating disorders.

Binge Eating Disorder

BED is recognized as an increasingly common eating disorder. BED was initially considered an atypical eating disorder (Patrick, 2002). Characterized by recurrent episodes of binge eating, BED is not associated with compensatory episodes of purging, fasting, or excessive exercise, as is typical with bulimia nervosa. Individuals suffering from BED tend to eat more rapidly, until uncomfortably full, without physical hunger, alone, and with tremendous feelings of guilt and disgust after overeating (ADA, 2001). A diagnosis is given when someone partakes in this behavior more than two days a week over a six-month period. BED is typically seen in the obese population and can impede weight loss due to its psychopathology.

Despite the consequent feelings of guilt and disgust following an episode, individuals with BED often seek comfort or attempt to dull feelings of **anxiety** and **depression** with bouts of overconsumption. Often a stressful situation or day will provoke an episode that is used as a means to cope. BED has therefore been described as a psychological dependence on food, as well as an addiction.

The etiology of BED continues to be investigated. Individuals suffering from BED are suspected to be unable to properly deal with their feelings or stressful situations. To cope with issues, they resort to overeating, and the cycle of binging and guilt/disgust persists. One area of interest is the impact that cortisol may have on the development of BED. Cortisol plays a role in the regulation of appetite, in addition to being released during stress. There is speculation that a chronic rise in cortisol may contribute to the consumption, or overconsumption, of "comfort foods" that are high in sugar and fat (Gluck, 2006).

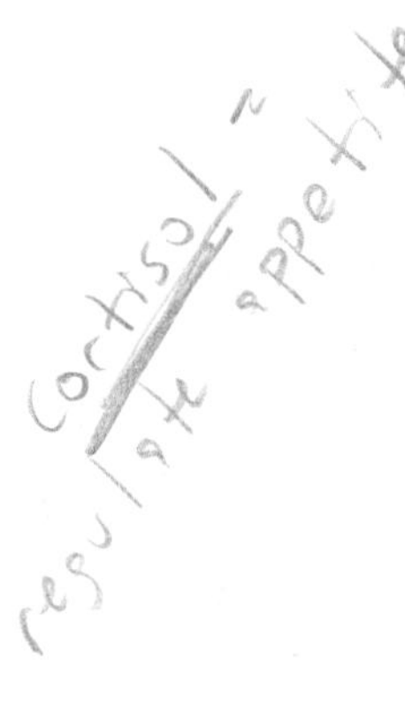

The health consequences and psychological impact of BED mirror those of overweight and obesity. BED often prohibits success in weight-loss programs, because the reason for consumption is not being addressed. In addition, individuals with BED are unable to detect hunger. They are encouraged to seek assistance in dealing with their emotions and the underlying disturbance, while also learning to read hunger and respond to feelings of fullness. Many self-help and support groups are available for BED, such as Overeaters Anonymous. Pharmaceutical interventions may also be warranted to relieve anxiety and/or depression.

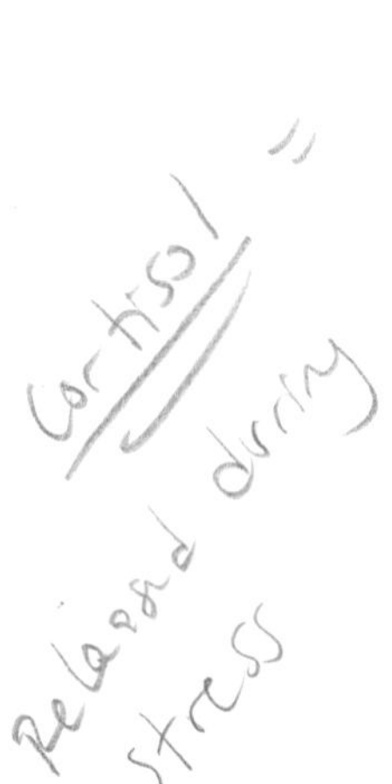

Bulimia Nervosa

Like BED, bulimia nervosa (BN) is characterized by recurrent episodes of binge eating and feelings of a loss of control. Unlike BED, BN includes compensatory behavior such as vomiting, excessive exercise, fasting, or laxative use (despite its ineffectiveness in controlling calorie intake). The concern for weight gain and/or drive to lose weight is also a feature of BN, along with a preoccupation with food and an extreme desire to eat.

The *International Classification of Diseases,* 10th edition (ICD-10) and *Diagnostic and Statistical Manual of Mental Disorders,* 4th edition, (DSM-IV) Diagnostic Criteria for BN outlined by the American Psychiatric Association and the World Health Organization's ICD classifications include the following (Patrick, 2002):

- Recurrent episodes of overeating in a short period of time, at least two times per week over three months
- Sense of a loss of control during episodes in combination with a strong desire to eat
- Recurrent, inappropriate compensatory behavior following overeating to prevent weight gain, including food restriction, self-induced vomiting, laxative or diuretic misuse, enemas, appetite suppressants, thyroid preparations, or medications to prevent weight gain. Diabetics with bulimia may modify their insulin treatment.
- Self-perception of being overweight and a morbid fear of becoming fat
- Behavior does not occur exclusively during episodes of BN
- Specific type: purging, as described above

The risk factors for BN range from a potential genetic link to a personality type. As with anorexia nervosa, family studies have identified an increase in lifetime risk for females with a family history of eating disorders (Klein & Walsh, 2003). Pinpointing the genetic marker for BN has yet to be done with consistency in the research, but is likely to be determined as investigations persist.

Personality, temperament, and environment each play a major role in the development of BN. It is quite common for people with BN to have a history of childhood obesity, as well as having experienced critical feedback from family regarding weight and body shape at an early age (Klein & Walsh, 2004). In a review of factors that make a person vulnerable to BN, Klein and Walsh (2004) point out the correlation between BN and anxiety and mood disorders, as well as personality traits common among patients. People with BN tend to be novelty-seeking and impulsive, and have a propensity for high negative emotionality and stress reactivity. Similarly, there is a three- to fourfold higher risk for substance abuse, and an increased rate of self-cutting and suicide attempts (Patrick, 2002; Klein & Walsh, 2004).

The health complications of BN far surpass the issue of weight loss. Individuals engaging in frequent vomiting or abuse of laxatives and diuretics are at risk for electrolyte disturbances, dehydration, muscle weakness, cardiac and kidney dysfunction, and gastrointestinal problems (ADA, 2001; Patrick, 2002). Of particular concern is the loss of potassium (**hypokalemia**), which can result in cardiac problems, as well as constipation, muscle myopathy, and kidney dysfunction. Cardiac abnormalities vary in severity, but can include **bradycardia** (heart rate below 60 beats per minute), low blood pressure (**hypotension**) leading to dizziness or fainting, electrocardiographic changes, and the potential for congestive heart failure, arrhythmias, and sudden death (ADA, 2001; Patrick, 2002). During recurring episodes of vomiting, the **esophagus** can become damaged and gastroesophageal reflux disease (GERD) may develop, as well as dental erosion (ADA, 2001).

The potential for serious medical complications with BN is high. Therefore, multidisciplinary intervention is imperative. Treatment varies, with many patients succeeding with outpatient care and others requiring hospitalization. The initial objectives are to control the compensatory behavior, especially the vomiting, and normalize eating behaviors. Medications may be prescribed for BN, and cognitive-behavioral therapy has been shown to be effective in treating individuals with BN.

Anorexia Nervosa

Cases of anorexia nervosa have been documented since the late 1800s (Klein & Walsh, 2003). Extreme weight loss and a drive for thinness are hallmark features of the disorder, and individuals with AN can suffer from myriad serious medical complications. More women are afflicted with AN than men—at a 10–20:1 ratio (females to males). An association with dance, fashion modeling, and some "weight-conscious" sports show greater numbers in both genders (Klein & Walsh, 2003). Of grave concern is the mortality rate for AN, as it is the highest among psychiatric disorders. In a review by Patrick (2002), AN is sited as a leading cause of death among females between the ages of 15 and 24 years, with suicide, infection, or chronic starvation being at fault.

The ICD-10 and DSM-IV Diagnostic Criteria for AN outlined by the American Psychiatric Association and the World Health Organization's ICD classifications include the following (Patrick, 2002):

- Weight is at least 15% below normal for age/height or failure to gain weight during periods of growth, leading to less than 85% of expected weight
- Self-induced weight loss secondary to avoidance of high-calorie foods, impaired perception of body weight or shape, and intense fear of gaining weight accompanied by denial of the seriousness of low body weight
- In postmenarcheal females, presence of **amenorrhea** (absence of at least three consecutive menstrual cycles). In males, the hypothalamic-pituitary gonadal axis disturbance manifests as a loss of sexual interest and potency.

The development of AN is multifactorial. Genetics has emerged as a contributing factor to the risk for, and development of, AN. It is estimated that approximately 58 to 76% of variance in the occurrence of AN is due to genetic factors (Klein & Walsh, 2004). Environmental and personality factors explain the remainder of AN's development, with keynotes being socio-cultural influences and perfectionism. The impact of puberty is considered in the development of AN, as it rarely occurs prepuberty and may be the psychological response to the "growing pains" associated with the maturing body (Klein & Walsh, 2004).

A culture that accepts and promotes "dieting" has long been considered a contributing factor. Young women and men are influenced by the barrage of advertisements, discussions, and media attention on the topics of dieting and body shape. During vulnerable years, in combination with any emotional instability and/or genetic factors, the socio-cultural influence can be great.

Typically, the first sign of AN to family and friends is weight loss. However, there are behavioral changes that present before weight loss occurs. Common alterations in behaviors surrounding food include elimination of particular foods or food groups, focus on low- or no-calorie items, delineation of "safe" foods, and increased consumption of noncaloric beverages (Klein & Walsh, 2004). Early stages of AN combine the intense fear of fatness, a strong desire for thinness, hunger denial, and a focus on food as a mechanism of control. As the disorder progresses and the weight declines, individuals with AN will often mask their changes with loose-fitting clothing and withdrawal from social gatherings. The consequences of starvation will eventually lead to decreased mental acuity, difficulty concentrating, and mood swings.

The medical symptoms and consequences can be quite serious as the disorder progresses. The following list presents the potential and devastating results from untreated AN (ADA, 2001; Patrick 2002):

- *Physical changes:* Lanugo hair on the face and trunk, brittle hair, **cyanosis** of the hands and feet, and dry skin
- *Electrolyte disturbances:* As with BN, potassium levels can drop, accompanied by low magnesium. Resulting conditions include muscle weakness, loss of concentration, muscular cramping, arrythmias, and memory loss.
- *Cardiovascular abnormalities:* Bradycardia, hypotension, reduced heart mass, and postural hypotension. These effects can stem from electrolyte disturbances and can often lead to death.
- *Gastrointestinal issues:* When the gut is left unfed, it can **atrophy** and have reduced motility, incomplete gastric emptying, and constipation; increased transit time; diminished **peristalsis;** and irritable bowel syndrome
- Amenorrhea
- **Osteopenia** or osteoporosis
- Vitamin and mineral deficiencies

As with BN, a multidisciplinary approach to AN care is integral. Whether it is inpatient or outpatient care will depend on the severity of the disorder. Body weight is the primary outcome measure for AN treatment, but comprehensive care requires a behavioral, nutritional, and psychiatric approach. Careful attention needs to be paid to the refeeding component of the plan, as rapid refeeding can lead to deadly changes in phosphate levels, drops in potassium and magnesium, alterations in glucose tolerance, and diminished gastrointestinal and heart function.

If an LWMC suspects that a client has an eating disorder and requires a referral for both psychological and nutrition care, the Internet can provide some help if he or she is unaware of the experts in the area:

- www.edreferral.com: A continuously updated site of treatment centers and eating-disorder resources
- www.eating-disorder-referral.com: Lists treatment centers by location
- www.anred.com: A nonprofit organization dedicated to eating disorders
- www.nationaleatingdisorders.org: Provides information and referral services

Anxiety and Eating Disorders

The link between eating disorders and other psychiatric disorders has long been recognized. Obsessive-compulsive disorders have been linked to risk for, and progression of, both AN and BN. As mentioned previously, particular personality traits are associated with eating disorders, and family history of these traits is influential as well. Anxiety disorder has been associated with AN and BN, and its influence has been investigated. Kaye et al. (2004) sought to assess the frequency of anxiety disorders among individuals with AN and BN, and to characterize its influence. By interviewing 282 individuals with BN and 293 with AN with a standardized tool for measuring anxiety, perfectionism, and obsessionality, a significantly higher prevalence of anxiety disorder was detected among the AN and BN subjects than is found in the overall population. Researchers concur that anxiety disorder is not only linked to AN and BN, but may also be a warning sign for its development and should be considered during treatment.

Depression, Disordered Eating, and Obesity

Behavioral and social factors contribute to the development of obesity and eating disorders (Dubois & Girard, 2006). In addition, depression or self-esteem issues may play a role in the development and perpetuation of a disorder. The factors that affect weight status were evaluated in 2,101 tenth-grade Turkish adolescents (Ozmen et al., 2007). A self-esteem measurement and the Children's Depression Inventory revealed that body dissatisfaction was related to low self-esteem and depression, although not correlated with obesity or overweight. There was a relationship, however, between perceptions of being overweight and low self-esteem. A similar investigation of children between seven and 13 years of age showed that those that were overweight or obese were more concerned about their body weights and shapes than those with healthy weights, and had lower self-esteem ratings, greater body dissatisfaction, and higher depression ratings (Allen et al., 2006). Goodman and Whitaker (2002) discovered a similar result in a prospective study of the role of depression in the development and persistence of adolescent obesity, indicating that depressed mood at baseline was a predictor of obesity, whereas the participants that were obese at baseline did not predict depression. The researchers indicated that depressed adolescents are at an increased risk for developing obesity.

Psychological issues have been identified as co-morbidities for eating disorders such as BN and AN (Blinders, Cumella, & Sanathara, 2006). In a sample of 2,436 inpatient females with a primary diagnosis of BN, AN, or eating disorders not otherwise specified, it was found that those with BN were more likely to suffer from alcohol abuse and polysubstance abuse. Those with AN and binge-purge anorexia were more likely to suffer from obsessive-compulsive disorder, post-traumatic stress disorder, schizophrenia, and/or other psychoses. All of those individuals with eating disorders suffered from depression. The evidence has implications for the prevention and treatment of all types of eating disorders, and supports the use of a multidisciplinary team approach.

Summary

Weight management is largely a matter of energy intake versus energy output, and finding an appropriate long-term balance between the two will be the central challenge for most clients. It is important for LWMCs to understand the many diets and pharmacological agents that continue to flood the marketplace, including both the potential effectiveness and the health risks and side effects associated with each. Having a solid foundation of up-to-date knowledge in this area is essential for

LWMCs who wish to present themselves as experts to their clients. Finally, LWMCs must be able to identify the signs of various eating disorders and explain the associated health risks to their clients. While diagnosing and treating eating disorders falls outside of an LWMC's scope of practice, LWMCs are often among the first to discuss the topic with individuals who are at risk or are already coping with eating disorders, so it is vital for LWMCs to approach this topic with compassion and expertise.

References

Allen, K.L. et al. (2006). Why do some overweight children experience psychological problems? The role of weight and shape concern. *International Journal of Pediatric Obesity,* 1, 4, 239–247.

American Dietetic Association (2001). Position of the American Dietetic Association: Nutrition intervention in the treatment of anorexia nervosa, bulimia nervosa, and eating disorders not otherwise specified (EDNOS). *Journal of the American Dietetic Association*, 101, 7, 810–819.

Anderson, G.H. & Woodend, D. (2003). Effect of glycemic carbohydrates on short-term satiety and food intake. *Nutrition Reviews,* 61, 5, S17–S26.

Astrup, A., Larsen, T.M., & Harper, A. (2004). Atkins and other low-carbohydrate diets: Hoax or an effective tool for weight loss? *Lancet,* 364, 897–899.

Blinder B.J., Cumella E.J., & Sanathara V.A. (2006) Psychiatric comorbidities of female inpatients with eating disorders. *Psychosomatic Medicine,* 68, 3, 454–462.

Bravata, D.M. et al. (2003). Efficacy and safety of low-carbohydrate diets: A systematic review. *Journal of the American Medical Association,* 289, 14, 1837–1850.

Dubois, L. & Girard, M. (2006) Early determinants of overweight at 4.5 years in a population-based longitudinal study. *International Journal of Obesity* (Lond), 30, 4, 610–617.

Foster, G.D. et al. (2003). A randomized trial of a low-carbohydrate diet for obesity. *New England Journal of Medicine,* 348, 2082–2090.

Freedman, M.R., King, J., & Kennedy, E. (2001). Popular diets: A scientific review. *Obesity Research,* 9 (Suppl): 1S–40S.

Gluck, M.E. (2006). Stress response and binge eating disorder. *Appetite,* 46, 1, 26–30.

Goodman E. & Whitaker R.C. (2002). A prospective study of the role of depression in the development and persistence of adolescent obesity. *Pediatrics,* 110, 3, 497–504.

Halford, J. (2004). Clinical pharmacotherapy for obesity: Current drugs and those in advanced development. *Current Drug Targets,* 5, 637–646.

Halford, J. (2006). Pharmacotherapy for obesity. *Appetite,* 46, 1, 6–10.

Kaye, W.H. et al. (2004). Comorbidity of anxiety disorders with anorexia and bulimia nervosa. *American Journal of Psychiatry,* 161, 2215–2221.

Klein, D.A. & Walsh, B.T. (2003). Eating disorders. *International Review of Psychiatry,* 15, 205–216.

Klein, D.A. & Walsh, B.T. (2004). Eating disorders: Clinical features and pathophysiology. *Physiology and Behavior,* 81, 2, 359–374.

Krieger, J.W. et al. (2006). Effects of variation in protein and carbohydrate intake on body mass and composition during energy restriction: A meta-regression. *American Journal of Clinical Nutrition,* 83, 2, 260–274.

Kurpad, A.V., Muthayya, S., & Vaz, M. (2005). Consequences of inadequate food energy and negative energy balance in humans. *Public Health Nutrition,* 8, 7A, 1053–1076.

Last, A.R. & Wilson, S.A. (2006). Low-carbohydrate diets. *American Family Physician,* 73, 11, 1942–1948.

Liu, S. (2006). Lowering dietary glycemic load for weight control and cardiovascular health: A matter of quality. *Archives of Internal Medicine,* 166, 1438–1439.

McMillan-Price, J. et al. (2006). Comparison of four diets of varying glycemic load on weight loss and cardiovascular risk reduction in overweight and obese young adults: A randomized controlled trial. *Archives of Internal Medicine,* 166, 1466–1475.

Noakes, M. et al. (2005). Effect of an energy-restricted, high-protein, low-fat diet relative to a conventional high-carbohydrate, low-fat diet on weight loss, body composition, nutritional status, and markers of cardiovascular health in obese women. *American Journal of Clinical Nutrition,* 81, 6, 1298–1306.

Ozmen, D. et al. (2007). The association of self-esteem, depression and body satisfaction with obesity among Turkish adolescents. *BMC Public Health,* 16, 7, 80.

Patrick, L. (2002). Eating disorders: A review of the literature with emphasis on medical complications and clinical nutrition. *Alternative Medicine Review,* 7, 3, 184–202.

Saris, W.H.M. (2003). Glycemic carbohydrate and body weight regulation. *Nutrition Reviews,* 61, 5, S10–S16.

Shetty, P. (2005). Energy requirements of adults. *Public Health Nutrition,* 8, 7A, 994–1009.

Sloth, B. et al. (2004). No difference in body weight decrease between a low-glycemic-index and a high-glycemic-index diet but reduced LDL cholesterol after 10-wk ad libitum intake of the low-glycemic-index diet. *American Journal of Clinical Nutrition,* 80, 2, 337–347.

Stein, K. (2000). High-protein, low-carbohydrate diets: Do they work? *Journal of the American Dietetic Association,* 100, 760–761.

St. Jeor, S.T. et al. (2001). Dietary protein and weight reduction: A statement for healthcare professionals from the Nutrition Committee of the Council on Nutrition, Physical Activity, and Metabolism of the American Heart Association. *Circulation,* 104, 1869–1874.

Stubbs, R.J. & Tolkamp, B.J. (2006). Control of energy balance in relation to energy intake and energy expenditure in animals and man: An ecological perspective. *British Journal of Nutrition,* 95, 4, 657–676.

Wardlaw, G.M. & Hampl, J.S. (2006). *Perspectives in Nutrition* (7th ed.). New York: McGraw-Hill.

Wellman, P.J. & Maher, T.J. (1999). Synergistic interactions between Fenfluramine and Phentermine. *International Journal of Obesity,* 23, 723–732.

Wenk, C. (2004). Implications of dietary fat for nutrition and energy balance. *Physiology and Behavior,* 83, 4, 564–571.

Westerterp-Plantenga, M.S. (2004). Fat intake and energy-balance effects. *Physiology and Behavior,* 83, 4, 579–585.

Westerterp-Plantenga, M.S. & Lejeune, M.P. (2005). Protein intake and body-weight regulation. *Appetite,* 45, 187–190.

Suggested Reading

American Heart Association (2005). *American Heart Association No-Fad Diet: A Personal Plan for Healthy Weight Loss*. New York: Clarkson Potter/Publishers.

Bauer, J. (2005). *The Complete Idiot's Guide to Total Nutrition* (4th ed.). Indianapolis, Ind.: Alpha Books.

Consumer Reports (June 2005). Rating the diets from Atkins to the Zone. 18–22.

Dansigner, M.L. et al. (2005). Comparison of the Atkins, Ornish, Weight Watchers, and Zone diets for weight loss and heart disease risk reduction: A randomized trial. *Journal of the American Medical Association,* 293, 1, 43–53.

Duyff, R.L. (2002). *American Dietetic Association Complete Food and Nutrition Guide* (2nd ed.). Indianapolis, Ind.: Wiley Higher Education.

Howard, B.V. et al. (2006). Low-fat dietary pattern and weight change over seven years: The Women's Health Initiative Dietary Modification Trial. *Journal of the American Medical Association,* 295, 39–49.

Nordmann, A.J. et al. (2006). Effects of low-carbohydrate vs. low-fat diets on weight loss and cardiovascular risk factors: A meta-analysis of randomized controlled trials. *Archives of Internal Medicine,* 166, 285–293.

Parikh, P. et al. (2005). Diets and cardiovascular disease: An evidence-based assessment. *Journal of the American College of Cardiology*, 45, 9, 1979–1987.

Sports, Cardiovascular and Wellness Nutritionists DPG & Dunford, M. (2006). *Sports Nutrition: A Practice Manual for Professionals* (4th ed.). Chicago, Ill.: American Dietetic Association.

Whitney, E.N. & Rolfes, S.R. (2007). *Understanding Nutrition.* (11th ed.). Belmont, Calif.: Wadsworth Publishing Company.

Yager, J. & Anderson, A. (2005). Anorexia nervosa. *New England Journal of Medicine,* 353, 14, 1481–1488.

Part IV

Screening, Assessment, and Referral

Chapter 9
Screening and Assessment

Chapter 10
Body-composition Assessment and Evaluation

Chapter 11
Referral

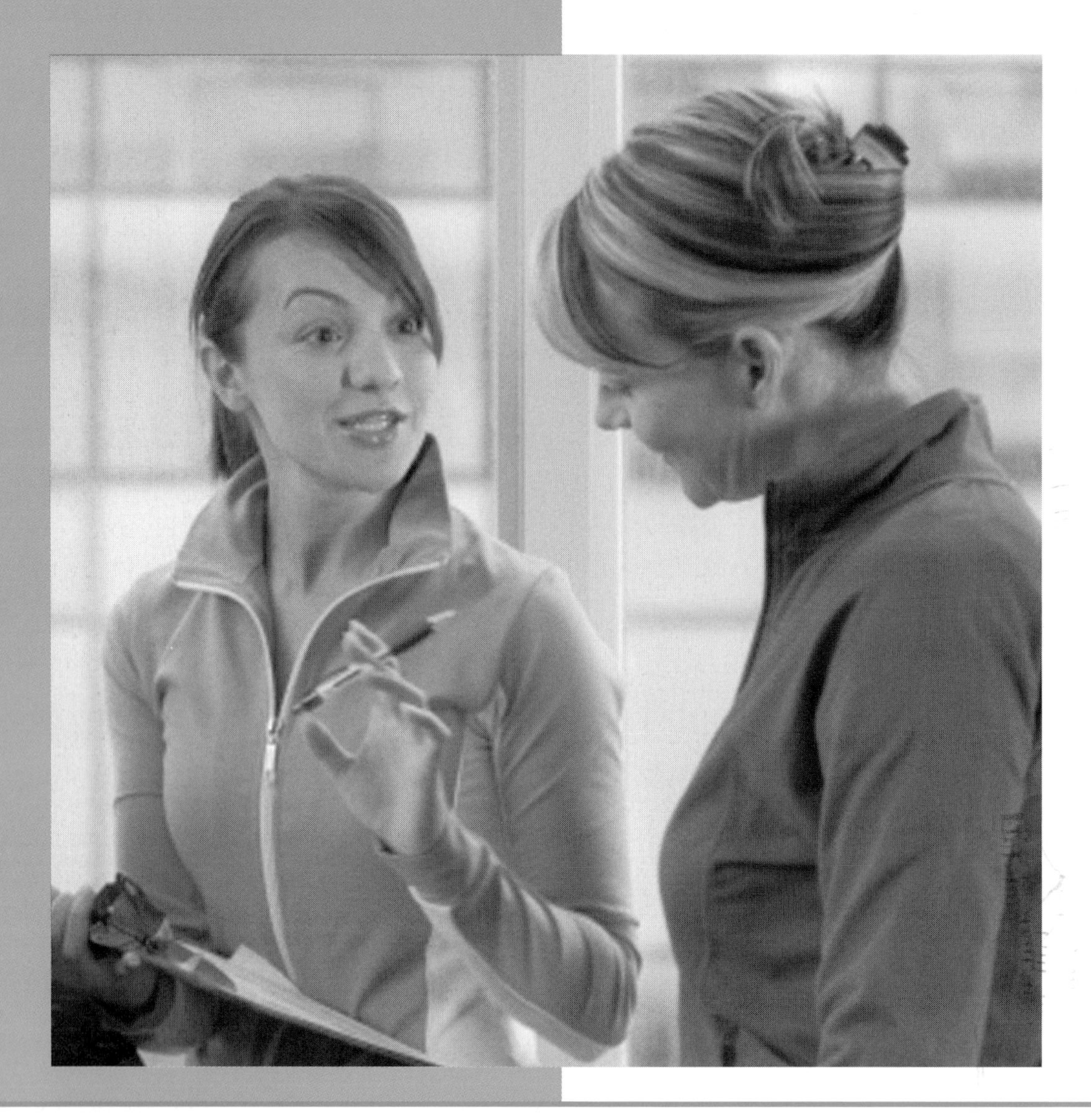

Susan Bartlett, Ross Andersen, and Richard T. Cotton

Susan Bartlett, Ph.D., is associate professor of medicine at the Johns Hopkins School of Medicine in Baltimore, Md. Dr. Bartlett is a licensed clinical psychologist and faculty member in the Division of Rheumatology and Johns Hopkins Arthritis Center. Her primary research and clinical interests focus on the effect of weight loss and exercise on arthritis, the mind-body effects of physical activity, and how psychosocial factors influence adherence to medical treatments.

Ross Andersen, Ph.D., is associate director of fellowship training in the Division of Geriatric Medicine at Johns Hopkins Medical Center. Since 1993, he has been conducting clinical trials examining the long-term effects of diet and exercise in helping people manage their weight. In addition, he has published several reports that have shaped current thinking about exercise for overweight individuals. For 10 years, Dr. Andersen operated community-based weight-loss programs in health clubs, and he is the author of The Health and Fitness Club Leader's Guide: Administering a Weight-Management Program. *He is a fellow of the American College of Sports Medicine (ACSM) and a member of the North American Association for the Study of Obesity (NAASO).*

Richard T. Cotton, M.A., is the national director of certification for the American College of Sports Medicine (ACSM). Before joining ACSM, he was the chief exercise physiologist at MyExercisePlan.com. Cotton is the former chief exercise physiologist for the Scripps Clinic & Research Foundation as well as for the American Council on exercise, where he also served as a media spokesperson and technical editor. He is certified by ACSM as both a Preventive and Rehabilitative Program Director and Exercise Specialist.

Chapter 9

Screening and Assessment

IN THIS CHAPTER:

Obesity is a serious threat to an individual's health and well-being. Medical risks associated with being overweight include **diabetes, hypercholesterolemia,** gallbladder disease, arthritis, **hypertension,** and some forms of cancer and cardiovascular disease (see Chapter 18). The most recent estimates from the National Health and Nutrition Examination Survey (NHANES) 2003–2004 suggest that the prevalence of overweight and obesity continues to grow (Ogden et al., 2006). Among adults aged 20 years and older, 66.3% are overweight or obese. Overweight and obesity rates among adults aged 40 to 59 have climbed to 73.1%. Significant differences are evident when the statistics are broken down by race and ethnicity. In adults 20 years and older, rates of overweight and obesity are lowest in non-Hispanic whites (64.2%), and higher among non-Hispanic blacks (76.1%) and Mexican-Americans (75.8%). The economic, medical, and psychological costs to society are staggering.

A record number of individuals are attempting to control their weight. In 2000, 46% of women and 33% of men reported that they were trying to lose weight (Bish et al., 2000). Notably, most adults trying to lose weight do not increase their level of physical activity as part of their weight-loss program (Gordon et al., 2000). Dieting and weight-loss practices have important health and economic implications. The pervasiveness of dieting in American culture has led to a multibillion dollar weight-loss industry and sparked congressional investigations into the activities and efficacy of many commercial programs.

Lifestyle & Weight Management Consultants (LWMCs) offer a valuable service, combining information from nutritional, behavioral, and exercise sciences to help clients manage their weight. The hallmark of ACE-certified LWMCs is their ability to promote safe and effective lifestyle changes for a wide variety of individuals. However, not all clients who seek the services of an LWMC can and should be treated by one. The purpose of this chapter is to assist LWMCs in screening for potential contraindications to weight-loss treatment and provide a framework for the assessment of potential clients.

The Importance of a Thorough Screening and Assessment

Many factors influence whether an individual will become overweight. Identifying underlying contributors to a client's weight problem is important, because they will influence the type of recommended treatment. Consider the following example: Joe is the chief counsel in a large firm of attorneys. His work takes him on the road often and for several weeks at a time. Before a trial, Joe works long days for weeks and doesn't get to relax until a couple of weeks after a trial. Though once a highly fit, athletic individual, Joe has gained about 50 pounds (23 kg) over the past 10 years. It is likely that Joe's long work hours, high stress level, frequent meals in restaurants, and lack of regular exercise are major contributors to his weight-management problems.

On the other hand, consider Sam, who is the chief operating officer of a major manufacturing plant. Recently separated from his wife, he is finding it increasingly difficult to return to an empty apartment each evening and has begun to work longer hours each day without taking a break for lunch or dinner. Once home, he finds himself consumed with thoughts of eating and binges nearly every night on food and alcohol. As a result, he has gained nearly 50 pounds (23 kg) in nine months. He confides that his eating is out of control and he feels powerless to stop his destructive behavior.

Both Joe and Sam need to lose similar amounts of weight. The excess 50 pounds (23 kg) each man carries confer a significant health risk, and their weight gain is likely to continue unless specific changes are made.

Joe's lifestyle is clearly affecting his weight. More appropriate food choices and behavioral strategies to reduce his calorie and fat consumption, combined with a regular program of physical activity, will be the cornerstone of his weight-management program. By contrast, Sam's weight difficulties appear more complex. His weight problem results from more than careless eating patterns or a **sedentary** lifestyle (though these may be important factors for later weight maintenance). The LWMC may suspect that Sam has high levels of depressive symptoms in response to his current stressors (the separation), which express themselves in a nightly pattern of excessive eating and drinking. Depression, current major stressors, and uncontrolled binging are potential contraindications for weight loss and may require the assistance of a mental-health professional before attempting weight-loss strategies. To best meet the needs of an overweight client, it is important to match his or her needs with the appropriate level of care.

Types of Obesity-treatment Programs

Many clients will require minimal direct involvement from healthcare professionals. However, to work with some clients, an LWMC may need to seek support from healthcare providers, such as physicians, mental health specialists (e.g., psychologists, psychiatrists, or social workers), dietitians, or physical therapists.

To understand when outside help is needed and who to involve in a client's care, it is helpful to be familiar with the spectrum of services available for treating overweight persons. The various approaches to obesity treatment can be broadly broken down into three categories: self-help programs, nonclinical programs, and clinical approaches [Institute of Medicine (IOM), 1995]. While clients without special medical or psychological issues can be treated within the parameters of any of these three categories, some clients may be better served by working with licensed professionals in more intensive clinical programs.

Self-help programs are widely used and vary in format. Examples may include the use of meal-replacement shakes or frozen entrees, participation in support or self-help groups (e.g., Overeaters Anonymous, church-based groups), popular diet books, manuals, magazine articles, or increased exercise. The safety, effectiveness, and quality of such approaches vary greatly. In general, in self-help programs, one basic approach is recommended for everyone, with little or no individualization.

Nonclinical programs are typically more structured and tailored than self-help programs. Most nonclinical programs are commercial-based franchises. The parent company provides the structure, materials and, in some cases, the food for clients to utilize. Consultants are then employed to present the program to participants. The training levels of these consultants vary widely. In some cases, counselors are simply program graduates who have received additional training from the company. Consultants may or may not be supervised by experienced weight-loss professionals. While some attempts may be made to individualize treatment programs, most allow only minimal deviation from a well-defined plan.

In clinical programs, treatment is provided largely by licensed professionals, such as psychologists, registered dietitians, and physicians. The clinician may work alone and refer patients to allied health professionals as needed, or, more often, be a part of a multidisciplinary team. Clinical programs are typically affiliated with a hospital or university. They generally begin with a thorough medical and psychological assessment and are best suited to treat complicated or severe cases of obesity. Treatment may be highly individualized to meet the unique medical and psychological needs of the participants.

Standards of Care for Weight-management Programs

New "diets" that promise fast, easy, and significant weight loss have been a part of American culture for decades. A quick, informal survey of the cover of top health and fitness and women's magazines shows that they all feature at least one article about diet and weight loss. New weight-loss books are often found among the top 10 best-sellers. Clearly, the weight-loss industry has grown tremendously, and with this growth has come the need to oversee the safety and efficacy of various approaches. Several regulatory bodies have developed guidelines to regulate the practices and advertising claims of weight-loss providers.

The Department of Consumer Affairs (DCA) of New York City was the first agency to document the deceptive practices of many rapid-weight-loss centers. These practices range from working with inappropriate candidates (i.e., underweight individuals) and offering false and misleading claims to outright quackery (Winner, 1991). The result was the first "Truth-in-Dieting" regulation, which mandated specific requirements for all centers promoting rapid weight loss [e.g., more than 1.5 to 2 pounds (0.7 to 0.9 kg) per week, or the loss of more than 1% of body weight per week after the second week of participation]. Specifically, such centers were required to post a "Weight-Loss Consumers' Bill of Rights" and provide all consumers with a wallet-size card outlining them (Table 9-1). In addition,

Table 9-1
The Weight-loss Consumers' Bill of Rights

- WARNING: Rapid weight loss may cause serious health problems. (Rapid weight loss is weight loss of more than 1½ to 2 pounds per week, or weight loss of more than 1% of body weight per week after the second week of participation in a weight-loss program.)
- Only permanent lifestyle changes—such as making healthful food choices and increasing physical activity—promote long-term weight loss.
- Consult your personal physician before starting any weight-loss program.
- Qualifications of this provider's staff are available upon request.
- You have a right to
  - Ask questions about the potential health risks of this program, its nutritional content, and its psychological support and educational components
  - Know the price of treatment, including the price of extra products, services, supplements, and laboratory tests
  - Know the program duration that is being recommended for you

Source: New York Department of Consumer Affairs

programs were required to disclose all costs and the recommended length of treatment.

At about the same time, the Michigan Department of Public Health developed its own set of guidelines for weight-loss programs (Drewnowski, 1990). The Michigan Guidelines applied to all nonclinical and clinical programs and were even more detailed than those developed in New York City. The Michigan Guidelines made these key recommendations:

- All clients must be screened to verify that they have no medical or psychological conditions that could make weight loss inappropriate. Depending on the client, such screening would range from a simple health checklist to a complete physical exam.
- All clients must be classified not only by excess body weight, but also by overall health risks, to ensure that the individual receives the appropriate level of care. Level I is intended for low-risk clients, Level II is for moderate-risk clients who require medical monitoring, and Level III is reserved for very obese or high-risk individuals.
- Care should be given by trained individuals. The qualifications of weight-loss staff should be commensurate with the health-risk level of the client. Thus, programs that accept clients with high health risks require highly trained healthcare professionals.

Specific recommendations were made concerning daily caloric intake, dietary composition, use of appetite-suppressant drugs, and the inclusion of exercise. An emphasis was also placed on individualizing the programs and including a maintenance phase to promote long-term weight management.

At a national level, the Food and Nutrition Board of the Institute of Medicine (IOM) of the National Academy of Sciences commissioned a committee to develop criteria for evaluating the effectiveness of weight-loss approaches to prevent and treat obesity. World-renowned researchers in nutrition, psychology, medicine, and exercise science sat on the committee. The book summarizing their results, *Weighing the Options: Criteria for Evaluating Weight-Management Programs* (IOM, 1995), set forth three primary criteria (Table 9-2).

Criterion 1 of the IOM recommendations—the match between program and consumer—addresses the importance of matching individuals to appropriate treatment strategies. Treatment for weight disorders range from the least invasive and most economical strategies to those requiring intensive and/or expensive professional care. To better match their specific needs and treatment options, a **stepped-care model** was developed (IOM, 1995). Stepped-care models are widely used in medicine and are based on the premise that treatment can be cumulative or incremental.

As shown in Figure 9-1, step 1 utilizes a low-fat diet, physical activity, and lifestyle change to promote a healthy and reasonable weight loss of up to 10 pounds (4.5 kg). Step 2 involves a more detailed assessment of health risks and utilizes more intensive efforts to help clients change their lifestyles while promoting a larger weight loss. When

Table 9-2
Criteria for Evaluating Weight-management Programs

Criterion	Program	Person
The match between program and consumer	Who is appropriate for this program?	Should I be in this program given my goals and characteristics?
The soundness and safety of the program	Is my program based on sound biological and behavioral principles, and is it safe for its intended participants?	Is the program safe for me?
Outcomes of the program	What is the evidence of success of my program?	Are the benefits I am likely to achieve from the program worth the effort and cost?

Source: Institute of Medicine (1995). *Weighing the Options: Criteria for Evaluating Weight-Management Programs.* Washington, D.C.: National Academy Press.

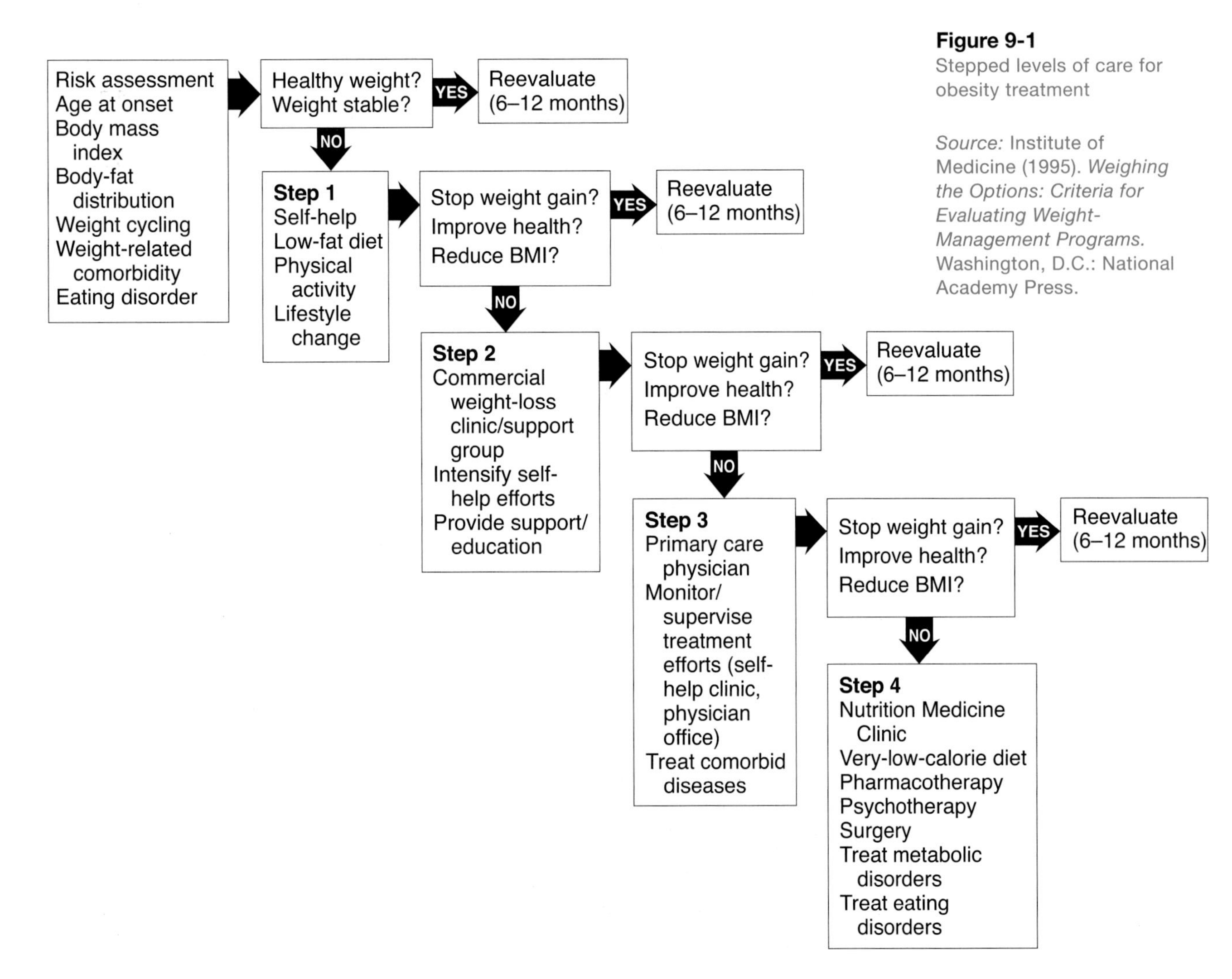

Figure 9-1
Stepped levels of care for obesity treatment

Source: Institute of Medicine (1995). *Weighing the Options: Criteria for Evaluating Weight-Management Programs.* Washington, D.C.: National Academy Press.

individuals are diagnosed with comorbid disease or are at a high risk for weight-related diseases, more intensive monitoring of the individual is required, as shown in step 3. The client's primary care physician may also participate more actively in the weight-management program through supervision and monitoring. Step 4 provides the most intensive and aggressive interventions for weight loss, including the use of **very-low-calorie diets**, medication, psychotherapy, and even surgery as indicated. Step 4 incorporates all of the goals of steps 1 through 3, while maximizing the loss of excess body fat and enhancing metabolic fitness.

Where does the work of an LWMC fit within the stepped model? It is possible that an LWMC may work with clients through all four steps, depending on the setting, the level of professional support available, and the LWMC's level of education and experience. However, an LWMC is ideally suited to promote lifestyle change in steps 1, 2, and 3 through education, support, and structure. Also, as healthcare becomes increasingly oriented toward the prevention of illness, an LWMC can potentially assume a primary role in working with individuals at step 1—that is, clients who are at risk for becoming overweight and developing obesity-related illnesses, but are currently free of such problems.

Criterion 2 of the IOM recommendations—the soundness and safety of the program—proposes **standards of care,** or minimum expectations of a credible weight-loss approach. Specifically, the following four areas are identified:

- Assessment of physical health and psychological status (including assessment of a client's knowledge and attitudes related to weight and a periodic reassessment to see if the client is still committed to losing weight and learning the needed information and skills to succeed)
- Attention to diet
- Attention to physical activity
- Ensuring program safety

The IOM offers two additional recommendations supporting the importance of small weight losses to reduce health risks while emphasizing long-term maintenance of weight loss. "We recommend that...the goal of obesity treatment should be refocused from weight loss alone, which is often aimed at appearance, to weight management, [or] achieving the best weight possible in the context of overall health. [Weight-loss programs] should be judged more by their effects on the overall health of participants than by their effects on weight alone" (IOM, 1995, p. 5). Similar recommendations were incorporated into the 2003 guidelines for healthcare providers on the Identification, Evaluation, and Treatment of Obesity developed by the National Heart, Lung, and Blood Institute (NHLBI) of the National Institutes of Health (NIH).

How can an LWMC ensure the soundness and safety of his or her program for potential clients? A structured guideline-based assessment of physical and psychological health (which may or may not involve the client's personal physician) is an important beginning. Attention needs to be given to dietary intake and physical activity to safely promote either an appropriate energy deficit (for weight loss) or **energy balance** (for weight maintenance). The IOM and NIH recommend that reassessment of diet and activity patterns be conducted at the beginning and end of the weight-loss phase of treatment, and every six months during the maintenance phase.

An LWMC must also be aware of the known and potential risks associated with any weight-loss attempt. In general, the more restrictive the diet, the greater the associated risks. For example, the risk of gallbladder disease is greatest with low-calorie diets and rapid weight loss. Diets with a caloric intake of fewer than 1,200 kcal/day may not meet nutritional guidelines, have not been shown to have long-term efficacy, and should not be promoted. Very-low-calorie diets of fewer than 800 kcal/day must only be used under a physician's supervision (IOM, 1995). For significantly obese individuals [i.e., **body mass index (BMI)** >40 or BMI >35 in the presence of additional risk factors], bariatric surgery appears to offer the best long-term results (NIH, 1998).

Criterion 3 of the IOM recommendations—outcomes of the program—focuses on four components of a successful program (IOM, 1995):

- Long-term weight loss
- Improvement in obesity-related risk factors
- Improved health practices (e.g., increased physical activity, improved eating habits)
- Monitoring of adverse effects that might result from the program

To successfully monitor outcome, it is critical that the initial and subsequent client assessments are thorough and well-documented. In the interest of consumer protection, the IOM suggests that all details of a weight-loss program be disclosed. This includes rate of weight loss, an outline of the treatment plan, cost estimates, the professional credentials of program staff, and the risks associated with treatment. Claims that weight losses will be maintained over time should be backed up with scientifically valid documentation, not "satisfied client" claims.

Screening Issues

Many factors must be considered when assessing the suitability of a potential client, including medical and psychological status, motivation, readiness to change, and timing. For example, think back to the examples of Joe and Sam. Even though Joe (the lawyer) appears to be a good candidate for the services of an LWMC, if the timing is inappropriate (e.g., he is just beginning a lengthy trial out of town), the lack of control over his environment and an inability to meet frequently are significant barriers to success. Certain factors may clearly signal that a potential client is not well-suited for the services of an LWMC. (For a more thorough review of an LWMC's **scope of practice,** refer to Chapter 19.) It is important that an LWMC carefully screens, assesses, and documents the relevant components of physical and psychological health in all clients with whom he or she plans to work.

The initial screening process allows an LWMC to separate individuals who may benefit from his or her services from those who clearly will not. The LWMC uses the process of assessment to determine the significance or importance of various factors that contribute to, or complicate, a client's weight-management needs. A thorough screening and assessment process protects both the LWMC and the consumer. It ensures that the needs of a potential client can be met by the services that an LWMC can legitimately and ethically provide.

Is This Client Appropriate for This Setting?

The degree of overweight, the type of treatment or program, and client characteristics are all factors to be considered when matching individuals with treatment protocols (IOM, 1995; NIH, 1998). A chief responsibility of an LWMC is to be able to determine the appropriateness of a program for a client. Though LWMCs may be found in all types of settings, the greatest responsibility lies with the LWMC who is essentially practicing without the formal support of an allied healthcare professional. Examples of this situation include LWMCs who work independently or provide services in a health club or commercial franchise setting.

Assessment Issues

An assessment of medical and psychological status, diet, and activity level is strongly advised for all clients. The scope and depth of the assessment will vary with the program setting and the level of care provided. This section presents information on the basic or minimum evaluation of physical and psychological health, readiness to exercise, fitness parameters, and motivation or readiness to change (see Chapter 12).

Assessing Physical Health

Since weight-management practices can potentially help or harm the health of clients (IOM, 1995), some type of physical and psychological health assessment is required for all individuals with whom an LWMC will work. Physical health can only be assessed by a physician. Physicians, physician assistants, and nurse practitioners are best trained to review a health history and conduct a physical exam to detect obesity-related illnesses and suitability for a diet and exercise program.

Criteria for Medical Clearance

Though it is recommended that all clients receive a physician's clearance before beginning a weight-management program, it is especially important for individuals with the following health conditions:

- Hypertension
- Elevated **cholesterol** or **triglyceride** levels
- **Diabetes**
- Significant emotional problems
- BMI greater than 30
- Chronic kidney failure
- Cardiovascular disease, including **angina, arrhythmias,** and congestive heart failure
- Liver disease
- Pregnancy—present or planned
- **Hyperthyroidism** or **hypothyroidism**
- Substance abuse
- Extreme obesity

The Basic Health Screen

For apparently healthy clients who report no significant current or past medical problems, it may be sufficient to obtain the following health data:

- BMI or body composition (percent body fat)
- **Waist circumference**
- Blood pressure and resting heart rate
- Current medications
- History of chronic illnesses
- Current medical history
- Family health history
- Health habits (e.g., cigarette, alcohol and recreational drugs)
- Assessment of obesity-related risk factors (NIH, 1998; National Task Force on the Prevention and Treatment of Obesity, 2000)

Height–weight tables are sometimes used to get a rough estimate of "ideal" body weight. A more useful estimate of appropriate body weight can be obtained by adjusting weight for height or stature and calculating a height-normalized index called the body mass index. Body mass index is highly predictive of the relative health risk associated with a person's body weight. (See Chapter 10 for information on the calculation and interpretation of body mass index and other body-composition testing methods.) A simple health-history checklist, including current medications and current and past illnesses, and a family health history should be included in the client's application forms (Figure 9-2). Dr. Nicholas DiNubile, in his book *FrameWork: Your 7-Step Program for Healthy Muscles, Bones, and Joints*, provides a self-test to determine an individual's musculoskeletal fitness and uncover what he terms "potential time bombs." LWMCs can use this book as a source when working with clients to assess their musculoskeletal health. In addition, Figure 9-3 presents a musculoskeletal health questionnaire that should be used as part of every client's initial assessment. Having clients complete such forms and obtain physician clearance (if necessary) prior to the first meeting saves time during the initial consultation. LWMCs must review all of this information with the client present to ensure that nothing has been omitted. This meeting also provides an excellent opportunity to identify and record risk factors of which the client may or may not be aware.

Measuring Blood Pressure and Resting Heart Rate

The LWMC can also effectively screen for two more components: resting blood pressure and resting heart rate. Blood pressure reflects the force of the heartbeat and the resistance of the arteries to the pumping action of the heart. It should be measured using a medical grade sphygmomanometer after a client has been seated with both feet flat on the floor for at least two full minutes. The cuff is firmly wrapped around the arm, with its lower margin approximately one inch above the antecubital space. At least two measurements should be taken approximately five minutes apart. LWMCs must use an appropriate-sized cuff, as overweight clients may have falsely elevated blood-pressure readings when standard-sized cuffs are used. Normative values for blood pressure readings are presented in Table 9-3.

Health History Checklist

Place an X next to any of the following conditions that you have now or have ever had:

____ High blood pressure
____ Heart disease
____ Chest pain
____ Shortness of breath
____ Irregular heart beat
____ Dizziness or fainting spells
____ Stroke
____ Severe headaches
____ Seizures or convulsions
____ Numbness or tingling
____ Fainting
____ Indigestion
____ Liver disease (hepatitis)
____ Gallbladder disease
____ Diabetes
____ Hypoglycemia
____ Thyroid disease
____ High cholesterol level
____ High triglyceride level
____ Anemia
____ Arthritis
____ Gout
____ Pain/swelling in joints
____ Kidney disease
____ Chronic cough
____ Asthma
____ Swelling of feet/ankles
____ Difficulty breathing
____ Allergies
____ Depression
____ Anxiety
____ Use of laxatives or water pills
____ Psychological difficulties
____ Alcoholism/substance abuse
____ Other (please explain)
____
____
____

Figure 9-2
Sample health history checklist

Table 9-3
Classification of Blood Pressure for Adults Age 18 and Older*

Category	Systolic (mmHg)		Diastolic (mmHg)
Normal†	<120	and	<80
Prehypertension	120–139	or	80–89
Hypertension‡			
Stage 1	140–159	or	90–99
Stage 2	≥160	or	≥100

* Not taking antihypertensive drugs and not acutely ill. When systolic and diastolic blood pressures fall into different categories, the higher category should be selected to classify the individual's blood pressure status. For example, 140/82 mmHg should be classified as stage 1 hypertension, and 154/102 mmHg should be classified as stage 2 hypertension. In addition to classifying stages of hypertension on the basis of average blood pressure levels, clinicians should specify presence or absence of target organ disease and additional risk factors. This specificity is important for risk classification and treatment.

† Normal blood pressure with respect to cardiovascular risk is below 120/80 mmHg. However, unusually low readings should be evaluated for clinical significance.

‡ Based on the average of two or more readings taken at each of two or more visits after an initial screening.

Source: National Institutes of Health (2003). *The Seventh Report of the Joint Committee on Prevention, Detection, Evaluation, and Treatment of High Blood Pressure*. NIH Publication No. 03-5233.

Musculoskeletal Health Questionnaire

1. Have you had to see a doctor in the past three years for any bone, joint, or spine problems?
   - ☐ No
   - ☐ One or two visits, but no problems now
   - ☐ Do doctors give frequent-flyer miles?

2. Have you ever had an orthopedic injury severe enough to result in one of the following?
   - Kept you out of sports or exercise for a month?
   - Required crutches for two or more weeks?
   - Required surgery?

   ☐ No ☐ Yes (to any of the questions)

3. Have you ever dislocated or separated your shoulder?

   ☐ Yes ☐ No

   If yes, please explain. ____________________

4. Do you have joint swelling? ☐ Yes ☐ No

5. Have you lost mobility (range of motion) in any joint? For example, can you fully straighten (extend) and fully bend (flex)? Compare right to left.
   - ☐ No
   - ☐ A little stiff at times, but motion is full
   - ☐ Motion is limited in one or two major joints or the spine

6. Do you have stiffness in any joints associated with any of the following conditions?
   - Upon awakening (i.e., until showering or moving for about 15–20 minutes)
   - After sitting still for more than 30 minutes
   - For no apparent reason

   ☐ No
   ☐ Only the day after a hard workout
   ☐ Yes

7. Do your knees creak or make noise when you are going up or down stairs?
   - ☐ No
   - ☐ Yes, but no discomfort or pain
   - ☐ Yes, and does cause discomfort and/or pain

8. Do you have trouble actually ascending or descending stairs?
   - ☐ No
   - ☐ Only after going up and down multiple times, especially while carrying heavier items
   - ☐ Yes

9. Does high barometric pressure (i.e., damp, rainy weather) make your joints ache?
   - ☐ No
   - ☐ Rarely
   - ☐ Friends consult me instead of the weatherman

10. Have you ever had an episode of lower-back or neck pain or spasm?
    - ☐ No
    - ☐ Yes, it kept me off my feet for less than 24 hours
    - ☐ Yes, I miss work due to recurrent episodes

11. Do you have pain while lying on either shoulder at night in bed?
    - ☐ No
    - ☐ Rarely
    - ☐ Almost nightly; tossing and turning to get comfy

12. Do you have difficulty falling asleep at night or awaken during the night because of any joint or muscle discomfort?
    - ☐ No
    - ☐ Rarely or minor difficulty
    - ☐ Yes

13. Do you awaken at night with your hands or fingers "asleep"?
    - ☐ No
    - ☐ Rarely and I easily shake it off
    - ☐ My hands get more sleep than I do

Figure 9-3
Sample musculoskeletal health questionnaire

Resting heart rate also is considered to be a marker of physical health and cardiovascular fitness. The average resting heart rate is 72 beats per minute (bpm) with a range of 60 to 100 bpm. Generally, the more fit an individual is, the lower the resting heart rate. However, it is important to recognize that certain medications, such as **beta blockers,** may slow both resting and non-resting heart rates. The client should be quietly seated for two full minutes with both feet flat on the floor. The LWMC will either place a stethoscope firmly to the left of the sternum or feel for the pulse at the thumb side of the wrist. The heart rate can be determined using a 15-second count and multiplying this count by four to calculate the resting pulse in bpm.

In the event that the resting heart rate is above 100 bpm, the LWMC should wait another five minutes and take the pulse again. If it is still above 100 bpm, the LWMC must refer the client to his or her physician before any aerobic or muscular-endurance fitness tests are performed.

Determining a Reasonable Weight

For many significantly overweight individuals, lost weight is often regained. For example, in one controlled study, individuals who lost large amounts of weight regained approximately two-thirds of it within one year and almost all of it within five years (Wadden et al., 1989). In response to such disappointing outcomes, recommendations no longer focus on the attainment of an **ideal weight**.

Obesity experts have suggested a weight loss of 10% of body weight over six months as an initial goal (IOM, 1995; NHLBI, 1998). Once this goal has been achieved, clients can be encouraged to focus on maintaining the initial weight loss. Alternatively, individuals who remain motivated may set an interval goal of losing additional weight, with reevaluation after each successive interval. While in many cases modest losses will not bring clients to their ideal weight, even small losses (i.e., 10%) confer important health benefits and may be more likely to be sustained over time.

The results of body-composition testing can also be used to determine a reasonable weight or to set an initial goal based on lowering percent fat to a healthier level. For example, consider a 47-year-old man who weighs 212 pounds (96 kg) and has an estimated body-fat percentage of 21.3%. His goal is to reach a body-fat percentage of 14 to 17%, which is the range for men desiring optimal fitness. To calculate this man's weight for the desired range, his lean body weight must first be calculated. Since 21.3% of his body weight is fat weight, 78.7% of his weight is lean body mass (100% – 21.3% = 78.7%). The decimal form of the percentage figures are used to derive a lean body weight of 167 pounds (76 kg). To summarize:

Step 1: 100% – fat percentage = lean body percentage
100% – 21.3 = 78.7%

Step 2: body weight x lean body percentage = lean body weight
212 pounds x 0.787 = 167 pounds (76 kg)

A body weight for a desired percent fat is then calculated by first subtracting the desired percent fat from 100% and then dividing the lean body weight by the decimal form of this percentage:

Step 3: 100 – desired body fat = desired lean percent

Upper limit: 100% – 17% = 83%
Lower limit: 100% – 14% = 86%

Step 4: lean body weight/desired lean percentage = desired body weight 167/0.83 = 201 pounds (91 kg)
167/0.86 = 194 pounds (88 kg)

The weight range corresponding to a desired body fat of 14 to 17% is 194 to 201 pounds (88 to 91 kg). With regular aerobic activity, resistance training, and dietary management, this man would need to lose a minimum of 11 pounds (5 kg) of fat weight (212 – 201 = 11 pounds; 96 – 91 = 5 kg).

It is important to understand that muscle weight can increase even when exercise participation is limited to aerobic activity. Body composition should be assessed periodically throughout an exercise program. This can provide motivating information, especially when fat weight loss appears to have reached a plateau.

Assessing Psychological Health

The psychological health of all potential clients should be evaluated prior to beginning a weight-loss program. This is especially important since several psychiatric disorders, such as eating disorders, anxiety disorders, and clinical depression, can initially appear to be weight-related difficulties. In reality, though food is involved in the expression of symptoms (e.g., under- or overeating), eating disorders are classified as mental disorders that can be potentially life-threatening and require specialized interventions by skilled mental-health professionals.

Obtaining a psychological history is an important first step. An LWMC should ask all clients whether they have any concerns about how frequently they experience high levels of stress, worry excessively, or feel down for more than a few days at a time. For clients who admit having any of these feelings, it may be wise to ask if they would consider counseling, are currently in therapy, or have previously received counseling. Keep a record of all counseling experiences, including the therapist's name, dates of treatment, and reasons for seeking therapy. If the client is currently receiving counseling, it may be helpful to contact the therapist (after obtaining the client's written permission) and mutually determine whether weight loss is appropriate at this time. Review the list of medications that each client is presently taking. Certain **psychotropic medications,** such as antidepressants, anti-anxiety medications, or mood stabilizers all signal the presence of psychological conditions (Table 9-4), and many psychotropic medications may facilitate or significantly hamper weight loss.

Table 9-4
Common Psychotropic Medications

Drug Name	Trade Name(s)	Major Use
alprazolam	Xanax	Anti-anxiety
amitriptyline	Elavil	Antidepressant
amoxapine	Asendin	Antidepressant
bupropion	Wellbutrin	Antidepressant
buspirone	Buspar	Anti-anxiety
carbamazepine	Tegretol	Mood stabilizer, Anticonvulsant
chlordiazepoxide	Librium	Anti-anxiety
clomipramine	Anafranil	Antidepressant
clonazepam	Klonopin	Anti-anxiety
clonidine	Catapres	Anti-anxiety
desipramine	Norpramin, Pertofrane	Antidepressant
dexfenfluramine	Redux	Anti-appetite
diazepam	Valium	Anti-anxiety
doxepin	Sinequan, Adapin	Antidepressant
fenfluramine	Pondimin	Anti-appetite
fluvoxamine	Luvox	Antidepressant
fluoxetine	Prozac	Antidepressant
haloperidol	Haldol	Antipsychotic
imipramine	Tofranil	Antidepressant
lithium	Eskalith, Lithonate, Lithobid	Mood stabilizer
lorazepam	Ativan	Anti-anxiety
nefazodone	Serzone	Antidepressant
nortriptyline	Pamelor, Aventyl	Antidepressant
oxazepam	Serax	Anti-anxiety
paroxetine	Paxil	Antidepressant
phenelzine (MAO inhibitor)	Nardil	Antidepressant
phentermine	Fasting Lonamin	Anti-appetite

Continued on next page

Table 9-4, continued

Drug Name	Trade Name(s)	Major Use
sertraline	Zoloft	Antidepressant
triazolam	Halcion	Anti-anxiety, Hypnotic
valproate	Dapakene, Depakote	Mood stabilizer
mirtazapine	Remeron	Antidepressant
duloxetine	Cymbalta	Antidepressant
citalopram	Celexa	Antidepressant
venlafaxine	Effexor	Antidepressant
escitalopram	Lexapro	Antidepressant

Note: This list is not intended to be exhaustive. LWMCs must always consult with the client's physician (with the client's written permission) if they have any questions regarding medication use.

Specific training in psychology, psychiatry, medicine, or social work is required to adequately evaluate psychological symptoms. However, by exploring their current sense of well-being with potential clients, an LWMC can obtain some indication of the person's likelihood of succeeding at weight loss and determine whether a more comprehensive psychological evaluation is indicated. Several psychological conditions, such as clinical depression and eating disorders (i.e., **anorexia nervosa, bulimia nervosa,** and **binge eating disorder**), are clear contraindications for weight loss (see Chapter 8).

Depression

Depression is a psychological disorder in which the person experiences pervasive feelings of sadness, hopelessness, helplessness, and worthlessness. Signs of depression include sleep disturbance (e.g., hypersomnia or **insomnia**), eating difficulties (overeating or lack of interest in eating), excessive guilt, and tearfulness or crying spells. Individuals who are depressed also may have difficulty concentrating, remembering, or thinking clearly [American Psychiatric Association (APA), 1994].

Depression is increasingly viewed, in part, as being related to a chemical imbalance in the brain. Effective treatments for depression include psychotherapy alone or in combination with medication and exercise. Weight loss is never an appropriate treatment for depression and, in fact, most obesity specialists believe that depression is a contraindication for weight-loss treatment (IOM, 1995; NHLBI, 1998). Some persons who are both overweight and depressed believe that the former causes the latter, but that would be oversimplifying potentially serious underlying problems. It is important to be able to identify signs of clinical depression and refer the individual to a mental-health specialist for further evaluation.

Eating Disorders

Anorexia nervosa is characterized by the refusal to maintain a minimally healthy body weight (i.e., at least 85% of ideal body weight), a morbid fear of gaining weight, **amenorrhea,** and disturbances in the way in which weight and shape are experienced or evaluated by the individual (APA, 1994). Bulimia nervosa is characterized by recurrent episodes of binge eating in which the individual experiences a loss of control over eating, followed by compensatory behaviors aimed at avoiding weight gain (e.g., vomiting, **laxative** or **diuretic** abuse, fasting, or excessive exercise) (APA, 1994). As with anorexia nervosa, self-evaluation is unduly influenced by weight and shape. Individuals with bulimia nervosa are often of normal weight or slightly overweight. In binge eating disorder (BED), which is classified as "eating disorder not otherwise specified" (EDNOS), the individual also experiences episodes of bingeing coupled with a sense of loss of control over eating. However, there is no active attempt at compensating for the binges (APA, 1994). Individuals with binge eating disorder tend to be overweight or obese. In clinical settings, 25 to 33% of individuals seeking weight-loss treatment suffer from BED (Spitzer et al., 1993). Table 9-5 presents screening questions to help detect binge eating disorder.

It is important to identify eating disorders in potential clients, because these individuals are more likely to suffer from

Table 9-5
Screening Questions to Detect Binge Eating

- Are there times during the day when you could not have stopped eating, even if you had wanted to?
- Do you ever find yourself eating unusually large amounts of food in a short period of time?
- Do you ever feel extremely guilty or depressed afterward?
- Do you ever feel even more determined to diet or eat healthier after the eating episodes?

Source: Reprinted from *Journal of the American Dietetic Association*, Vol. 96, Bruce, B. & Wilfley, D. Binge eating among the overweight population: A serious and prevalent problem. 58–61, 1996, with permission from Elsevier.

other psychological disorders as well (Bruce & Wilfley, 1996). Weight loss or maintenance of an abnormally low body weight is never appropriate for an individual with anorexia nervosa. This is important to remember when working with athletes by whom a low body weight is coveted, such as bodybuilders, gymnasts, dancers, and runners. Weight loss is only appropriate in individuals with bulimia when it is accompanied by ongoing psychotherapy (or follows a successful course of therapy). Recovery from binge eating disorder also appears to require psychotherapy specifically aimed at reducing binge eating (Bruce & Wilfley, 1996). It is unclear whether dieting complicates or facilitates recovery from binge eating disorder. If an LWMC suspects that a potential client may suffer from BED, it is important to consider referral to an eating disorders specialist before starting to train the individual. Cognitive behavioral psychotherapy may increase the client's ability to lose weight and maximize the likelihood of successful maintenance of a lower body weight.

Assessing Exercise Readiness

The American College of Sports Medicine (ACSM) has established recommendations concerning the need for a medical examination and exercise testing prior to participation in an exercise program (ACSM, 2006). Historically, many sedentary adults have been sent for a complete physical exam and stress test before beginning an exercise program. Unfortunately, the cost of such assessments, along with fears of conveying the erroneous message that all exercise is dangerous, may have prevented many adults from adopting a more active lifestyle. Thus, it is important for LWMCs to clearly understand who does and does not require a thorough medical screening before beginning an exercise program.

ACSM classifies adults into three levels of risk: low-risk, moderate-risk, and high-risk (Tables 9-6 through 9-9). Low-risk individuals may begin an unrestricted exercise program without a physician's approval. These people do not require physician supervision for maximal treadmill testing.

Individuals over the age cut-offs listed in Table 9-8 who are asymptomatic can also begin a moderate-intensity exercise program without a physician's approval. ACSM defines moderate-intensity exercise as 40 to 60% of $\dot{V}O_2R$ ($\dot{V}O_2R$ is the difference between $\dot{V}O_2$**max** and resting $\dot{V}O_2$). Moderate intensity can also be defined as exercise well within the individual's current exercise capacity that can be comfortably sustained for extended periods of time (i.e., 60 minutes) and is noncompetitive.

Healthy, asymptomatic women over 55 and men over 45 years of age should seek medical approval if they wish to exercise vigorously. ACSM defines vigorous exercise as being equal to or greater than 60% of $\dot{V}O_2R$. If actual exercise intensity is uncertain, vigorous exercise can be defined as an intensity that challenges the aerobic system or results in fatigue after 20 minutes of participation. Physician supervision is required for maximal exercise testing in asymptomatic older adults, but is not necessary for submaximal assessments.

Individuals who are considered moderate risk but have no symptoms may begin a moderate-intensity exercise program without physician approval; however, these persons require a medical exam and an exercise test before exercising vigorously. Persons with any

Table 9-6
Coronary Artery Disease Risk-factor Thresholds for Use With ACSM Risk Stratification

Positive Risk Factors	Defining Criteria
Family History	Myocardial infarction, coronary revascularization, or sudden death before 55 years of age in father or other male first-degree relative, or before 65 years of age in mother or other female first-degree relative
Cigarette smoking	Current cigarette smoker or those who quit within the previous 6 months
Hypertension	Systolic blood pressure ≥140 mmHg or diastolic ≥90 mmHg, confirmed by measurements on at least two separate occasions, or on antihypertensive medication
Dyslipidemia	Low-density lipoprotein (LDL) cholesterol >130 mg/dL (3.4 mmol/L) or high-intensity lipoprotein (HDL) cholesterol <40 mg/dL (1.03 mmol/L), or on lipid-lowering medication. If total serum cholesterol is all that is available, use >200 mg/dL (5.2 mmol/L) rather than low-density lipoprotein (LDL) >130 mg/dL
Impaired fasting glucose	Fasting blood glucose ≥100 mg/dL (5.6 mmol/L) confirmed by measurements on at least two separate occasions
Obesity*	Body mass index >30 kg/m^2 or Waist girth >102 cm (40 in) for men and >88 cm (35 in) for women or Waist/hip ratio: ≥0.95 for men and ≥0.86 for women
Sedentary lifestyle	Persons not participating in a regular exercise program or not meeting the minimal physical activity recommendations† from the U.S. Surgeon General's Report

Negative Risk Factor	Defining Criteria
High-serum HDL cholesterol‡	>60 mg/dL (1.6 mmol/L)

Hypertension threshold based on National High Blood Pressure Education Program. *The Seventh Report of the Joint National Committee on Prevention, Detention, Evaluation, and Treatment of High Blood Pressure* (JNC7). 2003. 03-5233.

Lipid thresholds based on National Cholesterol Education Program. *Third Report of the National Education Program (NCEP) Expert Panel on Detection, Evaluation, and Treatment of High Blood Pressure in Adults (Adult Treatment Panel III).* NIH Publication No. 02-5215, 2002.

Impaired FG threshold based on Expert Committee on the Diagnosis and Classification of Diabetes Mellitus. Follow-up report on the diagnosis of diabetes mellitus. *Diabetes Care 2003*; 26:3160–3167.

Obesity thresholds based on Expert Panel on Detection, Evaluation, and Treatment of Overweight and Obesity in Adults. National Institutes of Health. Clinical guidelines on the identification, evaluation, and treatment of overweight and obesity in adults—the evidence report. *Arch Int Med* 1998; 158:1855–1867.

Sedentary lifestyle thresholds based on United States Department of Health and Human Services. *Physical Activity and Health: A Report of the Surgeon General*. 1996.

* Professional opinions vary regarding the most appropriate markers and thresholds for obesity and therefore allied health professionals should use clinical judgment when evaluating this risk factor.

† Accumulating 30 minutes or more of moderate physical activity on most days of the week.

‡ It is common to sum risk factors in making clinical judgments. If HDL is high, subtract one risk factor from the sum of positive risk factors, because high HDL decreases CAD risk.

Source: Reprinted with permission from American College of Sports Medicine (2006). *ACSM's Guidelines for Exercise Testing and Prescription* (7th ed.). Philadelphia: Lippincott Williams & Wilkins.

Table 9-7

Major Symptoms and Signs Suggestive of Cardiopulmonary Disease

- Pain, discomfort (or other anginal equivalent) in the chest, neck, jaw, arms, or other areas that might be ischemic in nature
- Shortness of breath at rest or with mild exertion
- Dizziness or syncope (fainting spells)
- Orthopnea (shortness of breath when lying flat—often report sleeping on more than one pillow) or paroxysmal sudden onset nocturnal dyspnea (labored breathing)
- Ankle edema (swelling)
- Palpitations or tachycardia (racing heart)
- Claudication (intermittent leg pain) that occurs with walking
- Known heart murmur
- Unusual fatigue or shortness of breath with usual activities

These symptoms must be interpreted in the clinical context in which they appear, since they are not all specific for cardiopulmonary or metabolic disease.

Source: Reprinted with permission from American College of Sports Medicine (2006). *ACSM's Guidelines for Exercise Testing and Prescription* (7th ed.). Philadelphia: Lippincott Williams & Wilkins.

Table 9-8

ACSM Risk Stratification Categories

Low risk	Men <45 years of age and women <55 years of age who are asymptomatic (major symptoms are presented in Table 9-7) and meet no more than one risk-factor threshold from Table 9-6
Moderate risk	Men ≥45 years and women ≥55 years *or* those who meet the threshold for two or more risk factors from Table 9-6
High risk	Individuals with one or more signs and symptoms *or* known cardiovascular,* pulmonary,† or metabolic‡ disease

* Cardiac, peripheral vascular, or cerebrovascular disease

† Chronic obstructive pulmonary disease, asthma, interstitial lung disease, or cystic fibrosis (see American Association of Cardiovascular and Pulmonary Rehabilitation. *Guidelines for Pulmonary Rehabilitation Programs*. 2nd ed. Champaign, Ill.: Human Kinetics, 1998; 97–112.

‡ Diabetes mellitus (IDDM, NIDDM), thyroid disorders, renal, or liver disease.

Source: Reprinted with permission from American College of Sports Medicine (2006). *ACSM's Guidelines for Exercise Testing and Prescription* (7th ed.). Philadelphia: Lippincott Williams & Wilkins.

Table 9-9

ACSM Pre-participation Screening Algorithm—Level 3: Exercise Test Considerations

Low Risk	Moderate Risk	High Risk
Further medical examination and exercise testing not necessary* prior to initiation of exercise training	Medical examination and exercise testing recommended prior to initiation of vigorous exercise training	Medical examination and exercise testing recommended prior to initiation of moderate or vigorous exercise training
Medical supervision for submaximal or maximal exercise testing not necessary	Medical supervision† recommended for maximal exercise testing	Medical supervision† recommended for maximal or submaximal exercise testing

* The designation of "not necessary" reflects the notion that a medical examination, exercise test, and medical supervision of exercise testing would not be essential in the pre-activity screening; however, they should not be viewed as inappropriate.

† When medical supervision of exercise testing is "recommended," the physician should be in proximity and readily available should there be an emergent need.

Source: Reprinted with permission from American College of Sports Medicine (2006). *ACSM's Guidelines for Exercise Testing and Prescription* (7th ed.). Philadelphia: Lippincott Williams & Wilkins.

symptoms suggestive of cardiopulmonary or metabolic disease should seek physician approval before beginning either a moderate or vigorous exercise program. Physician supervision is required for maximal exercise testing in adults with moderate risk.

Individuals with known cardiopulmonary or metabolic disease should consult a physician prior to beginning an exercise program. Physician supervision is also required for both maximal and submaximal exercise testing in persons with known disease.

Clinical Exercise Testing vs. Aerobic Fitness Evaluation

Two types of testing are usually used to evaluate readiness to exercise: clinical exercise testing (or stress tests) and aerobic fitness evaluations. Clinical exercise testing is more sophisticated and is typically used to diagnose or rule out cardiopulmonary problems. In addition, persons with known disease often undergo clinical exercise testing to determine levels of **ischemia** and establish whether an increase in physical activity is safe. Maximal-capacity clinical exercise tests are typically administered by highly trained personnel in such settings as human performance laboratories or hospitals. Blood pressure, heart rate (via electrocardiogram), **rating of perceived exertion (RPE),** and expired gases are monitored continuously throughout a clinical exercise test.

Contrary to clinical exercise testing, aerobic fitness evaluations are not used to diagnose disease or establish whether exercise is safe. Some aerobic-fitness evaluations can be readily administered by an LWMC and will provide important information on baseline fitness levels to create an appropriate and safe exercise program. Furthermore, knowledge of baseline oxygen capacity ($\dot{V}O_2max$) can help both the LWMC and the client in setting realistic, attainable goals.

Traditionally, an individual's $\dot{V}O_2max$ has been used as the marker of aerobic fitness. The most accurate assessment of $\dot{V}O_2max$ is obtained by measuring the volume of expired gases during a maximal-effort, progressive exercise test. However, maximal aerobic testing has three notable drawbacks: It requires highly trained personnel, is time-consuming, and poses a higher risk to a sedentary client, since most exercise-related complications occur during attempted maximum exercise intensity.

As a result, submaximal exercise tests were developed. $\dot{V}O_2max$ can be estimated by knowing the oxygen cost of a given workload. A fundamental assumption of submaximal exercise testing is the existence of a linear relationship between work and heart rate or $\dot{V}O_2$. By plotting two or more workloads on a graph, an LWMC can interpolate and predict what a maximal effort would be based on a predicted maximal heart rate.

A simple way to evaluate fitness improvement is to measure submaximal heart-rate response repeatedly to a given workload. Thus, if the heart-rate response to a fixed workload decreases after training, it is likely that physical fitness has improved.

For safety, LWMCs should only use submaximal assessments when determining aerobic fitness in sedentary adults. It is beyond the LWMC's scope of practice to monitor an ECG (electrocardiogram) for arrhythmias during a fitness evaluation. An ECG should be used to monitor heart rate only. ECG traces should only be interpreted by a physician or an appropriately trained healthcare professional.

Assessing Fitness

Experts have had a difficult time agreeing on a definition of physical fitness over the years. However, most exercise scientists agree that four components are involved in physical fitness:

- Aerobic fitness
- Muscle and joint **flexibility**
- Muscle strength and endurance
- Body composition (see Chapter 10)

A fitness assessment provides the opportunity to analyze each of these components and is used for any or all of the following:

- To assess current fitness levels in relation to age and sex

- To aid in the development of exercise programs
- To identify areas of health and injury risk and the need for possible referral to the appropriate healthcare professional
- To establish realistic, attainable goals and provide motivation
- To educate the client about physical fitness
- To evaluate the success of the fitness program through follow-up assessments

Many clients may request that a fitness evaluation be part of their work with an LWMC. Others may feel frightened or embarrassed to undergo such an assessment. Still others may be overwhelmed and discouraged by the potentially negative feedback of baseline testing results. It is important to respect a client's sensitivity to, and interest in, a thorough fitness assessment. However, the minimum evaluation that the LWMC should undertake in assessing readiness for aerobic exercise involves assessing cardiovascular risk factors and measuring resting heart rate and resting blood pressure. LWMCs should also explore each client's activity history, attitudes toward exercise, and stated fitness goals. A sample Exercise History and Attitude Questionnaire is shown in Figure 9-4.

Figure 9-4
Sample exercise history and attitude questionnaire

Exercise History and Attitude Questionnaire

Name ______________________ Date ______________

General Instructions: Please fill out this form as completely as possible. If you have any questions, DO NOT GUESS; ask your consultant for assistance.

1. Please rate your exercise level on a scale of 1 to 5 (5 indicating very strenuous) for each age range through your present age:

   15–20 ______ 21–30 ______ 31–40 ______ 41+ ______

2. Were you a high school and/or college athlete? ☐ Yes ☐ No

   If yes, please specify. ______________________

3. Do you have any negative feelings toward, or have you had any bad experiences with, physical-activity programs? ☐ Yes ☐ No

   If yes, please explain. ______________________

4. Do you have any negative feelings toward, or have you had any bad experiences with, fitness testing and evaluation? ☐ Yes ☐ No

   If yes, please explain. ______________________

5. Rate yourself on a scale of 1 to 5 (1 indicating the lowest value and 5 the highest).

	Circle the number that best applies to you.				
Characterize your present athletic ability.	1	2	3	4	5
When you exercise, how important is competition?	1	2	3	4	5
Characterize your present cardiovascular capacity.	1	2	3	4	5
Characterize your present muscular capacity.	1	2	3	4	5
Characterize your present flexibility capacity.	1	2	3	4	5

6. Do you start exercise programs but then find yourself unable to stick with them? ☐ Yes ☐ No

Figure 9-4
continued

7. How much time are you willing to devote to an exercise program?
 _______ minutes/day _______ days/week

8. Are you currently involved in regular endurance (cardiovascular) exercise? ☐ Yes ☐ No
 If yes, specify the type of exercise(s) ______________________________
 _______ minutes/day _______ days/week
 Rate your perception of the exertion of your exercise program (circle the number):
 (1) Light (2) Fairly light (3) Somewhat hard (4) Hard

9. How long have you been exercising regularly? _____ months _____ years

10. What other exercises, sports, or recreational activities have you participated in?
 In the past 6 months? ______________________________
 In the past 5 years? ______________________________

11. Can you exercise during your workday? ☐ Yes ☐ No

12. Would an exercise program interfere with your job? ☐ Yes ☐ No

13. Would an exercise program benefit your job? ☐ Yes ☐ No

14. What types of exercise interest you?

☐ Walking	☐ Jogging	☐ Swimming	☐ Cycling
☐ Aerobics	☐ Strength training	☐ Stationary biking	☐ Rowing
☐ Racquetball	☐ Tennis	☐ Other aerobic activity	☐ Stretching

15. Rank your goals in undertaking exercise: What do you want exercise to do for you?
 Use the following scale to rate each goal separately.

	Not at all important				Somewhat important			Extremely important		
a. Improve cardiovascular fitness	1	2	3	4	5	6	7	8	9	10
b. Facilitate body-fat weight loss	1	2	3	4	5	6	7	8	9	10
c. Reshape or tone my body	1	2	3	4	5	6	7	8	9	10
d. Improve performance for a specific sport	1	2	3	4	5	6	7	8	9	10
e. Improve moods and ability to cope with stress	1	2	3	4	5	6	7	8	9	10
f. Improve flexibility	1	2	3	4	5	6	7	8	9	10
g. Increase strength	1	2	3	4	5	6	7	8	9	10
h. Increase energy level	1	2	3	4	5	6	7	8	9	10
i. Feel better	1	2	3	4	5	6	7	8	9	10
j. Increase enjoyment	1	2	3	4	5	6	7	8	9	10
k. Other	1	2	3	4	5	6	7	8	9	10

16. By how much would you like to change your current weight?
 (+) _______ lb (–) _______ lb

Assessing Aerobic Fitness

Two submaximal tests that are easily administered, readily interpreted, and recommended for assessing aerobic fitness are the YMCA Step Test and the Rockport Walking Test. Though both tests require little or no equipment, they are not as accurate as cycle ergometer or treadmill tests. Also, little comparative data are available. (For more information on administering cycle ergometry and treadmill assessments, see the *ACE Personal Trainer Manual.*)

YMCA Step Test

Developed by Dr. Fred Kasch of San Diego State University, the YMCA Step Test requires clients to step on and off a 12-inch-high step bench to a standardized cadence for three minutes (YMCA of the USA, 2000). Although this test does not result in an estimation of maximal oxygen consumption, it gives an estimation of cardiorespiratory fitness in comparison to established norms.

Required items:

- Step bench (12 inches in height)
- Metronome set at 96 bpm
- Stopwatch

Procedure:

Clients should perform a light warm-up prior to testing. Before beginning the test, the LWMC should demonstrate the correct stepping procedure. The LWMC should set the metronome to 96 bpm and start stepping to a four-beat cycle (up, up, down, down). Both feet should come in complete contact with the top of the bench during the up portion of the cycle and touch the floor during the down portion of the cycle. Allow clients an opportunity to practice the movement cycle along with the metronome. It is acceptable for participants to change the lead foot during the test. Just before administering the test, the LWMC must notify participants that they will step continuously for three minutes and be seated immediately afterward for a one-minute pulse count.

The LWMC places the metronome in a location where it may be easily heard by all participants. The clients start by simply marching on the floor in front of the bench to the rhythm provided by the metronome. The LWMC should remind the clients that they may use either foot to start the cycle and instruct them to begin stepping as the stopwatch is started. The LWMC checks their stepping rhythm throughout the test and announces when one minute, two minutes, and two minutes and 30 second has elapsed. Immediately after completing three minutes of stepping, clients should be instructed to sit down on their benches and count their pulses for one minute. The one-minute post-exercise heart rate is used to score the test (Tables 9-10 and 9-11).

Rockport Fitness Walking Test

The Rockport Fitness Walking Test is routinely used to assess the cardiovascular fitness of those with a low-to-moderate aerobic fitness level (Howley & Franks, 2007). The test involves a timed one-mile walk on a smooth and level surface (preferably a quarter-mile running track). The only other equipment necessary is a timing device and a form for recording results.

Whereas lab tests measure parameters (e.g., estimated $\dot{V}O_2$ workload or heart rate) that give a very good indication of how well an individual will perform during aerobic activity, the Rockport Fitness Walking Test directly evaluates performance. This test is also excellent for mass testing. It does, however, have its limits. Pacing ability and body-fat weight may adversely affect performance, and because the test requires the mile to be walked as fast as possible, lack of motivation may result in an underestimation of cardiovascular fitness.

Before beginning the test, the LWMC has the clients warm up by walking and performing light stretching exercises. The LWMC explains that while this test requires a near-maximal effort, clients should not walk to exhaustion and should stop at any time if necessary. Elapsed times should be announced with every lap. After completing the test, the clients should take a 10-second pulse. This 10-second value and its corresponding per-minute pulse (the 10-second pulse multiplied by six) should be

Table 9-10
Post-exercise Heart-rate Norms for the Three-minute Step Test (Men)

		Age (years)					
Rating	**% Rating**	**18–25**	**26–35**	**36–45**	**46–55**	**56–65**	**66+**
Excellent	100	50	51	49	56	60	59
	95	71	70	70	77	71	74
	90	76	76	76	82	77	81
Good	85	79	79	80	87	86	87
	80	82	83	84	89	91	91
	75	84	85	88	93	94	92
Above average	70	88	88	92	95	97	94
	65	90	91	95	99	99	97
	60	93	94	98	101	100	102
Average	55	95	96	100	103	103	104
	50	97	100	101	107	105	106
	45	100	102	105	111	109	110
Below average	40	102	104	108	113	111	114
	35	105	108	111	117	115	116
	30	107	110	113	119	117	118
Poor	25	111	114	116	121	119	121
	20	114	118	119	124	123	123
	15	119	121	124	126	128	126
Very poor	10	124	126	130	131	131	130
	5	132	134	138	139	136	136
	0	157	161	163	159	154	151

Source: YMCA Fitness Testing and Assessment Manual (4th ed.). © 2000. Reprinted and adapted with permission of the YMCA of the USA, 101 N. Wacker Drive, Chicago, Ill. 60606.

Table 9-11
Post-exercise Heart-rate Norms for the Three-minute Step Test (Women)

		Age (years)					
Rating	**% Rating**	**18–25**	**26–35**	**36–45**	**46–55**	**56–65**	**66+**
Excellent	100	52	58	51	63	60	70
	95	75	74	77	85	83	85
	90	81	80	84	91	92	92
Good	85	85	85	89	95	97	96
	80	89	89	92	98	100	98
	75	93	92	96	101	103	101
Above average	70	96	95	100	104	106	104
	65	98	98	102	107	109	108
	60	102	101	104	110	111	111
Average	55	104	104	107	113	113	116
	50	108	107	109	115	116	120
	45	110	110	112	118	118	121
Below average	40	113	113	115	120	119	123
	35	116	116	118	121	123	125
	30	120	119	120	124	127	126
Poor	25	122	122	124	126	129	128
	20	126	126	128	128	131	129
	15	131	129	132	132	135	133
Very poor	10	135	134	137	137	141	135
	5	143	141	142	143	147	145
	0	169	171	169	171	174	155

Source: YMCA Fitness Testing and Assessment Manual (4th ed.). © 2000. Reprinted and adapted with permission of the YMCA of the USA, 101 N. Wacker Drive, Chicago, Ill. 60606

recorded, along with the time it took to complete the one-mile walk. After test completion, all clients should walk for at least five minutes to cool down.

In addition to completion time and immediate postexercise heart rate, a maximal perceived exertion also can be recorded to provide an indication of effort and a comparison to subsequent tests. Completion time and minute pulse rate are used to score the test on the proper chart for age and sex (Table 9-12).

Table 9-12
Estimated Maximal Oxygen Uptake (mL/kg/min) for Men and Women, 20–69 Years Old

	Minutes/Mile										
	10	11	12	13	14	15	16	17	18	19	20
Heart Rate	**Men (20–29)**										
120	65.0	61.7	58.4	55.2	51.9	48.6	45.4	42.1	38.9	35.6	32.3
130	63.4	60.1	56.9	53.6	50.3	47.1	43.8	40.6	37.3	34.0	30.8
140	61.8	58.6	55.3	52.0	48.8	45.5	42.2	39.0	35.7	32.5	29.2
150	60.3	57.0	53.7	50.5	47.2	43.9	40.7	37.4	34.2	30.9	27.6
160	58.7	55.4	52.2	48.9	45.6	42.4	39.1	35.9	32.6	29.3	26.1
170	57.1	53.9	50.6	47.3	44.1	40.8	37.6	34.3	31.0	27.8	24.5
180	55.6	52.3	49.0	45.8	42.5	39.3	36.0	32.7	29.5	26.2	22.9
190	54.0	50.7	47.5	44.2	41.0	37.7	34.4	31.2	27.9	24.6	21.4
200	52.4	49.2	45.9	42.7	39.4	36.1	32.9	29.6	26.3	23.1	19.8
Heart Rate	**Women (20–29)**										
120	62.1	58.9	55.6	52.3	49.1	45.8	42.5	39.3	36.0	32.7	29.5
130	60.6	57.3	54.0	50.8	47.5	44.2	41.0	32.7	34.4	31.2	27.9
140	59.0	55.7	52.5	49.2	45.9	42.7	39.4	36.1	32.9	29.6	26.3
150	57.4	54.2	50.9	47.6	44.4	41.1	37.8	34.6	31.3	28.0	24.8
160	55.9	52.6	49.3	46.1	42.8	39.5	36.3	33.0	29.7	26.5	23.2
170	54.3	51.0	47.8	44.5	41.2	38.0	34.7	31.4	28.2	24.9	21.6
180	52.7	49.5	46.2	42.9	39.7	36.4	33.1	29.9	26.6	23.3	20.1
190	51.2	47.9	44.6	41.4	38.1	34.8	31.6	28.3	25.0	21.8	18.5
200	49.6	46.3	43.1	39.8	36.5	33.3	30.0	26.7	23.5	20.2	16.9
Heart Rate	**Men (30–39)**										
120	61.1	57.8	54.6	51.3	48.0	44.8	41.5	38.2	35.0	31.7	28.4
130	59.5	56.3	53.0	49.7	46.5	43.2	39.9	36.7	33.4	30.1	26.9
140	58.0	54.7	51.4	48.2	44.9	41.6	38.4	35.1	31.8	28.6	25.3
150	56.4	53.1	49.9	46.6	43.3	40.1	36.8	33.5	30.3	27.0	23.8
160	54.8	51.6	48.3	45.0	41.8	38.5	35.2	32.0	28.7	25.5	22.2
170	53.3	50.0	46.7	43.5	40.2	36.9	33.7	30.4	27.1	23.9	20.6
180	51.7	48.4	45.2	41.9	38.6	35.4	32.1	28.8	25.6	22.3	19.1
190	50.1	46.9	43.6	40.3	37.1	33.8	30.5	27.3	24.0	20.8	17.5
Heart Rate	**Women (30–39)**										
120	58.2	55.0	51.7	48.4	45.2	41.9	38.7	35.4	32.1	28.9	25.6
130	56.7	53.4	50.1	46.9	43.6	40.4	37.1	33.8	30.6	27.3	24.0
140	55.1	51.8	48.6	45.3	42.1	38.8	35.5	32.3	29.0	25.7	22.5
150	53.5	50.3	47.0	43.8	40.5	37.2	34.0	30.7	27.4	24.2	20.9
160	52.0	48.7	45.4	42.2	38.9	35.7	32.4	29.1	25.9	22.6	19.3
170	50.4	47.1	43.9	40.6	37.4	34.1	30.8	27.6	24.3	21.0	17.8
180	48.8	45.6	42.3	39.1	35.8	32.5	29.3	26.0	22.7	19.5	16.2
190	47.3	44.0	40.8	37.5	34.2	31.0	27.7	24.4	21.2	17.9	14.6

	Minutes/Mile										
	10	11	12	13	14	15	16	17	18	19	20
Heart Rate Men (40–49)											
120	57.2	54.0	50.7	47.4	44.2	40.9	37.6	34.4	31.1	27.8	24.6
130	55.7	52.4	49.1	45.9	42.6	39.3	36.1	32.8	29.5	26.3	23.0
140	54.1	50.8	47.6	44.3	41.0	37.8	34.5	31.2	28.0	24.7	21.4
150	52.5	49.3	46.0	42.7	39.5	36.2	32.9	29.7	26.4	23.1	19.9
160	51.0	47.7	44.4	41.2	37.9	34.6	31.4	28.1	24.8	21.6	18.3
170	49.4	46.1	42.9	39.6	36.3	33.1	29.8	26.5	23.3	20.0	16.7
180	47.8	44.6	41.3	38.0	34.8	31.5	28.2	25.0	21.7	18.4	15.2
Heart Rate	**Women (40–49)**										
120	54.4	51.1	47.8	44.6	41.3	38.0	34.8	31.5	28.2	25.0	21.7
130	52.8	49.5	46.3	43.0	39.7	36.5	33.2	29.9	26.7	23.4	20.1
140	51.2	48.0	44.7	41.4	38.2	34.9	31.6	28.4	25.1	21.8	18.6
150	49.7	46.4	43.1	39.9	36.6	33.3	30.1	26.8	23.5	20.3	17.0
160	48.1	44.8	41.6	38.3	35.0	31.8	28.5	25.2	22.0	18.7	15.5
170	46.5	43.3	40.0	36.7	33.5	30.2	26.9	23.7	20.4	17.2	13.9
180	45.0	41.7	38.4	35.2	31.9	28.6	25.4	22.1	18.9	15.6	12.3
Heart Rate	**Men (50–59)**										
120	53.3	50.0	46.8	43.5	40.3	37.0	33.7	30.5	27.2	23.9	20.7
130	51.7	48.5	45.2	42.0	38.7	35.4	32.2	28.9	25.6	22.4	19.1
140	50.2	46.9	43.7	40.4	37.1	33.9	30.6	27.3	24.1	20.8	17.5
150	48.6	45.4	42.1	38.8	35.6	32.3	29.0	25.8	22.5	19.2	16.0
160	47.1	43.8	40.5	37.3	34.0	30.7	27.5	24.2	20.9	17.7	14.4
170	45.5	42.2	39.0	35.7	32.4	29.2	25.9	22.6	19.4	16.1	12.8
Heart Rate	**Women (50–59)**										
120	50.5	47.2	43.9	40.7	37.4	34.1	30.9	27.6	24.3	21.1	17.8
130	48.9	45.6	42.4	39.1	35.8	32.6	29.3	26.0	22.8	19.5	16.2
140	47.3	44.1	40.8	37.5	34.3	31.0	27.7	24.5	21.2	17.9	14.7
150	45.8	42.5	39.2	36.0	32.7	29.4	26.2	22.9	19.6	16.4	13.1
160	44.2	40.9	37.7	34.4	31.1	27.9	24.6	21.3	18.1	14.8	11.5
170	42.6	39.4	36.1	32.8	29.6	26.3	23.0	19.8	16.5	13.2	10.0
Heart Rate	**Men (60–69)**										
120	49.4	46.2	42.9	39.6	36.4	33.1	29.8	26.6	23.3	20.0	16.8
130	47.9	44.6	41.3	38.1	34.8	31.5	28.3	25.0	21.7	18.5	15.2
140	46.3	43.0	39.8	36.5	33.2	30.0	26.7	23.4	20.2	16.9	13.6
150	44.7	41.5	38.2	34.9	31.7	28.4	25.1	21.9	18.6	15.3	12.1
160	43.2	39.9	36.6	33.4	30.1	26.8	23.6	20.3	17.0	13.8	10.5
Heart Rate	**Women (60–69)**										
120	46.6	43.3	40.0	36.8	33.5	30.2	27.0	23.7	20.5	17.2	13.9
130	45.0	41.7	38.5	35.2	31.9	28.7	25.4	22.2	18.9	15.6	12.4
140	43.4	40.2	36.9	33.6	30.4	27.1	23.8	20.6	17.3	14.1	10.8
150	41.9	38.6	35.3	32.1	28.8	25.5	22.3	19.0	15.8	12.5	9.2
160	40.3	37.0	33.8	30.5	27.2	24.0	20.7	17.5	14.2	10.9	7.7

Note: Calculations assume 170 lb for men and 125 lb for women. For each 15 lb beyond these values, subtract 1 mL. Adapted from Kline et al. (1987).

Source: Reprinted, with permission, from E.T. Howley and B.D. Franks, *Health Fitness Instructor's Handbook,* 2nd ed, (Champaign, IL: Human Kinetics), page 158–160.

The values in Table 9-12 are derived from the following formulas:

Women
$\dot{V}O_2$ (mL/kg/min) = 132.85 – (0.388 x age) – (0.077 x weight) – (3.265 x mile walk time) – (0.156 x exercise HR)

Men
$\dot{V}O_2$ (mL/kg/min) = 139.168 – (0.388 x age) – (0.077 x weight) – (3.265 x mile walk time) – (0.156 x exercise HR)

Note: weight is expressed in pounds; time is expressed in minutes.

The standard error of the estimate of maximal oxygen uptake from the Rockport Walking Test is 5.0 mL O_2/kg_{BW}/min. This is about 1.0 mL O_2/kg_{BW}/min better than most submaximal bike, treadmill, or step tests.

Assessing Muscle and Joint Flexibility

Flexibility is a measure of the range of movement on a joint or group of joints, and is often the most neglected component of physical fitness. However, significant improvements in flexibility can be achieved by following a sound training program.

Sit-and-Reach Test

The sit-and-reach test is used to assess low-back and hip-joint flexibility. Due to the possibility of injury to the low back and hamstrings, clients should refrain from fast jerky movements during this assessment. Instead, they should perform the test trials slowly and with control. Clients with a history of low-back dysfunction and/or pain should avoid performing this test.

Required items:

- Exercise mat
- Tape
- Yardstick

Procedure:

Clients should perform a light warm-up prior to testing. However, if this test follows a cardiorespiratory-fitness test, clients may proceed without a warm-up. Additional light stretching of the low back and hamstrings (e.g., modified hurdler stretch) is recommended before test administration. The LWMC places a yardstick on the floor and puts a piece of tape at least 12 inches long on the 15-inch mark on the yardstick. The LWMC then reviews and demonstrates the proper execution of the test. With shoes off, he or she sits on the floor with the yardstick parallel between extended legs. The zero mark of the yardstick should be toward the body. The feet should be placed approximately 12 inches part, with the heels aligned with the tape at the 15-inch mark. The LWMC then extends the arms in front of the chest and places one hand on top of the other, with fingertips aligned. Inhaling in the upright position and exhaling while leaning forward, he or she drops the head toward or between the arms. The fingers should maintain contact with the yardstick and the knees should remain in full extension (Figure 9-5).

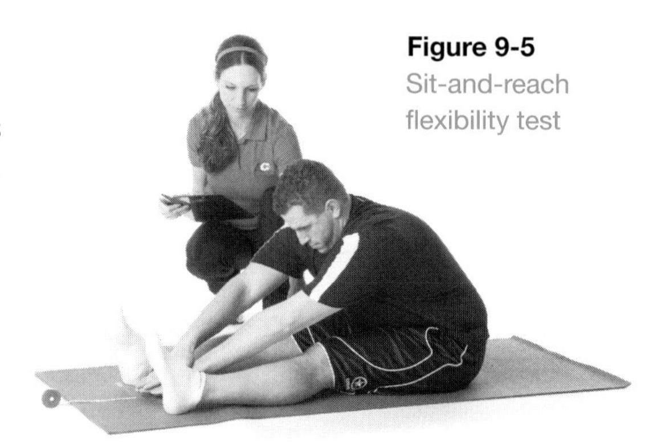

Figure 9-5
Sit-and-reach flexibility test

The LWMC should instruct clients to begin the test by slowly reaching forward with both hands as far as possible, holding this position for approximately two seconds. Clients must be reminded to keep their hands parallel and not to lead with one hand. The score is the furthest point on the yardstick reached after three trials (Table 9-13).

Assessing Muscle Strength and Endurance

The two components of muscular-fitness testing are muscular strength and muscular endurance. Adequate muscular strength and endurance are necessary for optimal health and to enhance quality of life.

Table 9-13
Norms for Trunk-flexibility Test Fitness Categories

Men						
Ages	18–25	26–35	36–45	46–55	56–65	>65
% Rating						
90	22	21	21	19	17	17
80	20	19	19	17	15	15
70	19	17	17	15	13	13
60	18	17	16	14	13	12
50	17	15	15	13	11	10
40	15	14	13	11	9	9
30	14	13	13	10	9	8
20	13	11	11	9	7	7
10	11	9	7	6	5	4

Women						
Ages	18–25	26–35	36–45	46–55	56–65	>65
% Rating						
90	24	23	22	21	20	20
80	22	21	21	20	19	18
70	21	20	19	18	17	17
60	20	20	18	17	16	17
50	19	19	17	16	15	15
40	18	17	16	14	14	14
30	17	16	15	14	13	13
20	16	15	14	12	11	11
10	14	13	12	10	9	9

Muscle strength is measured by the amount of force that can be produced by a single maximal effort. Strength historically has been assessed using maximal lifts such as the bench press or leg squat in the weight room. This type of assessment would not be practical or safe to use with overweight, sedentary adults. Two reasonable alternatives are the push-up and half sit-up tests, which measure both muscle strength and endurance.

Push-up Test

The push-up test is used to evaluate upper-body muscular strength and endurance (e.g., pectoralis major, anterior deltoids, triceps). The protocol calls for two different positions based on the sex of the client. Men are required to perform the test in the standard position with the hands and toes in contact with the floor. Women are required to use the modified position with the hands and knees in contact with the floor. Women who choose the standard push-up position (i.e., with the hands and toes in contact with the floor) must be notified that their scores will not be comparable to the standardized norms because the data represented in the norm table were produced from research using only the modified position for women.

Required items:

- Exercise mat
- Rolled towel (approximately 3 inches in height)

Procedure:

Participants should perform a light warm-up prior to testing. However, if this test follows a cardiorespiratory-fitness test, clients may proceed without a warm-up. A rolled towel should be placed on the center of the mat. Review the correct counting procedure—the push-up is complete when the chest touches the towel and returns to the start position with arms fully extended. Inform them of the proper breathing technique—to exhale with the exertion (when pushing away from the floor). Have clients assume the proper push-up position with the hands at, or slightly wider than, shoulder-width apart and their chests centered above the towel. Allow them to practice the push-up if they would like. Instruct them to begin the test by flexing the elbows and lowering the chest to the towel. This modified technique, which limits the depth of elbow flexion to 3 inches above the mat, has been provided to allow participation by more individuals. The traditional protocol (i.e., lowering the chest to the floor) puts undue stress on the glenohumeral joints, especially for individuals with a history of shoulder dysfunction. The score is the total number of push-ups completed without rest before the client reaches exhaustion (Table 9-14).

Half Sit-up or Partial Curl-up Test

The half sit-up test is used to evaluate abdominal muscle strength and endurance. It was developed to replace the traditional full sit-up test so that potential low-back

Table 9-14
Push-up Test Fitness Categories

	Age									
	20–29		30–39		40–49		50–59		60–69	
Gender	M	F	M	F	M	F	M	F	M	F
Excellent	36 or more	30 or more	30 or more	27 or more	25 or more	24 or more	21 or more	21 or more	18 or more	17 or more
Very Good	35 29	29 21	29 22	26 20	24 17	23 15	20 13	20 11	17 11	16 12
Good	28 22	20 15	21 17	19 13	16 13	14 11	12 10	10 7	10 8	11 5
Fair	21 17	14 10	16 12	12 8	12 10	10 5	9 7	6 2	7 5	4 2
Needs improvement	16 or fewer	9 or fewer	11 or fewer	7 or fewer	9 or fewer	4 or fewer	6 or fewer	1 or fewer	4 or fewer	1 or fewer

Source: The Canadian Physical Activity, Fitness, & Lifestyle Approach (3rd ed.). © 2003. *CSEP-Health & Fitness Program's Health-related Appraisal and Counseling Strategy* Reprinted with permission from the Canadian Society for Exercise Physiology.

problems could be eliminated and to better assess abdominal muscle function.

Required items:

- Exercise mat
- Stopwatch
- Tape
- Ruler
- Metronome set at 50 bpm

Procedure:

Participants should perform a light warm-up prior to testing. However, if this test follows a cardiorespiratory-fitness test, clients may proceed without a warm-up. Place two strips of masking tape parallel to each other on a mat 10 cm apart. Review and demonstrate the proper half sit-up technique. Assume a supine position with the feet flat on the floor, shoulders relaxed, and knees flexed at approximately 90 degrees. The arms are at the sides, palms facing down with the middle fingers of each hand touching the first strip of masking tape. Alternative hand positions include: (a) having the hands held across the chest or (b) placing the hands on the thighs and curling up until the hands reach the knee caps. Instruct clients that regardless of the hand position chosen, elevation of the trunk to 30 degrees is the important aspect of the movement.

Set the metronome to 50 bpm and instruct clients to perform slow, controlled curl-ups to lift the shoulder blades off the mat (the trunk makes a 30-degree angle with the mat) in time with the metronome (i.e., 25 curl-ups per minute).

If using the tape method, instruct them to curl the upper spine until the fingertips touch the second strip of tape. Finally, instruct them to return to the original position with the shoulders touching the mat.

Place the metronome in a location where it may be easily heard by all clients. Allow clients an opportunity to practice the movement along with the metronome. Inform clients of the correct counting procedure—one curl-up is counted each time their shoulders return to the mat. Instruct clients to begin curling the trunk as the stopwatch is started. The score is the number of curl-ups performed in one minute (maximum of 25) without pausing (Table 9-15).

Readiness to Change

A key factor to assess is whether a client is at the right time in life to make a serious attempt at losing weight. Readiness to change is a complex phenomenon that encompasses an individual's motivation to lose weight, commitment to restructuring his or life, and surrounding circumstances. Chances for success increase when a client's readiness to change is high (Brownell, 2000). Ideally, clients have carefully thought through these issues before meeting the LWMC. Realistically, however, many factors will lead people to seek help, including the need to please others (e.g., spouse, physician) or to find a quick fix for major problems.

Readiness to change can be assessed in several ways. The simplest way is to have clients evaluate what benefits may be obtained through weight loss against the sacrifices they need to be make. Two psychologists, Dr. James Prochaska and Dr. Carlo DiClemente, have developed a sophisticated model in which they identify discrete stages of change (see Chapter 12). The **stages-of-change model** suggests that a complicated

Table 9-15
Half Sit-up Test Fitness Categories

Norms for Men

Ages	20–29	30–39	40–49	50–59	60–69
Excellent	25 or more	25 or more	25 or more	25 or more	25 or more
Very Good	21–24	18–24	18–24	17–24	16–24
Good	16–20	15–17	13–17	11–16	11–15
Fair	11–15	11–14	6–12	8–10	6–10
Needs Improvement	10 or fewer	10 or fewer	5 or fewer	7 or fewer	5 or fewer

Norms for Women

Ages	20–29	30–39	40–49	50–59	60–69
Excellent	25 or more	25 or more	25 or more	25 or more	25 or more
Very Good	18–24	19–24	19–24	19–24	17–24
Good	14–17	10–18	11–18	10–18	8–16
Fair	5–13	6–9	4–10	6–9	3–7
Needs Improvement	4 or fewer	5 or fewer	3 or fewer	5 or fewer	2 or fewer

Source: The Canadian Physical Activity, Fitness, & Lifestyle Approach (3rd ed.). © 2003. *CSEP-Health & Fitness Program's Health-related Appraisal and Counseling Strategy* Reprinted with permission from the Canadian Society for Exercise Physiology.

period of psychological preparation precedes true readiness to commit to lifestyle change. Thus, even though clients may not be fully committed to losing weight, for many their motivation increases early on from seeing success and witnessing the benefits of making a lifestyle change. The American Dietetic Association has developed a Weight-Loss Readiness Quiz that addresses attitudes toward weight loss (Figure 9-6).

It is important to recognize that for most clients, change is never easy. In his book, *The 9 Truths About Weight Loss,* psychologist Dr. Daniel Kirschenbaum reviews some startling statistics surrounding the difficulty of making lifestyle changes, even when one's life may depend on it (Kirschenbaum, 2000). For example, when physicians prescribe medications for their patients, approximately 33% are never even filled. Parents fail to ensure that their children complete a directed course of medications 50% of the time. Approximately 70% of people with high blood pressure do not follow their physician's advice. And statistics show that 65% of Americans fail to use seat belts properly. Thus, it is very important to carefully review with clients the natural tendency to resist change. Kirschenbaum argues that a strong commitment and persistence is needed to make change possible. LWMCs must talk candidly with clients about their previous attempts at making lifestyle changes to ensure that their readiness is not merely a reflection of superficial enthusiasm or wishful thinking that their lifestyle could be different.

Summary

LWMCs offer an important service that encompasses principles of nutrition, exercise science, and behavior modification to promote lifestyle change for a wide variety of clients. LWMCs have an ethical and professional responsibility to adequately screen clients to see if they are suitable for treatment, assess relevant medical and psychological factors and fitness parameters, and refer clients to allied health professionals when indicated. In addition, the information that is gathered during the assessment phase provides an important foundation for establishing an individualized, safe, and effective weight-management program.

Figure 9-6
Sample weight-loss readiness quiz

Weight-loss Readiness Quiz

Are you ready to lose weight? Your attitude about weight loss affects your ability to succeed. Take this Readiness Quiz to learn if you need to make any attitude adjustments before you begin. Mark each item true or false. Be honest! It's important that these answers reflect the way you really are, not how you would like to be. A method for interpreting your readiness for weight loss follows:

1. ___ I have thought a lot about my eating habits and physical activities to pinpoint what I need to change.
2. ___ I have accepted the idea that I need to make permanent, not temporary, changes in my eating and activities to be successful.
3. ___ I will only feel successful if I lose a lot of weight.
4. ___ I accept the idea that it's best if I lose weight slowly.
5. ___ I'm thinking of losing weight now because I really want to, not because someone else thinks I should.
6. ___ I think losing weight will solve other problems in my life.
7. ___ I am willing and able to increase my regular physical activity.
8. ___ I can lose weight successfully if I have no "slip-ups."
9. ___ I am ready to commit some time and effort each week to organizing and planning my food and activity programs.
10. ___ Once I lose some initial weight, I usually lose the motivation to keep going until I reach my goal.
11. ___ I want to start a weight-loss program, even though my life is unusually stressful right now.

Scoring the Weight-loss Readiness Quiz

To score the quiz, look at your answers next to items 1, 2, 4, 5, 7, and 9. Score "1" if you answered "true" and "0" if you answered "false."

For items 3, 6, 8, 10, and 11, score "0" for each true answer and "1" for each false answer.

To get your total score, add the scores of all questions.

No one score indicates for sure whether you are ready to start losing weight. However, the higher your total score, the more characteristics you have that contribute to success. As a rough guide, consider the following recommendations:

1. If you scored 8 or higher, you probably have good reasons for wanting to lose weight now and a good understanding of the steps needed to succeed. Still, you might want to learn more about the areas where you scored a "0" (see "Interpretation of Quiz Items").
2. If you scored 5 to 7, you may need to reevaluate your reasons for losing weight and the methods you would use to do so. To get a start, read the advice given below for those quiz items where you received a score of "0."
3. If you scored 4 or less, now may not be the right time for you to lose weight. While you might be successful in losing weight initially, your answers suggest that you are unlikely to sustain sufficient effort to lose all the weight you want, or keep off the weight that you do lose. You need to reconsider your weight-loss motivations and methods and perhaps learn more about the pros and cons of different approaches to reducing. To do so, read the advice below for those quiz items where you marked "0."

Interpretation of Quiz Items

Your answers to the quiz can clue you in to potential stumbling blocks to your weight-loss success. Any item score of "0" indicates a misconception about weight loss, or a potential problem area.

Figure 9-6
continued

While no individual item score of "0" is important enough to scuttle your weight-loss plans, you should consider the meaning of those items so that you can best prepare yourself for the challenges ahead. The numbers below correspond to the question numbers.

1. It has been said that you can't change what you don't understand. You might benefit from keeping records for a week to help pinpoint when, what, why, and how much you eat. This tool also is useful in identifying obstacles to regular physical activity.

2. Making drastic or highly restrictive changes in your eating habits may allow you to lose weight in the short-run, but be too hard to live with permanently. Similarly, your program of regular physical activity should be one you can sustain. Both your food plan and activity program should be healthful and enjoyable.

3. Most people have fantasies of reaching a weight considerably lower than they can realistically maintain. Rethink your meaning of "success." A successful, realistic weight loss is one that can be comfortably maintained through sensible eating and regular activity. Take your body type into consideration. Then set smaller, achievable goals. Your first goal may be to lose a small amount of weight while you learn eating habits and activity patterns to help you maintain it.

4. If you equate success with fast weight loss, you will have problems maintaining your weight. This "quick fix" attitude can backfire when you face the challenges of weight maintenance. It's best—and healthiest—to lose weight slowly, while learning the strategies that allow you to keep the weight off permanently.

5. The desire for, and commitment to, weight loss must come from you. People who lose and maintain weight successfully take responsibility for their own desires and decide the best way to achieve them. Once this step is taken, friends and family are an important source of support, not motivation.

6. While being overweight may contribute to a number of social problems, it is rarely the single cause. Anticipating that all of your problems will be solved through weight loss is unrealistic and may set you up for disappointment. Instead, realize that successful weight loss will make you feel more self-confident and empowered, and that the skills you develop to deal with your weight can be applied to other areas of your life.

7. Studies have shown that people who develop the habit of regular, moderate physical activity are most successful at maintaining their weight. Exercise does not have to be strenuous to be effective for weight control. Any moderate physical activity that you enjoy and will do regularly counts. Just get moving!

8. While most people don't expect perfection of themselves in everyday life, many feel that they must stick to a weight-loss program perfectly. This is unrealistic. Rather than expecting lapses and viewing them as catastrophes, recognize them as valuable opportunities to identify problem triggers and develop strategies for the future.

9. Successful weight loss is not possible without taking the time to think about yourself, assess your problem areas, and develop strategies to deal with them. Success takes time. You must commit to planning and organizing your weight loss.

10. Do not ignore your concerns about "going the distance," because they may indicate a potential problem. Think about past efforts and why they failed. Pinpoint any reasons, and work on developing motivational strategies to get you over those hurdles. Take your effort one day at a time; a plateau of weight maintenance within an ongoing weight-loss program is perfectly okay.

11. Weight loss itself is a source of stress, so if you are already under stress, it may be difficult to successfully implement a weight-loss program at this time. Try to resolve other stressors in your life before you begin a weight-loss effort.

Source: Reprinted with permission from Duyff, R.L. (2006). *ADA Complete Food and Nutrition Guide* (3rd ed). New York: John Wiley & Sons.

References

American College of Sports Medicine (2006). *ACSM's Guidelines for Exercise Testing and Prescription* (7th ed.). Baltimore: Lippincott Williams & Wilkins.

American Psychiatric Association (1994). *Diagnostic and Statistical Manual of Mental Disorders* (4th ed.). Washington, D.C.: American Psychiatric Association.

Bish, C.L. et al. (2000). Diet and physical activity behaviors among Americans trying to lose weight 2000: Behavioral risk factor surveillance system. *Obesity Research,* 13, 596–607.

Brownell, K.D. (2000). *The LEARN Program for Weight Control* (10th ed.). Dallas: American Health.

Bruce, B. & Wilfley, D. (1996). Binge eating among the overweight population: A serious and prevalent problem. *Journal of the American Dietetic Association,* 96, 58–61.

DiNubile, N.A. & Patrick, W. (2005). *FrameWork: Your 7-Step Program for Healthy Muscles, Bones, and Joints*. Emmaus, Pa.: Rodale Press.

Drewnowksi, A. (1990). *Toward safe weight loss: Recommendations for adult weight loss programs in Michigan. Final Report of the Task Force to Establish Weight Loss Guidelines.* East Lansing, Mich.: Michigan Health Council.

Gordon, P.M. et al. (2000). The quantity and quality of physical activity among those trying to lose weight. *American Journal of Preventive Medicine,* 18, 83–86.

Howley, E.T. & Franks, B.D. (2007). *Health Fitness Instructor's Handbook* (5th ed.). Champaign, Ill.: Human Kinetics.

Institute of Medicine (1995). *Weighing the Options: Criteria for Evaluating Weight-Management Programs*. Washington, D.C.: National Academy Press.

Kirschenbaum, D.S. (2001). *The 9 Truths About Weight Loss*. New York: Henry Holt.

National Institutes of Health (2003). The Seventh Report of the Joint Committee on Prevention, Detection, Evaluation, and Treatment of High Blood Pressure. NIH Publication No. 03-5233.

National Institutes of Health (1998). Clinical guidelines on the identification, evaluation, and treatment of overweight and obesity in adults: The evidence report. *Obesity Research,* 6 (Suppl.), 51S–209S.

National Task Force on the Prevention and Treatment of Obesity (2000). Overweight, obesity, and health risk. *Archives of Internal Medicine,* 160, 898–904.

Ogden, C.L. et al. (2006). Prevalence of overweight and obesity in the United States, 1999–2004. *Journal of the American Medical Association,* 295,1549–1555.

Spitzer, R.L. et al. (1993) Binge eating disorder: A multi-site field trial of the diagnostic criteria. *International Journal of Eating Disorders,* 11, 191–203.

Wadden, T.A. et al. (1989). Treatment of obesity by very-low-calorie diets, behavior therapy, and their combination: A five-year perspective. *International Journal of Obesity,* 13, 2, 39–46.

Winner, K. (1991). *A Weighty Issue: Dangers and Deceptions of the Weight Loss Industry.* New York: Department of Consumer Affairs.

YMCA of the USA (2000). *YMCA Fitness Testing and Assessment Manual* (4th ed.). Champaign, Ill.: Human Kinetics.

Suggested Reading

Heyward, V.H. (2006). *Advanced Fitness Assessment & Exercise Prescription* (5th ed.). Champaign, Ill.: Human Kinetics.

Bryant, C.X., Franklin, B.A., & Newton-Merrill, S. (2007). *ACE's Guide to Exercise Testing and Program Design: A Fitness Professional's Handbook* (2nd ed.). Monterey, Calif.: Healthy Learning.

Morrow, J.R. et al. (2005). *Measurement and Evaluation in Human Performance* (3rd ed.). Champaign, Ill.: Human Kinetics.

Hoffman, J. (2006). *Norms for Fitness, Performance, and Health.* Champaign, Ill.: Human Kinetics.

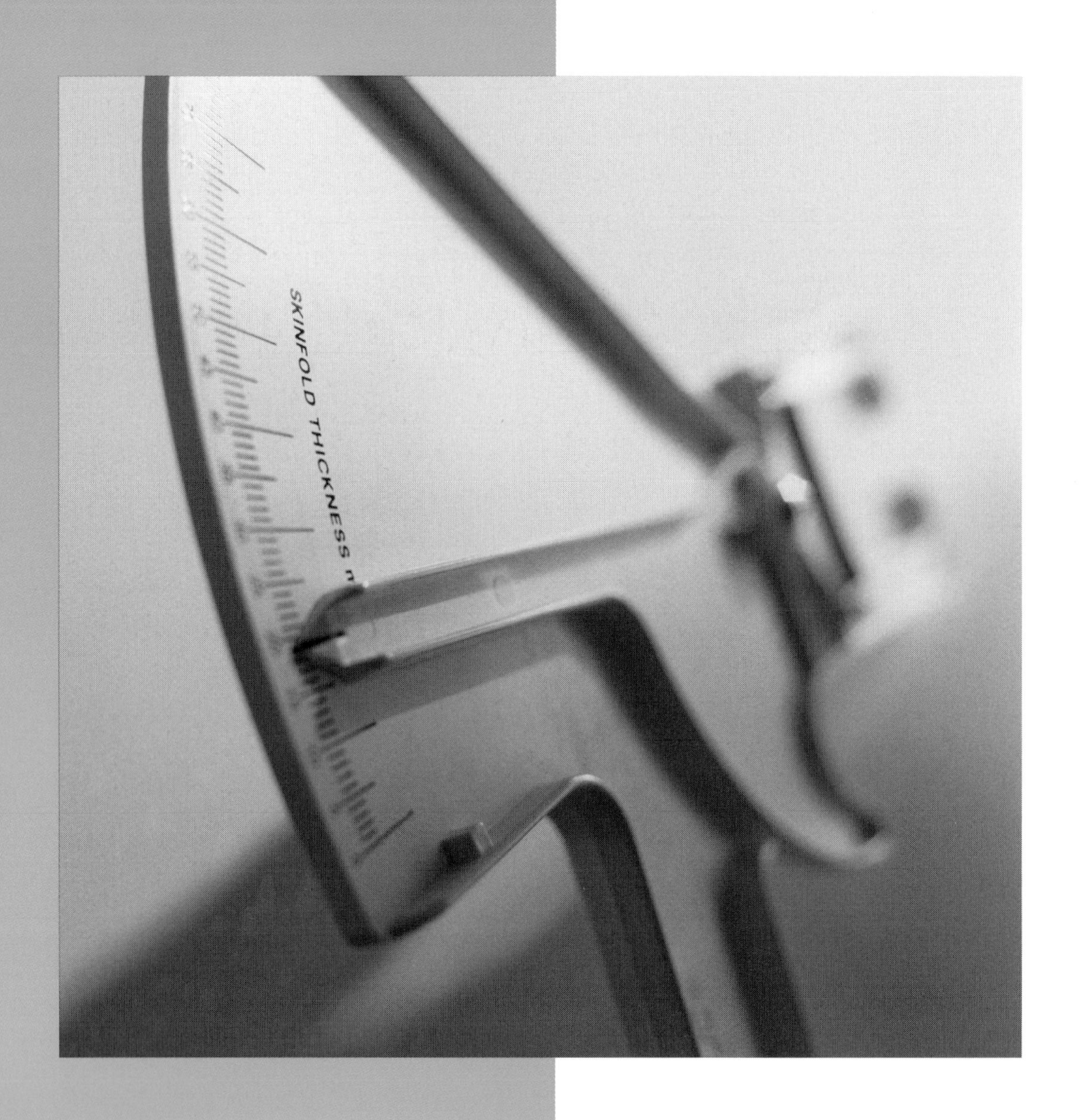

Scott Roberts

Scott Roberts, Ph.D., is an associate professor and program coordinator for the Exercise Physiology Program at California State University, Chico. He is a fellow of both the American College of Sports Medicine and the American Association of Cardiovascular and Pulmonary Rehabilitation. He is a widely published author and coauthor and an editor for several publications. Dr. Roberts authored the chapter "Exercise Guidelines for Individuals with Pacemakers and AICDs" and served as the section editor for the cardiovascular disease chapters in ACSM's Exercise Management for Persons With Chronic Diseases and Disabilities, *2nd edition. He also coauthored* Clinical Exercise Testing and Prescription: Theory and Application.

ACE would like to acknowledge the contributions to this chapter made by Cedric X. Bryant, Ph.D., FACSM, Chief Science Officer of the American Council on Exercise.

Chapter 10

Body-composition Assessment and Evaluation

IN THIS CHAPTER:

Achieving and maintaining a healthy body weight and **body composition** are central goals of good health. This issue also has become a national public-health priority, as an estimated 66% of American adults and nearly 20% of American children and adolescents are either **overweight** or obese. **Obesity** reduces quality of health and life, and increases the risk for developing numerous **chronic diseases,** including heart disease, **stroke, hypertension, type 2 diabetes,** certain types of cancer, gout, sleep apnea, and **osteoarthritis.** Many Americans are becoming more skeptical of bathroom scales and **body mass index (BMI)** charts. Most people understand that there is a difference between fat weight and body weight, and that the only way to find out the difference is to have their body composition analyzed.

The term body composition refers to the ratio of the various components of the body that, when combined, make up a person's total **body mass (BM).** Body-composition analysis is a process used to determine the percentage of an individual's total body weight that is composed of **fat mass (FM)** versus **fat-free mass (FFM).** Body composition is typically expressed as **percent body fat (%BF),** or the ratio of fat mass to BM. Scales and charts can only determine whether someone is above or below a recommended weight for his or her age, sex, and/or height, but can't determine the percentage of body weight that is accounted for by FM versus FFM. Without a body-composition assessment, it is impossible to know whether weight lost or gained after starting a diet or exercise program is the result of a change in FM or FFM.

Discussing Body Composition Using Non-scientific Language

Terms such as mass, densitometry, and lean body tissue may sound like a foreign language to many people. At the same time, Lifestyle & Weight Management Consultants (LWMCs) have to project a strong sense of professionalism, expertise, and knowledge in what they say and do to attract and keep good clients. The key is in learning how to communicate with clients based on their education levels, fitness knowledge, and previous exercise experiences. A good rule is to assume that new clients have little, if any, fitness and exercise background, and proceed from there.

Before defining body composition, make certain that clients understand that weight scales, height–weight charts, and BMI charts only consider total body weight, or total body weight in proportion to height, to indicate if individuals are of ideal weight, overweight, or obese. Anyone trying to lose weight needs to understand that they are really trying to lose fat, not necessarily weight. Charts are not a good indication of **ideal body weight (IBW)** for general health or for athletic performance. During a weight-loss program combining diet and exercise, there are going to be times when the rate or amount of weight loss slows, stops, or even reverses, and yet individuals can still be losing fat and gaining **lean body mass (LBM).** The only way to know for sure is through periodic body-composition assessments.

There are several ways to define body composition using non-scientific language. Clients should continually be reeducated about exercise-science principles and terminology as they become more comfortable and experienced with their training. Using the classic two-component model, body composition is typically defined as the ratio of fat mass or fat-free body mass to total body mass. LBM is sometimes used in place of FFM. Both versions are correct, with the only difference being that LBM includes a small amount of essential lipids, whereas FFM does not.

The following examples are ways to explain body composition in lay terms:

- "Body-composition testing measures how much body fat you have in proportion to the weight of your muscles, bones, and other tissues."
- "Body-composition testing is an estimate of the percentage of your weight that is fat, compared to "fat-free" weight, which makes up muscles, bones, and organs."

Understanding Body Composition

For the average person, the most common way to monitor body weight, not body composition, is to step on the bathroom scale. Scales, however, only measure the mass (weight in pounds or kilograms) of a person, and are unable to differentiate between FM and FFM. Using scale weight alone, some people appear overweight, even if they are not necessarily overfat. Conversely, a person could appear to be normal weight, but have a high %BF level. The only way to know for sure if a person's body weight reflects an ideal %BF level is to assess body composition.

Having an understanding of, and being able to accurately determine, a person's body composition is especially useful if that individual is dieting to lose weight. Simply knowing how many pounds an individual has lost does not reveal a full or meaningful picture, because dieting frequently results in a loss of significant amounts of fat-free weight and water. Considerable research suggests, however, that individuals who are trying to lose weight should focus their efforts on losing body fat—as opposed to fat-free weight and/or water. As such, a sound weight-control program must involve modifying an individual's physical-activity and dietary habits to reach an appropriate level of body fat. In that regard, one of the critical steps is to be able to accurately assess an individual's body-fat level to determine changes in body composition.

Body composition, as an important part of a comprehensive fitness assessment, helps establish the degree of risk associated with being under or over the ideal body weight or of having a body composition that is not considered optimal for health, fitness, and athletic performance. Routine assessment of body composition is perhaps in the most effective way of showing clients how effective changes in lifestyle can be (Table 10-1).

Table 10-1
Purpose of Body-composition Assessment

- To get baseline information
- To document for program assessment
- To use as a motivational tool
- To monitor development- and age-related changes in body composition
- To help formulate dietary recommendations
- To monitor changes in body composition that are associated with certain diseases
- To identify a client's health risk for excessively high or low levels of body fat
- To promote a client's understanding of body fat
- To monitor changes in body composition
- To assess the effectiveness of nutrition and exercise choices
- To help estimate healthy body weight for clients and athletes
- To assist in exercise programming

Body-composition Models

Body-composition analysis divides the human body into different components. The two-component model of body composition divides total body weight into FM and FFM. FM includes fat stored in the body, including both essential and non-essential body fat. **Essential fat** is fat that is necessary for normal functioning of the body and is incorporated into the nerves, brain, heart, lungs, liver, and mammary glands. Normal values for essential fat are 2 to 5% for men and 10 to 13% for women. Non-essential fat is composed mainly of **triglycerides,** which can be stored around vital organs and within muscle tissue, as well as directly beneath the skin. FFM includes chemicals, tissues, water, muscle, bone, connective tissues, and internal organs.

Determinants of Body Composition

Genetics, heredity, bone structure, and body type explain most of the variation in body weight and body composition among people. **Energy balance** (caloric intake versus caloric expenditure) plays a significant role in regulating body composition. A healthy diet and daily exercise are the two most important habits affecting the ability to reach and sustain an ideal body weight and %BF level. Genetics, however, plays the most significant role in the extent to which body composition can be changed. Unfortunately, most people simply do not possess "media-body" genes, nor do they have the fortitude and time to develop a lean, muscular body with "six-pack abs," no matter how hard they try. Therefore, the primary focus of body-composition assessment should be to establish realistic and achievable goals that lead toward a healthy body weight, image, and composition.

Body Composition and Health Risks

Overweight refers to a total body weight above the recommended range for good health, whereas obesity refers to severe overweight and a high body-fat percentage. Both overweight and obesity increase the risk of **diabetes,** heart disease, and hypertension, as well as other chronic health conditions (Table 10-2). When reviewing an individual's health-assessment data, it is important to consider what proportion of a person's total body weight is fat (%BF).

Table 10-2
Increased Risk of Obesity-related Diseases with Higher BMI

	BMI			
DISEASE	<25	25–30	30–35	>35
Arthritis	1.00	1.56	1.87	2.39
Heart disease	1.00	1.39	1.86	1.67
Diabetes (type 2)	1.00	2.42	3.35	6.16
Gallstones	1.00	1.97	3.30	5.48
Hypertension	1.00	1.92	2.82	3.77
Stroke	1.00	1.53	1.59	1.75

Note: A value of 1.00 equals a standard level of risk, while values exceeding 1.00 represent increased risk. For example, a value of 1.87 means that the individual is at an 87% greater level of risk.

Source: Centers for Disease Control and Prevention. Third National Health and Nutrition Examination Survey. Analysis by The Lewin Group, 1999.

The location of excess storage fat is also significant. People who gain weight in the abdominal area (i.e., **android obesity** or "apple-shaped") are at an increased risk of developing coronary heart disease, high blood pressure, diabetes, and stroke compared to people who gain weight in the hip area (i.e., **gynoid obesity** or "pear-shaped").

Assessing body composition provides additional information that **waist circumference** and **waist-to-hip ratio (WHR)** can't measure, such as FM, FFM, and %BF level. Waist circumference and WHR are simple ways to assess fat distribution.

Desirable Body Weight and Percent Body Fat

Many clients will ask LWMCs to define what percentage of BF is acceptable, too low, or too high. A person's %BF will vary depending on his or her sex, age, race, physical-activity level, and health status. In addition, hormonal changes in women due to pregnancy, menopause, and menstruation can cause water retention that can account for variations in outcomes between tests. The minimum %BF that is essential for normal physiological functioning is roughly 5% for males and 13% for females. Some athletes get close to or below minimal ranges for %BF for brief periods due to their training and higher-than-average FFM. Low %BF levels may be appropriate for some athletes, as long as they are otherwise in good health and are getting all of their daily nutritional requirements. However, a low %BF alone is not a guarantee of athletic success. Female athletes with very low %BF levels are at risk for developing **osteoporosis,** eating disorders, and **amenorrhea,** which are together known as the athletic triad. To try to achieve a low %BF level just to "look good" has potentially serious long-term physiological and psychological health risks.

Table 10-3 provides established %BF norms for men and women based on various categories of health and fitness. Whether someone's %BF is too high for good health depends on a number of variables. For example, some people may fall into in the high range of acceptability for %BF, but otherwise be healthy and physically active. Others may have acceptable %BF levels, but have an elevated risk for chronic illness and disease due to poor lifestyle choices. A person's overall health and lifestyle choices should be taken into account before making a decision about whether their %BF is acceptable or unacceptable. There is a large and convincing body of literature that confirms an increased risk of chronic illness and disease with high %BF levels of ≥32% in women and ≥25% in men (Wolf, 2002).

Table 10-3
Percent Body Fat Norms for Men and Women

DESCRIPTION	WOMEN	MEN
Essential fat	10–13%	2–5%
Athletes	14–20%	6–13%
Fitness	21–24%	14–17%
Acceptable	25–31%	18–24%
Obesity	≥32%	≥25%

How Often Should Body-composition Assessment Be Performed?

Assessing body composition on a frequent basis does not necessarily improve accuracy, and may cause more apprehension than motivation once people figure out that changes in body composition occur slowly. There are no definitive guidelines on how often body composition should be performed in a given population, because there are simply too many variables to consider. Practically speaking, there is little value in having it performed more frequently than monthly. For most people, two or three times a year should be adequate. Body composition may need to be assessed on a more frequent basis with a client who has a chronic disease or an eating disorder. In such cases, monitoring weight and lean body mass is essential to the medical therapy and treatment goals.

Calculating Ideal Body Weight

Once %BF has been determined, ideal body weight (IBW) can be predicted. For example, a 200-pound man (91-kg) with 25% BF has 50 pounds (23 kg) of fat (200 lb x 0.25) and 150 pounds (68 kg) of LBW (200 lb x 0.75). His goal is to reduce his BF to 18%, so that his LBW would then represent 82% of his total weight (150/0.82) or 183 pounds (83 kg). Thus, to reach his IBW, he would have to lose 17 (8 kg) pounds of fat (200 – 183).

Body-composition Assessment of Morbidly Obese Clients

Body-composition assessment equipment and the associated prediction equations are limited in terms of use with severely obese clients. In addition, issues such as self-esteem and body image play a role in deciding when, if, and how to assess body composition in this population. In some situations, it is not practical or possible to assess body composition in severely obese clients. Alternatives to body-composition assessment include weight and circumference measurements. Before deciding on an assessment method, LWMCs must ensure that there are published prediction equations available, and that the equipment selected has been validated for use with a particular client. **Bioelectrical impedance analysis (BIA)** would seem like a good choice to use with obese clients, but most of the research published using BIA with this population tends to underestimate %BF. Carella and colleagues (1997) measured body composition using BIA and **hydrostatic weighing** in obese patients who were enrolled in a weight-loss study and found that BIA tended to overestimate FFM (i.e., underestimate %BF) relative to hydrostatic weighing. In many cases, an accurate measurement of body composition is not needed, nor a priority, in severely obese clients.

Body-composition Assessment Techniques

Most adults initiate an exercise program in an attempt to lose weight. Accordingly, it is important to be able to accurately assess a person's body composition to determine a reasonable body-weight goal and to develop a safe and effective exercise program to reach it. An accurate body-composition assessment measures the relative percentages of fat-free and fat mass within a particular individual.

The misunderstood term "ideal body weight" has historically been determined without concern for body composition and has involved the use of the standardized height–weight tables. In these circumstances, ideal body weight is estimated only from height and frame size, without consideration of the composition of the weight. As a result, a muscular athlete would most likely be considered overweight, while another person could fall within the accepted "ideal" body weight range and actually be overfat according to reasonable body-composition criteria.

Furthermore, it is not uncommon for an exerciser to lose fat weight and gain muscle weight without any change in total body weight. In reality, such a transformation would be very favorable from an overall health perspective. On the other hand, without an accurate assessment of a person's level of body composition, this positive change could go undetected and possibly lead to frustration on the part of the exerciser. A number of body-composition assessment techniques for identifying such a change are available. Among the more commonly used methods of estimating or assessing body composition are height–weight measurements, BMI, anthropometric measurements, BIA, and hydrostatic weighing.

Height and Weight Tables

Again, the usual way that weight-conscious people track their body weight (not body composition) is to step on the bathroom scale. If the scale reads less than the last time, most people feel relieved. If the scale reading is higher than before, which is often the case, most people decide that they may be overweight. Periodically weighing oneself on a scale can help track weight gain or loss over time, but doing so provides no information about fat-mass or lean-body-mass changes over time.

In 1943, the Metropolitan Life Insurance Company gave scale weight more meaning when they published desirable weight tables for men and women (Metropolitan Life Insurance Company, 1959). The tables, which are based on people who applied for life insurance policies, identify desirable weights based on height and frame size. For the Metropolitan Life Insurance Company, the tables determined the policy applicants with the lowest mortality rates. The tables became known as height–weight tables, and eventually became a universal standard for deciding desirable weight for anyone, not just life insurance applicants. When the tables were revised in 1983, all of the weight ranges increased (Metropolitan Life Insurance Company, 1983). The term ideal weight gradually became associated with these tables, although the word "ideal" was never specifically published in this context.

Body Mass Index

More useful estimates of body composition can be obtained by adjusting weight for height or stature and calculating a height-normalized index. The most commonly used index is BMI, which is calculated as follows:

BMI = Weight (kg)/Height^2 (m)
Example:
Convert weight from pounds to kilograms by dividing by 2.2:
Weight = 209 lb
209 lb/2.2 = 95 kg
Convert height from inches to centimeters, and then to meters, by multiplying by 2.54 and then dividing by 100:
Height = 68 inches
68 inches x 2.54 = 173 cm
173 cm/100 = 1.73 m

BMI = 95/(1.73)^2 = 31.7

Use Table 10-4 to determine body mass index. People in a normal weight range usually have a BMI between 18.5 and 24.9 (Table 10-5). According to NHANES 2003–2004 data, 66.3% of U.S. adults aged 20 years and older are either overweight or obese; 34.1% are overweight, defined as having a body mass index (BMI) of 25.0 to 29.9 kg/m^2; and 32.2% are obese with a BMI of 30 kg/m^2 (see Table 17-1, page 376).

Since BMI uses total body weight (i.e., not estimates of fat and lean body mass separately) in the calculation, it does not discriminate between the overfat and the athletic or more muscular body type. Therefore, BMI should ideally be used in conjunction with other body-composition assessments.

Anthropometric Measurements

Anthropometric assessments of body composition are perhaps the easiest and least expensive methods for assessing body composition. These include circumference and skinfold measures, which are readily used in the field. Anthropometric measures also can be used to estimate body fat and its distribution (i.e., central vs. peripheral, upper body vs. lower body).

Circumference Measures

Circumference measures can easily be used to assess body composition, even with significantly overweight clients. However, to ensure accuracy, the LWMC must use exact anatomical landmarks for taking each circumference measurement (Table 10-6 and Figures 10-1 through 10-4). A thorough review of anthropometric measurement sites and techniques for optimizing accuracy is presented in Lohman, Roche, & Martorelli (1988).

A cloth or fiberglass (i.e., non-elastic) metric measurement tape must be used. The tape should be periodically calibrated against a meter stick to ensure that it has not been stretched. When assessing significantly overweight clients, be sure to use a long enough tape. Pull the tape tight enough to keep it in position without causing an indentation of

Table 10-4
Body Mass Index

	19	20	21	22	23	24	25	26	27	28	29	30	35	40
Height (inches)							Weight (pounds)							
58	91	95	100	105	110	115	119	124	129	134	138	143	167	191
59	94	99	104	109	114	119	124	128	133	138	143	148	173	198
60	97	102	107	112	118	123	128	133	138	143	148	153	179	204
61	100	106	111	116	121	127	132	137	143	148	153	158	185	211
62	104	109	115	120	125	131	136	142	147	153	158	164	191	218
63	107	113	118	124	130	135	141	146	152	158	163	169	197	225
64	110	116	122	128	134	140	145	151	157	163	169	174	203	233
65	114	120	126	132	138	144	150	156	162	168	174	180	210	240
66	117	124	130	136	142	148	155	161	167	173	179	185	216	247
67	121	127	134	140	147	153	159	166	172	178	185	191	223	255
68	125	131	138	144	151	158	164	171	177	184	190	197	230	263
69	128	135	142	149	155	162	169	176	182	189	196	203	237	270
70	132	139	146	153	160	167	174	181	188	195	202	209	243	278
71	136	143	150	157	165	172	179	186	193	200	207	215	250	286
72	140	147	155	162	169	177	184	191	199	206	213	221	258	294
73	144	151	159	166	174	182	189	197	204	212	219	227	265	303
74	148	155	163	171	179	187	194	202	210	218	225	233	272	311
75	152	160	168	176	184	192	200	208	216	224	232	240	279	319
76	156	164	172	180	189	197	205	213	221	230	238	246	287	328

Note: Find the client's height in the far left column and move across the row to the weight that is closest to the client's weight. His or her body mass index will be at the top of that column.

Table 10-5
BMI Reference Chart

Weight Category	BMI Range
Underweight	<18.5
Normal weight	18.5–24.9
Overweight	25.0–29.9
Grade I Obesity	30.0–34.9
Grade II Obesity	35.0–39.9
Grade III Obesity	>40

Table 10-6
Anatomic Locations of Circumference Measurement Sites

Circumference	Anatomic Site
Abdomen	At the level of the umbilicus
Hips	The largest circumference at the posterior extension of the gluteals
Iliac	Level with the iliac crests
Waist	The narrowest part of the torso

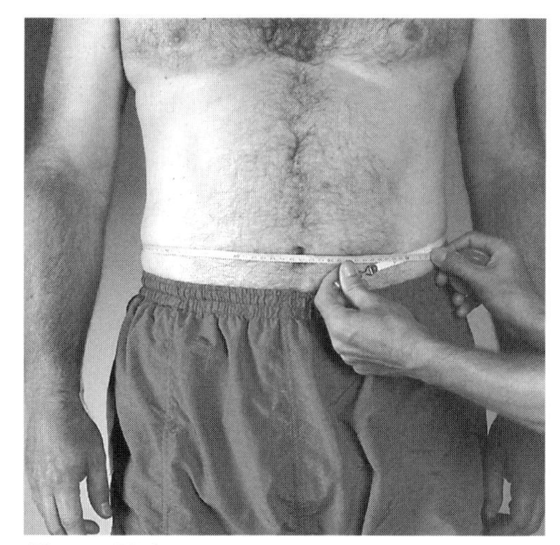

Figure 10-1
Abdominal circumference

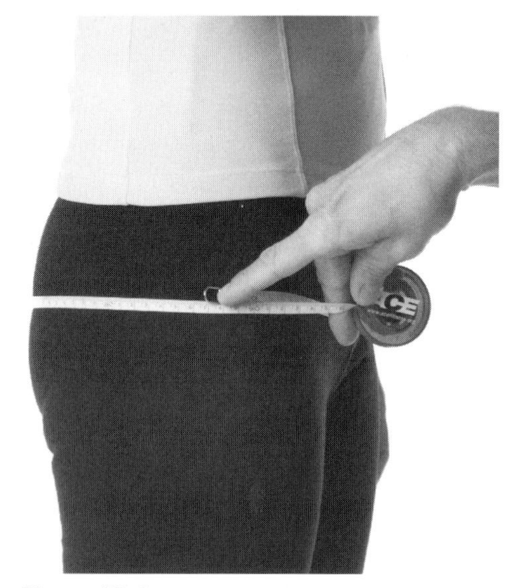

Figure 10-2
Hip circumference

the skin. There are tapes available that have a gauge that indicates the correct tension.

Estimating Body Fat from Circumference Measures

Body density (BD) for women and men can be predicted from generalized equations that use girth measurements (Tran & Weltman, 1989; Tran, Weltman, & Seip, 1988):

$$\text{BD for women} = 1.168297 - (0.002824 \times \text{abdomen}_{cm}) + (0.0000122098 \times \text{abdomen}^2_{cm}) - (0.000733128 \times \text{hips}_{cm}) + (0.000510477 \times \text{height}_{cm}) - (0.000216161 \times \text{age})$$

$$\text{BD for men} = 1.21142 + (0.00085 \times \text{weight}_{kg}) - (0.00050 \times \text{iliac}_{cm}) - (0.00061 \times \text{hip}_{cm}) - (0.00138 \times \text{abdomen}_{cm})$$

Body density can then be converted to percent fat by using the following formula:

$$\text{Percent fat} = (495/\text{BD}) - 450$$

Estimating Body-fat Distribution

Upper-body or abdominal obesity is known to increase health risk (e.g., type 2 diabetes, hypertension, **hypercholesterolemia**). A

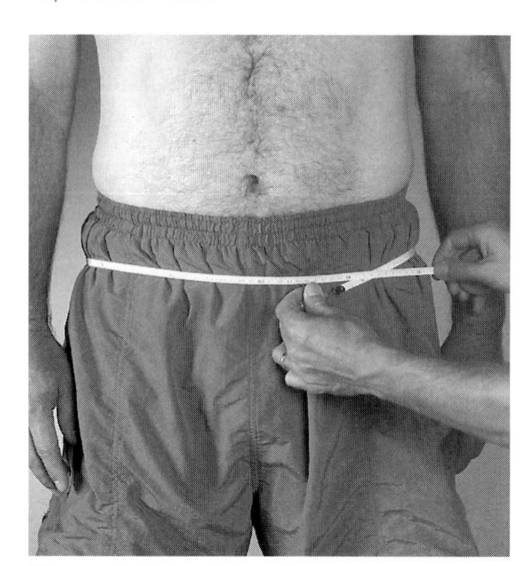

Figure 10-3
Iliac circumference

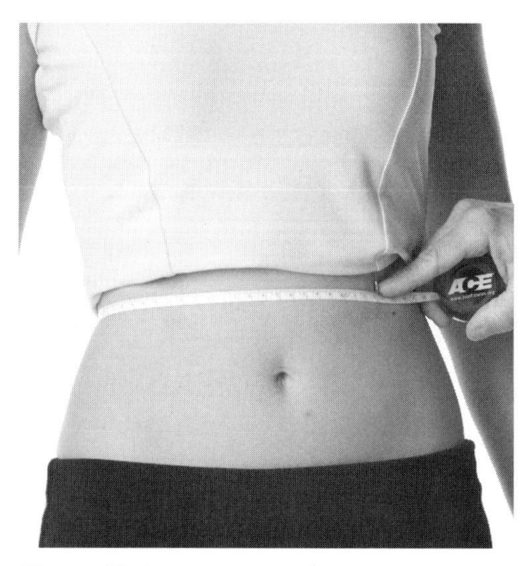

Figure 10-4
Waist circumference

quick and reliable technique for determining body-fat distribution is the waist-to-hip circumference ratio (WHR). To calculate WHR, divide the waist measurement by the hip measurement. Table 10-7 presents the relative risk ratings for WHR. It should also be noted that waist circumference is a reliable and easily measured indicator of abdominal obesity (NHLBI, 1998). Waist circumferences of greater than 40 inches (102 cm) in men and 35 inches (89 cm) in women are considered strong indicators of abdominal obesity.

Table 10-7
Waist-to-Hip Ratios and Associated Level of Health Risks

Classification	Men	Women
High risk	>1.0	>0.85
Moderately high risk	0.90–1.0	0.80–0.85
Lower risk	<0.90	<0.80

Reprinted with permission from Larsson B. et al. (1984). Abdominal adipose tissue distribution, obesity and risk of cardiovascular disease and death: 13-year follow-up of participants in the study of men born in 1913. *British Medical Journal*, 288, 1401–1404.

Skinfold Measurements

Skinfold measurements are a relatively inexpensive way to assess body composition, and, if the measurements are taken properly, the results are both valid and reliable. The standard error associated with this method is 3.5%, depending on the equation applied. This is compared to a 2.7% error for a hydrostatically determined measurement. Skinfold measurement is based on the belief that approximately 50% of total body fat lies under the skin, and involves measuring the thickness of the skinfolds at standardized sites. These measurements are summed and applied to one of many equations available. For the most part, the equations calculate body density, with percent fat being calculated from the same formula used for hydrostatic weighing. Calculation is often simplified through the use of a table or nomogram. Calipers specifically designed for skinfold measurement are the only equipment needed for this method of body-fat assessment, and range in cost from $3 to $300.

The procedure for measuring skinfolds is as follows:

- Identify the anatomical location of the skinfold. Take all measurements on the right side of the body. (Optional: Mark the site with a common eyebrow pencil to expedite site relocation in repeated measures.)
- Grasp the skinfold firmly with the thumb and index finger of the left hand.
- Holding the calipers perpendicular to the site, place the pads of the calipers approximately ¼ inch from the thumb and forefinger.
- Approximately one or two seconds after the trigger has been released, read the dial to the nearest 0.5 mm.
- A minimum of two measurements should be taken at each site, with at least 15 seconds between measurements to allow the fat to return to its normal thickness.
- Continue to take measurements until two measurements vary by less than 1 mm.

Improper site determination and measurement are the two primary sources of error when using this method. The technique is best learned by locating and measuring the standard sites numerous times and comparing results with those of a well-trained associate. Skinfold measurements should not be taken after exercise because the transfer of fluid to the skin could result in overestimations.

Of the many equations for estimating body composition, two developed by Jackson and Pollock (1985) have the smallest margin of error for the general population. These equations are based on the sum of measurements taken at three sites.

For men, the skinfold sites are as follows:

- Chest (Figure 10-5): A diagonal skinfold taken midway on the anterior axillary line (crease of the underarm and the nipple)
- Thigh (Figure 10-6): A vertical skinfold taken midway between the hip and knee joints on the front of the thigh
- Abdomen (Figure 10-7): a vertical skinfold taken 1 inch lateral to the umbilicus

Figure 10-5
Chest skinfold measurement for men:

Locate the site midway between the anterior axillary line and the nipple.

Grasp a diagonal fold and pull it away from the muscle.

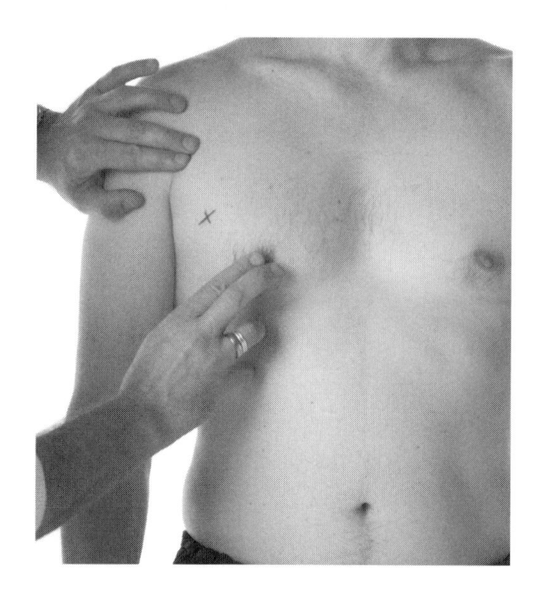

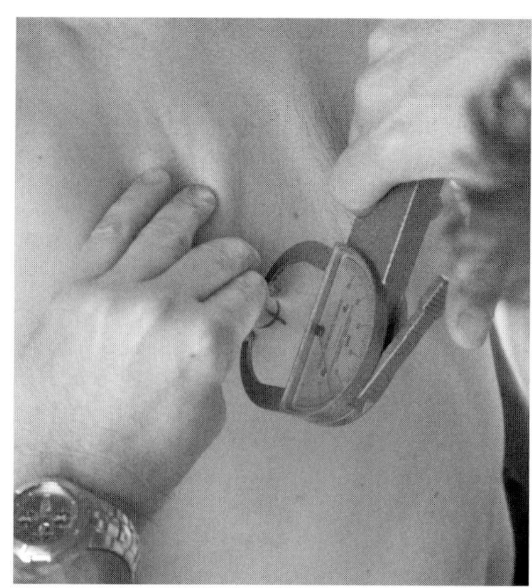

Figure 10-6
Thigh skinfold measurement for men:

Locate the hip and the knee joints and find the midpoint on the top of the thigh.

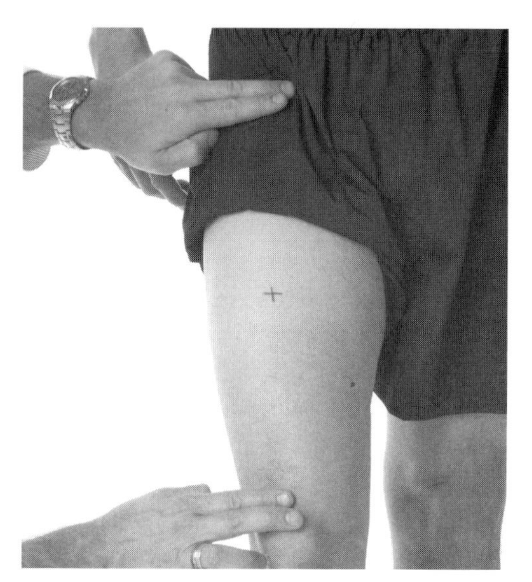

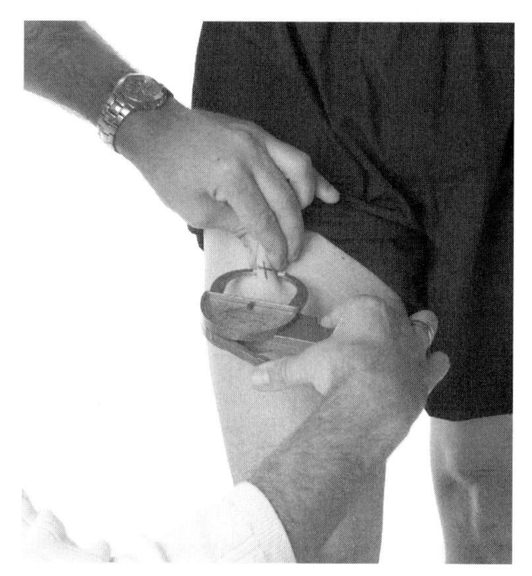

Figure 10-7
Abdominal skinfold measurement for men:

Grasp a vertical skinfold one inch to the right of the umbilicus.

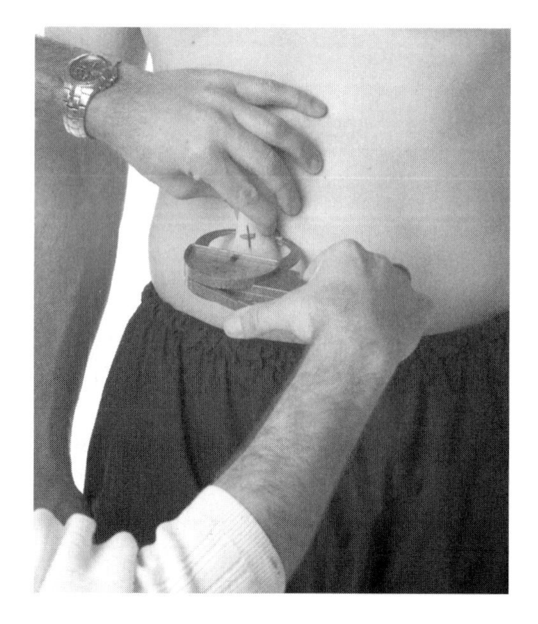

For women, the skinfold sites are as follows:

- Triceps (Figure 10-8): A vertical fold on the back of the upper arm taken halfway between the acromion (shoulder) and olecranon (elbow) processes
- Thigh (Figure 10-9): A vertical skinfold taken midway between the hip and knee joints on the front of the thigh
- Suprailium (Figure 10-10): A diagonal fold taken at, or just anterior to, the crest of the ilium

After obtaining three satisfactory measurements, add them and refer to Table 10-8 for men and Table 10-9 for women. For example, a 47-year-old man has the following

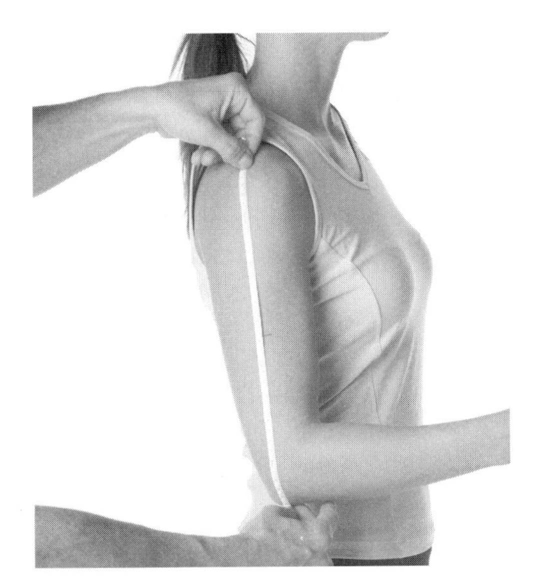

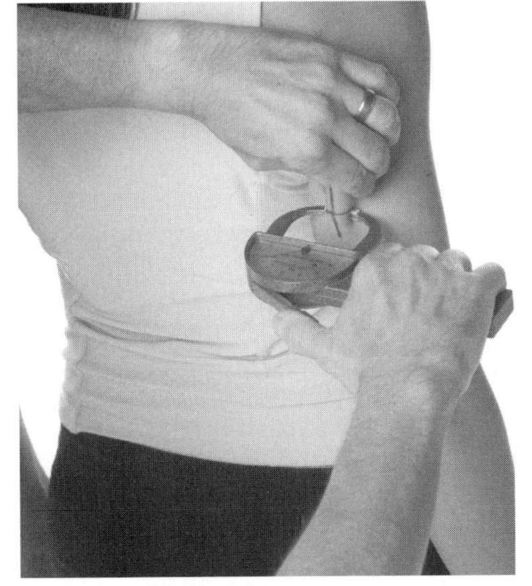

Figure 10-8
Triceps skinfold measurement for women.

Locate the site midway between the acromion: (shoulder) and olecranon (elbow) processes.

Grasp a vertical fold on the posterior midline and pull it away from the muscle.

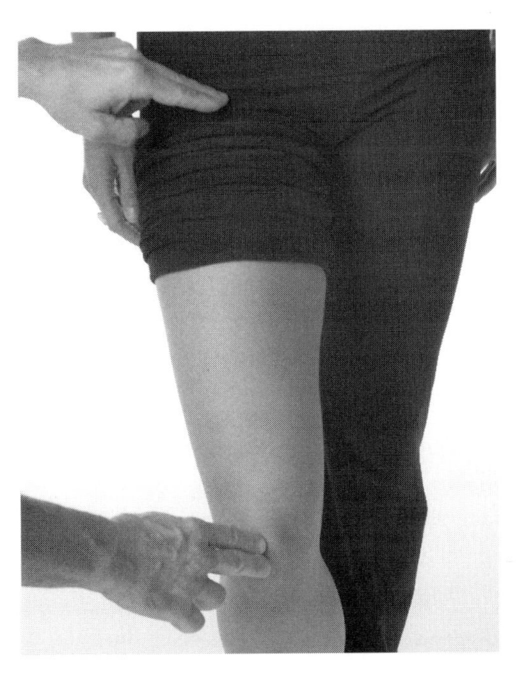

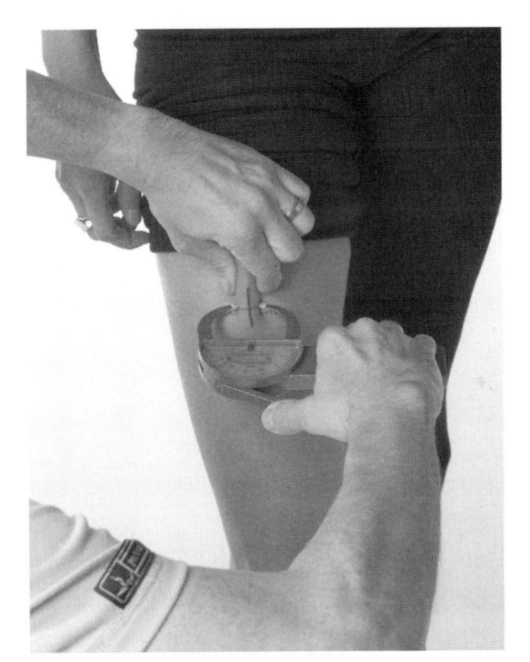

Figure 10-9
Thigh skinfold measurement for women:

Locate the hip and the knee joints and find the midpoint on the top of the thigh.

Grasp a vertical skinfold and pull it away from the muscle.

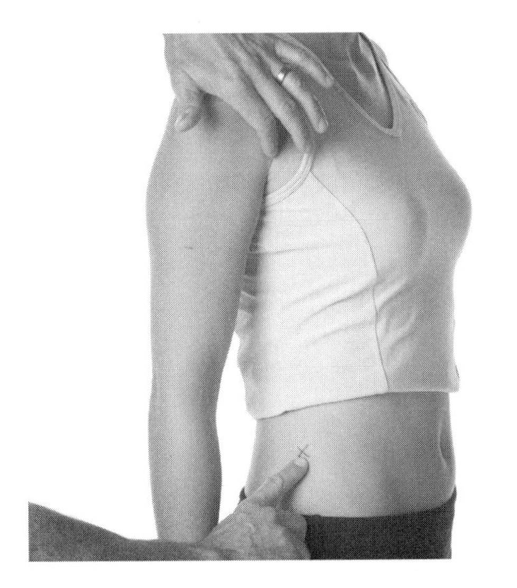

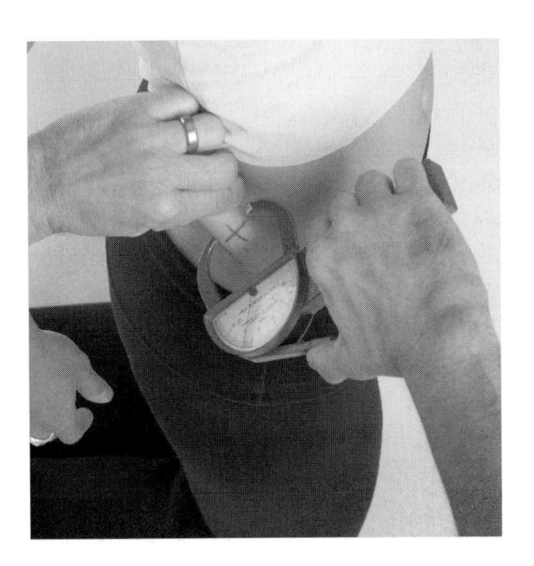

Figure 10-10
Suprailium skinfold measurement for women:

Grasp a diagonal skinfold just above, and slightly forward of, the crest of the ilium.

Table 10-8
Percent Body Fat Estimations for Men—Jackson and Pollock Formula

Sum of Skinfolds (mm)	Age Groups								
	Under 22	23–27	28–32	33–37	38–42	43–47	48–52	53–57	Over 57
8–10	1.3	1.8	2.3	2.9	3.4	3.9	4.5	5.0	5.5
11–13	2.2	2.8	3.3	3.9	4.4	4.9	5.5	6.0	6.5
14–16	3.2	3.8	4.3	4.8	5.4	5.9	6.4	7.0	7.5
17–19	4.2	4.7	5.3	5.8	6.3	6.9	7.4	8.0	8.5
20–22	5.1	5.7	6.2	6.8	7.3	7.9	8.4	8.9	9.5
23–25	6.1	6.6	7.2	7.7	8.3	8.8	9.4	9.9	10.5
26–28	7.0	7.6	8.1	8.7	9.2	9.8	10.3	10.9	11.4
29–31	8.0	8.5	9.1	9.6	10.2	10.7	11.3	11.8	12.4
32–34	8.9	9.4	10.0	10.5	11.1	11.6	12.2	12.8	13.3
35–37	9.8	10.4	10.9	11.5	12.0	12.6	13.1	13.7	14.3
38–40	10.7	11.3	11.8	12.4	12.9	13.5	14.1	14.6	15.2
41–43	11.6	12.2	12.7	13.3	13.8	14.4	15.0	15.5	16.1
44–46	12.5	13.1	13.6	14.2	14.7	15.3	15.9	16.4	17.0
47–49	13.4	13.9	14.5	15.1	15.6	16.2	16.8	17.3	17.9
50–52	14.3	14.8	15.4	15.9	16.5	17.1	17.6	18.2	18.8
53–55	15.1	15.7	16.2	16.8	17.4	17.9	18.5	19.1	19.7
56–58	16.0	16.5	17.1	17.7	18.2	18.8	19.4	20.0	20.5
59–61	16.9	17.4	17.9	18.5	19.1	19.7	20.2	20.8	21.4
62–64	17.6	18.2	18.8	19.4	19.9	20.5	21.1	21.7	22.2
65–67	18.5	19.0	19.6	20.2	20.8	21.3	21.9	22.5	23.1
68–70	19.3	19.9	20.4	21.0	21.6	22.2	22.7	23.3	23.9
71–73	20.1	20.7	21.2	21.8	22.4	23.0	23.6	24.1	24.7
74–76	20.9	21.5	22.0	22.6	23.2	23.8	24.4	25.0	25.5
77–79	21.7	22.2	22.8	23.4	24.0	24.6	25.2	25.8	26.3
80–82	22.4	23.0	23.6	24.2	24.8	25.4	25.9	26.5	27.1
83–85	23.2	23.8	24.4	25.0	25.5	26.1	26.7	27.3	27.9
86–88	24.0	24.5	25.1	25.7	26.3	26.9	27.5	28.1	28.7
89–91	24.7	25.3	25.9	26.5	27.1	27.6	28.2	28.8	29.4
92–94	25.4	26.0	26.6	27.2	27.8	28.4	29.0	29.6	30.2
95–97	26.1	26.7	27.3	27.9	28.5	29.1	29.7	30.3	30.9
98–100	26.9	27.4	28.0	28.6	29.2	29.8	30.4	31.0	31.6
101–103	27.5	28.1	28.7	29.3	29.9	30.5	31.1	31.7	32.3
104–106	28.2	28.8	29.4	30.0	30.6	31.2	31.8	32.4	33.0
107–109	28.9	29.5	30.1	30.7	31.3	31.9	32.5	33.1	33.7
110–112	29.6	30.2	30.8	31.4	32.0	32.6	33.2	33.8	34.4
113–115	30.2	30.8	31.4	32.0	32.6	33.2	33.8	34.5	35.1
116–118	30.9	31.5	32.1	32.7	33.3	33.9	34.5	35.1	35.7
119–121	31.5	32.1	32.7	33.3	33.9	34.5	35.1	35.7	36.4
122–124	32.1	32.7	33.3	33.9	34.5	35.1	35.8	36.4	37.0
125–127	32.7	33.3	33.9	34.5	35.1	35.8	36.4	37.0	37.6

Source: Jackson, A.S. & Pollock, M.L. (1985). *Practical Assessment of Body Composition*. Reprinted with permission of McGraw-Hill.

Table 10-9
Percent Body Fat Estimations for Women — Jackson and Pollock Formula

Sum of Skinfolds (mm)	Age Groups								
	Under 22	23–27	28–32	33–37	38–42	43–47	48–52	53–57	Over 57
23–25	9.7	9.9	10.2	10.4	10.7	10.9	11.2	11.4	11.7
26–28	11.0	11.2	11.5	11.7	12.0	12.3	12.5	12.7	13.0
29–31	12.3	12.5	12.8	13.0	13.3	13.5	13.8	14.0	14.3
32–34	13.6	13.8	14.0	14.3	14.5	14.8	15.0	15.3	15.5
35–37	14.8	15.0	15.3	15.5	15.8	16.0	16.3	16.5	16.8
38–40	16.0	16.3	16.5	16.7	17.0	17.2	17.5	17.7	18.0
41–43	17.2	17.4	17.7	17.9	18.2	18.4	18.7	18.9	19.2
44–46	18.3	18.6	18.8	19.1	19.3	19.6	19.8	20.1	20.3
47–49	19.5	19.7	20.0	20.2	20.5	20.7	21.0	21.2	21.5
50–52	20.6	20.8	21.1	21.3	21.6	21.8	22.1	22.3	22.6
53–55	21.7	21.9	22.1	22.4	22.6	22.9	23.1	23.4	23.6
56–58	22.7	23.0	23.2	23.4	23.7	23.9	24.2	24.4	24.7
59–61	23.7	24.0	24.2	24.5	24.7	25.0	25.2	25.5	25.7
62–64	24.7	25.0	25.2	25.5	25.7	26.0	26.7	26.4	26.7
65–67	25.7	25.9	26.2	26.4	26.7	26.9	27.2	27.4	27.7
68–70	26.6	26.9	27.1	27.4	27.6	27.9	28.1	28.4	28.6
71–73	27.5	27.8	28.0	28.3	28.5	28.8	29.0	29.3	29.5
74–76	28.4	28.7	28.9	29.2	29.4	29.7	29.9	30.2	30.4
77–79	29.3	29.5	29.8	30.0	30.3	30.5	30.8	31.0	31.3
80–82	30.1	30.4	30.6	30.9	31.1	31.4	31.6	31.9	32.1
83–85	30.9	31.2	31.4	31.7	31.9	32.2	32.4	32.7	32.9
86–88	31.7	32.0	32.2	32.5	32.7	32.9	33.2	33.4	33.7
89–91	32.5	32.7	33.0	33.2	33.5	33.7	33.9	34.2	34.4
92–94	33.2	33.4	33.7	33.9	34.2	34.4	34.7	34.9	35.2
95–97	33.9	34.1	34.4	34.6	34.9	35.1	35.4	35.6	35.9
98–100	34.6	34.8	35.1	35.3	35.5	35.8	36.0	36.3	36.5
101–103	35.3	35.4	35.7	35.9	36.2	36.4	36.7	36.9	37.2
104–106	35.8	36.1	36.3	36.6	36.8	37.1	37.3	37.5	37.8
107–109	36.4	36.7	36.9	37.1	37.4	37.6	37.9	38.1	38.4
110–112	37.0	37.2	37.5	37.7	38.0	38.2	38.5	38.7	38.9
113–115	37.5	37.8	38.0	38.2	38.5	38.7	39.0	39.2	39.5
116–118	38.0	38.3	38.5	38.8	39.0	39.3	39.5	39.7	40.0
119–121	38.5	38.7	39.0	39.2	39.5	39.7	40.0	40.2	40.5
122–124	39.0	39.2	39.4	39.7	39.9	40.2	40.4	40.7	40.9
125–127	39.4	39.6	39.9	40.1	40.4	40.6	40.9	41.1	41.4
128–130	39.8	40.0	40.3	40.5	40.8	41.0	41.3	41.5	41.8

Source: Jackson, A.S. & Pollock, M.L. (1985). *Practical Assessment of Body Composition*. Reprinted with permission of McGraw-Hill.

measurements: chest, 20; abdomen, 30; and thigh, 17, for a total measurement of 67. According to Table 10-8, at the intersection of the row corresponding to the sum of the skinfolds and the column corresponding to the age, his estimated body-fat percentage is 21.3%. This man is 5% above the upper limit of the 14 to 17% range for men desiring optimal fitness (see Table 10-3).

Bioelectrical Impedance

Bioelectrical impedance is a popular method for determining body composition. It is based on the principle that the conductivity of an electrical impulse is greater through lean tissue than through fatty tissue. An imperceptible electrical current is passed through two pairs of electrodes, which are placed on one hand and one foot. The analyzer, essentially an ohmmeter and a computer, measures the body's resistance to electrical flow and computes body density and body-fat percentage. The subject must lie still, with wrist and ankle electrodes accurately placed. The client should be well-hydrated and not have exercised in the past six hours or consumed any alcohol in the past 24 hours. Some research has shown the impedance method to be as accurate as the skinfold method, depending on the quality of the analyzer, the formula used to compute body density, and the adherence of the client to the aforementioned restrictions. Assessing body composition via bioelectrical impedance is both fast and easy and requires minimal technical training. The cost of the analyzers ranges from $300 to $5,000, depending on design and report-generation capabilities (from simple digital readouts to elaborate multipage reports).

Body-fat scales are available for around $100, though they are not accurate enough to be reliable measurement tools. The problem stems from the scales' inability to differentiate between body types and to provide consistent readings.

Hydrostatic Weighing

Hydrostatic weighing, also known as underwater weighing, is considered the "gold standard" of body-composition assessment. The test involves suspending a client, seated in a chair attached to a scale, in a tank of water. Body density is calculated from the relationship of normal body weight to underwater weight. Body-fat percentage is calculated from body density. This method is most accurate when combined with a measurement of residual volume (the amount of air left in the lungs after a complete expiration). When residual volume is estimated from a formula, the accuracy of the hydrostatic method can be significantly decreased. Though hydrostatic weighing is accurate, it is often impractical in terms of expense, time, and equipment.

Other Methods of Body-composition Assessment

The science of body-composition assessment is a relatively young discipline, but it is evolving rapidly due to the use of advanced technologies, such as **dual energy x-ray absorptiometry (DEXA)**, **air displacement plethysmography (ADP)**, and **near-infrared interactance (NIR).**

Dual Energy X-ray Absorptiometry

A relatively new technology that has been found to be very accurate and precise (an error rate of less than 1.5%), DEXA is based on a three-compartment model that divides the body into three components—total body mineral, fat-free soft (lean) mass, and fat tissue mass. This technique is based on the assumption that bone mineral content is directly proportional to the amount of photon energy absorbed by the bone being studied.

DEXA uses a whole-body scanner that has two low-dose x-rays at different sources that read bone and soft tissue mass simultaneously. The sources are mounted beneath a table with a detector overhead. The scanner passes across a person's reclining body with data collected at ½-cm intervals. A DEXA scan takes between three and five minutes, depending on the specific type of scanner used. This technique is safe and noninvasive, with little inconvenience to the individual (e.g., a person is not required to disrobe or monitor food or fluid consumption).

DEXA has become the "benchmark" for body-composition assessment techniques, because it has a higher degree of precision, while only involving one measurement, and has the ability to identify exactly where fat is distributed throughout the body (i.e., regional body-fat distribution). In fact, most clinical studies use DEXA to evaluate the accuracy of other body-composition assessment techniques. Research has shown DEXA to be a very reliable and useful tool for precisely measuring body-fat levels. Given its successful application in clinical settings and the increased awareness of the inherent dangers of excess body fat, the employment of DEXA in practical settings will undoubtedly become more commonplace in the near future.

Air Displacement Plethysmography

Air displacement plethysmography (ADP) is a relatively new, noninvasive, and rapid way to assess body composition that predicts %BF within 1 to 3% of hydrostatic weighing results (Fields, Goran, & McCrory, 2002). ADP equipment, such as the BOD POD,® uses whole-body air displacement instead of water to measure body volume and density. The BOD POD determines body volume by measuring the volume of air in the chamber while empty and then with a person inside.

Near-infrared Interactance

Near-infrared interactance (NIR) technology was developed by the USDA to measure the amount of fat contained in beef and pork carcasses following slaughter. NIR uses a small probe that emits an infrared light through the skin, fat, and lean tissues, and then records their optical densities (changes in color and tone) as the light is reflected off bone and back to the probe.

NIR equipment that has been adapted for use with humans, such as the Futrex® NIR model, is able to predict %BF based on the evidence that optical densities of FM and FFM are proportional to the amount of subcutaneous fat. By comparing known optical-density values for FM and FFM to the measured optical densities in subjects, one can estimate the amount of subcutaneous fat at the measured site. Most NIR equipment uses the anterior aspect of the biceps as the common NIR measurement site. Once the test is finished, NIR data is entered into a prediction equation based on the person's height, weight, frame size, and level of activity to estimate %BF.

Although NIR is an inexpensive and rapid way to measure %BF in humans, there has been significant debate over its reliability and validity. Factors such as probe pressure, skin color, and hydration status can affect results. Numerous studies using NIR produced mixed results. Mclean and Skinner (1992) found that skinfolds more accurately predicted body fat than NIR when underwater weighing was used as the criterion measure. When using NIR to estimate body composition, it is critical that an experienced technician who follows the manufacturer's recommended procedures perform the test. At best, NIR is a very general estimate of %BF, with an inherently high error rate.

Approaches to Discussing Results With Clients

Body-composition results should be used to help motivate clients and help them set realistic body-weight or fat-loss goals. They should never be used to humiliate, degrade, or categorize people. In addition, LWMCs must always use positive and encouraging language. Never say, "Mr. Jones, your body-composition results indicate that your percent body fat is high, which means that you fall into the obese category. Boy, we sure have a lot of work ahead of us, don't we?" While this statement may be true, LWMCs should be more encouraging: "Mr. Jones, your body-composition results indicate that you are above the range for good health, so I'm glad you made this appointment, and I'm excited to be working with you. I have set some very reasonable and attainable diet and exercise goals for you that I think will help bring your percent body fat down into a healthier range."

LWMCs must never focus on the numbers. Instead, they should consider the whole person when discussing the results of body-composition testing. When most people hear a number they think is too high, they tend to stop listening, because they have already made up their minds. For example, consider a client who is 5'7" and weighs 155 pounds (1.7 m; 70 kg), who tells you that he thinks he should weigh 135 pounds (61 kg) because he heard that a person can figure out his ideal weight by adding 5 pounds (2.3 kg) to a base of 100 for every inch of height over five feet. However, a body-composition test shows that 135 pounds (61 kg) would be unrealistic based on the client's amount of lean tissue (muscle). For example, if the client's body fat came out to 22%, then 78% of his weight, or 121 pounds (55 kg), is lean tissue. If he was to maintain that amount of lean tissue and lose 20 pounds (9.1 kg) of fat, he would weigh 135 pounds (61 kg), but his body composition would be down to 10% fat, which is too low for him.

Body-composition testing is only one tool to help guide a diet and exercise program. Body-composition results by themselves offer little value. In addition, body fat or weight is not the only measure of health. It is possible to be quite healthy by all other standards while exceeding a norm for body weight or body composition. LWMCs must discuss body-composition results by using phrases such as "within the desirable range," or "too high" or "too low," in addition to presenting the raw data. Saying that a body fat level is 28% likely means nothing to the client.

Summary

Body composition is an integral component of total health and physical fitness. Accordingly, fitness professionals have a responsibility to help educate those with whom they work and the general population regarding appropriate levels of body fat and how to safely and effectively achieve them. Not only can such an effort have a positive impact on the high prevalence of obesity in society, it can also help reduce the enormous healthcare costs that result from this very unhealthy condition. As such, a strong argument can be made that a body-composition evaluation should be included as an essential part of all health and fitness appraisals. The time for taking a more measured approached in the war on obesity and its related problems is now. Accurately assessing body composition and using that information to help design meaningful, personalized exercise regimens should serve as the foundation for that approach.

References

Carella, M.J. et al. (1997). Serial measurements of body composition in obese subjects during a very-low-energy diet (VLED) comparing bioelectrical impedance with hydrodensitometry. *Obesity Research,* 5, 250–256.

Fields, D., Goran, M., & McCrory, M. (2002). Body-composition assessment via air-displacement plethysmography in adults and children: A review. *American Journal of Clinical Nutrition,* 75, 453–467.

Jackson, A.S. & Pollock, M.L. (1985). Practical assessment of body composition. *The Physician and Sportsmedicine,* May, 76–90.

Lohman, T.G., Roche, A. F., & Martorell, R. (Eds.). (1988). *Anthropometric Standardization Reference Manual.* Champaign, Ill.: Human Kinetics.

Mclean, K.P. & Skinner, J.S. (1992). Validity of Futrex-5000 for Body Composition. *Medicine & Exercise in Sports & Exercise,* 2, 253–257.

Metropolitan Life Insurance Company (1959). New weight standards for men and women. *Statistics Bulletin Metropolitan Life Insurance Co.,* 40, 1–4.

Metropolitan Life Insurance Company (1983). 1983 Metropolitan height and weight tables. *Statistics Bulletin Metropolitan Life Insurance Co.,* 64, 1–19.

National Heart, Lung, and Blood Institute (1998). Clinical guidelines on the identification, evaluation, and treatment of overweight and obesity in adults: The evidence report. *Obesity Research,* 6 (Suppl. 2), 51S–209S.

Tran, Z. & Weltman, A. (1989). Generalized equation for predicting body density of women from girth measurements. *Medicine & Science in Sports & Exercise,* 21, 101–104.

Tran, Z. Weltman, A., & Seip, R. (1988). Predicting body composition of men from girth measurements. *Human Biology,* 8, 60, 167–176.

Wolf, A.M. (2002). Economic outcomes of the obese patient. *Obesity Research,* 10, 58S–62S.

Suggested Reading

Brozek, J. et al. (1963). Densitometric analysis of body composition: Revision of some quantitative assumptions. *Annals of the New York Academy of Sciences,* 110, 113–140.

Chan J.M. et al. (1994). Obesity, fat distribution, and weight gain as risk factors for clinical diabetes in men. *Diabetes Care,* 17, 9, 961–969.

Finkelstein, E.A. et al. (2005). Economic causes and consequences of obesity. *Annual Review of Public Health,* April, 26, 239–257.

Heymsfield, S.B. et al. (2005). *Human Body Composition* (2nd ed.). Champaign, Ill.: Human Kinetics.

Heyward, V.H. & Wagner, D.R. (2004). *Applied Body Composition Assessment.* Champaign, Ill.: Human Kinetics.

Jackson, A.S. & Pollock, M.L. (1978). Generalized equations for predicting body density. *British Journal of Nutrition,* 40, 497–504.

National Institutes of Health (1998). *The Practical Guide on Identification, Evaluation, and Treatment of Overweight and Obesity in Adults.* Bethesda, Md.: National Institutes of Health.

Siri, W.E. (1961). Body composition from fluid space and density. In: Brozek, J. & Hanschel, A. (Eds.). *Techniques for Measuring Body Composition* (pp. 223–244). Washington, D.C.: National Academy of Science.

Stunkard, A.J. & Wadden, T.A. (Eds.) (1993). *Obesity: Theory and Therapy* (2nd ed.). New York: Raven Press.

Thompson, D. et al. (1999). Lifetime health and economic consequences of obesity. *Archives of Internal Medicine*, 159, 2177–2183.

Wang, Y. et al. (2005). Comparison of abdominal adiposity and overall obesity in predicting risk of type 2 diabetes among men. *American Journal of Clinical Nutrition,* 81, 3, 555–563.

Yusuf, S. et al. on behalf of the INTERHEART Study (2005). Obesity and the risk of myocardial infraction in 27,000 participants from 52 countries: A case-control study. *The Lancet,* 366, 1640–1649.

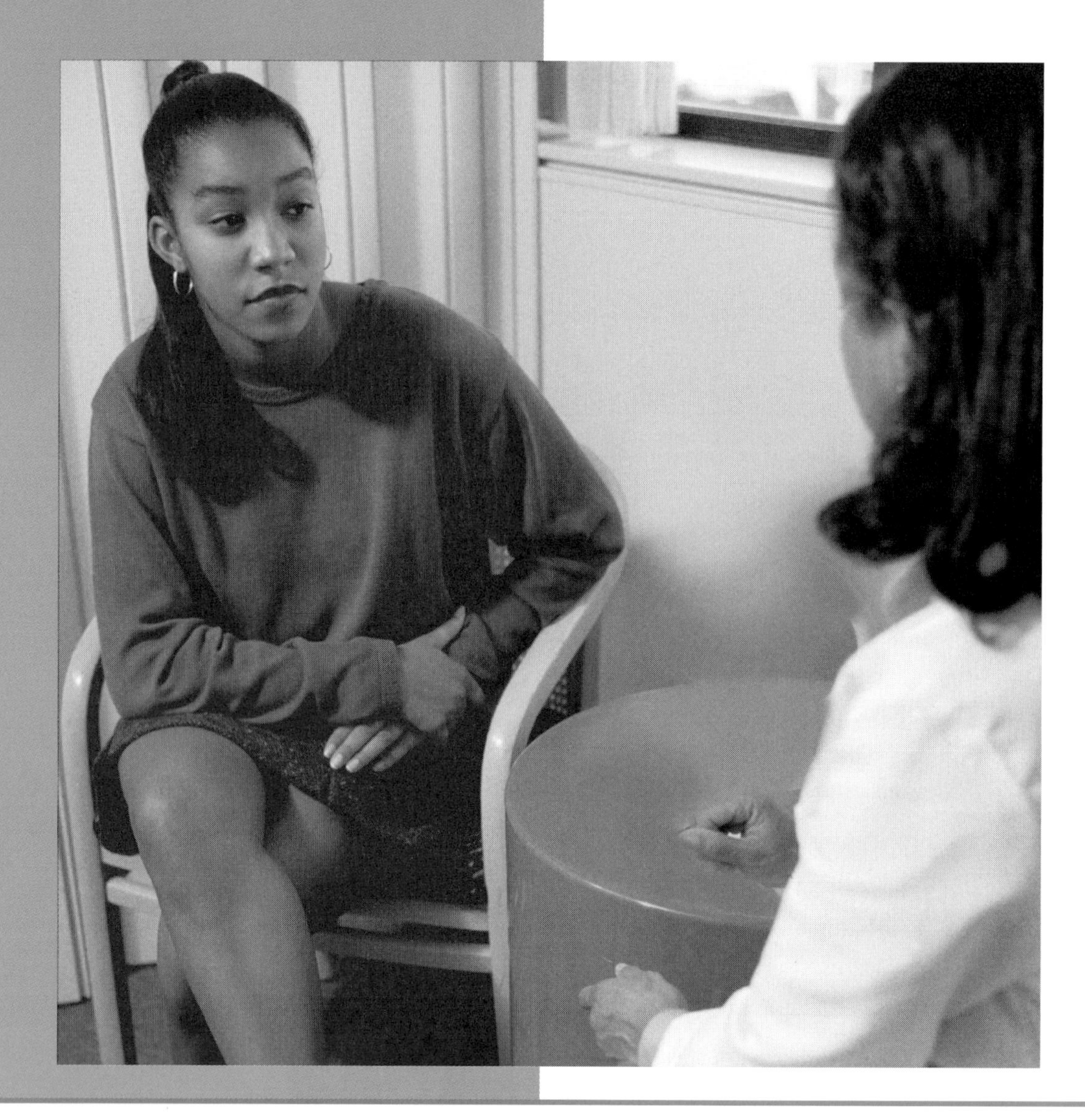

Susan Bartlett, Ross Andersen, and Richard T. Cotton

Susan Bartlett, Ph.D., is associate professor of medicine at the Johns Hopkins School of Medicine in Baltimore, Md. Dr. Bartlett is a licensed clinical psychologist and faculty member in the Division of Rheumatology and Johns Hopkins Arthritis Center. Her primary research and clinical interests focus on the effect of weight loss and exercise on arthritis, the mind-body effects of physical activity, and how psychosocial factors influence adherence to medical treatments.

Ross Andersen, Ph.D., is associate director of fellowship training in the Division of Geriatric Medicine at Johns Hopkins Medical Center. Since 1993, he has been conducting clinical trials examining the long-term effects of diet and exercise in helping people manage their weight. In addition, he has published several reports that have shaped current thinking about exercise for overweight individuals. For 10 years, Dr. Andersen operated community-based weight-loss programs in health clubs, and he is the author of The Health and Fitness Club Leader's Guide: Administering a Weight-Management Program. *He is a fellow of the American College of Sports Medicine (ACSM) and a member of the North American Association for the Study of Obesity (NAASO).*

Richard T. Cotton, M.A., is the national director of certification for the American College of Sports Medicine (ACSM). Before joining ACSM, he was the chief exercise physiologist at MyExercisePlan.com. Cotton is the former chief exercise physiologist for the Scripps Clinic & Research Foundation as well as for the American Council on exercise, where he also served as a media spokesperson and technical editor. He is certified by ACSM as both a Preventive and Rehabilitative Program Director and Exercise Specialist.

Chapter 11

Referral

IN THIS CHAPTER:

Making appropriate referrals is fundamental to the job of a Lifestyle & Weight Management Consultant (LWMC). The challenge lies in the scope of the job of an LWMC and how it can potentially overlap with other health professionals, especially medical doctors, dietitians, and psychologists. Knowing when and how to refer to other health professionals is an essential skill for an LWMC.

Making Appropriate Referrals

The referral process starts with the assessment of the client. In fact, the determination of the need to refer is one of the primary reasons for performing an assessment. Timing and personal needs are important considerations when attempting to lose weight, and therefore should be part of the information-gathering process. For some individuals, personal or professional circumstances are likely to become barriers to success if they are not addressed effectively. For others, certain personal characteristics may suggest that the individual needs further evaluation by a healthcare specialist before attempting to lose weight and beginning to exercise. Table 11-1 presents a list of potential candidates for referral, along with possible referral sources. Table 11-2 presents a brief description of various healthcare specialties.

Table 11-1
Individuals Requiring Further Evaluation by Healthcare Professionals

Candidates	Potential Referral Sources
Pregnant and lactating women	Primary care provider (obstetrician, family practitioner, nurse practitioner, midwife), dietitian
Anorexia, bulimia, and problems with frequent binge-eating episodes	Psychologist, psychiatrist, social worker (preferably specializing in eating disorders), primary care provider
Children	Primary care provider, dietitian, clinical weight-loss program specializing in children
Significant psychological distress such as frequent bouts of anxiety, persistent sadness, panic attacks, or excessive worrying	Psychologist, psychiatrist, social worker, or primary care provider
Any significant medical condition (e.g., cardiovascular problems, renal problems, diabetes, arthritis)	Primary care provider, dietitian, clinical weight-loss program

It is critical for an LWMC to be aware of who is truly qualified to practice nutrition or dietetics, a specialized field that allows individuals who have completed their studies to take a national registration examination to become a registered dietitian (R.D.) or licensed dietitian (L.D.). R.D. and L.D. are well-recognized designations that are protected from use by unqualified practitioners. However, self-proclaimed nutritionists or nutrition counselors often provide advice and counseling to those willing to pay for it. Unqualified practitioners can place their clients at risk for adverse health effects and make themselves targets of lawsuits (see Chapter 19). The public deserves to be protected from such unqualified practitioners.

Registration and licensure of nutrition professionals exist to protect the public from people who are not qualified to practice as nutrition professionals, just as licensure of physicians protects the public from people who are not qualified to practice medicine. Forty-six states have their own form of licensure or credentialing for nutrition professionals. There are commonly three credentials that allow people to legally practice as a nutrition or dietetics professional: registered dietitian, licensed dietitian/nutritionist (L.D./N.), and licensed dietitian.

It is very important that LWMCs know their state laws before making referrals for dietary support—both for the safety of their clients and for their own risk management.

Scope of Practice

LWMCs have an obligation to be knowledgeable in a wide variety of areas, including nutrition, psychology, behavior change, exercise programming, and counseling. There will likely be instances in which an LWMC will not be qualified to support a client who is facing a specific psychological or physical challenge. For example, LWMCs are not equipped to deal with psychological or psychiatric illnesses such as eating disorders (e.g., anorexia and bulimia nervosa) or depression. Also, while general nutritional recommendations related to decreasing fat consumption and eating more complex carbohydrates do not violate laws, the prescribing of a specific diet detailing food, vitamin, and calorie consumption may be regulated by the state and require the license of a registered dietitian or nutritionist. Laws vary from state to state. LWMCs must know the scope and limits of their practice and refrain from practicing in areas in which they have no formal training.

Table 11-2
Allied Healthcare Professionals

Primary Health

Primary healthcare providers include physicians, physician assistants, and nurse practitioners. They are licensed by state boards of professional standards to provide medical care.

- Physicians hold a doctoral degree, M.D. or D.O., and receive the most extensive training.
- Physician assistants (PA) work under the supervision of a physician. PA training programs usually last at least two years; admission requirements vary by program, but many require at least two years of college and some healthcare. They must pass a national exam to obtain a license to practice as a PA. Some PAs are able to prescribe medications under the direction of the supervising physician.
- Nurse practitioners (NP) are registered nurses who have at least two years of additional training and supervised experience at the master's level. In many states, NPs are licensed to practice medicine in a limited fashion independently of a physician and may prescribe certain types of medications.

Nutrition

There are several levels of specialization in the field of dietetics.

- The doctoral-level nutrition practitioner may be a physician with board certification in nutrition or a registered dietitian (RD) with a doctoral degree.
- The specialist RD has earned a master's degree in nutrition and/or has three to five years of experience.
- The generalist RD holds a bachelor's degree in nutrition. In some states, these individuals are licensed by the state's board of dietetics. The American Dietetic Association maintains a listing of registered dietitians in the United States (800-877-1600).
- The dietetic technician, registered (DTR) holds an associate's degree in nutrition and works under the supervision of a registered dietitian.

Mental Health

- Psychologists have completed doctoral-level training in clinical or counseling psychology and have passed both national and state exams certifying their competence. Only psychologists who are licensed to practice psychology may legally use the title "psychologist." In some states, master's-level practitioners who have completed additional training and field supervision in addition to the other requirements have been "grandfathered" and are able to use the title of licensed psychologist. Ethical standards of practice are set forth by the American Psychological Association. The State Board of Psychology for each state maintains a listing of all licensed psychologists, along with their areas of expertise.
- Psychiatrists are physicians who have completed a residency in psychiatry. Board-certified psychiatrists have met additional requirements set forth by the American Board of Psychiatry and Neurology. Some psychiatrists also have received additional specialized training in the treatment of eating disorders.
- Social workers have completed bachelor's-, master's-, or doctoral-level training in social work at an accredited college or university and have passed a licensure examination. The State Board of Social Work Examiners maintains a list of licensed social workers, including their level of specialization. A licensed certified social worker also has obtained significant training and supervision.

Exercise

At this time, there is no recognized registry or licensure of fitness professionals. LWMCs should look for instructors who are certified and experienced in working with clients with weight-management challenges. There are a number of certifications a fitness instructor may earn. The most credible are those from certification organizations that are accredited by the National Commission for Certifying Agencies (NCCA). The NCCA is an independent agency that accredits certifications in a variety of professions, including, for example, nursing and athletic training. The NCCA reviews the certification organization's procedures, protocols, and operations, and determines if the certification properly discriminates between those who are qualified and those who are not qualified to be awarded the respective credential. The ACE LWMC Certification Program is NCCA-accredited.

Therapist, Psychotherapist, Counselor, Nutritionist, Exercise Physiologist

These titles are not protected and have no governing bodies. Anyone may use these titles freely, as they do not reflect training, experience, or adherence to a set of ethical principles. *Note:* The title of nutritionist is limited in some states.

Establishing a Referral Network

For LWMCs who work relatively independently, establishing a network of allied healthcare professionals to whom they can refer clients is essential to managing risk and operating a successful business. LWMCs also have an ethical responsibility to ensure that the professionals to whom they refer their clients are appropriately qualified to treat the problem. For example, if an LWMC identifies elevated blood pressure in a client, the appropriate referral is to the primary healthcare provider. If the client does not have a provider, the LWMC can assist him or her in finding one, taking into consideration any restrictions related to health insurance.

It is always best for LWMCs to refer clients to professionals they personally know and trust. A referral for dietary counseling to, "Sarah Jones, a registered dietitian who specializes in weight management and has worked with previous clients," is always preferable to a referral to "the dietary department" at the local hospital. When establishing a referral network, LWMCs should try to speak directly to the professional to whom they wish to refer their clients, rather than to the receptionist. This direct contact will help the LWMC determine whether the healthcare provider's views on the importance of lifestyle change compliment his or her own. LWMCs and healthcare providers should collaborate to support and reinforce the efforts that the client is making in attempting to change lifestyle behaviors. For example, a brief comment by a doctor during an office visit about weight lost can boost a client's confidence and morale.

A referral network will also be supported by the creation of a professional network. LWMCs should contact local professional associations that are related to their work. Many national organizations have regional chapters that meet on a periodic basis. LWMCs can also start regular local meetings of weight-management professionals to exchange knowledge and share ideas. An LWMC's referral network does not have to be limited to his or her community. By attending professional meetings, LWMCs will meet other health professionals that can provide a wealth of support for many years to come.

There are also other creative ways to develop a referral network. Newsletters are an excellent way for an LWMC to keep his or her name and services visible. Providing educational talks and "brown bag lunch" discussions, both on and off the worksite, can introduce an LWMC to a wide range of professionals and potential clients. An LWMC may even be able to secure a regular spot on a local morning TV news show or local newspaper, where he or she can review principles of lifestyle change. While the LWMC may not be paid to provide any of these services, these opportunities can provide a wealth of exposure.

Working in a Supporting Role

Lifestyle-related behaviors are now the largest contributor to illness and disability in the United States. LWMCs are an important source for ongoing guidance and support to help clients initiate and maintain positive lifestyle changes. LWMCs should work with the referring professional to ensure that the programs they design complement the medical treatment the client is currently receiving. LWMCs should always send a letter to the professionals to whom they are referring their clients. In this letter, the LWMC should introduce the client and summarize the reasons for the referral. For example, the LWMC should spell out if the client is being referred for a long overdue health physical or because the LWMC has specific concerns about whether it is appropriate for the client to begin exercising at this time. The LWMC should indicate in the letter that he or she would appreciate the provider's recommendations related to the lifestyle changes that the client proposes to make (Figure 11-1).

The establishment and maintenance of a referral network is both a professional responsibility and an effective marketing strategy. LWMCs will find it is time well spent, especially as professionals in their communities begin referring clients to them. When this happens,

Figure 11-1
Sample Letter to Physician

Reprinted with permission from www.MyExercisePlan.com

Dear Dr. Smith,

Your patient, Richard Conrad (DOB: 08/17/1956), has contracted with me to provide services as an American Council on Exercise-certified Lifestyle & Weight Management Consultant (LWMC). As an LWMC, I design exercise programs and provide basic nutrition information and ongoing support to assist clients in adhering to their weight-management programs. All of the programs I develop are based on my clients' health status, fitness goals, and personal preferences.

I follow the pre-exercise health assessment standards developed by the American College of Sports Medicine, American Heart Association, and the Canadian Society for Exercise Physiology and offer recommendations to help minimize the risk for exercise-related illness and/or injury.

I have recommended that your patient, Richard Conrad, be evaluated by you prior to beginning an exercise program. This recommendation is based on the following findings:

- Age greater than or equal to 45 years old
- Total cholesterol greater than 200 mg/dL or HDL cholesterol less than 40 mg/dL
- Reports a bone, joint, or muscle problem that could be exacerbated with physical activity
- Reported an injury that could be made worse with exercise, specifically to the knee

To use my services, Richard Conrad has agreed to seek clearance from his or her personal physician.

Richard Conrad has also agreed to incorporate modifications that you suggest to the attached exercise program. To assist in the development and implementation of his exercise program, please check one of the following statements:

☐ I concur with Richard Conrad's exercise participation with no restrictions
☐ I concur with Richard Conrad's exercise participation with the following restrictions:

____

____

____

☐ I do not concur with Richard Conrad's participation in an exercise program.

____

____

Physician's name (type or print)________________________

Physician's signature____________________________

Date______________

Thank you for your assistance in helping to keep the exercise program safe and effective for Richard Conrad.

Sincerely,

Sally Samuelson
ACE-certified Lifestyle & Weight Management Consultant

LWMCs must send "thank you" letters summarizing the results of their initial meeting with the client and providing the results of any fitness evaluation. LWMCs should also periodically send a follow-up letter indicating each client's progress toward reaching his or her goals. All correspondence should be brief—ideally one page or less.

It is critical to obtain a client's written permission to both obtain information from, and release information to, healthcare providers. LWMCs should always tell the professionals they are calling that written permission to speak with them has been received from the client. Also, LWMCs should be prepared to fax or mail a copy of this permission form to professionals who wish to have it in their records before talking further.

SOAP Notes

SOAP is an acronym for subjective, objective, assessment, and plan. A **SOAP note** is intended to improve communication among all those caring for a given client and to communicate pertinent characteristics and provide the assessment, problems, and plans in an organized format to facilitate the care of the client. Depending upon the facility, they may also be used for record review and quality control.

Documentation of a client's characteristics, concerns, and related plans must be consistent, concise, and comprehensive. As such, SOAP notes are commonly written by physicians and other licensed healthcare providers, such as a physician's assistant (PA), physical therapist, or licensed nurse practitioner. Many medical offices use the SOAP note format to standardize medical-evaluation entries made in clinical records. Given this standard, SOAP notes provide an excellent method for LWMCs to gather information and communicate client status during the referral process.

The Components of a SOAP Note

- Subjective—The initial portion of the SOAP note format consists of subjective observations. These are symptoms verbalized by the client or by a significant other. These subjective observations include the client's descriptions of pain or discomfort, the presence of shortness of breath on exertion, or dizziness, along with a multitude of other descriptions of any dysfunction, discomfort, or illness.
- Objective—The next part of the format is the objective observation, which includes symptoms that can actually be measured, seen, heard, touched, or felt. Objective observations include vital signs such as resting heart rate, blood pressure, body weight, percent body fat, waist circumference, and the results of any other related tests or evaluations.
- Assessment—Assessment follows the objective observations. The assessment is a statement of the client's condition. In some cases, this statement may be clear, such as "moderately obese." However, an assessment may not be so clear and can include several possibilities.

Note: The word "statement" is used quite intentionally in this description. In the medical field, the assessment is usually a "diagnosis." The scope of practice of an LWMC does not include making a medical diagnosis. Therefore, any reference to a diagnosis should be avoided.

- Plan—The last part of the SOAP note is the plan. The plan may include further fitness testing or other testing (e.g., **DEXA scan**). This is where a referral to another healthcare professional would be noted. This is also the section where an LWMC would record his or her appropriate plan in terms of exercise, nutrition, and adherence strategies.

Remember, the SOAP note is not supposed to be as detailed as a progress report. Complete sentences are not necessary and abbreviations are appropriate. However, LWMCs should avoid using abbreviations until they have a thorough knowledge of how they are used. Abbreviations differ for each specialty and should be consistent within the facility in which the LWMC works.

The length of the note will differ depending on the use. SOAP notes that follow each client session will likely be shorter than ones that accompany a referral letter. SOAP notes can be flexible. LWMCs often develop their own styles as they accommodate varied preferences.

SOAP Note Case Examples

The following are three examples of individuals who may seek an LWMC's help with a weight-loss program.

Janet

Janet is 35 years old, married without children, and works as a secretary for a cardiologist. She is 5′8″ tall and weighs 260 pounds (1.73 meters; 118 kg). She is coming to see the LWMC at the insistence of her family, who are worried about her health. She says she is in good health at the present time, although she takes medication to control her blood pressure and chronic heartburn. During the assessment, she tells the LWMC that she has been on "every diet known to man." She does well on a diet for the first three to four months, but then returns to her old eating habits, only to regain all the weight she had lost, and often gain some more. She has exercised on occasion to facilitate weight loss, but has never stuck with any program of activity for more than a few weeks. She confides during the interview that she is very unhappy about her weight, as her husband makes frequent reference to it. To avoid his criticism, she eats very little in front of him, and then sneaks out to fast-food restaurants or convenience stores to get, "what I really want to eat" (e.g., ice cream, fried foods, candy bars). She has gained 20 pounds (9 kg) in the past six months. When the LWMC asks about her perceptions of eating, she replies, "Of course I'm out of control. If I was in control, would I eat this way?" She denies that she is depressed, but is tearful at times during the meeting.

Associated SOAP Note

Patient Name: Janet Smith
DOB: 09/17/1972
Date: 10/4/07
S—seeking assistance at the insistence of her family, has been on "every diet known to man," exercises occasionally, is unhappy about her weight, husbands makes frequent references to it, was tearful during intake evaluation, but denies depression
O—35-year-old female, 68″, 260 pounds (1.73 m, 118 kg), married, no children, taking blood pressure and heartburn medications
A—basically healthy, likely depressed, healthy body weight would fall within a range of 125 to 151 pounds (57 to 69 kg)
P—refer to mental-health professional for further evaluation, begin program based on input received

Approach to Referring Janet

The LWMC needs to find out more information about a number of things, including several red flags that Janet's eating may be especially problematic. The LWMC should:

- Explore Janet's motivation very carefully. Is she coming to the LWMC out of desperation, or to appease her husband?
- Carefully explore with Janet the burden of attempting lifestyle change at this time and mutually determine if she is really ready to undertake this challenge, especially if pleasing others is a major factor.
- Assess the presence of potential binge eating very carefully. Ask her to review several days of eating, noting what she ate and drank and the times and places associated with eating.
- Explore the secretive eating. Is she doing this out of shame and embarrassment, or to avoid criticism? Is she unhappy about her eating? Does she really "lose" control when she is eating, or does she simply eat on impulse (i.e., without thinking about what she is eating and why)?
- Talk about the tearfulness. Does this happen frequently when she thinks about herself, her weight, and her eating?

It is important that the LWMC has a good understanding of each of these issues to help determine whether Janet needs additional evaluation from her primary care provider or a mental-health specialist.

Billy

Billy is a 25-year-old lean construction worker who would like advice on how to optimize his training program and weight for bodybuilding competitions. He has been lifting weights for about a year in his basement and is satisfied with his progress. His maximal bench press is 255 pounds (116 kg) and he can squat 375 pounds (170 kg). Billy feels that his strength improvement has plateaued over the past two months. He would like the advice of an LWMC on how to get past this plateau to prepare for an upcoming show. He also would like a spotter when he is lifting heavier weights, since he sometimes feels dizzy during, or immediately after, his heavy lifts.

Associated SOAP Note

Patient Name: Billy Crawford
DOB: 09/17/1982
Date: 10/4/07
S—lean construction worker, seeking services to optimize training program and weight for bodybuilding competitions, states that strength improvements have plateaued over the past two months, is sometimes dizzy during and/or following heavy lifting
O—25 years old, male, bench presses 255 pounds (116 kg), squats 375 pounds (170 kg)
A—25-year-old bodybuilder, excellent strength fitness, dizziness a concern
P—secure client's permission to refer him to his personal physician, make referral

Approach to Referring Billy

Billy's youth and active lifestyle may be somewhat deceptive. Billy's dizziness may be an important warning sign of underlying cardiopulmonary disease (see Table 9-7, page 216). Thus, in spite of his age and apparent fitness, according to the ACSM recommendations (see Table 9-9, page 216), individuals with any major symptoms of disease should undergo a medical exam and exercise testing before beginning an exercise program under an LWMC's supervision. It will be important not to scare Billy, but the LWMC will have to let him know that he needs to meet with his primary care provider to talk about the dizziness he is experiencing during exercise as soon as possible. The LWMC can tell him that this is not a normal response to exercise, and that it is best to be cautious and certain that he can safely train for the upcoming event.

The LWMC may also want to ask Billy for permission to contact his primary care provider before proceeding any further. Permission must be in writing and filed in the LWMC's chart notes. When speaking with or writing to Billy's primary care provider, the LWMC must outline his or her concerns, including the intensity of Billy's program, his current response to exercise, and his stated goals. The LWMC must ask Billy's primary care provider to send a letter providing medical clearance to exercise and any recommendations related to exercise.

Mary

Mary is a 52-year-old single lawyer who has come to the LWMC for help with improving her health and losing weight. Her blood pressure is 138/88 mmHg and her body fat is 37% of her total weight. She has never been physically active and feels that, in general, she isn't well-coordinated. Furthermore, she is wary about exercising since her 62-year-old uncle died suddenly while shoveling snow last winter.

Associated SOAP Note

Patient Name: Mary Lucas
DOB: 09/17/1955
Date: 10/4/07
S—attorney, self-referred for health improvement and weight-loss assistance, no history of regular physical activity, says she is not well-coordinated, concerned about exercise safety based on her uncle's sudden cardiac death at 62 years old while shoveling snow

O—female, 52 years old, BP = 138/88, percent body fat = 37%
A—inactive, obese
P—begin moderate-intensity aerobic exercise program based on current weight, personal preferences, and concerns

Approach to Referring Mary

It is probably safe for the LWMC to begin working with Mary, since she is under 55 years of age, and her sedentary lifestyle and obesity are her only major risk factors. Her uncle was 62 and not a first-degree relative. She does have important potential risk factors to note. Her blood pressure is "high-normal" and her body composition places her in the obese category. However, these do not qualify as risk factors that would prevent her from beginning a moderate exercise program without her doctor's clearance. The LWMC could have Mary perform an aerobic fitness test [e.g., the YMCA Step Test or the Rockport Walking Test (see Chapter 9)] to establish her baseline fitness level and determine an appropriate starting point for exercise. When administering a submaximal aerobic fitness test, the LWMC should monitor heart rate to ensure that the activity remains "moderate."

It is important to work carefully with Mary to alleviate her low **self-efficacy** regarding exercise. It will be important for her to begin exercising gradually with activities that require little athletic skill. Outdoor walking and stationary cycling are good modes of activity to train the aerobic system. Stair-climbing machines, rowing ergometers, aerobic step classes, and cross-country ski machines can be introduced as physical fitness and self-confidence improve. She will no doubt benefit from and appreciate the LWMC's direct supervision when acquiring the necessary skills to begin using fitness equipment. Resistance training on machines is also an excellent way for individuals with no history of programmed exercise to train the musculoskeletal system, since it requires less skill or technique than free-weight options.

Summary

Proper referral is fundamental to the job of an LWMC. Knowing when and how to refer is better for the clients, as well as an integral component of an LWMC's risk-management practices. All LWMCs need written procedures and a system in place for evaluating their clients to determine suitability for referral, as well as for making the actual referral.

Suggested Reading

American College of Sports Medicine (2006). *ACSM's Guidelines for Exercise Testing and Prescription* (7th ed.). Baltimore: Lippincott Williams & Wilkins.

American College of Sports Medicine (2006). *ACSM's Exercise Management for Persons with Chronic Diseases and Disabilities* (2nd ed.). Champaign, Ill.: Human Kinetics.

American Council on Exercise (2003). *ACE Personal Trainer Manual* (3rd ed.). San Diego: American Council on Exercise.

American Council on Exercise (1999). *Clinical Exercise Specialist Manual.* San Diego: American Council on Exercise.

Andersen, R.E. (Ed.). (2003). *Obesity: Etiology, Assessment, Treatment, and Prevention.* Champaign, Ill.: Human Kinetics.

Brooks, D.S. (1998). *Program Design For Personal Training: Bridging Theory Into Application.* Champaign, Ill.: Human Kinetics.

Part V

Program Design and Implementation

Chapter 12
Weight-management Programming

Chapter 13
Exercise Programming

Chapter 14
Nutritional Programming

Chapter 15
Lifestyle Modification and Behavior Change

Chapter 16
Adherence to Physical Activity and Weight-loss Behaviors

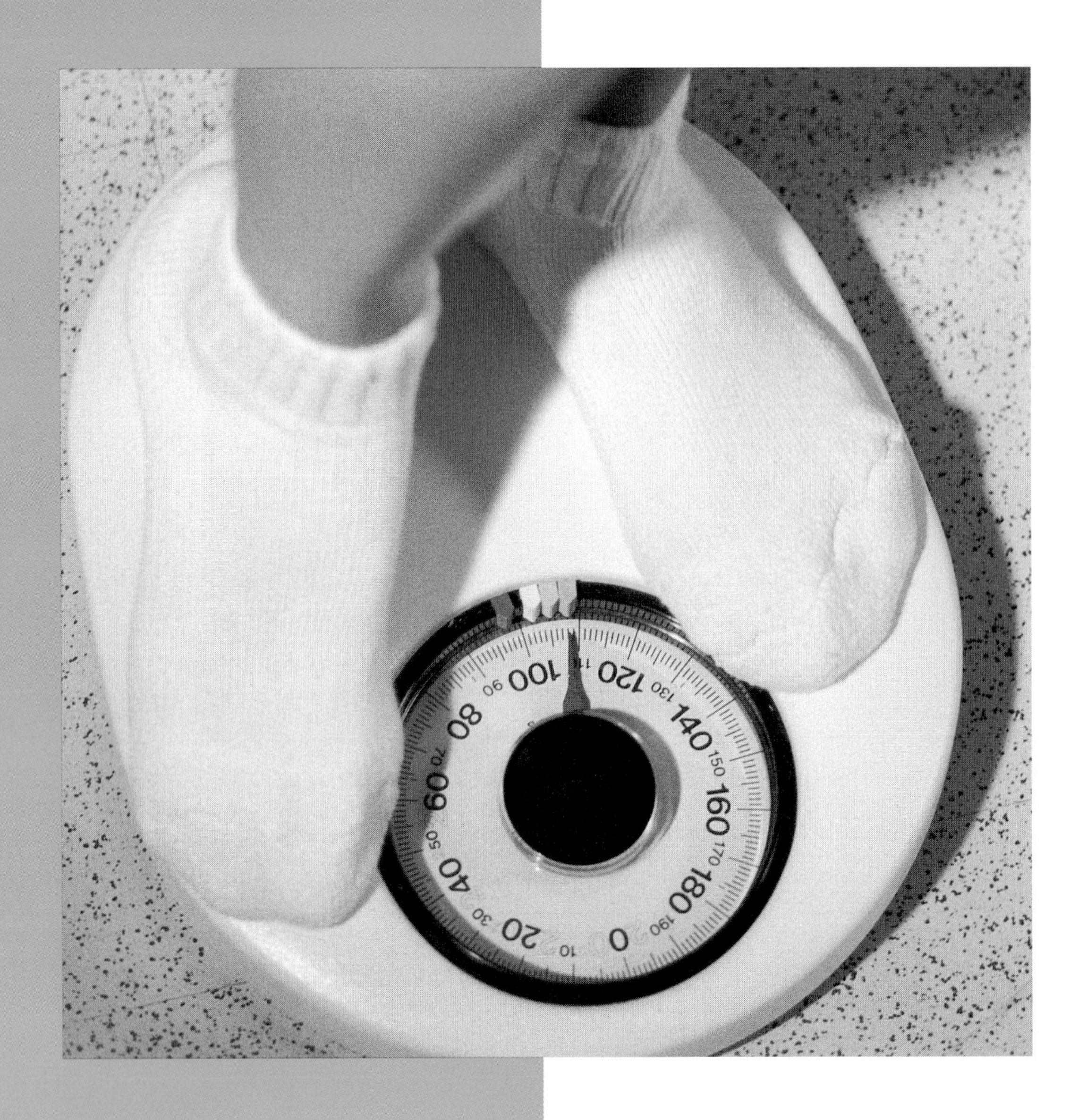

Fabio Comana

Fabio Comana, M.A., M.S.,is an exercise physiologist, research scientist, and spokesperson for the American Council on Exercise. He also currently teaches courses in exercise science and nutrition at the University of California, San Diego and San Diego State University. Comana regularly presents and writes on many topics related to exercise, fitness, and nutrition, and has authored or co-authored more than three dozen articles and chapters in various publications. He has master's degrees in exercise physiology and nutrition, and currently holds certifications from ACE, the American College of Sports Medicine (ACSM), the National Strength and Conditioning Association (NSCA), and the International Society of Sports Nutrition (ISSN).

Chapter 12

Weight-management Programming

In 2004, 71 million American dieters spent $46.3 billion in the weight-loss market, and forecasts estimate that amount to reach $61 billion by 2008 (Marketdata Enterprises, Inc., 2005). According to the Centers for Disease Control and Prevention (CDC), there has been a rising trend of Americans considered **overweight** and obese: from 65.7% and 30.6% in 2001–2002 to 66.3% and 32.2% in 2003–2004, respectively (Table 12-1).

An effective weight-management program involves a multidisciplinary team approach that includes a physician, registered dietitian, exercise physiologist, and behavioral therapist. Through this team approach, the three critical areas—behavior and lifestyle modification, nutrition, and physical activity—can be coordinated. While this approach is ideal, the cost of employing a team of healthcare experts, combined with the lack of third-party reimbursement, creates potential barriers. Hence, overweight or obese clients may instead opt to seek the services of competent allied health professionals who are experienced in all three disciplines and have an established referral network in place.

The success of a Lifestyle & Weight Management Consultant (LWMC) necessitates proven competencies in these areas and the ability to address the individualized needs of clients. The science behind each area is discussed earlier in this book, while the subsequent chapters focus on programming guidelines and strategies.

IN THIS CHAPTER:

Introduction to Effective Weight Management

Components of an Effective Weight-management Program

LWMCs can expect to encounter obstacles, either identified or reported by their clients, during the early stage of their relationship. During the interview and information-gathering stage, LWMCs may identify internal and external barriers. Internal barriers could be anxieties, ambivalence, or defensive avoidance, such as rationalizing a decision to delay starting a program. External barriers could be the inconvenience of the program, lack of time, or lack of support (Griffin, 2006).

While LWMCs have the best intentions for their clients, they must act ethically and responsibly to determine what is appropriate, given the client's current stage of behavioral change. LWMCs must never assume that a meeting with a client means that he or she has entered the preparation or action stage of behavioral change, and is therefore ready to move forward. LWMCs must be skilled in identifying a client's current stage of change and have the ability to implement or recommend the appropriate strategies. This is a critical first step toward facilitating a more permanent lifestyle change. Time and money invested in a nutritional or activity/exercise program may be wasted if the client's underlying psyche is not addressed first. The subsequent chapters address individual programming components of lifestyle and behavioral modification, exercise, and nutrition.

In general, the design of effective weight-management programs for clients requires that LWMCs gain a working knowledge of the following skill sets.

Lifestyle and behavior modification:

- Readiness to change behavior and identification of current stage of change
- Processes of change (cognitive and/or behavioral) and the shifting of a client's decisional balance toward change (Prochaska & Marcus, 1994)
- Self-esteem, **self-efficacy,** and self-efficacy-building strategies
- Acknowledgement of, and reframing of, current attitudes, perceptions, apprehensions, and belief systems
- Value of cognitive techniques, such as goal-setting
- Rapport building and maintenance
- Effective verbal and nonverbal communication, and good listening skills
- Different personality styles (e.g., technical, sociable, or assertive) and appropriate communication styles (Griffin, 2006)
- Support systems
- Internal and external barriers and obstacle management
- Appropriate cognitive, motor-skill, and affective learning techniques
- Motivational strategies, including reinforcements, antecedents, rewards (extrinsic to intrinsic), personal contracts, stimulus control, and self-talk

Exercise programming:

- Exercise science
- Health-risk assessments and risk stratification
- Referrals to appropriate professionals, confidentiality, and **SOAP note** format
- Exercise and testing contraindications
- Physiological assessments and termination criteria
- Limitations of assessments and the interpretation of criterion-referenced or norm-referenced data
- Program design and implementation
- Environmental effects
- Reevaluation and modification/progression

Nutritional programming:

- Nutrition (**macronutrient** and **micronutrient** function) and digestion
- Nutritional assessments
- Caloric balance and weight-management-program design

- Dietary guidelines, labels, and portions sizes
- Weight-loss diets and supplements
- Dietary needs for special populations, women, and vegetarians

Prevalence of Obesity

Population Statistics

The National Health and Nutrition Examination Survey (NHANES), which is conducted every 10 years by the National Center for Health Statistics (NCHS) and the CDC, assesses the health and nutritional status of adults and children in the United States. It is arguably the largest and longest-running longitudinal health survey of the U.S. population and provides valuable information on important health indicators. The prevalence of overweight and **obesity** has been tracked since 1971, and a rising trend is evident within the U.S. population. In 2002, an estimated 115 million adults were overweight or obese; among women 20 years and older, more than 64 million were overweight, and more than 34 million were obese.

According to the CDC, the average male weighed 166.3 pounds (75.5 kg) in 1960–1962, while the average female weighed 140.2 pounds (63.7 kg). By contrast, in 1999–2002, the average male weighed 191.0 pounds (86.7 kg), while the average female weighed 164.3 pounds (74.6 kg) (Table 12-1). The increased incidence of obesity is attributed to decreasing levels of activity and increasing access to, and consumption of, food. Physical-activity statistics from the Department of Health and Human Services and the Centers for Disease Control and Prevention in 2003 indicated that only 45.9% of U.S. adults were achieving the recommended physical-activity levels consistent with the U.S. Surgeon General's report; 38.4% were insufficiently active (defined as more than 10 minutes total per week of moderate- or vigorous-intensity lifestyle activities, but less than the recommended level of activity); 15.6% of adults were inactive (defined as less than 10 minutes total per week of moderate- or vigorous-intensity lifestyle activities). Likewise, the average consumption of calories in adults has increased by 12%, or 300 kcal, between 1985 and 2000.

Being overweight or obese significantly increases the risk of developing serious disease and health conditions, including the following:

- Hypertension
- Dyslipidemia
- Type 2 diabetes
- Coronary heart disease
- Stroke
- Gallbladder disease
- Osteoarthritis
- Sleep apnea and respiratory problems
- Some cancers (endometrial, breast, and colon)

Table 12-1
Age-adjusted Prevalence of Overweight and Obesity Among U.S Adults, Ages 20–74

	NHANES II (1976–1980) (n = 11,207)	NHANES III (1988–1994) (n = 6,679)	NHANES (1999–2000) (n = 4,117)	NHANES (2001–2002) (n = 4,413)	NHANES (2003–2004) (n = 4,431)
Overweight or Obese (BMI ≥25.0)	47.0%	56.0%	64.5%	65.7%	66.3%
Obese (BMI ≥30.0)	15.0%	22.9%	30.5%	30.6%	32.2%

* Age-adjusted by the direct method to the year 2000 U.S. Bureau of the Census estimates using the age groups 20–39, 40–59, and 60 years and over.

Source: National Center for Health Statistics, Centers for Disease Control and Prevention

The Centers for Disease Control and Prevention had previously reported that obesity is responsible for more than 356,000 deaths a year, a number that has increased by 33% over the past decade and may soon overtake tobacco as the leading preventable cause of death among Americans. More recently, a study based on a nationally representative sample of U.S. adults estimated that approximately 112,000 deaths are associated with obesity each year in the United States (Mokdad et al., 2004; 2005). There are two main reasons for the difference in the estimated number of obesity deaths—newer data and different methods of analyzing the data. Because obesity has many different effects on numerous diseases, doctors have difficulty reliably identifying obesity-related deaths based on death certificates. Scientists are now using more complex modeling techniques to estimate deaths related to obesity. Regardless, obesity shortens the average lifespan of an adult by four to nine months, and in a child, the lifespan may be cut by two to five years, given the current childhood obesity rates.

Obesity-attributable medical expenditures have been estimated to be $117 billion in the U.S. (Finkelstein, Fiebelkorn, & Wang, 2003). In 2002, the cost difference between treating a normal-weight person and an obese individual was $1,244, up from $272 in 1987. In general, the annual medical costs for overweight and obese individuals (under the age of 65 years) is 14.5% and 36–37.4% higher compared to normal-weight individuals, respectively (Segel, 2006). Weight loss can reduce lifetime medical costs by $2,200 to $5,300 per person.

In the corporate world, the impact can be significant. The hospital inpatient utilization rate for workers with unhealthy weights was 143% higher than for normal-weight workers. In March of 2005, the annual premium for an employee averaged $6,281.

Since 2000, employment-based health insurance premiums have risen 73% (The Henry J. Kaiser Family Foundation, 2005). Meanwhile, the average employee contribution to health insurance grew more than 143%, with employees paying $1,094 more in annual premiums for family coverage (Smith et al., 2006).

Health Objectives

Given the rising obesity and inactivity levels and correlating higher healthcare costs, being proactive in weight-management is critical. These issues are also being addressed at a federal level, which could affect corporations and consumers working with LWMCs.

The mission of the Center for Nutrition Policy and Promotion, an entity within the U.S. Department of Agriculture (USDA), is to improve the nutrition and well-being of Americans. In support of these objectives, the center offers several core resources, including the following:

- Dietary Guidelines for Americans
- My Pyramid Food Guidance System
- Healthy Eating Index
- U.S. Food Plans
- Nutrient Content of the U.S. Food Supply
- Expenditures on Children by Families

The USDA Dietary Guidelines are published every five years by the USDA. The guidelines provide educational material on good dietary habits to promote healthy living and reduce the risk for developing major chronic diseases for all Americans (from age two to aging adults).

In 1979, the U.S. Surgeon General established national health objectives that served as the basis for the development of state and community health plans (U.S. Department of Health and Human Services, 2000). The objectives were developed through a broad consultation process, derived from current scientific knowledge, and designed to measure programs over time. *Healthy People,* the statement of these national health objectives, is designed to identify the most significant preventable threats to health, and to establish a national consensus of how to reduce them. The current version, *Healthy People 2010,* contains 467 objectives in 28 focus areas (U.S. Department of Health and Human Services, 2000). Under focus area number 19, entitled

"Overweight and Obesity," specific objectives include the following:

- *Objective 19-1:* Increase the proportion of healthy-weight adults to at least 60%
- *Objective 19-2:* Reduce the proportion of obese adults to less than 15%

The National Institutes of Health (NIH) in 2005 developed a strategic plan for obesity research, earmarking a budget of $440.3 million. The NIH recognizes the multifaceted variables that affect obesity. Its plan to fight obesity is organized into four major themes related to obesity prevention and treatment:

- Lifestyle modification
- Pharmacologic, surgical, or other medical approaches
- The link between obesity and associated health conditions
- Crosscutting research topics, including health disparities and technology

The Food and Drug Administration's (FDA) Obesity Working Group released its final report in 2004 (U.S. FDA, 2004). The group's long- and short-term proposals are based on the scientific knowledge that weight control is primarily a function of caloric balance. Consequently, the FDA focuses on calorie counting in its obesity campaign. The FDA's ongoing actions include the following:

- *Labeling:* Enhancing food labels to display the calorie count more prominently, and implementing more meaningful serving sizes
- *Enforcement agencies:* Collaborating with the Federal Trade Commission (FTC) to increase enforcement against weight-loss products that have false or misleading claims, and products that declare inaccurate serving sizes
- *Educational partnerships:* Working cooperatively with other government agencies, nonprofits, industry, and academia to educate Americans on the dangers of obesity and the importance of leading healthier lives through better nutrition
- *Restaurants:* Encouraging the restaurant industry to launch a nationwide, voluntary, and point-of-sale nutrition-information campaign for consumers
- *Therapeutics:* Revising FDA guidance for developing obesity drugs and addressing challenges and gaps in knowledge about existing drug therapies for treating obesity
- *Research:* Supporting others and collaborating (with others, such as the NIH) on obesity-related research

Safe and Effective Weight Loss

Lifestyle changes, including modifications of food intake and physical activity to establish a daily negative caloric balance, remain the hallmarks of effective programming. It can be difficult to accurately estimate weight-loss rates for clients given the numerous factors influencing weight loss. Additionally, using weight-loss rate is not recommended for long-term weight management, because of the potential lean body mass gain that accompanies overload with resistance training. Instead, it is best to focus the client's attention on the perceived benefits of accomplishing various program-related goals, such as changes in body shape and image, and self-efficacy.

Modest and realistic expectations include achieving an initial 5 to 10% reduction in body weight, as this range is consistent with improved overall health benefits, increased self-efficacy, and improved adherence [American College of Sports Medicine (ACSM), 2006]. Always follow a prudent plan with a weight-loss goal that is consistent with the most current dietary guidelines, unless clients are medically supervised by a licensed physician or registered dietitian. The 2005 USDA Dietary Guidelines and the 2006 ACSM guidelines recommend a weekly weight loss of 0.5 to 1.0 kg (1.1 to 2.2 pounds) per week, which necessitates a negative caloric balance of 3,850 to 7,700 kcal weekly, or 550 to 1,100 kcal daily. A more conservative approach of 0.5 to 1.0 pounds (0.23 to 0.45 kg) per week, necessitating a negative caloric balance of 1,750 to 3,500 kcal weekly, or 250 to 500 kcal daily, may be more suitable for some clients. Ultimately, the weight-loss goal must be safe, satisfy the needs and desires of the client, and include the following considerations:

- Age
- Target weight (or amount of weight to be lost)
- Current physical-activity level
- Medical concerns
- History of dieting
- Emotional and psychological state

Individuals do not need to lose weight if their weight is within the healthy range represented in Table 12-2, if they have gained less than 10 pounds since reaching their adult height, or are otherwise healthy (USDA, 2005). Weight losses of only 5 to 10% may greatly diminish any health concerns associated with being overweight, but even smaller losses can make a difference. Weights above the ranges shown in Table 12-2 are considered less healthy for most people. The greater the margin of difference between actual body weight and the healthy weight range for height, the higher the risk of weight-related health disorders.

A more useful estimate of quantifying a healthy weight in relation to height can be obtained by calculating a height-normalized weight index. The **body mass index (BMI)** is the most commonly used indicator (Table 12–3). While the BMI has limited applications for athletes, seniors, and children, research points to a strong relationship between BMI and mortality rates. In a research study following 1 million adults for 14 years, the lowest BMI-mortality rates were BMI scores between 23.5 and 24.9 for men and 23.0 and 23.4 for women.

Table 12-2
Healthy Weight Ranges for Men and Women

Height	Weight (pounds)	Weight (kg)
4'10" (1.47 m)	91–119	41.4–54.1
4'11" (1.50 m)	94–124	42.7–56.4
5'0 " (1.52 m)	97–128	44.1–58.2
5'1" (1.55 m)	101–132	45.9–60.0
5'2" (1.57 m)	104–137	47.2–62.2
5'3" (1.60 m)	107–141	48.6–64.1
5'4" (1.62 m)	111–146	50.5–66.4
5'5" (1.65 m)	114–150	51.8–68.2
5'6" (1.67 m)	118–155	53.6–70.5
5'7" (1.70m)	121–160	55.0–72.7
5'8" (1.73 m)	125–164	56.8–74.5
5'9" (1.75 m)	129–169	58.6–76.8
5'10" (1.77 m)	132–174	60.0–79.1
5'11" (1.80 m)	136–179	61.8–81.4
6'0" (1.83 m)	140–184	63.6–83.6
6'1" (1.85 m)	144–189	65.5–85.9
6'2" (1.87 m)	148–195	67.3–88.6
6'3" (1.90 m)	152–200	69.1–90.1
6'4" (1.93 m)	156–205	70.9–93.2
6'5" (1.95 m)	160–211	72.7–95.9
6'6" (1.98 m)	164–216	74.5–98.2

Source: United States Department of Agriculture (2005). *USDA Dietary Guidelines for Americans.* www.health.gov/dietaryguidelines.

Understanding Behavioral Change

People make choices and decisions based on how they feel and think (Figure 12-1). Everyone's belief system is based on past and present experiences. These belief systems drive people's thought processes and feelings, and the decisions and choices they make. To influence desired behaviors, LWMCs must work with clients to help them think about ways to achieve desirable behaviors and talk to them about their feelings about those desired behaviors. LWMCs may successfully alter unfounded belief systems to influence decisions and choices. Additionally, these experiences should be engaging, positive, and memorable, and build self-efficacy to empower clients to want to stop unhealthy behaviors, while also enhancing their confidence in their abilities to initiate change.

Using a weight-management example to illustrate this point, imagine a client with an estimated caloric intake of 2,000 kcal, who would like to lose 1 pound (0.45 kg) per week. Long-term weight-loss success typically involves modest caloric reductions of 10 to

Table 12-3
Body Mass Index

	19	20	21	22	23	24	25	26	27	28	29	30	35	40
Height (inches)	**Weight (pounds)**													
58	91	95	100	105	110	115	119	124	129	134	138	143	167	191
59	94	99	104	109	114	119	124	128	133	138	143	148	173	198
60	97	102	107	112	118	123	128	133	138	143	148	153	179	204
61	100	106	111	116	121	127	132	137	143	148	153	158	185	211
62	104	109	115	120	125	131	136	142	147	153	158	164	191	218
63	107	113	118	124	130	135	141	146	152	158	163	169	197	225
64	110	116	122	128	134	140	145	151	157	163	169	174	203	233
65	114	120	126	132	138	144	150	156	162	168	174	180	210	240
66	117	124	130	136	142	148	155	161	167	173	179	185	216	247
67	121	127	134	140	147	153	159	166	172	178	185	191	223	255
68	125	131	138	144	151	158	164	171	177	184	190	197	230	263
69	128	135	142	149	155	162	169	176	182	189	196	203	237	270
70	132	139	146	153	160	167	174	181	188	195	202	209	243	278
71	136	143	150	157	165	172	179	186	193	200	207	215	250	286
72	140	147	155	162	169	177	184	191	199	206	213	221	258	294
73	144	151	159	166	174	182	189	197	204	212	219	227	265	303
74	148	155	163	171	179	187	194	202	210	218	225	233	272	311
75	152	160	168	176	184	192	200	208	216	224	232	240	279	319
76	156	164	172	180	189	197	205	213	221	230	238	246	287	328

Note: Find the client's height in the far left column and move across the row to the weight that is closest to the client's weight. His or her body mass index will be at the top of that column.

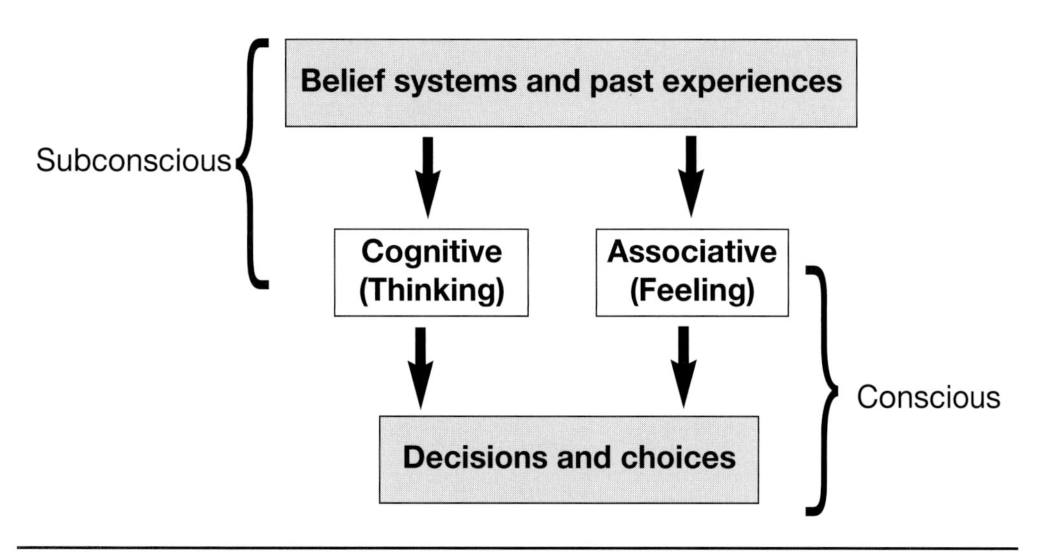

Figure 12-1
Influences on decisions and choices

15% initially, although some studies do demonstrate long-term success with initial caloric reductions of 20 to 25%. Using a modest reduction of 300 kcal of intake leaves a balance of 200 kcal that must be expended via physical activity and exercise. Most overweight clients tend to be deconditioned and are better suited to walking or performing walk-jog intervals for exercise that burns between 5 and 9 kcal per minute (for a 165-pound or 75-kg individual). To expend 200 kcal, the individual needs to participate in 23 minutes of jogging or 40 minutes of walking. Considering that only 46% of the U.S adult population meets minimum recommendations of the U.S Surgeon General, 38% participate in 10 to 30 minutes of physical activity, and 16% participate in less than 10 minutes of physical activity daily, the likelihood of success in expending 200 kcal is low. More importantly, the individual may potentially have a negative and unenjoyable experience that might prove to be disengaging. Remember that the initial few weeks of a program have a high risk of dropout. A viable option may be to increase daily physical activity levels to expend 75 to 100 kcal, leaving the balance to structured exercise, but keep in mind that too many lifestyle changes may negatively impact long-term adherence. Consider the following strategy to enhance the overall experience, engage the individual, and promote self-efficacy:

- Focus the initial two to four weeks on building self-efficacy and program compliance and creating an enjoyable experience.
- De-emphasize numbers temporarily until attitudes toward regular exercise and activity appear positive and the desired behaviors occur frequently with minimal resistance.

Transtheoretical Model of Change (Stages of Behavioral Change)

This model was developed as a framework to describe the different stages of acquiring and maintaining healthy behavior. It provides a premise to understand lifestyle modification based upon readiness for change, making the assumption that people progress through stages of behavioral change at varying rates (Prochaska & Marcus, 1994). To adopt or engage in new behaviors, individuals must first move in an orderly progression through a number of stages. The model also takes into account that lapses are inevitable and part of the process of working toward lifelong change. Hence, it is possible for an individual to move in either direction along this continuum. The four components of this model, which are constructs hypothesized to influence behavior, are as follows:

- Stages of change
- Processes of change
- Decisional balance
- Self-efficacy

Stages of Change

There are five stages of change described in the transtheoretical model (Table 12-4 and Figure 12-2):

Precontemplation:

- The individual has no plans or thoughts to improve or change behavior within the next six months.
- The individual is neither engaged in change, nor contemplating it.
- The individual may have lapsed or is in denial at this level. He or she is resigned to the unhealthy behavior because of previous failed efforts and no longer believes that he or she can control change.

Contemplation:

- The individual is somewhat ambivalent toward changing behavior and weighs the costs and benefits of making the lifestyle modification.
- The individual is not engaged, but is contemplating improving or changing behavior within the next six months ("thinking about it").
- Low self-efficacy levels increase the resistance to changing behavior.

Preparation:

- The individual has taken some steps toward healthier behavior and intends to commit within the next 30 days, or has already begun to make some changes, but demonstrates inconsistent behavior (irregular activity patterns). There is, however, greater determination to achieve change.
- The individual is mentally and physically preparing and may ask questions, seek information, or make purchases (of equipment, etc.) as an incentive to commit.

Table 12-4
The Stages of Behavioral Change

Stage	Traits	Goals	Strategies
Precontemplation	Unaware or under-aware of the problem, or believe that it cannot be solved (e.g., latent pain)	Increase awareness of the risks of inactivity, and of the benefits of activity Focus on addressing something relevant to them Have them start thinking about change	Validate lack of readiness to change and clarify that this decision is theirs Encourage reevaluation of current behavior and self-exploration, while not taking action Explain and personalize the inherent risks Utilize general sources, including media, Internet, and brochures to increase awareness
Contemplation	Aware of the problem and weighing the benefits versus risks of change Have little understanding of how to go about changing	Inform them of available options Provide cues to action and some basic structured direction	Validate lack of readiness to change and clarify that this decision is theirs Encourage evaluation of the pros and cons of making change Identify and promote new, positive outcome expectations and boost self-confidence Offer invitations to become more active (e.g., free trials)
Preparation	Seeking opportunities to participate in activity (combine intent and behavior with activity)	Structured, regular programming with frequent positive feedback and reinforcements on their progress	Verify that the individual has the underlying skills for behavior change and encourage small steps toward building self-efficacy Identify and assist with problem-solving obstacles Help the client identify social support and establish goals
Action	Desire for opportunities to maintain activities Changing beliefs and attitudes High risk for lapses or returns to undesirable behavior	Establish exercise as a habit through motivation and adherence to the desired behavior	Behavior-modification strategies Focus on restructuring cues and social support toward building long-term change Increase awareness to inevitable lapses and bolster self-efficacy in coping with lapses Reiterate long-term benefits of adherence Require continual feedback on progress
Maintenance	Empowered, but desire a means to maintain adherence Good capability to deal with lapses	Maintain support systems Maintain interest and avoid boredom or burnout	Reevaluate strategies currently in effect Plan for contingencies with support systems, although this may no longer be needed Reinforce the need for a transition from external to internal rewards Plan for potential lapses Encourage program variety
Lapse	Encounter lapses that they are unable to overcome	Return to action	Identify reasons for lapse Identify current stage of change to progress once again toward action Maintain existing systems and relationships and offer appropriate support

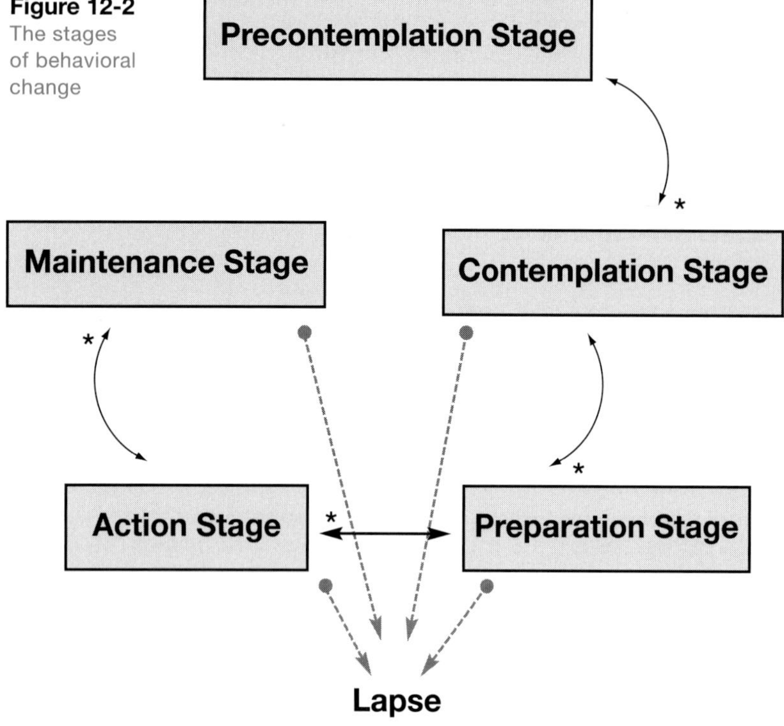

Figure 12-2
The stages of behavioral change

Action:

- The individual has shown improved behavior, and has been participating in regular activity for less than six months.
- The individual demonstrates the desire to change his or her beliefs and attitudes, and should be supported as much as possible.
- The individual is still considered to be at a high risk for **relapse.**

Maintenance:

- Practices have been sustained for more than six months. The person demonstrates adherence and higher levels of self-efficacy.
- The individual has successfully developed strategies to cope with lapses.
- Discouragement with occasional slips or lapses may hamper maintenance within this phase and result in the individual reversing into unhealthy behaviors. A typical pattern involves cycling through the stages of change several times before the change becomes truly established as a lifelong endeavor.

Individuals progress through these stages at different rates, sometimes remaining in one stage or relapsing to earlier stages for extended periods of time. Never assume that someone is in the action stage because he or she joined a club or fitness center or purchased personal-training sessions. LWMCs must identify the stage of change before starting to plan programs and then implement appropriate strategies to move a client toward the action phase. For example, a new member might be offered an orientation with a basic personal-fitness plan and receive instructions on using equipment. While this may be appropriate for an individual in the action stage, LWMCs may need to adopt a different strategy for an individual in the **contemplation stage.** Such an individual may require education on the benefits of lifestyle change, diet, and physical activity.

After successfully developing a **rapport** so that a client feels comfortable opening up, LWMCs should assess the client's readiness to change a negative behavior. During the initial interviews, LWMCs should ask the following questions to assess a client's readiness for change:

- Are you making the decision to change a behavior for yourself?
- Will your friends, family, or loved ones support you in this endeavor?
- Besides possible health improvements, what other reasons do you have for wanting to change this behavior?
- Do you believe that you are susceptible to injury or illness, or that you may compromise your health by continuing your current behavior?
- Are you willing to make the commitment to this change, even through very tough and challenging times?
- Are you willing to make the desired change a top priority?
- Have you ever tried to change this or a similar behavior before?

- Are you committed to being patient with yourself and persistent when and if you encounter obstacles?

The more "yes" answers the client provides, the more ready he or she is to make the commitment to change. A client who answers "no" to most questions, by contrast, is less likely to make the commitment and adhere to a program. LWMCs should identify the current stage and develop appropriate strategies to move the client toward the action stage.

Processes of Change

Individuals use certain strategies as they move between stages. These strategies are divided into cognitive (or experiential) and behavioral categories:

- Cognitive processes (CP) are defined as those that gather relevant information on the basis of one's own experiences.
- Behavioral processes (BP) are defined as those that gather relevant information via events from the environmental and experienced behaviors.

Some examples of the processes of change include the following:

- Consciousness raising is the act of increasing knowledge and awareness of healthy behaviors.
- Helping relationships feature caring and understanding, and include gaining the trust and acceptance of others as the individual assumes healthy behaviors.
- Counter-conditioning is the act of changing one's response to a particular stimuli with the objective of substituting healthy behaviors for unhealthy ones.
- Stimulus control is the act of changing one's environment by removing cues that trigger unhealthy behaviors and adding prompts to entice healthier alternatives.
- Social liberation is the act of increasing social opportunities to make healthy choices.
- Self-evaluation is the act of assessing or critically reviewing one's image and performance after engaging in unhealthy and healthy behaviors.
- Environmental evaluation is the act of assessing what effect unhealthy behavior may have on one's own environment.
- Self-liberation is the belief that a person has to change his or her life from within and is driven by self-efficacy.
- Dramatic relief is the act of experiencing negative emotions associated with engaging in unhealthy behavior.

Within each stage, individuals can and will utilize various processes of change to move toward the next stage. Transitions between stages can be facilitated with stage-specific interventions. For example, during the **precontemplation stage,** consciousness-raising is an effective process. During the action stage, self-liberation, stimulus control, and helping relationships are effective processes.

Decisional Balance

Decisional balance is the third component of this model. It assumes that decision-making regarding healthier behavior involves weighing the risks and benefits of changing behavior (i.e., measuring the benefits to be attained against the potential losses involved with making the change) (Table 12-5). Differences exist among the individual stages with regard to benefit–risk analysis and subsequently, individuals' likelihood to change. During the precontemplation and contemplation stages, individuals typically perceive more risks than benefits regarding change, and therefore remain resistant or ambivalent. During the **preparation stage,** the benefits and risks appear equal, which explains why individuals are often stuck in this stage. During the action and **maintenance stages,** the benefits outweigh the risks, and therefore, the individual continues to move toward desired behaviors. LWMCs should attempt to shift the decisional balance and influence the client's perceptions of the potential benefits vs. risks (e.g., diffuse anxieties and irrational beliefs) without being confrontational.

Self-efficacy

Self-efficacy is defined as the belief in one's capability to complete a task. Like

Table 12-5
Decision Balance Worksheet

Instructions:
- Work with the client to document the gains and potential losses that he or she might experience when making a lifestyle change.
- Identify and list the recommended implementation strategies needed to achieve the gains and list coping strategies that can be used to deal with the potential losses or obstacles associated with the change.

Decision Balance Worksheet	
Perceived gains associated with adopting desired behaviors	**Perceived losses associated with adopting desired behaviors**
1.	1.
2.	2.
3.	3.
4.	4.
Strategies to maximize potential for achieving gains	**Strategies to minimize potential of perceived losses**
1.	1.
2.	2.
3.	3.
4.	4.

self-confidence, this terms deals with a belief in one's self. While self-confidence is more global, self-efficacy is more task-specific, and is influenced by the following:

- Past performance and experiences (successes and failures, and the experience itself)
- Vicarious experiences (successes and failures of others who are similar to the individual and are seen as role models)
- Verbal persuasion (support offered by others—credible sources—that build trust and rapport)
- Physiological responses (responses of heart rate, sweat rate, ratings of perceived exertion, etc., and the perception of these responses as positive or negative)
- Emotional responses (the feelings and impressions associated with the task, both positive and negative)
- Imagery experiences (the experience one envisions, both positive or negative)

The more capable a person feels regarding his or her ability to engage in a task and successfully accomplish it, the more likely he or she is to adhere. Improvements in self-efficacy occur naturally as a person progresses through the stages. The level of self-efficacy is lowest in the earlier stages of behavioral change. Establishing challenging, but manageable, tasks is an effective strategy in building self-efficacy.

Self-efficacy will influence task choice or complexity. Individuals with lower levels of self-efficacy tend to select easier tasks to ensure success or difficult tasks to ensure failure. Individuals with higher levels of self-efficacy typically select appropriate task complexities. Self-efficacy also influences effort. People with lower levels will put forth minimal effort, as they have a higher perception of failure. Self-efficacy will also influence persistence. Those with higher levels of self-efficacy tend to persevere in spite of obstacles or minor setbacks. Finally, self-efficacy can be a determinant as well as an outcome of activity. Success in accomplishing a task or successfully performing an activity raises self-efficacy levels. Therefore, working to improve a client's self-efficacy level will improve the probability of achieving a desired behavior.

Tracking Progress and Keeping Records

Effective goal-setting will improve adherence and performance. Goals clarify expectations and provide feedback, and are a means to evaluate progress. If appropriately set, they establish appropriate challenges for individuals to strive for, which in turn improves self-efficacy and confidence. Additionally, effective goals can focus the client's attention more intently and motivate the client to take action. Establishing goals is the basis and justification for maintaining participation and activity logs. Logs are discussed in the next section of this chapter, while goal-setting strategies are discussed in Chapter 13.

Participation and Activity Logs

LWMCs can empower clients to have more self-control and self-management, and create a need within clients to assume more responsibility for making a lifestyle change. One simple technique to achieve these objectives involves maintaining activity or participation logs, a responsibility that the LWMC should share with the client. Keeping activity records and logs of the measurable programming parameters provides the following:

- A means to evaluate program adherence and efficacy
- Information for program progression, modification, and continued education
- Effective feedback for clients

Record-keeping is an invaluable component of a client's weight-management program, especially during the first six months, when the individual is considered at high risk for noncompliance and prone to dropout. It is best to record some data after workout sessions or meals (e.g., heart rates, sets and repetitions, meal composition), while other information needs to be tracked over a longer period of time (e.g., changes in behavior, attitudes). Compliance with maintaining records is contingent upon convenience; the more accessible and simplistic the modality, the more likely the client is to comply. Given the widespread advances in technology and portability in communications, LWMCs should determine the medium that suits each client's lifestyle. Simple log forms and diaries can be created electronically or in the traditional paper-and-pencil format. Textbooks and health clubs typically offer numerous examples of such templates. They may also be created by LWMCs to suit the specific needs of their clients. Activity logs can be created to use a variety of formats for recording events, ranging from simply recording the completion of an event to earning points or mileage for activities or events that accumulate toward an end goal or reward. Ultimately, LWMCs and their clients should agree on a format that facilitates the achievement of specific goals and lifestyle changes. Figure 12-3 is an example of an activity log that utilizes a points system.

Emotional Association With Programming

Any positive emotional change associated with the client's program can be leveraged for adherence-support purposes. Strategic use of the positive emotional feelings associated with activity will promote a client's continued desire to participate. Normally, a client will experience a positive mood change after just a few weeks or months of regular activity. This results from changes in circulating endorphins, serotonin and norepinephrine levels, or the increased self-efficacy that comes from accomplishing tasks or achieving some initial short-term goals. Arm clients with the knowledge that continued exercise and activity will likely benefit their stress levels, energy levels, moods, and feelings of self-worth and self-efficacy, in addition to bringing about positive physical changes.

Leverage emotional change by recommending exercise types, amounts, and

Figure 12-3
Example of an activity log that utilizes a points system

GOAL:____

Log Instructions: Complete this electronic log daily and award yourself points as follows:

- Every 10 minutes of continuous moderate-intensity activity = 2 points
- Every 10 minutes of incremental or less-than-moderate-intensity activity = 1 point
- Every flight of stairs substituted for an elevator or escalator = 1 point
- Submitting your weekly totals to your trainer = 1 point

	Week 1	Week 2	Week 3	Week 4	Week 5	Week 6
Sunday	Points: ___	Points: ___	Points: ___	Points: ___	Points: ___	Points: ___
Monday	Points: ___	Points: ___	Points: ___	Points: ___	Points: ___	Points: ___
Tuesday	Points: ___	Points: ___	Points: ___	Points: ___	Points: ___	Points: ___
Wednesday	Points: ___	Points: ___	Points: ___	Points: ___	Points: ___	Points: ___
Thursday	Points: ___	Points: ___	Points: ___	Points: ___	Points: ___	Points: ___
Friday	Points: ___	Points: ___	Points: ___	Points: ___	Points: ___	Points: ___
Saturday	Points: ___	Points: ___	Points: ___	Points: ___	Points: ___	Points: ___
Total Points	Points: ___	Points: ___	Points: ___	Points: ___	Points: ___	Points: ___

intensities that promote positive after-session feelings. A slow start with moderate progression ensures positive after-session feelings that promote long-term maintenance. However, it is prudent that LWMCs always investigate a client's aversion to physical stress and discomfort prior to implementing this strategy.

An effective means to evaluate emotional change is through verbal or documented feedback from the client. This allows LWMCs to assess the emotional perceptions of the recently completed activity.

The exercise-induced feeling inventory (EFI) is a survey administered after an exercise or activity session that seeks to identify the individual's after-session impressions (Gauvin & Rejeski, 1993) (Figure 12-4). The use of such an inventory can facilitate the establishment of baseline emotional states

Figure 12-4
Exercise-induced feeling inventory (EFI) survey

Instructions: Please use the following scale to indicate the extent to which each word describes how you feel at this moment in time. Record your responses by checking the appropriate box next to each word.

0 = Do not feel
1 = Feel slightly
2 = Feel moderately
3 = Feel strongly
4 = Feel very strongly

	0	1	2	3	4		0	1	2	3	4
1. Refreshed	☐	☐	☐	☐	☐	**7. Happy**	☐	☐	☐	☐	☐
2. Calm	☐	☐	☐	☐	☐	**8. Tired**	☐	☐	☐	☐	☐
3. Fatigued	☐	☐	☐	☐	☐	**9. Revived**	☐	☐	☐	☐	☐
4. Enthusiastic	☐	☐	☐	☐	☐	**10. Peaceful**	☐	☐	☐	☐	☐
5. Relaxed	☐	☐	☐	☐	☐	**11. Worn out**	☐	☐	☐	☐	☐
6. Energetic	☐	☐	☐	☐	☐	**12. Upbeat**	☐	☐	☐	☐	☐

Source: Reprinted, with permission, from L. Gauvin & W.J. Rejeski, 1993, "The exercise-induced feeling inventory: development and initial validation," *Journal of Sport & Exercise Psychology* 15(4): 409.

and opinions regarding previous exercise experiences when administered prior to activity in the new program. Additionally, it provides a means to track emotional change and offers valuable feedback to evaluate the program design. The information collected over time can be effectively used as a tool to empower clients into self-direction as the LWMC works to wean them toward self-sufficiency and independence.

During the interview or information-gathering stage with a client, consider administering the survey while discussing previous experiences and preferences, which will help to establish an emotional baseline. During the initial stages of working with a new client or any time significant changes are made to a program, LWMCs should administer the survey with some frequency. However, it is important to taper the frequency within a few weeks to minimize the chances of desensitization and maintain the learning effects associated with the survey.

The key objective of collecting aggregated data is to track changes over time by monitoring whether there is an upward trend of positive subscales or a downward trend of negative subscales. This information provides insight into long-term adherence to programming and efficacy of a particular program design. The culled information can also be compiled and presented in a graphic format to illustrate changes to clients. Figure 12-5 shows a graphic representation of aggregated scores on the EFI over a 12-week period.

Strategies for Overcoming Obstacles

Barriers to Participation

Of new and returning exercisers, 50 to 65% will cease their activity within three to six months, although it is estimated that working with personal trainers can increase adherence by 40% over a 24-week period (Annesi, 2000; Pronk et al., 1994). Clients often have a history of unsuccessful weight loss or temporary weight-loss success. These perceived

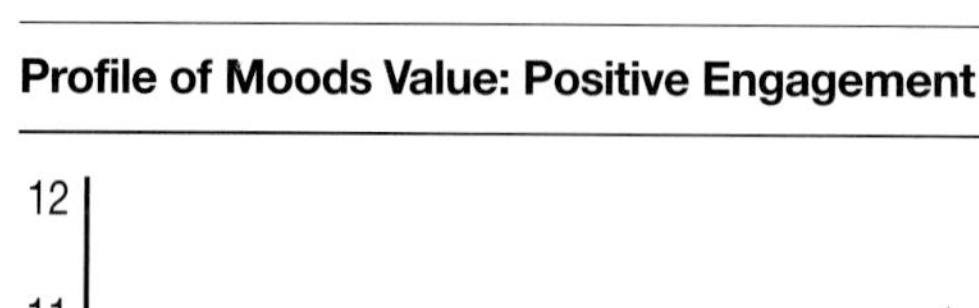

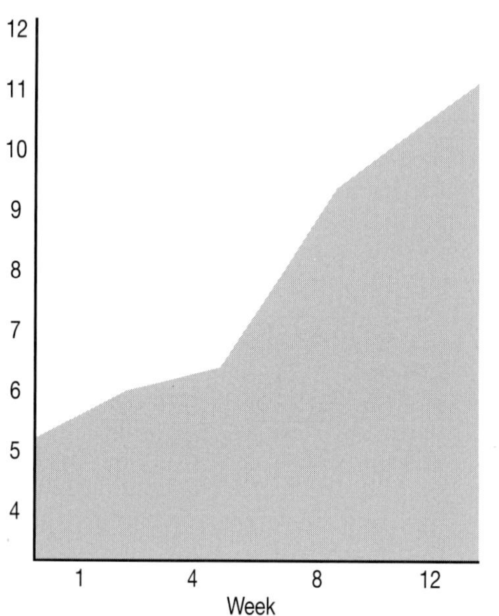

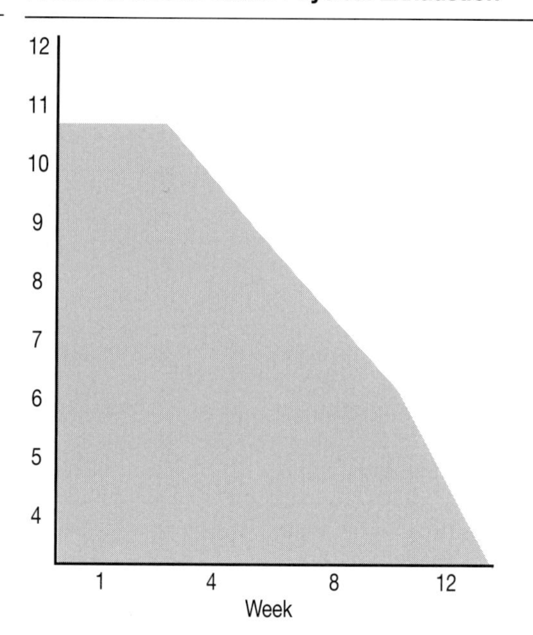

Figure 12-5
Examples of aggregated data for subscales of positive engagement and physical exhaustion over 12 weeks

failures certainly present themselves as barriers to future success. It is the responsibility of LWMCs to diffuse clients' anxieties and discuss existing belief systems. Many clients, based on experience, have unfounded beliefs and misconceptions regarding foods, physical activity, and dietary practices. While LWMCs must never devalue a client's belief systems, the goal is to identify misconceptions without being insensitive.

Obstacles to participation and long-term adherence are inevitable and should be acknowledged. These potential barriers are considered high-risk situations and can challenge the client's confidence in adhering to the desired behavior (Buckworth & Dishman, 2002). They most often occur during the action stage of change. Consequently, LWMCs must increase the clients' awareness of this likelihood and work with them to achieve the following four objectives:

- Recognize that lapses are inevitable
- Restructure the perception of lapses (as slips instead of failures)
- Identify barriers or sources of potential lapses
- Anticipate barriers and potential lapses, and develop effective coping strategies

Appropriate coping strategies lead to increased self-efficacy and a decreased probability of a relapse. Inappropriate coping strategies, or the absence of any coping strategies, will decrease self-efficacy, as well as the positive expectations regarding adherence. Figure 12-6 provides an example of a worksheet that LWMCs can use to help identify high-risk situations and document coping strategies to circumvent barriers. Barriers manifest themselves as a product of environment and lifestyle. They may also appear due to an internal process (Griffin, 2006). These environment and lifestyle factors are called external barriers and include:

- Lack of convenience
- Financial limitations
- Increased work demands
- Increased family demands
- Lack of support
- Inclement weather
- Injury or medical issues
- Overtraining
- Lack of time
- Lack of interest in programs (boredom)
- Lack of available childcare
- Lack of transportation
- Unrealistic goals

Indicate which of the following obstacles deter you from participation:

☐ Busy work schedule	☐ Busy home/family schedule	☐ Gym/club environment
☐ Lack of convenience	☐ Lack of available childcare	☐ Financial constraints
☐ Lack of activity partner(s)	☐ Insufficient activities or amenities	☐ Lack of support
☐ Scheduling conflict with partner	☐ Lack of self-motivation	☐ Lack of confidence in my ability
☐ Scheduling conflict with activities	☐ Lost interest in keeping records	☐ Failure to reach goals
☐ Unrealistic goals	☐ Goals too challenging	☐ Inclement weather
☐ Physical injury	☐ Health concerns/problems	☐ Other ________________

For each identified obstacle, devise a primary coping strategy to overcome the obstacle. In the event that your primary coping strategy may not prove successful, consider an alternative plan of action.

Obstacle	Primary Coping Strategy	Secondary Coping Strategy
☐		
☐		
☐		
☐		
☐		
☐		
☐		

Figure 12-6
Worksheet: High-risk situations and effective coping strategies

- Educational, socioeconomic, and cultural issues

Internal barriers are personal thoughts, perceptions, and feelings that individuals have about themselves, or about the exercise program itself, that reduce adherence. These barriers may include:

- Anxieties regarding one's physique or the perception of one's physique by others
- Intimidation in the gym environment
- Self-esteem
- Self-efficacy

Relapse Prevention

The major challenge of weight maintenance is to avoid regaining lost fat. The limited follow-up data on weight-loss programs indicate low (3 to 6% of initial weight) to no sustained levels of weight loss after four to five years. A successful program is often defined as maintaining fat losses of at least 5% of body weight (Anderson et al., 2001).

The National Weight Control Registry is the largest prospective investigation of long-term successful weight-loss maintenance. It monitors individuals who have lost at least 30 pounds (13.6 kg) and sustained the loss for a minimum of one year, although registrants often have achieved greater losses and sustained the losses for more than five years. A majority of the success stories within the registry attribute ongoing maintenance to reduced-calorie and low-fat diets and increased levels of physical activity. While it has not been established whether these behaviors represent minimal competence for weight-loss maintenance, these modifications have produced successful long-term weight-loss maintenance.

Textbooks present models to explain the environmental, emotional, and behavioral aspects of relapse. Still, researchers do not fully understand the biological impact of metabolic rate, hunger, and satiety, which are all factors contributing to regained weight. Therefore, LWMCs should continue to:

- Address the risks of relapse as part of the overall program
- Exert leadership in combating weight-management relapse

- Emphasize long-term change as the overall lifestyle goal
- Educate clients that regained weight is not a failure, but rather an indicator to start another phase of active management

A more systematic approach, assuming the LWMC first identified high-risk situations and developed appropriate coping strategies, is to:

- Teach the client that temporary breaks or slips from regular activity are acceptable and should not to be viewed as failures. If these relapses are anticipated or structured, a client should look at such incidents as deserved or programmed breaks.
- Identify in which stage of change the relapse occurred in the past
- Identify potential new barriers or obstacles, and evaluate why previous coping strategies, if any, were not effective for clients
- Develop new coping strategies in anticipation of future barriers
- Identify the most effective start-up strategies to initiate a return to an activity that is appropriate given the current stage of change
- Inquire about strategies that have proven successful before moving to the action phase

Summary

As the number of overweight and obese individuals grows, the need for qualified Lifestyle & Weight Management Consultants becomes more critical. Success as an LWMC requires knowledge and skills sets to address the three primary tenets of weight management: lifestyle and behavior modification; regular exercise; and sound nutritional programming. LWMCs must identify, understand, and develop programs around the intricate complexities of weight management. They need to demonstrate competency with behavioral change; implement effective strategies to facilitate the adoption of healthier behaviors; design and implement safe and effective exercise and dietary programs consistent with client goals; instill the philosophy of client ownership with this lifelong endeavor; recognize potential obstacles to success and develop coping strategies to overcome such barriers; and leverage all opportunities to associate positive emotion and thinking to the exercise experience. This involves a multifaceted approach with the three components, working independently with clients or as part of a team of health professionals while respecting scope of practice.

References

American College of Sports Medicine (2006). *Guidelines for Exercise Testing and Prescription* (7th ed.). Philadelphia: Lippincott, Williams & Wilkins.

Anderson, J.W. et al. (2001). Long-term weight-loss maintenance: A meta-analysis of U.S. studies. *American Journal of Clinical Nutrition,* 74, 579–584.

Annesi, J. (2000, July-August). Retention crisis? Exercise dropouts and adherents. *Fitness Business Canada,* pp. 6–8.

Buckworth, J. & Dishman, J.K. (2002). *Exercise Psychology*. Champaign, Ill.: Human Kinetics.

Finkelstein, E.A., Fiebelkorn, I.C., & Wang, G. (2003). National medical spending attributable to overweight and obesity: How much, and who's paying? *Health Affairs Web Exclusive,* W3, 219–226.

Gauvin, L. & Rejeski, W.J. (1993). The exercise-induced feeling inventory: Development and initial validation. *Journal of Sport and Exercise,* 15, 403–423.

Griffin, J.C. (2006). *Client Centered Exercise Prescription* (2nd ed.). Champaign, Ill., Human Kinetics.

Marketdata Enterprises, Inc. (2005). *The U.S. Weight Loss & Diet Control Market.*

Mokdad, A. et al. (2005). Correction: Actual causes of death in the United States, 2000 (letter). *Journal of the American Medical Association*, 293, 3, 293–294 (correction of original study).

Mokdad, A. et al. (2004). Actual causes of death in the United States. *Journal of the American Medical Association,* 291, 1238–1245 (original study).

Prochaska, J.O. & Marcus, B.H. (1994). The transtheoretical model: Applications to exercise. In: Dishman, R.K. (Ed.) *Advances in Exercise Adherence.* Champaign, Ill.: Human Kinetics.

Pronk, N. et al. (1994). Effects of Increased stimulus control for exercise through use of a personal trainer. *Annals of Behavioral Medicine,* 16: SO77.

Segel, J.E. (2006). Cost of Illness Studies—A Primer. RTI International.

Smith, C. et al. (2006). Health spending growth slows in 2004. *Health Affairs,* 25, 1, 186–196.

The Henry J. Kaiser Family Foundation (2005). *Employee Health Benefits: 2005 Annual Survey.*

United States Department of Agriculture (2005). *USDA Dietary Guidelines for Americans.* U.S. Department of Health and Human Services.

U.S. Department of Health and Human Services (2000). *Healthy People 2010: Understanding and Improving Health.* Washington, D.C.: U.S. Department of Health and Human Services, Government Printing Office.

United States Food and Drug Administration (12 March 2004). Calories Count: Report of the Working Group on Obesity. www.cfsan.fda.gov/~dms/owg-rpt.html.

Suggested Reading

Annesi, J. (August, 2001). Using emotions to empower members for long-term exercise success. *Fitness Management.*

Borger, C., et al. (2006). Health spending projections through 2015: Changes on the horizon. Health Affairs Web Exclusive, W61: 22 February 2006.

Canadian Society of Exercise Physiologists (2003). *Canadian Physical Activity, Fitness and Lifestyle Appraisal: CSEP's Plan for Healthy Active Living.*

Food and Drug Administration (2004). *Report of the Working Group on Obesity.*

Van Gaal L.F. (1998). Dietary treatment of obesity. In: Bray G.A., Bouchard, C., & James, W.P.T. (Eds.). *Handbook of Obesity.* New York: Marcel Dekker.

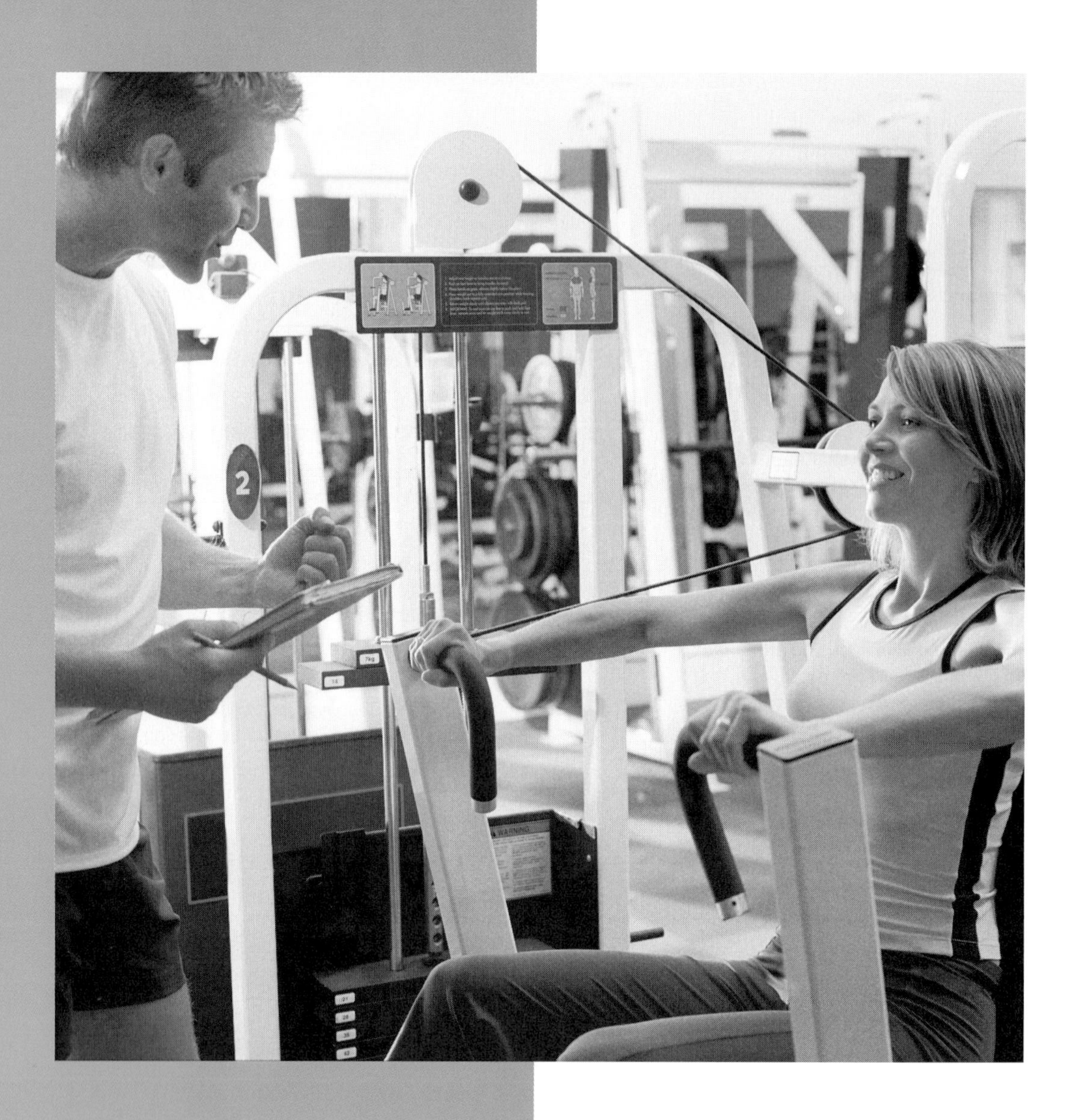

Len Kravitz

Len Kravitz, Ph.D., is an associate professor and the program coordinator of exercise science at the University of New Mexico, where he recently won the Outstanding Teacher of the Year award. Kravitz was honored with the 1999 Canadian Fitness Professional International Presenter of the Year and the 2006 Canadian Fitness Professional Specialty Presenter of the Year awards, as well as being named the ACE 2006 Fitness Educator of the Year.

Chapter 13

Exercise Programming

IN THIS CHAPTER:

All types of exercise, health, and weight-management programs need to begin with a goal-setting process. An invaluable way to manage the action steps in any behavioral-change process is to use the SMART goal-setting approach, which stands for specific, measurable, attainable, relevant, and time-bound. Each one of these components is an essential aspect of goal formation.

SMART Goal Setting

The SMART goal-setting system is an effective self-check tool for developing focused goals for clients. Many goals in resistance exercise, for example, are associated with improvements in **muscular strength, muscular endurance,** power, balance, speed, and **body composition.** Goals in cardiovascular exercise are often related to improvements in health, cardiorespiratory fitness, weight management, and body composition. Goals for some older clients may be associated with improving locomotion capabilities, balance, fall prevention, and muscle mass. The SMART goal-setting structure makes it easy to identify the correct action steps for developing a person's health, fitness, and weight-management plan for success.

Specific

The specificity of goal-setting involves answering most of the following questions.

- Why is this goal being created? Are there any benefits to accomplishing this goal?
- Who is involved in this goal? Does this goal involve one or more participants?
- What needs to be accomplished? What outcome or steps to the eventual outcome are desired?
- Where will the goal be accomplished? Is this a goal that needs to be completed at a gym, at home, at work, or throughout one's daily activities?

Measurable

As a person progresses in a goal behavior, there needs to be continual objective measurement to track progress. This measurement procedure will help evaluate whether a person is on track in attaining a specific goal, and will also indicate if modifications are needed for the goal to be reached.

Attainable

In the process of goal attainment, it is helpful to evaluate the necessary steps to achieve the goal. Thus, a person needs to assess his or her abilities, skills, and attitudes toward a particular outcome and truly determine if this goal is within reach. If a goal is realistic, a person will be able and willing to strive toward its accomplishment. Therefore, if a person "believes" that he or she can attain the goal, the motivation, drive, and perseverance to attain the goal will be available. It often helps to draw on past successes with goal-setting as a means of motivating an individual to work toward a new goal.

Relevant

Relevant goals are pertinent to the unique needs, interests, and abilities of the individual. If a goal is relevant, the individual will be motivated to strive toward its achievement.

Time-bound

When will the goal be accomplished? A schedule needs to be developed to put the overall goal and the incremental steps in attaining the goal into an appropriate timetable.

Using Health Screening and Assessment Data

For most people, physical activity will not pose any health problems. However, the primary purpose of any pre-exercise health screening is to identify individuals who may have health or medical conditions that could put them at risk during physical testing and exercise. The American Council on Exercise (ACE), the American College of Sports Medicine (ACSM), and other professional organizations for exercise professionals have determined that pre-exercise screening is an important part of the duties of a fitness professional. According to Heyward (2006), the pretest health screening of clients that a fitness professional should minimally complete before exercise testing and participation commence must include the following:

- The Physical Activity Readiness Questionnaire (PAR-Q)
- Identification of signs and symptoms of disease, if present
- Evaluation of the coronary risk profile
- Classification of heart disease risk factors

The Physical Activity Readiness Questionnaire (PAR-Q)

The PAR-Q has been designed to identify the small number of adults for whom physical activity might be inappropriate or those who should have medical advice concerning the type of activity most suitable for them (Figure 13-1, pages 286–287).

Identification of Signs and Symptoms of Disease, if Present

If any signs or symptoms of disease are present, the client should be referred to his or her physician for clearance prior to any exercise testing or participation. Figure 13-2 presents a checklist of some health-screening signs and symptoms (Heyward, 2006). If a client checks "yes" beside any of the conditions, he or she should be advised to obtain medical clearance and/or appropriate exercise guidelines prior to exercise testing and participation.

Evaluation of the Coronary Risk Profile

The coronary artery disease risk factor threshold is helpful in determining a client risk profile (Table 13-1, page 288).

Classification of Heart Disease Risk Factors

The following health-risk categories help determine a client's needs for further medical clearance or evaluation before beginning an exercise program.

Despite the recommendations provided in this section about a person's potential health risks regarding exercise, any individual who has the slightest reservations about his or her ability to undergo exercise testing or participate in exercise with minimal health risk should consult a physician. If a client's health status relative to any of the PAR-Q questions, coronary risk factors, or signs and symptoms of disease changes after starting or modifying an exercise program, it would be advisable to have the individual consult a physician.

Low Risk

A low-risk individual exhibits one or no risk factors, no signs or symptoms of cardiovascular disease, and is either a male under 45 years of age or a female under 55 years of age. While a physical examination within the last year would be appropriate, a low-risk client is considered safe to participate in exercise at all of the intensities described in the ACSM guidelines (ACSM, 2006).

Moderate Risk

A moderate-risk individual exhibits two or more of the risk factors or is either a male over 45 years of age or a female over 55 years of age, but has no signs or symptoms of cardiovascular or pulmonary disease. A prior physical examination is appropriate. However, only individuals who plan to participate in vigorous exercise training or competition need to obtain prior medical clearance.

Instructions: Please check all answers that apply.

Do you have any of the following musculoskeletal signs and symptoms?

- ❑ Artificial joints
- ❑ Low-back pain
- ❑ Osteoarthritis
- ❑ Osteoporosis
- ❑ Orthopedic pain
- ❑ Swollen joints

Do you have any of the following cardiovascular signs and symptoms?

- ❑ Abnormal cholesterol levels
- ❑ Ankle edema
- ❑ Chest pain
- ❑ Claudication
- ❑ Dizziness and/or fainting spells
- ❑ Heart attack
- ❑ Heart murmur
- ❑ Hypertension
- ❑ Ischemia
- ❑ Stroke

Do you have any of the following pulmonary signs and symptoms?

- ❑ Asthma
- ❑ Breathlessness during or after mild exercise
- ❑ Bronchitis
- ❑ Exercise-induced asthma
- ❑ Emphysema

Do you have any of the following metabolic signs and symptoms?

- ❑ Diabetes
- ❑ Cirrhosis
- ❑ Glucose intolerance
- ❑ Hypoglycemia
- ❑ McArdle's syndrome
- ❑ Thyroid disease

Figure 13-2
Health screening signs and symptoms questionnaire

High Risk

A high-risk individual exhibits one or more signs or symptoms of cardiovascular, pulmonary, or metabolic disease, or has a known cardiovascular, pulmonary, or metabolic disease. A physical examination and medical clearance is considered essential before anyone in this classification participates in exercise programs of any intensity.

Programming Components

Physical fitness is defined as a person's ability to perform daily, occupational, and recreational activities without becoming overly tired and weary. It may also be described as the ability of the body to

Figure 13-1
The Physical Activity Readiness Questionnaire

The Physical Activity Readiness Questionnaire—PAR-Q

(revised 2002)

PAR-Q & YOU (A Questionnaire for People Aged 15 to 69)

Regular physical activity is fun and healthy, and increasingly more people are starting to become more active every day. Being more active is very safe for most people. However, some people should check with their doctor before they start becoming much more physically active.

If you are planning to become much more physically active than you are now, start by answering the seven questions below. If you are between the ages of 15 and 69, the PAR-Q will tell you if you should check with your doctor before you start. If you are over 69 years of age, and you are not used to being very active, check with your doctor.

Common sense is your best guide when you answer these questions. Please read the questions carefully and answer each one honestly: check YES or NO.

YES	NO	
☐	☐	1. Has your doctor ever said that you have a heart condition *and* that you should only do physical activity recommended by a doctor?
☐	☐	2. Do you feel pain in your chest when you do physical activity?
☐	☐	3. In the past month, have you had chest pain when you were not doing physical activity?
☐	☐	4. Do you lose your balance because of dizziness or do you ever lose consciousness?
☐	☐	5. Do you have a bone or joint problem (for example, back, knee, or hip) that could be made worse by a change in your physical activity?
☐	☐	6. Is your doctor currently prescribing drugs (for example, water pills) for your blood pressure or heart condition?
☐	☐	7. Do you know of *any other reason* why you should not do physical activity?

If you answered YES to one or more questions:

✔ Talk with your doctor by phone or in person BEFORE you start becoming much more physically active or BEFORE you have a fitness appraisal. Tell your doctor about the PAR-Q and which questions you answered YES.

✔ You may be able to do any activity you want—as long as you start slowly and build up gradually. Or, you may need to restrict your activities to those that are safe for you. Talk with your doctor about the kinds of activities you wish to participate in and follow his or her advice.

✔ Find out which community programs are safe and helpful for you.

If you answered NO honestly to all PAR-Q questions, you can be reasonably sure that you can:

✔ Start becoming much more physically active—begin slowly and build up gradually. This is the safest and easiest way to go.

✔ Take part in a fitness appraisal—this is an excellent way to determine your basic fitness level so that you can plan the best way for you to live actively. It is also highly recommended that you have your blood pressure evaluated. If your reading is over 144/94, talk with your doctor before you start becoming much more physically active.

Delay becoming much more active:

- ✔ If you are not feeling well because of a temporary illness such as a cold or a fever—wait until you feel better; or
- ✔ If you are or may be pregnant—talk to your doctor before you start becoming more active.

Please note: If your health changes so that you then answer YES to any of the above questions, tell your fitness or health professional. Ask whether you should change your physical-activity plan.

Informed Use of the PAR-Q: The Canadian Society for Exercise Physiology, Health Canada, and their agents assume no liability for persons who undertake physical activity, and if in doubt after completing this questionnaire, consult your doctor prior to physical activity.

No changes permitted. You are encouraged to copy the PAR-Q but only if you use the entire form.

Note: If the PAR-Q is being given to a person before he or she participates in a physical-activity program or a fitness appraisal, this section may be used for legal or administrative purposes.

I have read, understood, and completed this questionnaire. Any questions I had were answered to my full satisfaction.

____

Name

____

Signature Date

____

Signature of Parent Witness
or Guardian (for participants under the age of majority)

Note: This physical activity clearance is valid for a maximum of 12 months from the date it is completed and becomes invalid if your condition changes so that you would answer YES to any of the seven questions.

Supported by: 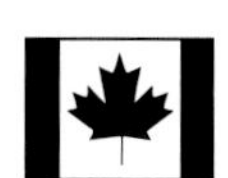 Health Canada Santé Canada

Table 13-1
Coronary Artery Disease Risk-factor Thresholds

Instructions:

Determine the total number of risk factors using the following risk-factor criteria, scoring a point for each risk factor identified. If high-density lipoprotein (HDL) levels exceed 60 mg/dL, subtract one point from the sum of positive risk factors, as high HDL levels lower the risk for coronary artery disease.

Positive Risk Factors

Family History +1
- Myocardial infarction, coronary revascularization, or sudden death before 55 years of age in father or other first-degree male relative
- Myocardial infarction, coronary revascularization, or sudden death before 65 years of age in mother or other first-degree female relative

Cigarette Smoking +1
- Current cigarette smokers or those who quit within the previous six months

Hypertension +1
- Systolic blood pressure ≥140 mmHg or diastolic blood pressure ≥90 mmHg, confirmed by measurements on at least two separate occasions, or on anti-hypertensive medications

Dyslipidemia +1
- Low-density lipoprotein (LDL) cholesterol ≥130 mg/dL or HDL cholesterol <40 mg/dL, or on lipid-lowering medication
- If serum cholesterol is all that is available, use serum cholesterol ≥200 mg/dL

Impaired Glucose Fasting +1
- Fasting blood sugar ≥100 mg/dL confirmed by measurements on at least two separate occasions

Obesity +1
- Body mass index of ≥30 kg/m^2
  or
- Waist girth >102 cm (40 inches) for men and ≥88 cm (35 inches) for women
  or
- Waist/hip ratio ≥0.95 for men and ≥0.86 for women

As professional opinions vary regarding the most appropriate markers and thresholds for obesity, use additional valid markers to evaluate obesity as a risk factor (this may include a valid measure of percent body fat).

Sedentary Lifestyle +1
- Persons not participating in a regular exercise program or not meeting the minimal recommendations from the Surgeon General's Report/USDA Guidelines

Negative Risk Factor

High serum HDL Cholesterol - 1
- Score >60 mg/dL

TOTAL SCORE ______

Source: American College of Sports Medicine (2006). *ACSM's Guidelines for Exercise Testing and Prescription* (7th ed.). Philadelphia: Lippincott Williams & Wilkins.

adjust to the stresses and demands of physical exertion. More specifically, it is the capacity of the heart, lungs, muscles, and bones to adapt to the challenges placed upon them.

Technology has advanced civilization to the point where a person no longer needs to do much physical effort to survive. Advanced transportation options, escalators and elevators in malls and businesses, and homes that are programmed by remote control are hallmarks of modern society. What might have once taken an hour to do physically can now be accomplished with the push of a button in a matter of seconds. Unfortunately, these timesaving amenities and other environmental factors have led many people to adopt sedentary lifestyles.

The human body is designed for movement and physical activity. To give the body the physical challenge it needs to be strong and healthy, a person must make a concerted effort to incorporate physical activity into his or her daily life. A lack of physical activity puts each person at a much higher risk for developing many diseases, such as heart disease, **hypertension,** high cholesterol, **obesity, diabetes,** and musculoskeletal disorders (Warburton, Nicol, & Bredin, 2006). A properly planned exercise program can play a critical role in combating obesity, heart disease, and musculoskeletal ailments. LWMCs must consider the following five key components of health-related physical fitness when developing personalized exercise programs.

Cardiorespiratory Endurance

Cardiorespiratory endurance, or aerobic conditioning, is the ability of the heart, lungs, and circulatory system to supply oxygen and nutrients to the working muscles. It involves the ability to persist in continuous rhythmic activities such as elliptical training, walking, jogging, cycling, step training, and other aerobic activities. Improved cardiorespiratory endurance is associated with decreased mortality and morbidity for both women and men (Warburton, Nicol, & Bredin, 2006).

Muscular Strength and Endurance

Muscular strength refers to the capacity of the muscles to exert maximal or near-maximal force against a resistance. The development of stronger muscles leads to the increased strength and integrity of the body's skeletal system. In the cycle of life, muscular strength may also lessen the chance of injury (Warburton, Gledhill, & Quinney, 2001).

Muscular endurance is the ability of the skeletal muscles to exert force, but not necessarily near-maximal force, for an extended period of time. The ability to increase muscular endurance is often associated with improved bodily posture, enhanced function in **activities of daily living (ADL)**, and a reduced potential for injury.

Flexibility

Flexibility is the **range of motion** of the muscles and joints of the body. It involves the muscles' normal and trained ability to extend beyond their natural resting length. Increasing and maintaining range of motion to readily perform activities of daily life is an appropriate goal for all individuals.

Body Composition

Body composition refers to the proportion of body fat and lean body tissue (i.e., muscle, bone, water, and vital organs). Being overfat is associated with a number of health problems (ACSM, 2006); however, aerobic exercise and resistance training are effective in positively altering body composition.

Mind/Body Vitality

This sixth component of physical fitness has received growing attention. **Mind/body vitality** refers to an individual's ability to minimize or alleviate unnecessary stress and tension from the body through the integration of physical exercise and mental focus. Popular classes such as yoga, tai chi, and Pilates present constructive means of harmonizing this union of the mind, body, and spirit.

Cardiorespiratory Training

Most of an LWMC's clients will be participating in some form of cardiorespiratory training, including group fitness classes. It is important to ask each client about what type of exercise he or she performs and to provide tips for reducing injury and maximizing results. Safety is especially important among overweight and obese participants, as they tend to be at a higher risk for injury and often struggle to keep up with the more fit participants. Diminished coordination is also a common problem in this population, which is another reason why safety and careful progression are so important. It is essential that LWMCs have detailed conversations with clients about their exercise participation. The following sections provide information that should be invaluable during consultation with clients.

According to fitness industry experts, to develop and maintain cardiorespiratory fitness, individuals should perform endurance exercise three to five days per week, using an exercise mode that involves the major muscle groups (in a rhythmic nature) for a prolonged time period (ACSM, 2006). This includes physical activities such as step aerobics, aquatic exercise, cardio-kickboxing, rowing, and walking. ACSM recommends an intensity of exercise between 55/65% and 90% of maximum heart rate (or 40/50% and 85% of oxygen uptake reserve), with a continuous duration of 20 to 60 minutes per session. Beginners who are in the lower cardiorespiratory fitness classification should begin with 10 to 20 minutes of aerobic conditioning. Very deconditioned individuals may be more suited for multiple sessions of short duration, such as five to 10 minutes. Inherent in the exercise design is the concept of individualizing the program for each person's fitness level, health, age, personal goals, risk-factor profile, medications, behavioral characteristics, and individual preferences.

ACSM (2006) recommends that the exercise design for optimizing weight loss should emphasize the duration and frequency of the aerobic exercise, keeping intensity moderate and progressing gradually. ACSM further suggests that the frequency of training should be five to seven days per week, with the goal of accumulating 200 to 300 minutes of aerobic activity per week (which is equivalent to ≥2,000 kilocalories of exercise per week). This can be accomplished with longer bouts of exercise or by performing shorter, 10-minute bouts of exercise spread out over the week.

These ACSM recommendations for the development and/or maintenance of cardiorespiratory fitness and for weight loss serve as the framework for the aerobic fitness designs that follow. A diverse number of both small and large group-exercise programs have emerged in an effort to meet the retention needs of regular exercisers, and to attract new fitness participants. Some of these programs are choreographed to accompanying music, while others use music as a background source of inspiration. Some clients may struggle with choreography, so LWMCs should be prepared to help them master basic movements. For example, an LWMC may teach a client that music is customarily arranged in units of two, alternating between emphasized and deemphasized beats, referred to as the **downbeat** and **upbeat,** respectively. Some programs, such as step aerobics, follow a specialized 32-beat phrasing, while other programs may easily incorporate a blend of music phrases. Regardless of the music phrasing, the music volume must not put any participants at risk for sustaining hearing loss.

Some of the most popular cardiorespiratory programs are described in the following sections—step aerobics, mixed-impact aerobics, mixed-martial arts exercise, indoor cycling, aquatic exercise, and aerobic interval training.

Step Aerobics

Step aerobics has long been a stronghold of cardiorespiratory teaching due to its widespread popularity and ease of use with the varying fitness abilities commonly seen in exercise classes. Step aerobics, or step training, can be a low-impact exercise program that provides high-intensity aerobic conditioning for participants (Kravitz, 2006). The workouts can be as challenging as a rigorous jogging workout, while producing impact forces that are generally as safe as walking. The cadence of step aerobics classes ranges from 118 to 126 beats per minute. The most widely used step platforms have adjustable heights from 4 to 12 inches (10 to 30 cm), with a stepping surface 14 (36 cm) inches wide and 42 inches long (107 cm). The progression of exercise intensity is best adjusted by modifying step height. The typical step platform risers allow for a 2-inch (5-cm) change in step height. Encourage participants to begin gradually by using a lower step height, and then to progressively increase the platform height as they become more comfortable performing the instructor-led workouts.

Step-training programs, for the most part, have been designed to include movements that are relatively easy to learn and follow. However, some participants will find the unfamiliarity of stepping on and off of the step to be a challenging motor skill. One option is to introduce many of the step combinations gradually and without musical accompaniment for these learners. LWMCs should review the following key safety tips regarding step-aerobics programs with their clients (Kravitz, 2006):

- Step entirely on the top part of the platform with each step; do not allow any part of the foot to hang over an edge.
- Avoid flexing the knees more than 90 degrees. Most participants find progressing up to a 6-inch (15-cm) step height to provide a satisfactory workout.
- When using handheld weights [up to 3 pounds (1.4 kg)], modify the arm choreography to slow, controlled, shorter-lever movements.
- To quickly lower the intensity of the workout, stop stepping and march in place on the ground.
- Be careful not to step too far back off the platform. This causes the body to lean slightly forward, placing extra stress on the Achilles tendon and the muscles of the calf.
- Use a good cross-training or indoor-fitness shoe for step workouts. The tread on most running shoes does not provide suitable support for the lateral pathways of step movements.
- Step training involves a stepping motion using the entire foot. Avoid pounding foot movements on the platform and bouncing actions onto and off of the floor.
- Steer clear of step combinations that travel forward and down off the bench.
- Be aware of the potential for overuse injury syndrome by participating in a variety of aerobic activities to allow for different stresses on the lower body.
- Always look at the step platform when doing step aerobics, but don't drop the head too far forward.
- The correct posture in step training involves standing tall and bending at the knees for the ascending and descending movements. Too much hip flexion while stepping may place unwanted stresses on the spine.
- Change the lead foot when doing step patterns to avoid overstressing one leg. A good rule of thumb is to change the lead foot at least every minute.
- Step-training choreography allows for some moves to be repeating actions. Avoid performing more than five consecutive repeating movements on the same leg.
- Explosive lunges off a step can provide high-intensity challenges, but are often performed incorrectly or too swiftly, with potential trauma to the lower leg from the ground impact. Take the time to learn safe lunges and be careful not to overperform them.
- Participants who complain of knee stress from a step class should be advised to seek help from their health practitioner. Step aerobics may not be a suitable exercise mode for all exercisers.

Mixed-impact Aerobics

Mixed-impact aerobics combines high-impact aerobic movements that are associated with greater stresses on the lower extremities (such as running and jumping) with low-impact aerobic movements (such as side lunges and step touches) that present minimal stress to the lower extremities. Movement phrases and sequences are choreographed to music that has approximately 130 to 150 beats per minute and incorporate a variety of arm and leg movements, traveling patterns, and directional turns. An advantage of mixed-impact aerobic classes is the ability to easily modify the intensity of the exercise. With all exercise programs, modification involves analyzing the movements or exercises and determining safe ways in which the exercise can be introduced to people of different fitness levels. The most common ways to modify any cardiorespiratory mixed-impact exercise design is to alter the speed of movement, modify the range of motion of the movement, vary the amount of traveling completed with a movement, and/or change the vertical direction of the movement.

With mixed-impact classes, there is no single, preferred method of combining the impact styles. Some classes alternate impact styles using the songs to mark the style changes. For example, some mixed-impact programs will alternate between high-impact and low-impact movement with every song change on a soundtrack (i.e., every three to five minutes). Other programs combine the impact styles within all sections of the choreography, interspersing the low-impact and high-impact movements throughout the program. It is essential that group fitness instructors determine how to best minimize injury risks while maximizing health benefits. LWMCs should review the following key safety tips regarding mixed-impact aerobics programs with their clients (Kravitz, 2006):

- Always wear good aerobic shoes in a mixed-impact class.
- Encourage all participants to exercise at their own preferred intensity.
- Regularly monitor exercise intensity with pulse-rate checks and/or **ratings of perceived exertion (RPE).**
- Do not hop on one foot more than four times in a row.
- Stay away from twisting hop variations that may lead to spinal stress.
- Drink water before, during, and after aerobic exercise workouts.
- Gradually slow down the aerobic section to a walking pace to ensure safe and proper recovery of heart rate, blood pressure, blood flow, and ventilation.

Mixed Martial Arts Exercise

Kickbox aerobics, aerobic kickboxing, cardio boxing, and aerobic boxing are just a few of the many mixed martial arts exercise formats that are now staples of the fitness industry. Enthusiasts appear to enjoy the exhilaration that comes from delivering kicks, punches, elbows, jabs, knee strikes, and combinations used in boxing and martial arts. The athletic drills in these classes are interspersed with recovery bouts of basic aerobic movements such as boxer-style rope skipping (with and without a rope), walking, and light jogging in place. Some mixed martial arts exercise programs involve authentic boxing gloves, punching bags, and martial arts equipment, whereas other programs incorporate a form of "shadowboxing," which involves no equipment. The majority of these classes are driven by moderately paced music (approximately 120 to 130 beats per minute), although the music in many instances is more for motivation, since the exercise program is not always performed to a specific tempo. Some of the classes are led exclusively by instructors, while others are taught in circuit formats, where each participant or group of participants rotates from station to station, performing different types of kicks, jabs, and punches at each station.

A primary concern with mixed martial arts exercise classes is the ability or qualifications of the instructor to properly teach the program. LWMCs should remind their clients that instructors must have proper knowledge of correct punching techniques and progressive teaching skills to help ensure that participants avoid any joint-related injuries. The challenge for these instructors is to create a motivating workout environment while progressively introducing safe, enjoyable, and challenging mixed martial arts exercise. As with all instructor-led classes, the effectiveness of a martial arts instructor largely depends on his or her ability to modify the movements to suit the needs and abilities of the class participants. LWMCs should review the following key safety tips regarding mixed martial arts programs with their clients (Olson & Williford, 1999):

- Perform a satisfactory warm-up to properly prepare the muscles and joints for the ensuing challenge of the workout.
- With all upper-body strikes and jabs, make sure the elbow is not taken past its normal extension range of motion.
- Avoid performing complex upper-body strike-and-kick combinations.
- Do not execute high repetitions of any one move.
- Do not do physical-contact exercises without proper skill progressions.

- Be careful not to kick beyond the normal range of motion.
- Be aware that martial-arts movements may lead to more **delayed onset muscle soreness (DOMS)** in individuals who are new to these types of workouts.

Indoor Cycling

Indoor cycling classes and sessions have attracted many devoted enthusiasts. Since most people know how to ride a bicycle, indoor cycling presents a cardiorespiratory-training format that may seem less intimidating. Because of its non-weightbearing nature, indoor cycling also offers some orthopedic advantages to those individuals who are unable to perform traditional weightbearing exercise.

Indoor cycling class formats often introduce a workout "journey" using instructor-led visualization and imagery to create the desired environment for participants (Sherman, 1997). Music selection in an indoor cycling class is geared toward enhancing the chosen mood of the "ride." No actual beats-per-minute guidelines have been established for indoor cycling classes. However, a variety of tempos are often used to increase or decrease the exercise intensity (Sherman, 1997). The success of an indoor cycling class largely depends on the instructor's knowledge of exercise program design and ability to create an effective workout using his or her leadership skills. In addition, soft-lighting room designs, with bikes placed close together, create an atmosphere similar to outdoor riding with a pack of cyclists. Naturally, due to the close environment of the exercisers, good air circulation is a must for indoor cycling classes.

Mainstreaming all fitness levels is easily accomplished with indoor cycling classes. Students can control their own workout intensity with cycling cadence (pedaling speed), cycle workload (wheel resistance), and body position (seated or standing position while cycling) (Sherman, 1997).

Aquatic Fitness

Aquatic fitness classes are popular among individuals of varying fitness levels. The resistance afforded by the water provides an effective environment to perform numerous exercise movements. Many exercise enthusiasts use the aquatic environment to complete a greater volume of work with less stress to the body's bones and joints. LWMCs should consider the following key benefits of aquatic exercise and review them with interested clients (Sanders, 1999):

- Water provides an adequate resistance overload for resistance training, as well as a sufficient stimulus for improving cardiovascular function.
- The minimal weightbearing environment allows for graded exercise intensities without risk to the lower extremities.
- The aquatic environment gives exercisers the ability to explore a variety of physical movements that are different than those imposed by gravity.
- The external pressure of the water medium may be suitable for individuals encumbered with blood circulation problems, as the external pressure of the water against the body will enhance venous return.
- The external pressure of the water may also provide a sufficient challenge for

Attire Suggestions for the Overweight Aquatic Exerciser

For some overweight individuals, exposing their bodies in the pool area may be the number-one deterrent or excuse for not participating in an aquatic exercise program. Fitness professionals need to dress professionally and appropriately, keeping the larger participants in mind. Inform overweight students of where they can find large Lycra™ bike shorts and supportive exercise bras that can be used in the water. Remind them that they can cover up their swimsuit with other clothing such as a T-shirt or towel when walking to and from the pool. Encourage them to focus on how good they will feel about themselves while they are in the water exercising and for the rest of the day after their workout. Lastly, suggest to them that they can always arrive a little early to class and stay a little later after class if they wish to avoid walking in front of the majority of students in the class.

individuals suffering from weakened respiratory muscle function.

- The aquatic medium provides a unique opportunity to modify the range-of-motion patterns of many exercises and movements.
- Functional balance and stabilization movement patterns may be improved and practiced in the water.
- Clients who fear falling on land may find the aquatic environment less intimidating.
- The frequently changing movement patterns in the water may translate to improved posture on land, as the trunk and abdominal muscles are regularly stimulated to maintain posture in the water.

Generally, the three water depths [in 81 to 84° F (27 to 29° C) water] used in aquatic-exercise classes are shallow, which is navel to nipple; transitional, which is nipple to neck; and deep, in which the feet are not touching the bottom of the pool (Sanders, 1999). In deep-water exercise, some type of buoyancy gear is required. The choice of water depth may be determined by what is accessible, the available aquatic equipment, the participants' fitness levels, and the desired amount of weightbearing movement. The shallow-water environment is ideal for mimicking movements on land without the impact. For some special populations and physically challenged individuals, deep-water exercise may be preferred due to its completely non-impact environment (Sanders, 1999).

Exercises in the water can be graded by the range of motion of performance, the speed of motion, and the lower-body load (Sanders, 1999). Lower-body load is higher at a shallow water level when incorporating more jumping and leaping movements. In deep-water exercise, the lower-body movements can be intensified with the use of aquatic exercise equipment such as giant aquatic sandals, which add more resistance to the movement. Finally, for exercise variety, numerous types of aquatic equipment, including webbed gloves, fins, and non-buoyant bells, can provide multiple training-stimulus options to an aquatic exercise program.

Aerobic Interval Training

Interval training has become a popular cardiovascular-training method. One of the major benefits of interval training is its adaptability to multiple fitness levels. Aerobic interval training is a form of conditioning that combines segments of high-intensity work with segments of moderate-to-light intensity work. This type of training systematically emphasizes the body's different energy systems (phosphagen, glycolytic, and mitochondrial respiration), thus effectively burning fat and carbohydrates. The incorporation of interval training with continuous aerobic programming optimizes the development of cardiorespiratory fitness and can help clients attain their body-composition goals. Terminology related to interval training and general interval-training guidelines for developing the various energy systems are summarized in Tables 13-2 and 13-3, respectively.

Although there are many types of interval-training programs, the following method has been scientifically tested with fitness enthusiasts (Kravitz et al., 1997). An aerobic interval workout should feature a modality that the client enjoys doing (e.g., walking, jogging, cycling, rowing, stair stepping, elliptical training). The aerobic exercise should always begin gradually with three to five minutes of low-intensity aerobic activity to prepare the heart, lungs, and musculoskeletal system for the challenging workout to follow. Following the warm-up, participants train for four minutes at a higher intensity, followed by four minutes at a moderate-to-light intensity. These four-minute intervals alternate for the duration of the workout. This program utilizes self-assessed ratings of perceived exertion to monitor workout intensity. For example, during the four-minute high-intensity interval, the participant should exercise at an intensity that he or she feels

Table 13-2
Terms Related to Interval Training

Term	Definition
Work interval	Time of work effort or work bout
Recovery interval	Time between work intervals. The recovery interval may consist of light activity such as walking (passive recovery) or mild-to-moderate exercise such as jogging (active recovery).
Work/recovery ratio	Time ratio of the work and recovery intervals. A work/recovery ratio of 1 to 3 means the recovery time is three times that of the work interval.
Cycle	One cycle includes a work and recovery interval.
Set	The number of cycles completed per workout

Table 13-3
General Interval-training Guidelines

Energy System	Work Time	Cycles	Sets	Work/Recovery Ratio	Recovery Time	Type of Recovery
ATP-PC	0–30 seconds	8–10	4–5	1/3	0–90 seconds	Passive
Glycolytic	30–120 seconds	5–6	1–3	1/2	60–240 seconds	Active
Oxidative	3–5 minutes	3–4	1–2	1/1	2–5 minutes	Active

Note: Passive recovery means very-low-intensity movement such as walking or even rest; active recovery involves mild-to-moderate intensity.

is "comfortably challenging"; during the moderate-intensity bout, the client should feel that the intensity level is "somewhat challenging." The alternating variations of workout intensity will enhance total caloric burning at the cellular level.

Depending on the individual's fitness level, the duration of the workout can gradually increase to 20 to 60 minutes. For cardiovascular maintenance and improvement, cardiovascular training should be done three to five times a week, combining the interval training with other aerobic workouts. To help a client achieve weight-management goals, aerobic exercise should be performed five to seven times per week, regularly alternating this interval-training workout with long, slow continuous aerobic training, fast continuous aerobic training, and **Fartlek training** (a form of randomly changing aerobic exercise intensities within the same workout). For variety and orthopedic-injury prevention, exercises should alternate all of these various aerobic-training schemes on different exercise modalities.

Resistance Training

Although resistance training is considered a valuable component of health and fitness program design, simply lifting weights does not ensure the desired outcome. Several factors related to the client or class must be considered to determine a physiologically sound approach to achieve the program's goals. Some of the basic elements of the resistance-training plan include:

- Assessing the initial fitness level of the client
- Setting short- and long-term goals
- Identifying specific muscle groups to work
- Choosing the type of exercise equipment
- Selecting the type and order of the exercises
- Manipulating the frequency, intensity, and duration of the workouts, as well as the number of repetitions, types of

contraction, rest periods, and sets during the workout
- Planning ahead for the progressive overload
- Motivating the client to comply to the program

Considering all of these factors, the likelihood of one training program meeting the needs of all participants is highly impractical. Resistance-training programs designed specifically to enhance musculoskeletal fitness have been effective in improving several indicators of health status, including bone health, glucose metabolism, overweight and obesity, the incidence of falling and associated injuries, activities of daily living, and/or psychological well-being (Warburton, Gledhill, & Quinney, 2001). In weight-management programs, resistance exercise is vital for helping to preserve muscle mass (which is metabolically active tissue) during the weight-loss process (Jackicic et al., 2001). Following are the answers to some key questions that LWMCs may hear about resistance training (Kravitz, 2006):

- *What is a concentric muscle action?* A **concentric** muscle action (or contraction) involves a muscle going through a shortening motion as it overcomes resistance.
- *What is an eccentric muscle action?* During **eccentric** muscle actions (or contractions), the muscle lengthens as it resists the load. During a biceps curl, for example, the upward phase of the movement is the concentric action and the lowering phase of the movement is the eccentric action.
- *What is an isometric action?* During **isometric** muscle actions (or contractions), a muscle is stimulated to develop tension, but no joint movement occurs. Isometric contractions represent the amount of strength an individual can exhibit at a fixed point in the range of motion. With isometric actions, there is no limb movement or change in the joint angle. Holding a weight in one position is an example of isometric strength.
- *What is speed strength?* Speed strength is a relatively new term that is interchangeable with the term power. Speed strength refers to the maximum force exhibited over a distance at a certain speed of movement. Examples of speed strength in sports include swinging a bat, throwing a javelin, and striking a punching bag.
- *What is absolute strength?* **Absolute strength** is the maximal amount of weight that an individual can lift one time. It is sometimes referred to as the **one-repetition maximum (1 RM).**
- *What is relative strength?* **Relative strength** compares the strength of different individuals. It is the ratio of the amount of weight lifted to the total body weight of the person. For example, if a 120-pound (54.5-kg) person can do a 1 RM biceps curl with a 50-pound (23-kg) weight, the relative strength of this muscle group can be determined as follows: 50 pounds/120 pounds (23 kg/54.5 kg) = 0.42. Relative strength is reported as a percentage; therefore, in this example, multiplying 0.42 by 100 means the relative strength of the biceps muscle is 42%.
- *What is functional strength?* Functional strength is a popular term used in both fitness and sports. In fitness, functional strength is often discussed in terms of doing exercises that will enhance a person's ability to execute everyday activities. Some experts describe this strategy as "meaningful exercise" to enhance daily physical tasks. With functional strength, exercises are chosen that are task-specific to help a person perform better in daily life.

  In sports, the term functional strength is used to describe applied strength that results in improved sports performance. For recreational and competitive athletes, trainers and coaches try to duplicate the range of motion (or a portion of the range) with an exercise. For example, a push-up is excellent for developing the strength of the shoulder joint, yet it is not the best functional exercise choice for training a golfer. When working with a golfer, a better option would be to design an exercise that goes through more of a diagonal pathway, which mirrors the motion of swinging a golf club.

- *What is core strength?* Core strength and core stability are relatively new concepts in strength training. Core-training exercises are designed to strengthen the deep spinal muscles—the deep abdominal and lower-back muscles surrounding the spine, often referred to as the intrinsic muscles. The purpose of core training is to spare the spine from damage. Core strength training creates a stable and mobile lower back, which may in turn improve exercise performance and enjoyment.

Resistance training is an effective method for maintaining and increasing lean body mass and improving muscular strength and endurance. Resistance-training programs should be designed to meet the needs and goals of the individual. All training programs need to be monitored and evaluated closely. LWMCs should be acutely aware of the many signs and symptoms of overtraining: muscle soreness, injury, fatigue, drops in exercise performance, attitude changes, unplanned drops in body weight, sickness, tiredness, and restlessness. If any one of these signs, or a combination of these signs, is observed, rest or a change in the training program is necessary. LWMCs can use the following checklist of questions as an effective needs analysis when designing a safe and appropriate resistance-training program for clients:

- What results does the client want to achieve?
- What component of muscular fitness (strength, endurance, speed, power, or some combination of these components) does the client want to improve?
- Are there any movement patterns that need to be developed?
- What muscle groups need to be developed?
- Are there any specific muscle imbalance concerns?
- How is the client's muscular fitness going to be assessed (e.g., 1 RM, 5 RM, 10 RM, trial-and-error method)?
- What is the client's health history? Are there any past injuries or chronic limitations that need to be addressed?
- Have the short- and long-term goals been collaboratively written with the client?
- Where will the workouts take place (e.g., class, gym, home facility)?
- What equipment is available or needed?
- What days/times are available and recommended for the client's workout?
- Approximately how long will each training session last?
- What methods of resistance training will be included in the program?
- What types of exercises will be predominantly chosen for the client?
- What order of exercises will be used in designing the workouts?
- What workout intensity will be used in the sessions?
- How many sets and repetitions will be utilized?
- How much rest will there be between sets and exercises?
- What type of a warm-up and cool-down will be utilized?
- How will the client's progress be monitored and evaluated?

ACSM recommends a minimum of one set of eight to 10 exercises (multijoint and single joint) that involve the major muscle groups (at a sufficient intensity to enhance the development and maintenance of muscular strength and endurance), performed two to three times a week for healthy participants of all ages. A more technical and advanced form of training known as **periodization** training is discussed in the following section.

Periodization

Periodization is a systematic approach to training that involves progressively cycling various aspects of a training program during a specific period of time. The roots of periodization come from Hans Selye's model, known as the general adaptation syndrome (Selye, 1976), which has been used by the athletic community since the late 1950s. Selye identified a source of biological stress referred to as eustress, which denotes beneficial muscular strength and growth, and a distress state, which is stress that can lead to tissue damage, disease, and death. Periodization is most widely used in resistance-training program design to avoid overtraining and to methodically alternate high loads of training with decreased loading phases to improve components of muscular fitness (e.g., strength, strength-speed, muscular endurance).

This system of training is traditionally divided up into three types of cycles: **microcycles, mesocycles,** and **macrocycles.** A microcycle generally lasts up to seven days. A mesocycle may last anywhere from two weeks to a few months and can be classified as a preparation, competition, peaking, or transition phase. The macrocycle refers to the overall training period, usually a year.

Periodization Models

Periodization, as it has been defined, refers to specific methods of manipulating the volume and intensity of the training. Traditional models of periodization describe a progression from high-volume and low-intensity work toward decreasing volume and increasing intensity during the different cycles (Table 13-4). Other periodization programs have been developed that also have potential advantages over nonperiodized approaches. A method that utilizes a reduction in volume and an increase in intensity in distinct steps during the training cycle is referred to as stepwise periodization. In the overreaching periodization model, there is a periodic short-term (one- to two-week) increase in volume or intensity, followed by a return to normal training. The newest concept in periodization is undulating periodization (Figure 13-4). With undulating periodization, training volume and intensity are increased and decreased during the course of a mesocycle (seven-day period).

While the body of research pertaining to periodization focuses on the effect of varying volume and exercise intensity, it should be clear that these are not the only variables that determine training adaptations. Other influential components that are addressed in program design include the following:

- Choice and number of exercises
- Order of exercises
- Resistance or load
- Number of sets per exercise
- Number of exercises per muscle group
- Repetition range(s)
- Type of contraction(s) emphasized and varied (i.e., concentric, eccentric, and isometric)
- Speed of movement
- Rest periods between sets
- Rest periods between training sessions
- Nutritional status of the client

Further research on periodized training programs is needed. However, for more advanced resistance-training designs, the evidence appears to strongly recommend utilizing a periodized approach as compared to constant repetition/set–type programs (Kraemer & Fragala, 2006).

Circuit Training

Circuit training is a popular resistance-exercise format that can be utilized with all populations and fitness levels, especially those in weight-loss programs. Circuit training was developed by R.E. Morgan and G.T. Anderson in 1953 at the University of Leeds in England (Kravitz, 1996). The term "circuit" refers to a number of carefully selected exercises arranged successively. In the original format, nine to 12 stations comprised the circuit, but this number may vary according to the design goals of the program. Each partici-

Table 13-4
Traditional Periodization Design

	Hypertrophy	Strength & Hypertrophy	Strength	Transition
Sets	1–5	1–5	1–5	1–2
Reps	9–12	6–8	1–5	13–20
Weeks	2–3	2–3	2–3	1–2

Note: For each period, the "rep zone" represents the intensity at which all exercises are performed to momentary muscular fatigue. Daily workout decisions are made regarding the type and number of exercises, order of exercises, loads to attain muscular fatigue in the rep zone, number of sets per exercise, number of exercises per muscle group, type of contraction(s) emphasized (i.e., concentric, eccentric, and isometric), speed of movement, rest periods between sets, and rest periods between training sessions.

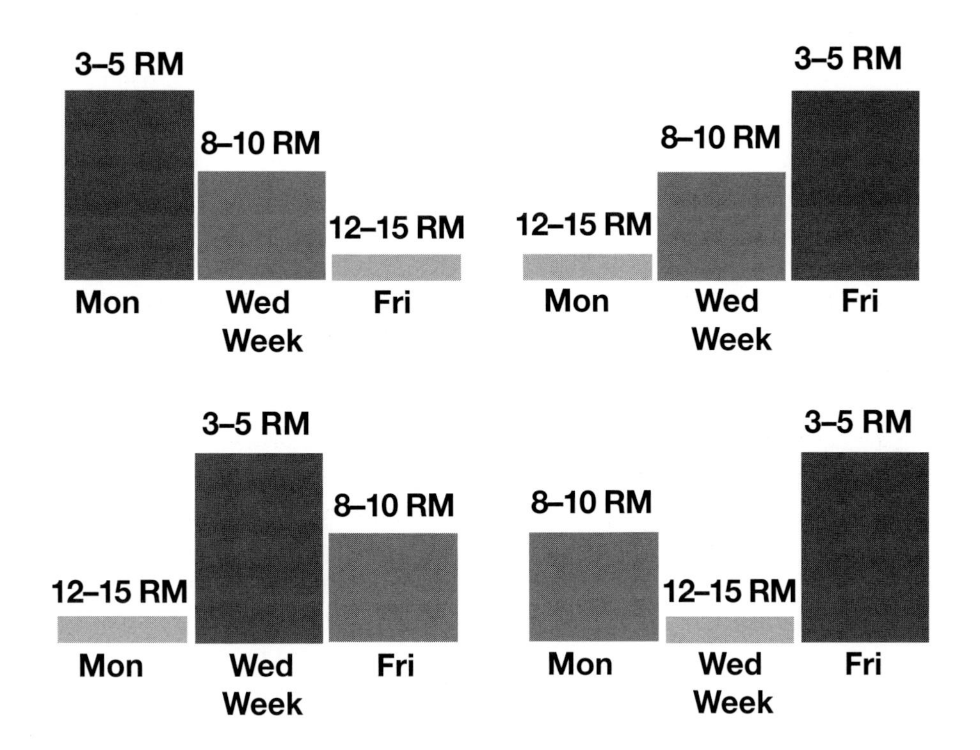

Figure 13-4
Undulating periodization design

Note: Typically, this method is utilized as a total-body workout scheme with seven to 10 exercises for the major muscle groups performed during each workout. Daily workout decisions are made regarding the type and number of exercises, order of exercises, loads to attain muscular fatigue in the "rep zone," number of sets per exercise, number of exercises per muscle group, type of contraction(s) emphasized (i.e., concentric, eccentric, and isometric), speed of movement, rest periods between sets, and rest periods between training sessions.

pant moves from one station to the next with little (15 to 30 seconds) or no rest, performing a 15- to 45-second set of eight to 20 repetitions at each station (using a resistance of about 40 to 60% of 1 RM). The program may be performed using one or more of the following: exercise machines, hand-held weights, elastic resistance, or calisthenics. The circuit is often repeated one to four times, depending on the fitness level and goals of the client.

Adding a 30-second to three-minute (or longer) cardio station between each resistance station (referred to as aerobic circuit training) promotes greater energy expenditure, which is desirable in weight-loss programs. One variation of this aerobic circuit-training model involves performing two, three, or four or more exercise stations consecutively, and then performing the cardio station. Table 13-5 presents a sample aerobic circuit-training workout that features a cardio station interspersed between every two resistance-exercise stations. Note the use of different aerobic modes for variety in this aerobic circuit design.

Table 13-5
Sample Aerobic Circuit-training Workout

- Chest fly
- Leg press
- 3-minute session on cycle ergometer
- Row pull
- Traveling lunge
- 3-minute session on treadmill
- Lat pull-down
- Shoulder press
- 3-minute session on elliptical trainer
- Triceps extension
- Biceps curl
- 3-minute session on cycle ergometer
- Heel raise
- Squat
- 3-minute session on rowing ergometer

Lifestyle Fitness Activities

Spontaneous physical activity is defined as the physical activity in a person's daily life that is not purposely structured. Researchers have begun to study the role that daily spontaneous standing, walking, and fidgeting movements play in combating weight gain and obesity; spontaneous physical activity is currently gaining great attention and scientific support as a possible (and novel) approach to combating the rise of obesity in children and adults (Levine et al., 2005). From this research, scientists have defined a new component of energy expenditure called non-exercise activity thermogenesis (NEAT) (physiological processes that produce heat). Levine and colleagues have revealed some unexpectedly useful data in this area.

NEAT represents the energy expenditure of daily activities such as standing, walking, moving, and shifting while sitting—all activities that are not considered planned physical activity in a person's daily life. To measure NEAT, investigators utilize highly sensitive monitoring devices known as inclinometers and triaxial accelerometers that are worn on the hips and legs. These devices capture data on body-position movements in all planes of movement 120 times per minute. Combining this information with other laboratory measurements of energy expenditure leads to a calculation of NEAT. The following are some particularly interesting research highlights on NEAT that may better explain the efficacy of this approach in increasing lifestyle fitness and verify the practicality of its use by fitness professionals in helping clients battle overweight and obesity.

Levine and colleagues (2005) recruited 20 healthy volunteers, all of whom did no structured physical activity. Of the 20 volunteers, five men and five women had **body mass index (BMI)** measurements of 23 ± 2 kg/m^2 (classifying them as lean) and five men and five women had BMI measurements of 33 ± 2 kg/m^2 (classifying them as Grade I obese; see Table 17-3, page 378). The authors noted that such a population was selected because they were less likely to have medical impediments and orthopedic troubles as compared to a morbidly obese group. Each subject wore an inclinometer and triaxial accelerometer and data were collected every half-second for 10 days.

Researchers were looking for lifestyle physical activity clues that might explain why 10 non-exercising lean men and women varied from 10 non-exercising mildly obese men and women. They found that the obese subjects were seated for 164 minutes longer each day than the lean participants. Additionally, the lean participants were standing and moving for 153 minutes more per day than the obese subjects. Sleep times between the two groups did not vary at all. Thus, the lean subjects had significantly more total-body ambulatory movement, which consisted of standing and walking. Amazingly, this extra movement by the lean subjects averaged 352 ± 65 calories per day, which is equivalent to 36.5 pounds (16.6 kg) of fat in one year.

Despite the time and effort spent designing structured exercise programs for clients wishing to achieve fitness and weight-management goals, not all individuals will maintain their exercise program. According to ACSM (2006), approximately 50% of people drop out of exercise within one year. Therefore, another important key to helping people attain their fitness and weight-loss goals is to find new behaviors that encourage more mobility in their daily lives. The U.S. Department of Health & Human Services has established a "Get Active" website (www.SmallStep.gov) to help individuals increase their levels of spontaneous physical activity. Table 13-6 presents a few of the many suggestions provided at this website to help people get moving and become more physically active during the day. Teaching clients how to make small movement changes in their daily lives may significantly contribute to some desirable changes in their overall fitness and weight-management goals.

Table 13-6
Lifestyle Suggestions to Help Clients Be More Active During the Day

- Walk to work.
- Walk during your lunch hour.
- Walk instead of drive whenever you can.
- Take a family walk after dinner.
- Skate to work instead of driving.
- Mow the lawn with a push mower.
- Walk to your place of worship instead of driving.
- Walk your dog.
- Replace the Sunday drive with a Sunday walk.
- Get off the bus a stop early and walk.
- Work and walk around the house.
- Take your dog to the park.
- Wash the car by hand.
- Run or walk fast when doing errands.
- Pace the sidelines at your kids' athletic games.
- Take the wheels off your luggage.
- Walk to a coworker's desk instead of emailing or calling.
- Make time in your day for physical activity.
- If you find it difficult to be active after work, try to fit exercise in before work.
- Take a walk break instead of a coffee break.
- Perform gardening and/or easy-to-do home-repair activities.
- Bring your groceries (from your car) into your house one bag at a time.
- Play with your kids at least 30 minutes a day.
- Dance to music.
- Walk briskly in the mall.
- Take the long way to the water cooler or break room.
- Take the stairs instead of the escalator.
- Go for a hike.

The SPORT Principle

The body adapts to the demands placed upon it. It is important to follow some basic principles of exercise training and progression when designing an exercise program to improve a client's level of fitness. The following training tactics are known as the SPORT principle: specificity, progression, overload, reversibility, and training effect (Kravitz, 2006).

Specificity

Specificity takes the guesswork out of training. This training principle states that for an individual to become proficient at any given movement, that movement itself must be trained and practiced. The body will adapt to the specific type of training placed upon it. Marathons, for example, require long-distance or high-volume endurance training. LWMCs should keep specificity in mind when working with clients, as adherence to this principle will allow clients to develop fitness and movement strategies that will help them when the time comes to actually perform the goal movements.

Progression

The human body responds much more efficiently to gradual and progressive challenges. With each new physical challenge, the physiological systems of the body challenged by the exercise will adapt with improved functioning ability. Gradual progression is the key to a successful training program. The early research of Hans Selye (1976) demonstrated that for progression to continue and physical exhaustion to be avoided, the exercise stimulus must be regularly and gradually increased.

Overload

Overload is introduced by increasing the intensity, duration, or frequency of an established level of exercise. For example, a cardiovascular-training program may be overloaded by adding another training bout during the week, lengthening the training sessions, or training at a higher level of cardiovascular intensity. In resistance training, overload is easily introduced by using heavier weights or by doing more repetitions. In flexibility, overload is created by doing additional stretches or trying to stretch further than the previous limits. If the exercise program becomes too easy or somewhat routine, it may be appropriate to add exercise overload. The body will adapt and develop a new training threshold, beyond which new benefits occur.

Reversibility

Consistent exercise is essential for maintaining the benefits of exercise, because these benefits cannot be stored; instead, they are reversible. If a person stops exercising, the body will adapt to the decreased exercise demands and start to decline from the previous fitness level.

Training Effect

Fitness levels are improved with regular, progressively overloaded training programs. This is known as the training effect. How much a person can improve is closely associated with his or her initial level of fitness, lifestyle habits, motivation, time investment in exercise, and certain genetic endowments. Regularly evaluating a client's progress can provide the information needed to establish an appropriate **maintenance stage** that coincides with the client's desired health and fitness goals. At this stage, the goal is to maintain this training effect by continuing with the exercise program, not adding more overload.

Functional Exercise Progression

Yoke and Kennedy present a new method of exercise selection and progression in their book, *Functional Exercise Progressions* (2004). This novel design progresses from simple to complex exercises that strengthen the core muscles (i.e., internal obliques, tranverse abdominis, multifidus, quadratus lumborum). Yoke and Kennedy's six-step exercise design system consists of the following:

- *Step #1:* Isolate and educate. The student is learning how to focus on the muscle and movement. Exercises in this level are often performed in the supine or prone position.
- *Step #2:* Isolate, educate, and add resistance. Add resistance to the exercises used in Step #1.
- *Step #3:* Add a functional-training position. To better challenge the stabilizing muscles, clients can perform exercise in a seated or standing position (for the targeted muscles).
- *Step #4:* Combine the functional challenge with resistance. Add some type of overload (e.g., weights, tubing, bands) to challenge the body's stabilizers in the functional position.
- *Step #5:* Involve multiple muscle groups with increasing resistance and core challenge. Clients can perform more complex exercises (e.g., squats, lunge variations) that combine

muscular fitness, balance, coordination, and stability.

- *Step #6:* Add balance, increased functional challenge, speed, and/or rotational movements. Use stability balls, wobble boards, and/or spinal rotation with the exercise movements. Yoke and Kennedy (2004) note that some individuals may never reach this level due to their fitness level or health history.

Exercise Precautions and Modifications

Although there are many health benefits of exercise, there are also several precautions of which an LWMC must be aware to maximize exercise safety. This section presents general precautions, concerns for exercising outdoors or in hot environments, precautions for special populations and the elderly, and alert signs for a stroke or a heart attack.

General Precautions

- Advise clients to always warm up before exercise. Usually a five- to seven-minute general warm-up on a treadmill, stationary bike, elliptical cross-trainer, or other aerobic mode is sufficient to prepare the cardiorespiratory and metabolic systems of the body for the workout to follow. A specific muscle-joint warm-up of light overload exercises is also recommended before moderate-to-heavy physical activity.
- Make sure clients learn how to perform the correct movement techniques for all exercises before progressively overloading the musculoskeletal system. Teach clients to exhale on the exertion when lifting heavy weights to avoid the **Valsalva maneuver,** which occurs when the glottis restricts air through the trachea, dramatically increasing thoracic pressure.
- Exercising too soon after a meal may hamper oxygen and nutrient delivery to the working muscles, leading to gastrointestinal distress. Advise clients to wait at least 60 to 90 minutes after a complete meal before engaging in moderate-intensity exercise. As a general rule, the higher the exercise intensity, and/or the greater the amount food consumed, the longer the time should be between eating and exercising.
- Teach clients how to correctly stack weights on barbells and to always use safety pins when using free weights.
- Advise clients to wear well-fitting and appropriate workout shoes and comfortable-fitting fitness clothing that allows the body to readily dissipate heat. Encourage them to wear less jewelry during workouts, as it may be damaged from the physical movements of the exercise, or possibly injure someone.
- Many people starting an exercise program do "too much, too soon, too hard," leading to pointless muscle soreness and possible injury. Encourage clients to start slowly and to incrementally increase the intensity and duration of their workouts.
- Promote the concept of "comfortably challenging" workouts, as opposed to training sessions that achieve total exhaustion. "No pain, no gain" has no scientific substantiation.
- An adequate cool-down (or recovery) is necessary to bring the body's physiological processes to pre-exercise levels. Include stretching exercises to facilitate relaxation of the muscles that have been vigorously contracting.
- Urge clients to hydrate before, during, and after the workout. Also, it is advisable to avoid caffeine or alcohol before and during exercise, as they may further dehydrate the body. Alcohol may also substantially affect a person's balance and judgment.
- It is a good idea to vary the intensity of workouts. Performing two high-intensity workouts in a row may cause undue

exhaustion, leading to possible overtraining and overuse complications.

- When training during vigorous exercise, encourage clients to slow down if they feel out of breath. For most people, being able to talk while exercising is a good indicator of appropriate exercise intensity, while gasping for breath is a sign of exercising too strenuously.
- Teach clients how to listen to their bodies. The human body has a remarkable sensory message system that informs one if there is pain, discomfort, and injury. Pain is an important message that tells an exerciser to slow down and/or stop.
- Don't urge clients to push through injuries, as doing so can lead to greater health problems. If pain persists for more than a few days, clients may need to seek the advice of a qualified healthcare professional.

Concerns for Exercising Outdoors or in Hot Environments

Environmental pollutants can be a concern when exercising outdoors or in big cities. Have clients learn where these unsafe areas are in their city and have them keep away from them whenever possible.

Encourage clients to wear sunscreen when exercising outdoors, especially in sunny environments.

Exercising in hot weather increases the risk of injury and other complications. The following guidelines will help clients avoid heat stress (see Chapter 3 for more on these environmental considerations):

- Drink water before, during, and after exercise.
- Wear loose-fitting clothes that allow for evaporation of sweat from the body onto the clothes.
- Avoid training during the hottest part of the day, usually between 10 a.m. and 4 p.m. (during the summer).
- Allow one to two weeks for acclimatization to a hot environment.
- Decrease workout intensity in a hot environment if necessary.
- Remember that some people are more heat-sensitive than others; this includes those who are overweight, obese, unfit, older, or have any combination of these conditions.

Precautions for Special Populations and Older Adults

It is essential to be able to identify those clients who may not have normal joint integrity or have diseases or disorders that could alter exercise performance. Seek council from a healthcare professional to determine appropriate precautions and modifications for any exercise program (see Chapter 18). For example, 50 million Americans have high blood pressure and many are not aware of this health risk (which is why it is called the "silent killer"). Hypertensive persons should not engage in high-intensity resistance exercise, as the increase in thoracic pressure may dangerously elevate blood pressure.

Exercise is one of the best things that older adults can do to improve quality of life. However, in addition to the general precautions, older adults must adhere to the following safety measures:

- For some seniors, the body may not be as flexible or supple as it used to be. Therefore, range-of-motion exercises that help clients perform ADL should be included in the fitness program.
- A basic rule for initiating exercise programs with older adults is to start slowly and then progress very gradually. Help them learn to adjust progressively to the new requirements of daily exercise and physical activity.
- Seniors often take medications that affect heart rate, blood pressure, and standing balance. Discussing any concerns with an appropriate health practitioner will enable a fitness professional to properly design safe and effective workouts for these older clients.

- For seniors, a good warm-up includes adequately preparing the musculoskeletal and cardiorespiratory systems, as well preparing the mind to facilitate mental readiness of the upcoming exercises.
- Among older adults, falls are the leading cause of injuries, hospital admissions for trauma, and deaths due to injury. Fractures are among the most serious health consequence of falls. Many of these falls and their resulting injuries are preventable. Strategies for preventing falls in older adults include incorporating exercises to improve strength, balance, and flexibility; exercising close to grab bars; improving lighting; and removing items that may cause tripping.

Signs of Stroke or Heart Attack

The symptoms of stroke are distinct and happen quickly. If a client is exhibiting any of the following symptoms and appears to be having a stroke, the LWMC should call 911 immediately:

- Sudden numbness or weakness of the face, arm, or leg (especially on one side of the body)
- Sudden confusion and trouble speaking or understanding speech
- Sudden trouble seeing in one or both eyes
- Sudden trouble walking, dizziness, or loss of balance or coordination
- Sudden severe headache with no known cause

The American Heart Association (www.americanheart.org) and other medical organizations advise that heart attack victims will experience one or more of the following warning signals:

- Uncomfortable pressure, fullness, squeezing, or pain in the center of the chest lasting more than a few minutes
- Pain spreading to the shoulders, neck, or arms. The pain may be mild to intense and may be located in the chest, upper abdomen, neck, jaw, or inside the arms or shoulders
- Chest discomfort with lightheadedness, fainting, sweating, nausea, or shortness of breath
- Anxiety, nervousness, and/or cold, sweaty skin
- Irregular or abnormally accelerating heart rate
- A pale face

Not all of these signs occur with every heart attack. A doctor who has studied the results of several tests must make the actual diagnosis of a heart attack. However, if a client appears to be experiencing a heart attack, the LWMC should call 911 immediately.

Summary

Educating and motivating clients to make a commitment to a physically active lifestyle of exercise and spontaneous movement may very well contribute to some desirable and profound changes to their overall health and weight-management goals. LWMCs need to take the leadership role in helping clients help themselves to positive health through meaningful physical-activity programming. By successfully doing this, LWMCs will indeed be meeting "head on" some of the most difficult health challenges facing modern society, including diabetes and obesity.

References

American College of Sports Medicine (2006). *ACSM's Guidelines for Exercise Testing and Prescription* (7th ed.). Philadelphia: Lippincott Williams and Wilkins.

Heyward, V.H. (2006). *Advanced Fitness Assessment and Exercise Prescription* (5th ed.). Champaign, Ill.: Human Kinetics.

Jakicic, J.M. et al. (2001). Appropriate intervention strategies for weight loss and prevention of weight regain for adults. *Medicine & Science in Sports & Exercise,* 33, 2145–2156.

Kraemer, W.J. & Fragala, M.S. (2006). Personalize it: Program design in resistance training. *ACSM's Health & Fitness Journal,* 10, 4, 7–17.

Kravitz, L. (2006). *Anybody's Guide to Total Fitness* (8th ed.). Dubuque, Iowa: Kendall/Hunt Publishers.

Kravitz, L. (1996). The fitness professional's complete guide to circuits and intervals. *IDEA Today,* 14, 1, 32–43.

Kravitz, L. et al. (1997). Does step exercise with handweights enhance training effects? *Journal of Strength and Conditioning Research,* 11, 194–199.

Levine, J.A. et al. (2005). Interindividual variation in posture allocation: Possible role in human obesity. *Science,* 307, 584–586.

Olson, M.S. & Williford, H.H. (1999). Martial arts exercise: A T.K.O. in studio fitness. *ACSM's Health & Fitness Journal,* 3, 6, 6–13.

Sanders, M.E. (1999). Cross over to the water. *IDEA Health and Fitness Source,* 17, 3, 53–58.

Selye, H. (1976). Forty years of stress research: Principal remaining problems and misconceptions. *Canadian Medical Association Journal*, 115, 53–56.

Sherman, R.M. (1997). The indoor cycling revolution. *IDEA Today,* 15, 3, 30–39.

Warburton, D.E., Gledhill, N., & Quinney, A. (2001). The effects of changes in musculoskeletal fitness on health. *Canadian Journal of Applied Physiology,* 26, 161–216.

Warburton, D.E., Nicol, C.W., & Bredin, S.S. (2006). Health benefits of physical activity: The evidence. *Canadian Medical Association Journal,* 174, 801–809.

Yoke, M. & Kennedy, C. (2004). *Functional Exercise Progressions.* Monterey, Calif.: Healthy Learning.

Suggested Reading

American College of Sports Medicine (2006). *ACSM's Resource Manual for Exercise Testing and Prescription* (5th ed.). Philadelphia: Lippincott Williams & Wilkins.

Fleck, S.J. & Kraemer, W.J. (2004). *Designing Resistance Training Programs* (3rd ed.). Champaign Ill.: Human Kinetics.

Kennedy, C.A. & Yoke, M.M. (2005). *Methods of Group Exercise Instruction.* Champaign, Ill.: Human Kinetics.

U.S. Department of Agriculture (2005). Dietary Guidelines for Americans 2005. www.health.gov/dietaryguidelines

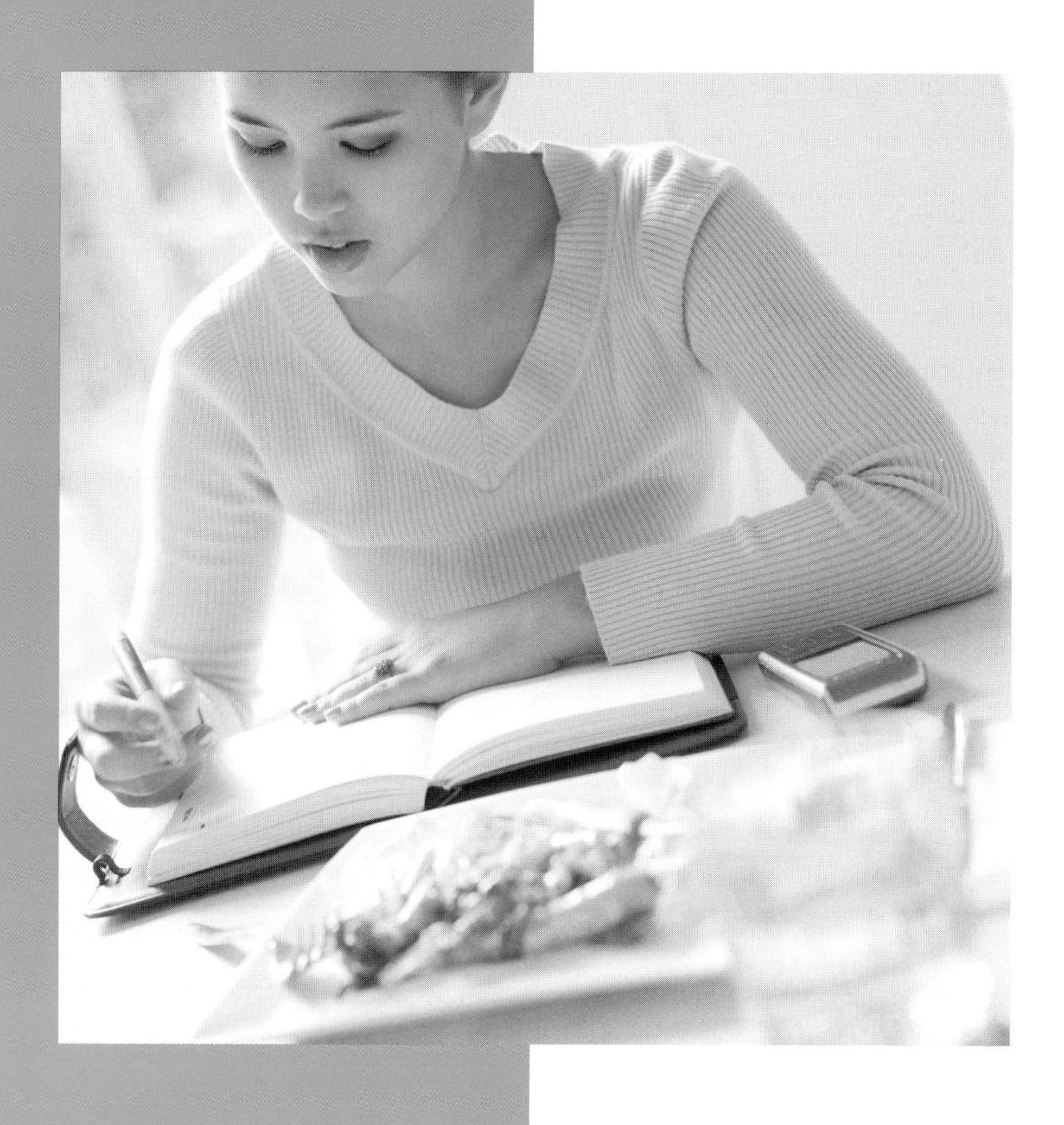

Debra Wein

Debra Wein, M.S., R.D., L.D.N., C.S.S.D., NSCA-CPT, is on the faculty at the University of Massachusetts Boston and Simmons College, and is the president of Sensible Nutrition, Inc. She has worked with the United States of America Track and Field Association, National Hockey League, Boston Ballet, and numerous marathon training teams.

Chapter 14

Nutritional Programming

Implementing a Nutrition Program

Clients will often describe schedules that barely allow them enough time to sleep, let alone eat healthy meals and exercise regularly. Grocery shopping and preparing meals are often out of the question. Even though they may be well aware that fueling their bodies with healthy foods is important, "life" often gets in the way.

It is important to help clients understand that they won't *find* the time to exercise and eat right—they must make the time. Contrary to popular belief (or popular excuses), eating a healthy diet is not impossible. Like anything else, it takes knowledge, practice, and planning to set goals and overcome barriers. (For more information on assessing a client's readiness for change, see Chapter 15.)

Eating behaviors, which are among the most complex of human behaviors, are learned habits that are deeply entrenched and strongly influenced by religious, ethnic, and family customs. Emotional influences also play an important role in why, when, and what people eat. But it is possible for people to "relearn" how to eat more healthfully. The processes of eating, cooking, and choosing foods are shaped by one's past, but these behaviors can be modified. Behavior modification, however, takes time. When working with clients, the focus should remain on gradually modifying eating and exercise behaviors, both of which are necessary for

IN THIS CHAPTER:

sustainable weight loss. Lifestyle & Weight Management Consultants (LWMCs) should remind clients that small, permanent changes in both behavior and weight loss are better than large, temporary ones.

Behavior modification involves the following:

- Modifying old ways of eating and developing healthier eating habits
- Taking small steps in a consistent direction
- Focusing on environmental or situational control of eating in a program that is designed to reduce the exposure, susceptibility, and response to environmental situations that result in high calorie intake and/or low energy expenditure
- Self-monitoring and self-management

The Nutrition Interview

Understanding a Client's Current Dietary Habits

An effective way to learn about a client's current dietary habits is to administer a lifestyle and health-history questionnaire (Figure 14-1), which may be used to identify clients whose needs fall outside the **scope of practice** of an LWMC. Alternatively, this questionnaire can be administered by the LWMC in an interview format, which might stimulate greater conversation and insight.

Several methods can be used to learn more about a client's eating and lifestyle patterns, including food diaries, food records, 24-hour recall, and food-frequency questionnaires. With practice, an LWMC may find that certain clients may be very likely to complete food records, while others may only be willing or able to give a 24-hour diet recall. Regardless of which method is used, the information gleaned from these tools will be invaluable in helping clients meet their goals.

Food Diary/Food Record

Keeping a food diary involves having clients describe a "typical" eating day, including all foods and beverages (Figure 14-2). Clients should be urged to be specific and estimate amounts as best they can. Be sure to discuss weekends versus weekdays. Space is provided in the food diary for the client to note how hungry he or she is when the food is consumed. Additional space could be added to include information on mood, location, and time of day for more detailed intake information.

One thing to consider is that people generally underestimate or under-report their caloric intake and tend to eat more salads, vegetables, and lower-calorie foods when using a food diary than their weight might suggest. Experience with probing the client, asking nonjudgmental questions, and offering a supportive environment is likely to reveal a more truthful picture of a client's eating pattern.

Proper instruction on how to keep food records will often yield better results than just handing a client a sheet of paper and telling him or her to "write down what you eat." LWMCs should share the following guidelines with clients to help them more accurately report their food intakes (Figure 14-3):

- Keep a record for three consecutive days, including one weekend day (for example, Thursday-Friday-Saturday or Sunday-Monday-Tuesday). Advise the client to choose three days that would be typical of his or her usual intake (to obtain the most accurate picture of the client's diet).
- The client should record everything he or she eats or drinks during those days, including water, any added salt, candies, gum, condiments, vitamin/mineral supplements, sports drinks, coffee, tea, medications, and alcoholic beverages.
- Use a separate sheet of paper for each day and create columns with the following titles: Meal/Snack Time, Food/Beverage & Amount, Food Group Servings, Hunger Level, and Location.
- In the first column, record whether the foods and/or beverages were part of a meal (and which one) or consumed as part of a snack.

Figure 14-1
Sample lifestyle and health-history questionnaire

Medical Information

1. How would you describe your present state of health?
   ❑ very well ❑ healthy ❑ unhealthy ❑ ill ❑ other:______________________
2. Are you taking any prescription medications? ❑ Yes ❑ No
   If yes, what medications and why?______________________
   Do these interact with foods or weight loss in any way?
3. Do you take any over-the-counter medications or supplements? ❑ Yes ❑ No
   If yes, what medications and why?______________________
4. When was the last time you visited your physician?______________________
5. Have you ever had your cholesterol checked? ❑ Yes ❑ No
   What were the results?______________________ Date of test:__________
   Total Cholesterol:________ HDL:________ LDL:________ TG:________
6. Have you ever had your blood sugar checked? ❑ Yes ❑ No
   What were the results?______________________ Date of test:__________
7. Please check those that apply to you and list any important information about your condition:

❑ Allergies (Specify: ____________)
❑ Amenorrhea
❑ Anemia
❑ Anxiety
❑ Arthritis
❑ Asthma
❑ Celiac disease
❑ Chronic sinus condition
❑ Constipation
❑ Crohn's disease
❑ Depression
❑ Diabetes
❑ Diarrhea
❑ Disordered eating
❑ Intestinal problems
❑ Gastroesophageal reflux disease (GERD)
❑ High blood pressure
❑ Hyper-/hypothyroidism
❑ Hypoglycemia
❑ Insomnia
❑ Intestinal problems
❑ Irritable bowel syndrome (IBS)
❑ Irritability
❑ Menopausal symptoms
❑ Osteoporosis
❑ Premenstrual syndrome (PMS)
❑ Polycystic ovary disease
❑ Pregnant
❑ Ulcer
❑ Skin problems
❑ Major surgeries:
❑ Past injuries:
❑ Describe any other health conditions that you have:______________
____
____
____

Family History

8. Has anyone in your immediate family been diagnosed with any of the following?
   ❑ Heart disease If yes, what is the relation:____________ Age of diagnosis:_____
   ❑ High cholesterol If yes, what is the relation:____________ Age of diagnosis:_____
   ❑ High blood pressure If yes, what is the relation:____________ Age of diagnosis:_____
   ❑ Cancer If yes, what is the relation:____________ Age of diagnosis:_____
   ❑ Diabetes If yes, what is the relation:____________ Age of diagnosis:_____
   ❑ Osteoporosis If yes, what is the relation:____________ Age of diagnosis:_____
9. What are your dietary goals?______________________
10. Have you ever followed a modified diet to manage a health condition? ❑ Yes ❑ No
    If so, describe:______________________
11. Are you currently following a specialized diet (e.g., low-sodium, low-fat)? ❑ Yes ❑ No
    If so, what type of diet?______________________
12. Why did you choose this diet?______________________
    Was the diet prescribed by a physician? ❑ Yes ❑ No
    How long have you been on the diet?______________________
13. Have you ever met with a registered dietitian? ❑ Yes ❑ No
    Are you interested in meeting with one? ❑ Yes ❑ No
14. What do you consider to be the major challenges/issues in your diet and eating plan (e.g., eating late at night, snacking on high-fat foods, skipping meals, lack of variety)?

Figure 14-1
Continued

15. How much water do you drink per day? ____8-ounce glasses
16. Do you have any food allergies or intolerance? ❑ Yes ❑ No
    If so, what?____________________
17. Who purchases and prepares your food?
    ❑ Self
    ❑ Spouse
    ❑ Parent
    ❑ Minimal preparation
18. How often do you dine out or purchase take-out? ____times per week
19. Please specify the type of restaurants for each meal:
    Breakfast:____________________
    Lunch:____________________
    Dinner:____________________
    Snacks:____________________

Habits

20. Do you crave any foods? ❑ Yes ❑ No
    If so, please specify:____________________
21. How is your appetite affected by stress?
    ❑ increased ❑ not affected ❑ decreased
22. Do you drink alcohol? ❑ Yes ❑ No
    How often? ____times per week
    Average amount? ____glasses
23. Do you drink caffeinated beverages? ❑ Yes ❑ No
    Average number per day ________
24. Do you use tobacco? ❑ Yes ❑ No
    How much (cigarettes, cigars, chewing tobacco per day)?
25. Do you take any vitamin, mineral, or herbal supplements? ❑ Yes ❑ No
    Please list type and amount per day:____________________
26. Do you currently participate in any structured physical activity? ❑ Yes ❑ No
    If so, please describe:
    ____minutes of cardiovascular activity, ____times per week
    ____strength-training sessions, ____times per week
    ____minutes of flexibility, ____times per week
    ____minutes of sports per week
    List sports:____________________
27. Have you experienced any injuries that may limit your activity?
    If so, please describe:____________________
28. On a scale of 1–10, how ready are you to adopt a healthier lifestyle?
    1 = very unlikely 10 = very likely __________

Weight History

29. What would you like to do with your weight?
    ❑ lose weight ❑ gain weight ❑ maintain weight
30. What was your lowest weight within the past five years? ____lb
31. What was your highest weight within the past five years? ____lb
32. What do you consider to be your ideal weight? ____lb ❑ don't know
33. What is your present weight? ____lb ❑ don't know
34. What are your current waist and hip circumferences? ________waist ________ hip
35. What is your present body composition? ____% body fat ❑ don't know

Food	Description	Amount	Level of Hunger (1–5)

Note: 1 = Not hungry at all; 5 = Very hungry

Figure 14-2
Sample food diary

Meal/Snack Time		Food/Beverage & Amount	Food Group Servings	Hunger Level	Location	Other Comments
BREAKFAST						
SNACK						
LUNCH						
SNACK						
DINNER						

Figure 14-3
Sample food log

- In the first column, the client should also record the time when all foods and beverages were consumed. The client should record everything immediately after each meal or snack so that he or she does not forget what was eaten.
- In the second column, the client should give as much specific information as possible:
  - Method of cooking (baked, broiled, fried, boiled, toasted)
  - Brand names of commercial products
  - Specific foods and drinks
    - Bread (whole wheat, white, rye; number of slices per loaf)
    - Milk (whole, low-fat, skim, protein-enriched)
    - Margarine (stick, tub, diet)
    - Vegetables (canned, fresh, frozen)
    - Meats (fat trimmed, weighed with bone, skinned)
    - Drinks (light, low-calorie, diet, low-fat), including additions such as cream and sugar
    - Snacks (pretzels, chips, nuts, dry roasted, raw)
    - Size of fruits or vegetables (small, medium, large, extra large)
    - Ingredients/condiments used in salads and sandwiches (e.g., mayo, ketchup, mustard, gravy, sauce, grated cheese, salad dressing, lettuce, and tomato)
- The client should also list the amount of food or beverage consumed, measured by a scale (for weight in ounces or grams), a ruler (for height, length, and width), or via a household measure (for volume: cups, tablespoons, or teaspoons). If possible, the client should weigh and measure foods after preparation and indicate when it was done. He or she can use package-label information on commercially made products.
- The client should also record any significant feelings or emotions he or she was experiencing before and after eating, his or her hunger level, where the food was eaten, and any obstacles that were faced when making decisions and choices.

Description and Procedure

Sources: Mahabir, 2006; Svendsen et al., 2006; Willet, 2001

- The client records intake throughout the day, including water and beverages. The client also records daily physical activity. The client is solely responsible for the foods consumed throughout the day, as well as for recording them.
- By reviewing food intake along with the calories and **fat** consumed, the LWMC can easily pinpoint any trouble spots with food (e.g., late-night eating, meal skipping).
- The client must be very specific. Instead of writing "ham sandwich," write down how much ham was actually on the sandwich. Was it 3 ounces or (88 mL) 8 ounces (237 mL)? Include what types of condiments were used, etc.

Necessary Components

- The client only needs to record his or her food intake in a food diary booklet, in a notebook, or on pieces of paper. LWMCs should teach clients that it is best to record food intake immediately after consumption, instead of writing it down at the end of the day when it is easy to forget foods consumed.

Pros

- Easy to administer
- Economical
- Increased awareness of habits and foods consumed

Cons

- Dependent on the literacy of the client
- Respondent burden
- Recall bias; records may not reflect "typical" intakes; interest in "pleasing" the facilitator may alter consumption or tracking

- Lack of knowledge on estimating portion sizes, calories, and fat content of foods consumed

24-hour Recall

The same tools used for the food diary can be used when administering the 24-hour recall (see Figures 14-2 and 14-3). Obviously, a major limitation of the 24-hour recall is that "yesterday" may not truly reflect the scope of a person's typical eating patterns. In addition, this tool relies heavily on memory.

Description and Procedure

Sources: Resnicow et al., 2000; Schatzkin et al., 2003

- Obtain information on food and fluid intake for the previous day or previous 24 hours.
- The 24-hour recall is based on the assumption that the intake described is typical of daily intake.
- A five-pass method can be used that includes the following
  - A "quick list" pass in which the respondent is asked to list everything consumed in the previous day
  - A "forgotten foods" pass in which a standard list of foods and beverages that are often forgotten is read to prompt recall
  - A "time and occasion" pass in which the time and name for each eating occasion is collected
  - A "detailed" pass in which the detailed descriptions and portion sizes are collected and the time interval between meals is reviewed to check for additional foods
  - The "final" pass—one last opportunity to recall the foods consumed

Necessary Components

- Time that the food or beverage was consumed
- The food or beverage item
- Serving size of the food or beverage item
- How the food was prepared
- Where the client consumed the food or beverage item
- Any relevant notes regarding the meal or food item

Pros

- Easy to administer
- Not dependent on the literacy of the respondent
- Precision and, when multiple days are assessed, validity
- Low administration costs

Cons

- The need to obtain multiple recalls to reliably estimate usual intake
- Participant burden
- Difficulty of the estimation of portion sizes
- Recall bias; records may not reflect "typical" intakes; interest in "pleasing" the facilitator may alter consumption or tracking

Food-frequency Questionnaire

Food-frequency questionnaires (FFQ) may be challenging for clients, as it can be difficult to truly estimate the number of times an individual food is eaten. However, the benefit of this tool is that the client is less likely to forget foods, because they are listed on the chart. It is also easy to identify the type of diet the client typically follows (e.g., low-fat/high-fiber, high-protein/high-fat). Figure 14-4 presents a portion of a sample food-frequency questionnaire.

Description and Procedure

Sources: Mahabir, 2006; Resnicow et al., 2000; Schatzkin et al., 2003; Svendsen et al., 2006; Willett, 2001

- The FFQ identifies foods that the client most commonly eats.
- The client indicates, on average, how much and how often he or she consumes different foods.
- Analysis of the FFQ data provides information about the daily intake of many nutrients.

Figure 14-4
Sample food-frequency questionnaire

Food	Every Day (Always)	3 or 4 Times/Week (Often)	Every 2 or 3 Weeks (Sometimes)	Don't Eat (Never)
Dairy Products				
Milk, whole				
Milk, reduced fat				
Milk, nonfat				
Cottage cheese				
Cream cheese				
Other cheeses				
Yogurt				
Ice cream				
Sherbet				
Puddings				
Margarine				
Butter				
Other				
Meats				
Beef, hamburger				
Poultry				
Pork, ham				
Bacon, sausage				
Cold cuts, hot dogs				
Other				
Fish				
Canned tuna				
Breaded fish				
Fresh or frozen fish				
Eggs				
Peanut butter				
Grain products				
Bread, white				
Bread, whole wheat				
Rolls, muffins				
Pancakes, waffles				
Bagels				
Pasta, spaghetti				
Pasta, macaroni and cheese				
Rice				
Crackers				
Other				

Food	Every Day (Always)	3 or 4 Times/Week (Often)	Every 2 or 3 Weeks (Sometimes)	Don't Eat (Never)
Cereals				
Sugar-coated				
High-fiber (bran)				
Natural (granola)				
Plain (e.g., Cheerios®)				
Fortified				
Other				
Fruits				
Oranges, orange juice				
Tomatoes, tomato juice				
Grapefruit, grapefruit juice				
Strawberries				
Cranberry juice				
Apples, apple juice				
Grapes, grape juice				
Fruit drink				
Peaches				
Bananas				
Other				
Vegetables				
Peppers				
Potatoes				
Lettuce				
Broccoli				
Spinach				
Carrots				
Corn				
Squash				
Peas				
Green beans				
Beets				
Other				
Snacks and Sweets				
Chips (potato, corn)				
Pretzels				
Popcorn				
French fries				
Cookies				
Pastries				
Candy				
Sugar, honey, jelly				
Soda, regular				
Soda, diet				
Cocoa				
Other				

Necessary Components

- Vary among FFQs, but typically include a large list of foods with their corresponding frequency of consumption

Pros

- Relatively low administrative costs
- Ability to assess usual and longer-term intake

Cons

- Inaccuracy of absolute nutrient values
- Fluctuation of nutrient values depending on instrument length and structure
- Lack of detail regarding specific foods
- General imprecision
- Recall bias; records may not reflect "typical" intakes; interest in "pleasing" the facilitator may alter consumption or tracking
- Seasonal variability
- Cultural/diet variability (e.g., vegetarians, individuals on therapeutic diets)

Food Models and Portion Estimates

A portion is the amount of food a person chooses to eat, while a serving is a standardized amount of a food used to estimate and/or evaluate one's intake. Portions are very difficult for some to estimate, and correct estimates could mean the difference between a 1,400-calorie diet and a 2,200-calorie diet.

LWMCs can assist clients in a number of ways when estimating their portions. The guidelines presented in Figure 14-5 can be used to help clients more accurately determine the amount of food that they are consuming (Wein, 2006).

In addition, there are a number of tools that can be purchased to help clients better understand their portion sizes. For example, the National Dairy Council sells paper cutouts of various foods with detailed nutrition information on the back. Also, various companies sell plastic food models that demonstrate average and large sizes. Food models range from $2 for a single food to $125 for an extensive package. Some of these companies also sell index cards with pictures of foods in specific serving sizes. The sizes range from 1-ounce servings to "supersize" servings, so clients can visualize the difference and understand how portion-size choices impact their diets.

Using the 2005 USDA Dietary Guidelines

The 2005 Dietary Guidelines for Americans provide science-based advice aimed at promoting health and reducing the risk for major chronic diseases through diet and physical activity (United States Department of Agriculture, 2005). The intent of the Dietary Guidelines is to summarize and synthesize knowledge regarding individual nutrients and food components into recommendations for a pattern of eating that can be adopted by the public.

These guidelines encourage most Americans to eat fewer calories, be more active, and make wiser food choices. A basic premise of the Dietary Guidelines is that nutrient needs should be met primarily through consuming foods. Foods provide an array of nutrients and other compounds that may have beneficial effects on health. In certain cases, fortified foods and dietary supplements may be useful sources of one or more nutrients that otherwise might be consumed in less than recommended amounts. Dietary supplements, while recommended in some cases, cannot replace a healthful diet. The following sections present recommendations for an active person or athlete. The complete guidelines can be found at www.health.gov/dietaryguidelines.

General Guidelines

LWMCs should review the following guidelines with their clients:

- Consume a variety of nutrient-dense foods and beverages from the basic food groups, while choosing foods that limit the intake of saturated and **trans fats, cholesterol,** added sugars, salt, and alcohol.

Figure 14-5
Guidelines for determining food portions

Source: Wein, D. (2006). *SNaC Pack: The Health Professional's Guide to Nutrition.* www.sensiblenutrition.com

Meat, Poultry, Fish

- ¾ ounce equals:
  - Amount in a chicken wing
- 1½ ounces equals:
  - Amount in a chicken thigh
- 3 ounces equal
  - Size of the palm of a woman's hand (3 x 3½ inches)
  - Amount in a small chicken breast
  - Size of a deck of cards
  - Size of a checkbook
- 4 ounces equals:
  - Amount in a sandwich
  - Amount in a quarter-pound hamburger
  - Amount in an Asian stir-fry
- 5 ounces equals:
  - Amount on an entree salad
- 6 ounces equals:
  - A restaurant chicken breast (6 inches across)
  - Typical lunch or cafeteria portion
- 8 to 12 ounces equals:
  - Common evening restaurant portion

Cheese

- 1 ounce equals:
  - One slice on a sandwich or hamburger
  - Amount on a small slice of pizza
  - 1-inch cube, one small wedge, or a strip the size of a pinky finger
  - 3 tablespoons of parmesan
  - 1 tablespoon of feta or shredded cheese (salad bar)
- 2 ounces equals:
  - Amount on a large slice of pizza

Vegetables

- ½ cup equals:
  - Cafeteria or restaurant portion
  - Size of one-half of a baseball
  - Coleslaw or beans at a barbeque restaurant
  - Amount in a bowl of vegetable soup
- 1 cup equals:
  - Amount in side dinner salad
  - Size of one baseball
- 2 to 4 cups equals:
  - Amount on a salad bar plate

Fruit

- One serving equals:
  - 60 calories, or the size of a fist
  - One large grapefruit
  - 15 grapes or cherries
  - One medium apple or orange (2½ inches across, or a little bigger than a tennis ball)
  - One small banana (6 inches, or the length of dollar bill)
  - 1 cup of pineapple, blackberries, or blueberries
  - 1½ cups of melon or strawberries
  - Four dried prunes
  - 3 tablespoons of raisins (⅛ cup or two miniature boxes)

Potato

- One small potato equals:
  - 70 calories (2½ inches long)
- One medium potato equals:
  - 110 calories (4 inches long)
- One large potato equals:
  - 140 calories (5 inches long)
  - Typical restaurant portion
- One extra-large potato equals:
  - 200 calories (6 inches long)

Fats

- One butter pat equals:
  - 45 calories
- 1 tablespoon of mayonnaise equals:
  - 100 calories (typical amount on a sandwich)
- 2 tablespoons of salad dressing equals:
  - 150 calories (typical amount on a dinner salad)
  - One small ladle (salad bar)
  - One-half large ladle (salad bar)

Beverages

- 1½ ounces equals one jigger of an alcoholic drink
- 4 to 6 ounces equals a typical juice portion (restaurant)
- 6 ounces equals a glass of wine (restaurant)
- 8 ounces equals a common milk portion or the size of one's fist (⅔ soda can)
- 12 ounces equals one can/bottle of beer or soda

Source: Wein, 2006

- To maintain body weight in a healthy range, balance calories from foods and beverages with calories expended.
- Meet recommended intakes within energy needs by adopting a balanced eating pattern, such as the USDA Food Guide or the **DASH eating plan** (see Chapter 7). In other words, maximize nutrient intake by choosing a wide variety of nutrient-dense foods. This is especially important for people who are restricting their caloric intake to lose weight. Choosing foods that are high in calories and low in nutrients may mean that the active individual is not adequately taking in appropriate nutrients for performance (i.e., **protein, complex carbohydrates,** B vitamins, iron, calcium, potassium).
- To prevent gradual weight gain over time, make small decreases in food and beverage calories and increase physical activity. Also be sure to include strength-training activities, which may help to prevent a decrease in metabolism over time.
- Individuals who need to lose weight should aim for a slow, steady weight loss by decreasing calorie intake while maintaining an adequate nutrient intake and increasing physical activity. A good goal is to decrease intake by 250 calories (e.g., 2½ tablespoons of butter or mayonnaise or a small order of french fries), while increasing expenditure by 250 calories. Doing so will promote a weight-loss goal of approximately 1 pound per week. Overweight adults and overweight children with chronic diseases and/or on medication should consult a healthcare provider about weight-loss strategies prior to starting a weight-reduction program to ensure appropriate management of other health conditions.

Food Groups to Encourage

LWMCs should review the following guidelines with their clients:

- Consume a sufficient amount of fruits and vegetables while staying within energy needs. Two cups of fruit and 2½ cups of vegetables per day are recommended for a 2,000-calorie intake, with higher or lower amounts depending on the calorie level. Fruits and vegetables are high in complex carbohydrates, **vitamins, minerals,** and **fiber.** Active people cannot train properly without adequate **carbohydrates** in the diet.
- Choose a variety of fruits and vegetables each day. In particular, select from all five vegetable subgroups (dark green, orange, legumes, starchy vegetables, and other vegetables) several times a week. Choosing a variety will allow an active person to maximize his or her nutrient intake, thereby reducing the need for supplements.
- Consume three or more ounce-equivalents of whole-grain products per day. In all, Americans are advised to eat 6 ounces of grains each day with at least half of the grains coming from whole grains, based on a 2,000-calorie diet. Whole-grain foods provide an active individual with the complex carbohydrates necessary to perform endurance activities such as running or biking and high-intensity activities such as strength training or sprinting. These foods also supply the B vitamins necessary for energy production. In addition, many of these products are fortified with iron, which also is important for an athlete. Diets rich in whole grains may reduce the risk of heart disease and diabetes and help with weight management.
- Consume three cups per day of fat-free or low-fat milk or equivalent milk products. These products are low-fat sources of protein, which is necessary to promote muscle growth, and are the most available sources of calcium, which is important for bone health.

Fats

LWMCs should review the following guidelines with their clients:

- Consume less than 10% of calories from **saturated fats** and animal fats and less than 300 mg/day of cholesterol, and keep trans fat consumption as low as possible. Saturated fats, trans fats, and cholesterol can clog arteries and affect long-term health and performance.
- Keep total fat intake between 20 and 35% of calories, with most fats coming from sources of **polyunsaturated** and **monounsaturated fatty acids,** such as fish, nuts, and vegetable oils. Active individuals need higher amounts of carbohydrates (55 to 65% of total calories) and protein (20 to 30% of total calories), so limiting fats in the diet is a good idea.
- When selecting and preparing meat, poultry, dry beans, and milk or milk products, make choices that are lean, low-fat, or fat-free. Low-fat sources of protein are the best choices for an active individual's long-term health.
- Limit intake of fats and oils high in saturated and/or trans fats, and choose products low in these fats and oils.

Carbohydrates

LWMCs should review the following guidelines with their clients:

- Choose fiber-rich fruits, vegetables, and whole grains at each meal and for snacks. Active individuals require 55 to 65% of total calories as carbohydrates, of which fiber-rich foods are excellent sources.
- Choose and prepare foods and beverages with little added sugars or caloric sweeteners. Added sugars may mean more fluctuations in glucose level (**hypoglycemia** or **hyperglycemia**), which may affect performance.

Sodium and Potassium

LWMCs should review the following guidelines with their clients:

- Consume less than 2,300 mg of sodium (approximately 1 teaspoon of salt) per day.
- Choose and prepare foods with little salt. At the same time, consume potassium-rich foods, such as fruits and vegetables. Highly active individuals may sweat out more electrolytes and need to replace them through their diet.

Alcoholic Beverages

LWMCs should review the following guideline with their clients:

- Those who choose to drink alcoholic beverages should do so sensibly and in moderation, which is defined as the consumption of up to one drink per day for women and up to two drinks per day for men. Alcohol may promote **dehydration,** which may result in poor exercise performance.

Addressing A Client's Nutritional Needs While Staying Within the LWMC's Scope of Practice

Making specific nutrition/nutrient recommendations and developing meal plans are beyond the scope of practice of an LWMC. However, providing general nutrition information on nutrition and weight management can be helpful and useful for clients. An LWMC must know when to tackle and when to refer nutrition issues, as doing so will help maintain professionalism as well as decrease the risk of liability (see Chapter 19 and Appendix A).

Table 14-1 features a list of issues that an LWMC might discuss with clients, as well as issues that are more appropriate for referral. Every LWMC must ultimately determine what topics are appropriate to discuss with the client. An LWMC should not hesitate to refer a client to a registered dietitian (R.D.) or more qualified individual if the client's needs exceed the LWMC's training and level of expertise. Refer to Chapter 11 for more information on making appropriate referrals.

Table 14-1
Scope of Practice Guidelines for Nutrition

Appropriate Nutrition Topics for an LWMC
- MyPyramid Guidelines
- Suggestions for weight loss
- Pre-evaluations and use of a food diary
- Lifestyle changes
- Hydration
- Recipes
- Support
- Basic pre- and post-exercise nutrition
- Weight-loss physiology

Nutrition Areas That Should Be Referred
- Specific meal plans
- Tailored plans
- Medications
- Diseases
  - Cardiovascular disease
  - Hypertension
  - Hyperlipidemia
  - Diabetes
  - Eating disorders
  - AIDS
- Medical diagnoses
  - Anemia
  - Osteoporosis
  - Polycystic ovary disease
- Post-op
- Yo-yo dieting
- Supplements
- Large weight loss or morbid obesity

Qualified registered dietitians can be located through the following organizations and channels:
- The American Dietetic Association (www.eatright.org)
- SCAN Sports, Cardiovascular, and Wellness Nutritionists (www.scan-dpg.org)
- Professional meetings
- Local fitness centers
- Medical professionals
- Professional networking

What do all of those terms and letters mean?
- Nutritionist—A general term that anyone can really use
- Registered dietitian (R.D.)—An R.D. is an individual who has completed certain related coursework, an undergraduate degree, and an approved internship, and has passed a national exam given by the Commission on Dietetic Registration (CDR). An R.D. also completes yearly continuing education requirements.
- Certified specialist in sports dietetics (C.S.S.D.)— An accreditation from the credentialing agency of the American Dietetic Association
- Licensed dietitian/nutritionist (L.D./N., L.D., or L.N.)—Requirements for these titles vary by state. California, for example, does not offer licensure to dietitians.
- Master of science or doctorate degree (M.S. or Ph.D.)—LWMCs should always check that the degree was earned in a related field (e.g., nutrition, exercise science, psychology) before making a referral.

What questions should the R.D. be asked?
- How does he or she stay up-to-date on the latest research?
- Which organizations does he or she belong to? What hospital or medical group is he or she affiliated with?
- What journals or research does he or she read?
- What are the fees? What is included in the appointment?
- What is his or her area of specialty or expertise (e.g., age groups, certain populations)?
- Does he or she sell vitamins, supplements, or foods?
- Discuss a current client situation with the R.D. to get a better idea of his or her approach or philosophy on nutrition.

Nutritional Program Planning for the Weight-loss Client

Estimating Caloric Needs

There are a variety of methods that can be used to estimate a client's daily calorie needs. Daily energy needs (caloric requirement) are determined by three factors:

- **Resting metabolic rate (RMR)**
- Thermogenesis (calories required for heat production)
- Physical activity

Resting metabolic rate is the amount of energy (measured in calories) expended by the body during quiet rest. RMR makes up between 60 and 80% of the total calories used daily. Physical activity is the second largest factor contributing to daily calorie requirements. This is the most variable component of RMR, as this number changes based on the frequency, intensity, and duration of an individual's workouts. Thermogenesis, also referred to as the **thermic effect of food,** is the smallest component. This is the amount of calories needed to digest and absorb the foods that are consumed. While certain diets claim to enhance this component (e.g., food-combining programs), no research exists to support that concept. The bottom line is that regular physical activity is the most effective way to increase the body's caloric expenditures.

The following section reviews methods for determining a client's energy needs. This information does not, however, take into account a client's disease risk in relation to his or her weight or nutritional habits. For more information on how to use tools such **waist-to-hip ratio** and **body mass index (BMI),** see Chapter 10.

Calculating Energy Needs

There are numerous ways to calculate a client's daily caloric needs. The simplest method is to multiply the client's weight (in pounds) by the appropriate conversion factor (Table 14-2). This calculation will yield an approximation of how many calories the individual needs to maintain his or her current weight, based on activity level and gender.

Table 14-2
Conversion Factors for Estimating Daily Caloric Requirements Based on Gender and Activity Level

	Activity Level		
	Light	Moderate	Heavy
Male	17	19	23
Female	16	17	30

Light activity level: Walking (level surface, 2.5–3.0 mph), housecleaning, child care, golf

Moderate activity level: Walking (3.5–4.0 mph), cycling, skiing, tennis, dancing

Heavy activity level: Walking with a load uphill, basketball, climbing, football, soccer

The Harris-Benedict equation for **basal metabolic rate (BMR)** takes into account the individual's weight, height, age, and gender. However, it has been shown to slightly underestimate BMR in females and slightly overestimate BMR in males (Harris & Benedict, 1919).

Harris-Benedict Equation

For men: BMR = [13.75 x weight (kg)] + [5.003 x height (cm)] – [6.775 x age] + 66.5

For women: BMR = [9.563 x weight (kg)] + [1.850 x height (cm)] – [4.676 x age] + 655.1

Note: To determine weight in kg, divide weight in pounds by 2.2. To determine height in cm, multiply height in inches by 2.54.

Incorporate an activity correction factor between 1.2 and 1.5 to account for the individual's average amount of physical activity.

Note: Multiply the BMR value derived from the prediction equation by the appropriate activity correction factor:

- 1.2 = bed rest
- 1.3 = sedentary
- 1.4 = active
- 1.5 = very active

Table 14-3 includes several RMR prediction equations that can be used to help clients understand how many calories they burn throughout the day while at rest. Some of these equations provide more accurate results for certain populations than others, so LWMCs must be sure to choose the most appropriate equation for each client.

Table 14-3
RMR Prediction Equations (kcal/day)

Mifflin-St Jeor Equations
(Mifflin et al., 1990; Frankenfield et al., 2003; Frankenfield, Roth-Yousey, & Compher, 2005)
Men: RMR = (9.99 x weight) + (6.25 x height) – (4.92 x age) + 5
Women: RMR = (9.99 x weight)+ (6.25 x height) – (4.92 x age) – 161
Multiply the RMR value derived from the prediction equation by the appropriate activity correction factor:
1.200 = sedentary (little or no exercise)
1.375 = lightly active (light exercise/sports one to three days per week)
1.550 = moderately active (moderate exercise/sports three to five days per week)
1.725 = very active (hard exercise/sports six to seven days per week)
1.900 = extra active (very hard exercise/sports and a physical job)
Note: This equation is more accurate for obese than non-obese individuals.

Schofield Equation
(Schofield, 1985; Harris & Benedict, 1919; Tverskaya et al., 1998)

Age	*Males*	*Females*
15–18	BMR = 17.6 x weight + 656	BMR = 13.3 x weight + 690
18–30	BMR = 15.0 x weight + 690	BMR = 14.8 x weight + 485
30–60	BMR = 11.4 x weight + 870	BMR = 8.1 x weight + 842
>60	BMR = 11.7 x weight + 585	BMR = 9.0 x weight + 656

Note: This equation slightly underestimates for women and slightly overestimates for men.

Owen Equation
(Owen et al., 1986; 1987)
Males: RMR = (10.2 x weight) + 879
Females: RMR = (7.18 x weight) + 795

Cunningham Equation
(Cunningham, 1991)
All subjects: REE (kcal/day) = (21.6 x FFM) + 370
Note: This is considered one of the better prediction equations for athletes because it takes into account fat-free mass.

Wang Equation
(Bauer, Reeves, & Capra, 2004)
All subjects: REE (kcal/day) = (21.5 x FFM) + 407
Note: This equation is potentially better for athletes because it takes into account fat-free mass.

Note: All methods of determining RMR are estimates only; Equations use weight in kilograms (kg) and height in centimeters (cm); REE = Resting energy expenditure; FFM = Fat free mass

In addition to the estimation equations presented in Table 14-3, another method called indirect calorimetry is used to predict resting metabolic rate. Since oxygen is used in the metabolic process to create energy, a person's metabolic rate can be determined by measuring how much oxygen he or she consumes when breathing. There is a relationship between the body's use of oxygen and the energy it expends, so scientists use formulas to convert gas usage into energy/calories used.

Historically, oxygen-consumption measurements were only performed with a medical device called a metabolic cart, which can cost between $20,000 and $50,000. Newer technology has made it possible to measure oxygen consumption using hand-held devices, making the analysis more accessible and affordable.

Using Caloric Information to Affect Weight

Once the client's daily caloric needs have been estimated, this information can be used to help the client lose, gain, or maintain weight. To change weight by 1 pound (0.45 kg), caloric intake must be decreased or increased by 3,500 calories. For weight loss, it is advisable to reduce daily caloric intake by 250 calories per day and to increase daily expenditure (through exercise) by 250 calories. This 500-calorie difference, when multiplied by seven, creates a weekly negative caloric balance that results in a loss of 1 pound (0.45 kg). These numbers may be doubled to achieve a loss of 2 pounds (0.91 kg) per week, but that may be too great a goal for some clients. Most health organizations recommend a weight-loss rate of 1 to 2 pounds (0.45 kg to 0.91 kg) per week.

To gain approximately a ½-pound (0.23 kg) of weight, clients can add 300 to 500 calories to the daily intake. It is crucial that the exercise routine be maintained so that additional calories are used to fuel muscles, rather than to simply store additional fat. Advise clients to follow this new calorie plan for a few months and make changes as needed (Baechle & Earle, 2004; American College of Sports Medicine, 2006).

Summary

The client interview is a time not only to assess a client's current dietary habits and readiness for change, but also to develop rapport and build a foundation for the LWMC–client relationship. LWMCs should understand which programming tools to use with each client, as well as how to modify those tools as needed. Finally, it is essential for the LWMC to stay within his or her scope of practice.

References

American College of Sports Medicine (2006). *ACSM's Resource Manual for Guidelines for Exercise Testing and Prescription* (6th ed.). Philadelphia, Pa.: Lippincott, Williams & Wilkins.

Baechle, T.R. & Earle, R.W. (2004). *Essentials of Strength Training and Conditioning* (2nd ed.). Champaign, Ill.: Human Kinetics.

Bauer, J., Reeves, M.M., & Capra, S. (2004). The agreement between measured and predicted resting energy expenditure in patients with pancreatic cancer: A pilot study. *Journal of the Pancreas*, 5, 1, 32–40.

Cunningham, J.C. (1991). Body composition as a determinate of energy expenditure: A synthetic review and a proposed general prediction equation. *American Journal of Clinical Nutrition*, 54, 963–969.

Frankenfield, D., Roth-Yousey, L., & Compher, C. (2005). Comparison of predictive equations for resting metabolic rate in healthy nonobese and obese adults: A systematic review. *Journal of the American Dietetic Association,* 105, 5, 775–789.

Frankenfield, D. et al. (2003). Validation of several established equations for resting metabolic rate in obese and nonobese people. *Journal of the American Dietetic Association,* 103, 9, 1152–1159.

Harris, J. & Benedict, F. (1919). A biometric study of basal metabolism in man. *Key Facts in Clinical Nutrition.* Washington, D.C.: Carnegie Institute of Washington.

Mahabir, S. (2006). Calorie intake misreporting by diet record and food frequency questionnaire compared to doubly labeled water among postmenopausal women. *European Journal of Clinical Nutrition,* 60, 561–565.

Mifflin, M.D. et al. (1990). A new predictive equation for resting energy expenditure in healthy individuals. *American Journal of Clinical Nutrition,* 51, 241–247.

Owen, C.E. et al. (1987). A reappraisal of caloric requirements of men. *American Journal of Clinical Nutrition,* 46, 75–85.

Owen, C.E. et al. (1986). A reappraisal of caloric requirements in healthy women. *American Journal of Clinical Nutrition,* 44, 1–19.

Resnicow, K. et al. (2000). Validation of three food frequency questionnaires and 24-hour recalls with serum carotenoid levels in a sample of African-American adults. *American Journal of Epidemiology,* 152, 11, 1072–1080.

Schatzkin, A. et al. (2003). A comparison of a food-frequency questionnaire with a 24-hour recall for use in an epidemiological cohort study: Results from the biomarker-based Observing Protein and Energy Nutrition (OPEN) study. *International Journal of Epidemiology,* 32, 1054–1062.

Schofield, R. (1985). Equations for estimating basal metabolic rate (BMR). *Human Nutrition: Clinical Nutrition,* 39C, 5–41.

Svendsen, M. et al. (2006). Accuracy of food intake reporting in obese subjects with metabolic risk factors. *British Journal of Nutrition,* 95, 640–649.

Tverskaya, R. et al. (1998). Comparison of several equations and derivation of a new equation for calculating basal metabolic rate in obese children. *Journal of the American College of Nutrition,* 17, 4, 333–336.

United States Department of Agriculture (2005). Dietary Guidelines for Americans 2005. www.health.gov/dietaryguidelines

Wein, D. (2006). *SNaC Pack: The Health Professional's Guide to Nutrition.* www.sensiblenutrition.com

Willett, W. (2001). Commentary: Dietary diaries versus food frequency questionnaires—a case of undigestible data. *International Journal of Epidemiology,* 30, 317–319.

Suggested Reading

Kiem, M.L. et al. (1997). A descriptive study of individuals successful at long-term maintenance of substantial weight. *American Journal of Clinical Nutrition,* 66, 239–246.

Wadden, T.A. et al. (2005). Randomized trial of lifestyle modification and pharmacotherapy for obesity. *New England Journal of Medicine,* 353, 2111–2120

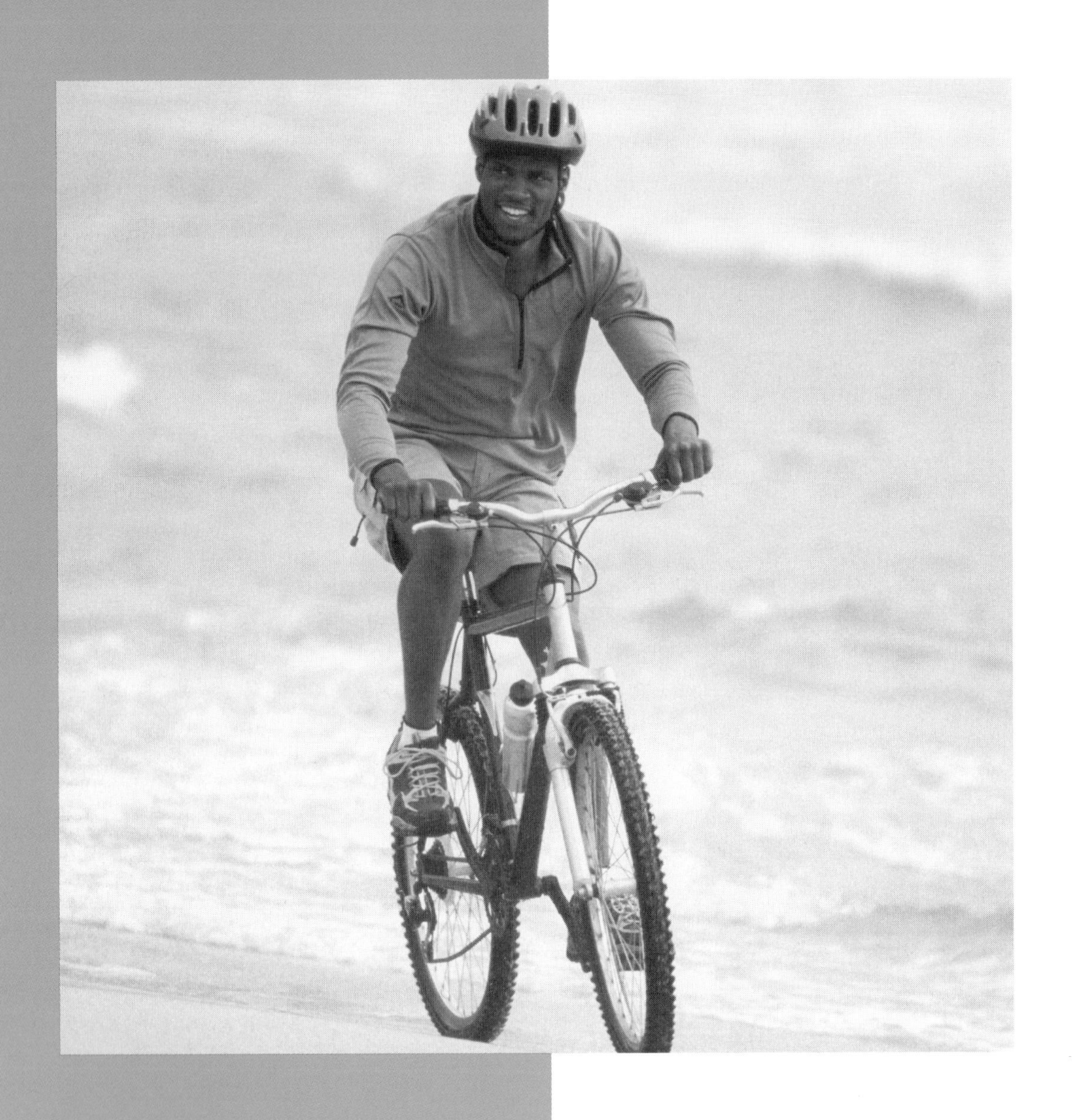

Barbara A. Brehm

Barbara A. Brehm, Ed.D., is professor of exercise and sport studies at Smith College, Northampton, Mass., where she teaches courses in nutrition, health, and stress management. She is also director of the Smith Fitness Program for Faculty and Staff and an instructor for the Smith College Executive Education Programs. She is the author of several books, including Successful Fitness Motivation Strategies, *and is a contributing editor for* Fitness Management *magazine.*

Chapter 15

Lifestyle Modification and Behavior Change

IN THIS CHAPTER:

Most clients will likely tell their Lifestyle & Weight Management Consultants (LWMCs) that designing a weight-loss plan is the easy part; sticking to the plan is the hard part. Clients often say, "I know what I am supposed to do. I just can't seem to do it."

For many health and fitness professionals, mastering the basics of good exercise and nutrition is fairly straightforward. Soon after developing this foundation, they become comfortable with recommending exercise programs, giving advice on preventing injury, and guiding clients on how to make good food choices. Helping clients stick with their plans, however, is often the biggest challenge.

Lifestyle modification and behavior change are simple in theory. First, LWMCs help clients figure out what lifestyle habits and other behaviors are problem areas. Then they come up with ways to replace them with behaviors that promote a healthier weight. Clients modify their lifestyles as planned, and they lose weight—simple!

Of course, if losing weight was really that simple, the United States would not face an **obesity** crisis. In reality, changing one's lifestyle is a complicated and difficult challenge. Lifestyles evolve for various reasons over many years, and people behave the way they do because their behaviors "work" for them. Clients' eating and activity patterns have adapted over the years, and have been influenced by such factors as family, culture, financial constraints, health, and work. Some clients may use eating and other behaviors to cope with negative moods, connect with family and friends, celebrate triumphs, and soothe jangled nerves.

While working with clients to implement lifestyle-modification and behavior-change programs, an LWMC must transition from being an expert to acting as a cheerleader and guide. While fitness professionals may know more about exercise and nutritional science than their clients, clients are ultimately in control of choosing a healthier lifestyle.

When studying lifestyle modification and behavior change, it is important to keep in mind the material presented in Chapter 5 on the importance of good communication. Good listening skills are essential. An LWMC must listen with **empathy** and keep an open mind when talking to clients about their lives and challenges.

An LWMC must try to understand the clients who come in for help. If a client's cultural background differs from that of the LWMC, it is the LWMC's responsibility to learn about the client's diets and traditions, belief system, and family structure. Advice on behavior change will not be relevant without an understanding of a client's lifestyle.

People generally do not like to be told what to do, especially by someone younger and less experienced than themselves. For LWMCs who have never had a weight problem, identifying with **overweight** or obese clients may be difficult. Clients do not want to be judged or criticized, especially by someone who "just doesn't understand." LWMCs must examine and correct their own prejudices regarding obese clients (Teachman & Brownell, 2001). LWMCs can use the suggested readings at the end of this chapter to learn more about the experiences of overweight people.

It is also important for LWMCs to let the clients take the lead in designing lifestyle-modification and behavior-change programs. Every person is different, and each client's life must be regarded with dignity and respect. Fitness professionals must combine their knowledge of behavior-change research with the emotional intelligence needed to respond with their hearts and minds to the individualized experiences of every client.

What Determines Behavior?

Chapter 4 presents an overview of the multiple factors that have been found somewhat predictive of exercise behavior. Several theories attempt to explain health behaviors. Keep in mind that theories are approximations that can help LWMCs better understand clients. Theories will not, however, always apply to every individual. Nevertheless, they give LWMCs a starting point for their work, from which they can make adjustments as they get to know their clients better.

Stages of Change

The **transtheoretical model (TTM)** of behavior change emphasizes the importance of determining a client's readiness for change. According to this model, people who change their behavior go through several stages, from **precontemplation** (not thinking about changing), to **contemplation** (weighing the pros and cons of changing), to **preparation** (getting ready to make a change), **action** (practicing the new behavior), and finally to **maintenance** (incorporating the new behavior into one's lifestyle). Refer to Table 12-4 on page 271 for a summary of the stages of change for exercise and a list of effective intervention approaches for clients in each stage.

When LWMCs begin a consultation with clients, determining where they are in the behavior-change process is key for designing effective interventions. Fitness professionals often assume that people come to them for exercise advice and are eager to begin an exercise program. While this is often the case, many times these people are still weighing the pros and cons of starting an exercise program and haven't yet formed a strong intention to commit to the class or regularly visit the fitness center. Yet fitness professionals plow ahead in designing a delightfully complicated, but effective exercise program for them—and then wonder why they stop attending after a few weeks.

Applying the stages-of-change model in a weight-management program is somewhat tricky, because it requires addressing different behaviors simultaneously. Some changes come more easily than others, and clients may be ready to change some behaviors, but not others. For example, a client might already be entering the action stage in terms of reducing empty-calorie foods, but have doubts about his or her ability to stick to an exercise program. This scenario is not uncommon for people with a history of obesity. They may have avoided exercise because physical activity was embarrassing or difficult for them, but may have had plenty of practice dieting. LWMCs should assess stages of exercise and diet readiness separately, and use appropriate intervention strategies according to the readiness for change.

Health Belief Model

The **health belief model** suggests that a person's health beliefs influence decisions about behavior change (see Chapter 4). Addressing health beliefs with overweight clients is especially important in the early stages of behavior change. LWMCs should discuss clients' beliefs about obesity, weight loss, nutrition, and physical activity and correct misperceptions with accurate information from handouts, pamphlets, websites, and other reputable sources. Useful information will help clients weigh the pros and cons of behavior change and create an incentive to modify their lifestyles.

According to this model, it is best if clients perceive obesity as a potential health problem so that they become motivated to do something about it. However, the health belief model falls short, because people who feel threatened and anxious, or are unable to deal with the health threat, may avoid the problem rather than address it (Witte & Allen, 2000). LWMCs should help clients understand that lifestyle modification is the best option for addressing obesity. Perceiving obesity as a health threat can motivate behavior change, as long as the change is perceived as feasible. LWMCs should also build clients' **self-efficacy,** so that they feel empowered to modify their lifestyles to reduce health risks.

Social Factors

Humans are social animals, and social factors affect behavior-change and lifestyle-modification success at every stage of the behavior-change process. Friends, family, coworkers, and acquaintances nudge people from stage to stage with their words and actions. A loved one expressing sincere concern can motivate a client to get up off the couch. Friends might decide to join a health club, and then sign up for the LWMC program together.

Social factors may also inhibit positive change. Spouses may miss sharing the ritual ice cream after dinner, friends may bring over a fattening treat to share, or coworkers may frown on someone using the lunch hour to exercise.

Social factors also affect a person's self-efficacy regarding behavior change. If clients see people similar to themselves exercising and eating well, they will feel more capable of performing similar behaviors. If a significant other scoffs at a client's attempts to modify his or her lifestyle, change will become even more challenging.

Principles of Lifestyle Modification

Health psychology research has clarified many helpful principles of lifestyle modification for LWMCs. While some of these principles may have intimidating names and terminology, they are congruent with common sense and should be remembered while working with clients to evaluate and guide their lifestyle-modification efforts.

Operant Conditioning

Operant conditioning examines the relationships among **antecedents** (situations and feelings that precede a certain behavior), behaviors, and consequences (see Chapter 4). For the purpose of weight control, fitness professionals should focus on factors that stimulate and reinforce exercise and eating behaviors. What factors shape these behaviors? In other words, what factors trigger both good and bad behaviors, and what reinforcements reward or punish eating and exercise behaviors?

In many cases, clients will state **triggers** that make them eat too much, or eat the wrong things. They may describe situations that cause them to skip an exercise session. LWMCs should take detailed notes, as this is the critical information that will enable LWMCs to help their clients make plans that will result in lifestyle modification.

In other cases, clients may overlook, or be in denial about, the factors and situations that trigger negative eating and exercise behaviors. Keeping a record of food intake that includes notes on reasons for eating and situations that trigger eating helps both the LWMC and the client take an objective look at a client's behavior and evaluate how it is influenced both positively and negatively by antecedents and consequences.

Principle of Limited Self-control

Clients will often say, "If only I had more willpower..." It takes effort to change one's lifestyle, exercise regularly, and change one's eating habits. Psychologists who study willpower refer to this concept as **self-regulation** or **self-control.** Their research has several applications for LWMCs.

First, psychologists believe that for each person, self-control is a limited resource (Muraven & Baumeister, 2000). While some clients have more self-control than others, no one has limitless self-control. The more LWMCs and clients can minimize the amount of self-control needed to maintain lifestyle modifications, the more successful they will be.

Second, habits are comfortable and require little self-control. The more quickly lifestyle modifications can become habits, the happier and more successful a client will be. People are creatures of habit and tend to settle into daily routines. Researchers who study self-control believe that most people are able to tolerate only a relatively small disruption in their daily routines before experiencing stress (Vohs & Heatherton, 2000).

Third, coping with stress requires self-control. This observation helps explain why it is more difficult to change a habit when under a lot of stress; energy for self-control gets used up when a person is dealing with stress. Encourage clients to begin a lifestyle-modification program when stress levels are relatively low, such as after, rather than during, the holidays. Managing stress and negative emotions must be an integral part of every lifestyle-modification program.

Lastly, self-control appears to be renewed daily. It is highest in the mornings, and then gradually diminishes as the day goes on. This observation helps explain why people who exercise in the morning tend to be most successful in sticking to their exercise programs. It also explains why dieters are "good" in the early part of the day, but often give in to temptation in the late afternoon and evening.

Many overweight people have a great deal of self-control, even though they often don't think so. A failure to lose weight is often chalked up to a failure of willpower rather than to the fact that diets are impossible to follow or that people establish totally unrealistic weight-loss goals.

One type of self-control that has been extensively studied is **dietary restraint** (Stice, Fisher, & Lowe, 2004). People who exert a great deal of self-control over their food intake, even though they are feeling hungry and unhappy about their diet, develop the ability to main dietary restraint for a certain period of time. However, high levels of dietary restraint cannot usually be sustained for very long. When the restraint is finally overwhelmed by the drive to eat, some people may go overboard, going "off" their restrictive diets and overeating. While people wanting to lose weight must exercise some dietary restraint, research suggests that very high levels of restraint may be counterproductive. LWMCs must help clients come up with realistic suggestions for modifying their lifestyles that do not require excessive levels of self-control.

The False-hope Syndrome and the Planning Fallacy

As Alexander Pope wrote, "Hope springs eternal in the human breast." This is a good thing, but psychologists have observed that hope can be problematic when it leads to unrealistic goals. People's tendency to set unrealistic goals is called the **false-hope syndrome** (Polivy & Herman, 2000). Setting ambitious goals makes people feel good. Their self-image improves, and they feel optimistic and in control. "I will lose 20 pounds before summer." But what happens as time goes by and goals are not reached? Clients are disappointed in themselves, feel bad, and discontinue their behavior-change programs.

The **planning fallacy** states that people consistently underestimate the time, energy, and other resources required to complete a given task (Buehler, Griffin, & Ross, 1994). Whether someone is building a space shuttle, remodeling the kitchen, starting an exercise program, or changing eating habits, most projects end up taking more money, time, and effort than anticipated. Clients often say that they will spend more time exercising or coming to LWMC meetings than they really can, or that they will change their eating habits more drastically than they can really tolerate.

Therefore, LWMCs must keep in mind the false-hope syndrome and planning fallacy when helping clients design lifestyle-modification programs. LWMCs must encourage clients to get positive results, but make them understand that changing habits takes a great deal of time and effort. It is important to help clients set modest goals and take small, doable steps that reinforce feelings of self-efficacy and the belief that they can stay with the program.

Self-efficacy

Self-efficacy refers to a person's belief that he or she can perform a given task (Bandura 1997). While self-efficacy is similar to self-confidence, it is always situation- or behavior-specific. For example, a client may be very confident in his ability to reduce calorie intake, but have low self-efficacy in terms of sticking to an exercise program.

Self-efficacy predicts how much effort clients will exert in sticking to their lifestyle-modification programs. Self-efficacy also predicts how hard clients will persist in their behavior-change efforts when facing difficulties (Bandura, 1997).

Strengthening self-efficacy is important at all stages of behavior change. That said, precontemplators and contemplators tend to have especially low self-efficacy in the realm of weight-control behaviors (see Chapter 4). Much of an LWMC's work with clients in these stages will be focused on helping them believe that they can modify their lifestyles and change problematic behaviors.

Stress Management and Negative Mood

Stress is the most common reason that people abandon their plans to change behavior. Stress depletes self-control and lowers feelings of self-efficacy. It zaps energy and motivation. Too much stress triggers negative emotions such as **anxiety**, anger, and sadness. When people feel bad, they look for ways to feel better. Coping with negative emotions is more important for most people than sticking to a lifestyle-modification program, especially if the lifestyle modifications are perceived to lead to future benefits, but feel like deprivation at the present time (Tice, Bratslavsky, & Baumeister, 2001).

Some people respond to feelings of stress and to negative and/or positive emotional states by eating, even when they're not hungry. **Emotional eating** refers to eating triggered by emotional states. This response is fairly widespread in the general population, not just in the overweight (Geliebter & Aversa, 2003). Emotional eating becomes a problem when people are trying to reduce food intake. The stress associated with lifestyle modification can compound the problem of emotional eating. In other words, eating less than normal causes stress, so what happens if a person responds to that stress by overeating?

Guiding clients to monitor and manage stress levels must be an integral and continuing component of all lifestyle-modification and behavior-change recommendations. Lifestyle modifications should create as little stress as possible, and clients, especially emotional eaters, must learn new ways of coping with stress and negative moods.

Lifelong Sustainability and Relapse Prevention

A sobering principle that all clients must face is that obesity is a chronic disease with no quick fix. The lifestyle modifications and behavior changes that lead to weight loss must be maintained to prevent weight regain. People who succeed in maintaining weight loss continue to exercise and watch their eating habits for a lifetime (Wing & Phelan, 2005). Successful weight control means lifelong lifestyle modifications.

A lifetime offers many opportunities for disruption to lifestyle-modification programs, even for people with the best of intentions. Clients must understand that achieving perfection is impossible, and that they may overeat or skip exercise sessions at times. The goal of relapse-prevention work is to prevent a lapse (i.e., a short-term disruption in a lifestyle-modification program) from turning into relapse (i.e., a return to one's former behaviors and the act of "giving up" on the lifestyle-modification program) (Marlatt & George, 1998).

Relapse-prevention discussions with clients can encourage them to anticipate and visualize occasions during which they may experience lapses in their behavior-change programs. LWMCs can help clients understand that lapses are normal and should be accepted and taken in stride. While feelings of disappointment may arise when lapses occur, it is important for clients to avoid feelings of failure and guilt, as these negative thoughts and emotions can deplete self-control energy, increase feelings of stress, and lead to total relapse and motivational collapse.

Lifestyle-modification Strategies

Successful lifestyle-modification strategies derive from an understanding of the principles presented earlier in this chapter. The following strategies may be incorporated into either individual or group formats.

Lead Educational Discussions Tailored for the Stage of Change

Weight-control groups usually meet weekly and follow a curriculum that includes educational discussions that address topics of interest to participants. LWMCs can also engage in educational discussions with individual clients. These discussions should be informational and motivational.

LWMCs should assess clients' readiness to change eating habits and engage in physical activity early on. Educational discussions should be designed to help clients form and strengthen their intentions to change behavior (Armitage, 2006). Clients in the earlier stages of behavior change, who are still weighing the pros and cons, should be given information on the dangers of obesity and the benefits of exercise and proper nutrition, as well as concrete ideas for implementing a lifestyle-modification program that will lead to weight loss. If LWMCs are leading group discussions, the group members will chime in and add to discussions. It is the LWMC's role to correct misinformation and give clients the take-home message that while lifestyle modification takes effort, it is the only way to achieve healthful, lifelong weight control.

As LWMCs discuss lifestyle-modification issues and assess clients, it is important to find out if clients are ready to make a change. Be sure that clients are at least in the preparation stage for lifestyle modification before asking too much of them.

Help Clients Set Realistic Goals

LWMCs should help clients set both weight-loss and lifestyle-modification/ behavior-change goals. Remembering that clients will tend to be overly ambitious, LWMCs should help clients set realistic goals.

While most clients will want to focus on weight loss, LWMCs should help them focus more on behavior. After all, they will have more control over their behavior than their weight. Simply adhering to their exercise and nutrition plans each day should be seen as reaching a goal.

When working with clients to devise healthy exercise and diet guidelines, LWMCs should focus on adherence. LWMCs should ask themselves, "Is this advice something the client can really follow?" Remember that the new behaviors the clients are adopting should require as little self-control as possible so that they can become habits as quickly as possible.

Advice on behavior change should include a great deal of structure for meals (Berkel et al., 2005). Meal structure decreases the effort required for meal planning and decision making, and reduces temptation and guesswork. Clients who quickly develop a daily routine for eating will be most successful in modifying their lifestyles.

Exercise recommendations can be somewhat more flexible, with some built-in choice to accommodate each client's schedule. Exercise recommendations that are too structured may make adherence difficult, and some researchers suggest helping people who are overweight develop more lifestyle activity, such as walking, doing yard work, and taking stairs (Andersen et al., 1999).

Encourage Clients to Modify Environmental Cues

Obesity has been called an environmental issue (Carlos Poston & Foreyt, 1999). Environmental cues encourage excessive calorie intake and low levels of physical activity. Clients will probably have a lot to say about how their environment encourages overeating and lack of exercise.

LWMCs should encourage clients to become aware of environmental cues that trigger food intake and physical activity. Many environmental factors will be out of a client's control. For example, a client will not be able to change the price of fresh fruits and vegetables, decrease restaurant portion sizes, or move to a new apartment to avoid living next door to the fast-food restaurant with delicious french fries.

One of the first steps many clients take, however, as they prepare to improve their eating habits, is to clean up their immediate environments at home and at work. They can give away (or stop purchasing) high-calorie, low-nutrition foods. They can keep food out of view, in cupboards or containers. These preparations help reduce cues for eating the wrong foods or eating when not hungry. Similarly, clients may prepare to become more active by buying exercise videos or exercise clothes, or checking out exercise opportunities near home or work.

Look for Ways to Increase Self-efficacy

Self-efficacy helps clients stick to their lifestyle-modification programs. Research suggests that fitness professionals can help clients build self-efficacy in several ways (McAuley & Blissmer, 2000).

As the old adage states, success breeds success. LWMCs can help clients achieve success early in their lifestyle-modification programs by setting reasonable goals that they can easily accomplish.

Clients should be exposed to role models. People of a similar age, gender, and ethnic background, who exercise regularly and have lost weight and maintained it, encourage the belief that, "If they can do it, so can I." If a client feels "different" from everyone else in the group or at the fitness center, self-efficacy may decline.

Social support enhances self-efficacy. Clients should be encouraged to join the program with a friend. That way they can exercise together and boost each other's self-confidence.

LWMCs must provide continued positive reinforcement. Self-efficacy is in the eye of the beholder. Clients must believe that they are being successful. LWMCs should help them find concrete evidence of success, such as their diet records or exercise log. In the early stages, the focus should remain on successful adherence to lifestyle-modification plans.

LWMCs should help clients feel comfortable in the exercise environment by advising them on what to wear, where to go, and how to act. They should also help clients find exercise opportunities that are not embarrassing and where they feel comfortable.

Discuss How to Manage Stress and Negative Moods

Most clients already have many stress-management strategies in place, as well as ways to cope with negative moods. In a group situation, clients can share the things they do to make themselves feel better when they are feeling bad. In one-on-one sessions, clients can brainstorm a list of things that they enjoy, such as listening to music, enjoying a cup of tea, reading a good book, talking to a friend, or watching a funny movie.

Reinforce the pleasures and psychological benefits of physical activity. Research shows that regular physical activity can reduce feelings of **depression,** stress, and anxiety, and improve mood and energy levels (Brehm, 2000). Help clients identify enjoyable activities, and encourage them to tune into the positive effects of exercise. If clients get "hooked" on exercise, they achieve three rewards: They accomplish the physical activity that is part of their weight-control programs; they reduce stress; and, by reducing stress, they increase the energy available for self-control.

Some clients find relaxation techniques, such as meditation and breathing exercises, helpful. Many techniques are simple to teach and learn (Brehm, 1998). Relaxation techniques can teach clients to be more mindful of their eating habits, to slow down and enjoy their food more, and to reduce emotional eating during stress.

Clients who confide that stress and negative moods are especially disruptive to their eating habits should be referred to a mental-health specialist, such as a psychotherapist or other licensed counseling professional (See "Knowing When to Refer," page 341).

Set Up Systems for Self-monitoring and Problem-solving

It is important to set up systems for self-monitoring of food intake and physical activity early in the working relationship with each client. LWMCs may ask clients to monitor themselves even before making diet and exercise recommendations to get a baseline for behaviors. Continuing to refine self-monitoring systems will help clients evaluate their lifestyle-modification plans.

Self-monitoring systems usually consist of written or computer forms in which clients record the behaviors they are working to change. Clients will need ways to record both food intake and physical activity. Clients may also want to record body weight daily or weekly. Once clients get used to recordkeeping, it is also useful to ask them to observe thoughts and feelings, both helpful and unhelpful, that precede eating and exercise behaviors.

Research has consistently shown that self-monitoring is one of the most important components of successful weight-control and weight-maintenance programs (Boutelle & Kirschenbaum, 1998). Self-monitoring systems help in several ways. First, they increase people's self-awareness. For example, clients may not realize how many extra calories they consume while nibbling as they cook dinner or snacking as they watch television. Self-monitoring acts as a mirror so that clients can get a more objective view of their behavior.

Second, self-monitoring systems forge a link between the LWMC and the client outside of sessions. Clients will anticipate careful surveillance of their records. Hopefully, they will stick to their lifestyle-modification and behavior-change programs and be proud of their accomplishments when the LWMC next reviews their records.

Third, self-monitoring systems will serve as an important tool for evaluating clients' lifestyle-modification and behavior-change successes and challenges. While reviewing clients' records each week, the LWMC can note occasions where challenges arose. Why did this occasion of overeating occur? What triggered this response? Clients and LWMCs can then brainstorm ways to eliminate negative triggers when possible and identify better responses to those situations to prevent relapses. Self-monitoring systems will reveal times when lifestyle-modification efforts are working. LWMCs should help clients analyze what works and what doesn't.

Lastly, self-monitoring records can serve as a form of positive reinforcement and increase self-efficacy. A completed exercise log or a chart showing a good daily intake of vegetables, for instance, shows clients that they are being successful in their lifestyle-modification and behavior-change programs.

Cognitive Restructuring: Thinking About Thinking

Consciously changing the way one perceives or thinks about something is called **cognitive restructuring.** Cognitive restructuring requires developing a mindful awareness of one's automatic thoughts, or self-talk, and consciously changing counterproductive thoughts. Over time, and with practice, clients can learn to change the way they think, and thus, the ways they feel and behave.

LWMCs can help clients apply cognitive restructuring when weighing the pros and cons of starting a weight-control program. As LWMCs educate clients about the benefits of exercise, the goal should be to make physical exercise appealing to them. This will be a continued effort while working with clients.

For example, clients who say they "hate" exercise should try to see physical activity in a more positive light. Cognitive restructuring may make them more aware of the things they say to themselves about exercise. This can be part of their self-monitoring routine. For example, they can make a note of the thoughts and feelings that occur as they get ready to participate in physical activity. Hopefully, as clients become aware of counterproductive thinking, they can learn to replace negative thoughts with more positive and realistic ones.

To continue this example, suppose a client associates exercise with being teased in school. The LWMC should explore this association and help the client understand that there are ways to be active that don't involve teasing. LWMCs should strive to help clients adopt new ways of thinking and create more positive feelings about physical activity. This means steering them away from any negative automatic thoughts relating to "exercise" and creating more positive associations.

Cognitive restructuring requires a great deal of practice and self-monitoring. It also requires the ability to observe one's own thinking, and to not accept one's immediate thoughts as "reality." Positive thinking alone is not enough; clients must restructure thoughts in ways that are believable, as well as positive. "I love exercise," may not ring true, but "I don't mind walking on the treadmill while I watch TV," might become true.

Implementing a Lifestyle-modification Program

The specifics of implementing a lifestyle-modification program will vary depending upon the work setting. LWMCs may lead lifestyle- and weight-management groups or work more as personal trainers with certain clients. The following suggestions may be incorporated into either individual or group work. Specific suggestions for group programs are included at the end of this section.

Many LWMCs make clients commit to a minimum timeframe for lifestyle- and weight-modification programs. Research suggests that programs should last at least 16 to 26 weeks to foster success (Renjilian et al., 2001). LWMCs must plan a general progression to the program that accommodates the timeframe in which they work, but allows for flexibility depending upon client needs and interests.

LWMCs should remain positive in all aspects of their work. Working with an LWMC must be a positive experience for clients, or they will go elsewhere. It is important to always be understanding and supportive of clients, even when questioning their behaviors. Remember that while the behavior may be a problem, these clients are doing the best they can. Therefore, LWMCs need to express confidence in every client's ability to change.

Lifestyle Assessment and Overview of the Program

Before diving into assessment procedures, LWMCs need to obtain health histories and get medical-clearance forms (when necessary) from their clients, and make sure that they are qualified to work with clients who have certain health conditions. They should also discuss the forms with clients to ensure that all health information is complete and accurate.

Most lifestyle-modification programs include exercise, nutrition, and behavior-change components. Advice in all of these areas will begin with the initial client assessment. Looking at current lifestyle behaviors is key. Exercise, diet, and weight history reveal a lot about a client's lifestyle and the various factors that account for the client's weight problems. LWMCs must be sure to discuss clients' past successes with diet, exercise, and weight loss. What worked in the past may work again, and discussing successful experiences will enhance clients' self-efficacy.

The big question that the LWMC and the client are trying to answer is as follows: Why is the client overweight? LWMCs must consider biological and environmental influences, including exercise, diet, and weight-loss history. LWMCs should also ask clients about social-support networks, stress levels, and stress-management techniques (Fabricatore & Wadden, 2005).

During the initial assessment, LWMCs should analyze the client's stage of change for physical activity and diet. Simply by coming to an LWMC, clients indicate that they are probably preparing to make changes in their behavior, either in diet or physical activity, or both. Keep in mind, however, that the stage of change may differ for exercise and diet. LWMCs can assess the stage of change by asking clients questions about their readiness, or by using a questionnaire (Brehm, 2004). If an LWMC senses that a client is not yet in the preparation stage for exercise or diet, he or she can spend more time on discussion and education to help the client form the intention to change.

LWMCs should initially ask clients to keep a daily food and activity log for one week. This log will help clients set lifestyle-modification goals. Be sure that the format of this log matches each client's specific interests and abilities. Keep logs simple at first to get clients into the self-monitoring habit. Recordkeeping can become more complex over time if necessary. Difficult logs should not be allowed to form a barrier to action. Computerized logs are fine, but only if a client uses a computer on a daily basis and finds computer use easy and convenient.

LWMCs should provide an overview of the program early in the relationship with each client. LWMCs should tailor programs to accommodate each client's needs and explain that losing weight and changing one's lifestyle take commitment, time, and effort.

Establish Goals for Interventions

After completing the initial exercise, diet, and lifestyle assessments, LWMCs should work with the client to establish program goals, including weight-loss and behavioral goals. Use the information from Chapters 13 and 14 to establish goals for physical activity and diet. Remember that goals must be specific, measurable, attainable, relevant, and time-bound (**SMART goals**). If the LWMC and client are meeting regularly, the LWMC can help the client create a specific guide to what should be accomplished during the week.

How elaborate should the goal-setting process be? It is easy to overwhelm clients with information and motivational suggestions during the first few weeks. Clients often come in very ambitious and willing to take it all on at once. LWMCs should err on the side of caution to be sure that clients are successful in meeting their lifestyle-modification goals early in the program. Suggest behavior changes that clients have successfully accomplished in the past and are willing to try again. Early weight-loss success is associated with adherence and long-term weight control (Renjilian et al., 2001).

Self-monitoring and Problem-solving: The Heart of Lifestyle Modification

At subsequent meetings, LWMCs should review clients' lifestyle-modification records. Did they meet their behavioral goals? Why or why not? Discuss both helping and hindering factors. Let the clients do most of the talking in problem-solving situations. Listen and ask questions, but try not to make suggestions right away. Remember that each client is the expert on his or her lifestyle.

Consider a client who is struggling with evening snacking. The LWMC must first understand what is causing the behavior. Is the client hungry? Maybe she needs more calories during the day—check her diet records. Is she eating for other reasons? Boredom? Stress? Habit? If she doesn't know why she eats in the evening, ask her to note the factors that seem to precede and follow the evening snacking during the coming week. Ask her to record her observations of her thoughts and feelings in her self-monitoring work. Her work in the program will hopefully help her uncover the antecedents and reinforcements to her problematic snacking behavior.

Once she understands some of the factors that contribute to the evening snacking, this client can try to design some ways to support a change in this behavior. Can she eliminate any of the factors that trigger the snacking? If she finds that she eats because she is bored, can she get out of the house, or stay busy and away from snacks? Can she get rid of the snack foods at home? If she can't stop snacking, can she snack on healthier foods? How can her friends and family help?

Problem-solving is about defining the problem, then brainstorming possible solutions. Clients should weigh the pros and cons of solutions, decide which ones to implement, and then evaluate their success during the next meeting. LWMCs and clients should revise tactics until they find workable solutions. Theoretically, this process should lead to behavioral changes, which become habits, and then result in a new, healthier lifestyle.

As clients weigh the pros and cons, LWMCs need to stay supportive, but also evaluate the likelihood that clients will adopt new behaviors. Asking the client if these new behaviors could really work for them, and defining strategies to achieve them, will be critical.

LWMCs should ask clients if self-talk has affected their eating and exercise behaviors and whether they have become more aware of thoughts and feelings that lead to overeating and negative self-talk.

Continue Education and Self-monitoring

Continue to review and discuss clients' lifestyle-modification records throughout the program's duration. Give clients educational material that addresses their questions and specific behavior-change issues. Most clients appreciate motivational reading and want to learn about physical activity, nutrition, and weight control. Topics typically included in weight-management curricula include eating out, managing the holidays, traveling, cooking, grocery shopping, reading food labels, managing stress, avoiding emotional eating, and preventing relapses.

Between sessions, the LWMC should think about each client and develop strategies that might be used to promote self-efficacy and behavior-change success. Review the material in this chapter on lifestyle-modification principles and strategies. While clients will take the lead, be prepared to make helpful suggestions, or ask new questions, at each session. Would the client like to try a new exercise class at the fitness center and ask a friend to join him? How will his exercise program change now that it is getting dark earlier in the day? How will he eat during the holidays? The LWMC should help clients anticipate and plan for challenges.

Relapse Prevention

People are creatures of habit, and most find it difficult to change habits. For this reason, most people experience lapses during their behavior-change efforts. Lifestyle-modification programs for weight loss can be especially difficult to maintain long-term, as they involve modification of many different behaviors and habits. Helping clients accept the difficulty of this work and anticipate factors that contribute to both success and relapse may help them stick to their weight-loss programs.

Most clients can identify high-risk situations and anticipate ways in which they might abandon their behavior-change programs. The LWMC's goal in discussing these situations is to help clients understand that it is human to make mistakes, and that self-forgiveness is the correct response, followed by continued efforts to resume a healthful lifestyle. A lapse need not be interpreted as a relapse.

High-risk situations are typically accompanied by feelings of stress and negative moods. Lapses are often preceded by such thoughts as, "I would feel a lot better if I had a milkshake." LWMCs should continue to encourage clients to monitor their thoughts and feelings, and to develop effective ways to cope with stressful situations.

Some people relapse because of the mistaken belief that behavior-change programs are "all-or-nothing" efforts. Consequently, when these clients "break their rules" about eating or exercise (for example, overeating one evening), they blame themselves, feel a loss of control, and fall into relapse. This tendency is called the **abstinence violation effect,** a term borrowed from addiction treatment programs to describe the behavior of people who resume alcohol or drug abuse after a period of abstinence (Witkiewitz & Marlatt, 2004). Dieting can be the same way. Once people "break" their diet, they often continue to overeat and lose all motivation to stick to a lifestyle-modification program. LWMCs need to step in and help clients break that vicious cycle. LWMCs can help clients see that lapses are solvable problems, not indicators of failure. Clients must avoid all-or-nothing thinking when it comes to lifelong behavior.

Technology and Lifestyle-modification Programs

Research suggests that keeping in touch with clients through telephone and computer contact can be very effective (Fabricatore & Wadden, 2005). Programs relying on technology seem to be more effective when participants can also contact a "live person," either in person or over the Internet, as compared to standardized programs that feature no personal interface (Tate, Jackvony, & Wing, 2003).

If an LWMC uses telephone or computer contact with clients, he or she must be sure that the clients agree to this contact ahead of time. Many clients are annoyed by telephone calls and emails that interrupt their day. LWMCs must make such contact part of the initial plan if they anticipate using technology as part of their programs.

Lifestyle and Weight-management Groups

Research suggests that lifestyle- and weight-management groups tend to be more effective than individual consultations, regardless of whether individuals say they prefer group or individual counseling (Renjilian et al., 2001). When it comes to working with groups, experienced LWMCs have often found that groups provide valuable support, motivation, and information.

Group members generally follow the same progression outlined earlier in this chapter, from assessment and goal-setting to self-monitoring and problem-solving. Most group programs follow a set curriculum that includes weekly readings and "homework"—self-monitoring assignments that focus on a particular behavior-change topic.

LWMCs with teaching experience may feel more confident in leading group discussions, as groups require good listening and observation skills. The role of a group leader is to ensure that discussions are not dominated by a few individuals, that individuals listen respectfully to each other, and that members feel comfortable. Before leading a lifestyle- and weight-management group, LWMCs should participate or assist in a group led by an experienced leader. See Chapter 5 for more information on working with groups.

Continuing Support

Weight-loss maintenance is enhanced when people have ongoing contact with their LWMCs and fellow group members (Renjilian et al., 2001). Consider offering ways to keep in touch with participants once the program has ended.

Knowing When to Refer

In general, if an LWMC has concerns about a particular client and wonders about whether to refer, then he or she should refer. LWMCs find themselves referring clients for many reasons.

Sometimes an LWMC will want to refer a client back to his or her healthcare provider because the LWMC can't figure out why the client is overweight. If the client already has a healthy lifestyle, exercises daily, and eats healthfully, LWMCs have little more to offer. If the client's behaviors are not the problem, then the LWMC doesn't have the solution. Perhaps the obesity has other causes that other providers can address.

Obese clients often have other health conditions such as **diabetes** and **hypertension.** If their healthcare providers permit them to exercise and work with an LWMC, then the LWMC should still proceed with caution. If clients complain of health symptoms that may indicate poor control of their medical conditions, the LWMC should refer them back to their providers. Such symptoms include chest pain, dizziness, and any new health symptoms that develop during the program. Orthopedic problems, such as knee or foot pain, may develop and should be referred as well.

LWMCs should immediately refer clients to an appropriate healthcare provider if there is any suspicion of an eating disorder. Excessive restricting (dieting), binging, and purging all indicate psychological problems that are outside the LWMC's **scope of practice.** Review the warning signs of eating disorders presented in Chapter 8. People with **binge-eating disorder** may continue to work with LWMCs to modify their behavior with their therapist's consent, since research shows that lifestyle modification is helpful for binge eaters (Gladis et al., 1998).

Sometimes clients struggle with addictions, which also translates into a needed referral. The underlying issue with a weight problem can be an alcohol or drug problem. Lifestyle modification can support recovery for certain addictions, but clients also need to be in therapy.

Mood disorders such as depression and anxiety also require referral. Research suggests that obese people seeking treatment report greater rates of mood disturbances than obese people who do not seek treatment (Fitzgibbon, Stolley, & Kirschenbaum, 1993). While everyone feels sad and anxious at times, clients who report ongoing negative feelings or symptoms that interfere with daily living need to be referred to a healthcare provider.

LWMCs need to establish a referral network early on in their careers. Follow the guidelines in Chapter 11 on how to create a referral network. LWMCs who make sound decisions regarding referrals will earn the respect of clients and coworkers, and lift the reputation of fitness professionals to a higher level.

Summary

Behavior change is essential for lifelong weight management. LWMCs should teach lifestyle-modification strategies throughout their work with weight-control clients, in addition to helping clients discover and address the specific causes of their obesity. LWMCs should understand the theories and principles that help explain health behavior, as well as the many variables that affect weight loss-success. Lifestyle-modification strategies built on self-monitoring can help LWMCs work with clients to address readiness to change, goal-setting, environmental cues, self-efficacy, stress management, cognitive restructuring, and problem-solving.

References

Andersen, R.E. et al. (1999). Effect of lifestyle activity vs. structured aerobic exercise in obese women. *Journal of the American Medical Association,* 281, 335–340.

Armitage, C.J. (2006). Evidence that implementation intentions promote transitions between the stages of change. *Journal of Consulting and Clinical Psychology,* 74, 1, 141–151.

Bandura, A. (1997). *Self-efficacy: The Exercise of Control.* New York: Freeman.

Berkel, L.A. et al. (2005). Behavioral interventions for obesity. *Journal of the American Dietetic Association,* 105, 5, Suppl. 1, 35–43.

Boutelle, K.N. & Kirschenbaum, D.S. (1998). Further support for consistent self-monitoring as a vital component of successful weight control. *Obesity Research,* 6, 219–224.

Brehm, B.A. (2004). *Successful Fitness Motivation Strategies.* Champaign, Ill.: Human Kinetics.

Brehm, B.A. (2000). Maximizing the psychological benefits of physical activity. *ACSM's Health & Fitness Journal,* 4, 6, 7–11, 26.

Brehm, B.A. (1998). *Stress Management: Increasing Your Stress Resistance.* New York: Addison, Wesley, Longman.

Buehler, R., Griffin, D., & Ross, M. (1994). Exploring the "planning fallacy": Why people underestimate their task completion times. *Journal of Personality and Social Psychology,* 67, 366–381.

Carlos Poston, W.S., II, & Foreyt, J.P. (1999). Obesity is an environmental issue. *Athlerosclerosis,* 146, 2, 201–209.

Fabricatore, A.N. & Wadden, T.A. (2005). Lifestyle modification in the treatment of obesity. In: D.J. Goldstein (Ed.). *The Management of Eating Disorders and Obesity* (2nd ed.). (pp 209–229). Totowa, N.J.: Humana Press.

Fitzgibbon, M.L., Stolley, M.R., & Kirschenbaum, D.S. (1993). Obese people who seek treatment have different characteristics than those who do not seek treatment. *Health Psychology,* 12, 342–345.

Geliebter, A. & Aversa, A. (2003). Emotional eating in overweight, normal weight, and underweight individuals. *Eating Behavior,* 3, 4, 341–347.

Gladis, M.M. et al. (1998). A comparison of two approaches to the assessment of binge eating in obesity. *International Journal of Eating Disorders,* 23, 17–26.

Marlatt, B.A. & George, W.H. (1998). Relapse prevention and the maintenance of optimal health. In: Shumaker, S.A. et al. (Eds.). *The Handbook of Health Behavior Change.* New York: Springer.

McAuley, E. & Blissmer, B. (2000). Self-efficacy determinants and consequences of physical activity. *Exercise and Sport Sciences Reviews,* 28, 2, 85–88.

Muraven, M. & Baumeister, R.F. (2000). Self-regulation and depletion of limited resources: Does self-control resemble a muscle? *Psychological Bulletin,* 126, 2, 247–259.

Polivy, J. & Herman, C.P. (2000). The false-hope syndrome: Unfulfilled expectations of self-change. *Current Directions in Psychological Science,* 9, 4, 128–131.

Renjilian, D.A. et al. (2001). Individual vs. group therapy for obesity: Effects of matching participants to their treatment preference. *Journal of Consulting and Clinical Psychology,* 69, 717–721.

Stice, E., Fisher, M., & Lowe, M.R. (2004). Are dietary restraint scales valid measures of acute dietary restriction? Unobtrusive observation data suggest not. *Psychological Assessment,* 16, 1, 51–59.

Tate, D.F., Jackvony E.H., & Wing, R.R. (2003). Effects of internet behavioral counseling on weight loss in adults at risk for type 2 diabetes. *Journal of the American Medical Association,* 289, 1833–1836.

Teachman, B.A. & Brownell, K.D. (2001). Implicit anti-fat bias among health professionals: Is anyone immune? *International Journal of Obesity,* 25, 1525–1531.

Tice, D.M., Bratslavsky, E., & Baumeister, R.F. (2001). Emotional distress regulation takes precedence over impulse control: If you feel bad, do it! *Journal of Personality and Social Psychology,* 80, 1, 53–67.

Vohs, K.D. & Heatherton, T.F. (2000). Self-regulatory failure: A resource-depletion approach. *Psychological Science,* 11, 3, 249–254.

Wing, R.R. & Phelan, S. (2005). Long-term weight loss maintenance. *American Journal of Clinical Nutrition,* 82, 1, 222S–225S.

Witkiewitz, K. & Marlatt, G.A. (2004). Relapse prevention for alcohol and drug problems: That was Zen, this is Tao. *American Psychologist,* 59, 4, 224–235.

Witte, K. & Allen, M. (2000). A meta-analysis of fear appeals: Implications for effective public health campaigns. *Health Education & Behavior,* 27, 5, 591–615.

Suggested Readings

Annesi, J.J. (2002).The exercise support process: Facilitating members' self-management skills. *Fitness Management,* 18, 10 (Suppl), 24–25.

Brehm, B.A. (2004). *Successful Fitness Motivation Strategies.* Champaign, Ill.: Human Kinetics.

Brehm, B.A. (2000). Maximizing the psychological benefits of physical activity. *ACSM's Health & Fitness Journal,* 4, 6, 7–11, 26.

Carlos Poston, W.S., II, & Foreyt, J.P. (2000). Successful management of the obese patient. *American Family Physician,* 61, 3615–3622.

Miller-Kovach, K. (2006). *Weight Watchers Family Power: 5 Simple Rules for a Healthy-Weight Home.* Hoboken, N.J.: John Wiley & Sons.

Rippe, J.M. and Weight Watchers (2005). *Weight Loss That Lasts: Break Through the 10 Big Diet Myths*. Hoboken, N.J.: John Wiley & Sons.

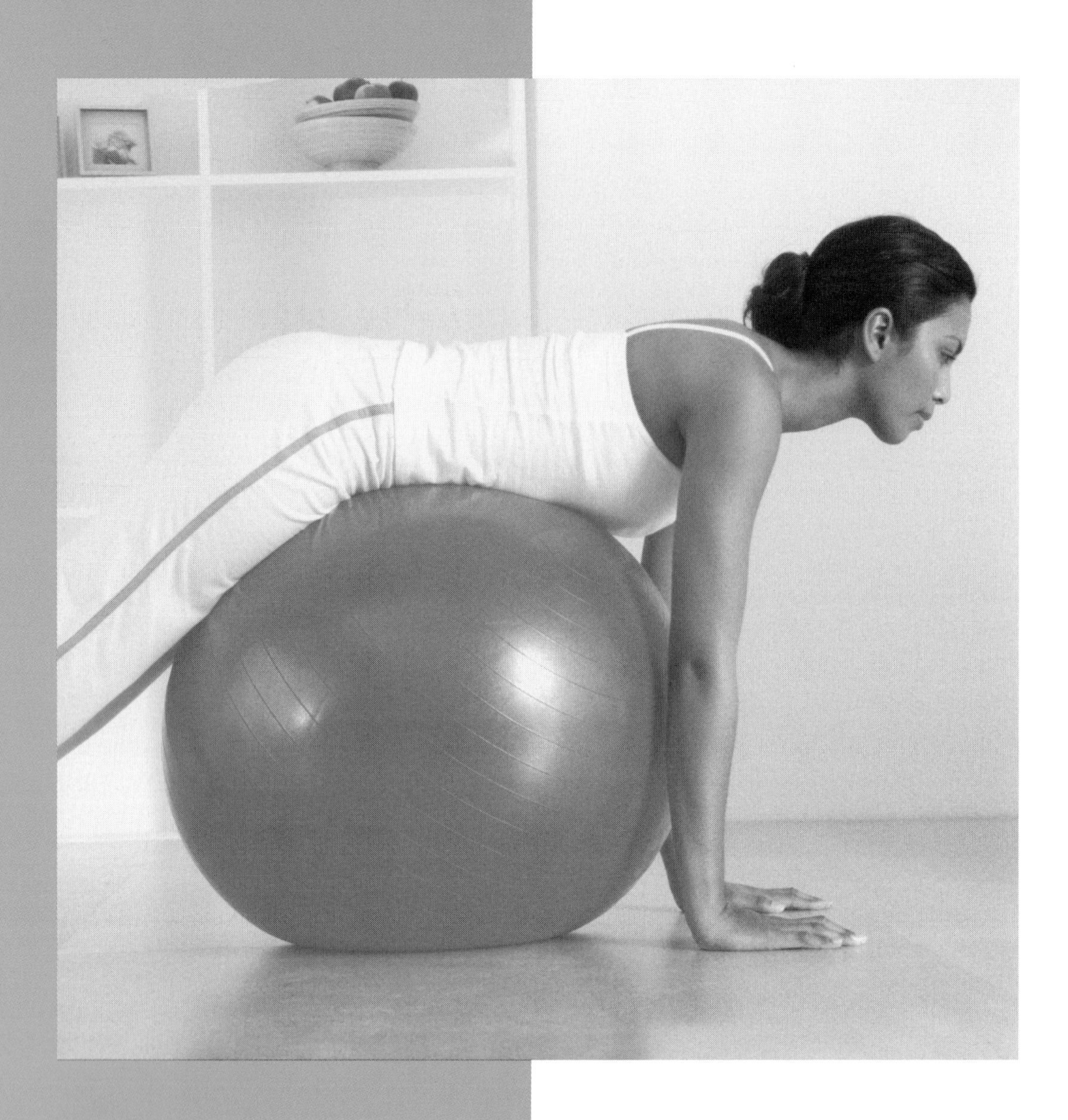

James J. Annesi

James J. Annesi, Ph.D., is director of wellness advancement for the YMCA of Metropolitan Atlanta. He is the principal architect of THE COACH APPROACH,® Youth Fit For Life,™ and The Health and Fitness Experience health-behavior-change initiatives. Dr. Annesi has held appointments with Rutgers University, the Veterans Affairs Health Care System, and the United States Sports Academy, and has consulted with numerous YMCAs and other health-promotion organizations in the U.S., United Kingdom, Canada, Italy, and Japan. He continues an active research program focused on exercise adherence, weight loss and maintenance, and the effects of physical activity on depression, anxiety, self-image, and other mental-health and quality-of-life factors.

Chapter 16

Adherence to Physical Activity and Weight-loss Behaviors

IN THIS CHAPTER:

The Problem of Adherence

Adherence to exercise and weight-loss programs is a problem. Although most overweight and sedentary people understand the need to lose weight and be more physically active, and are willing to give the requisite behaviors a try, long-term maintenance is extremely difficult for most. Studies on exercise adherence show that approximately 50 to 65% of new and returning participants drop out of physical-activity regimens within the initial three to six months (Annesi, 2003; Annesi & Unruh, 2007; Dishman, 1988). More than half of this attrition occurs within the first several weeks of initiating efforts and declaring a commitment. Even in fitness-center settings, drop-out rates approaching 80% within eight months are commonly found (Figure 16-1). Although considerable thought has been given to physiological issues such as recommended amounts of daily exercise, target heart rate, and optimal number of sets and repetitions, these issues may be of secondary concern when most people struggle with even short-term maintenance of very basic programs.

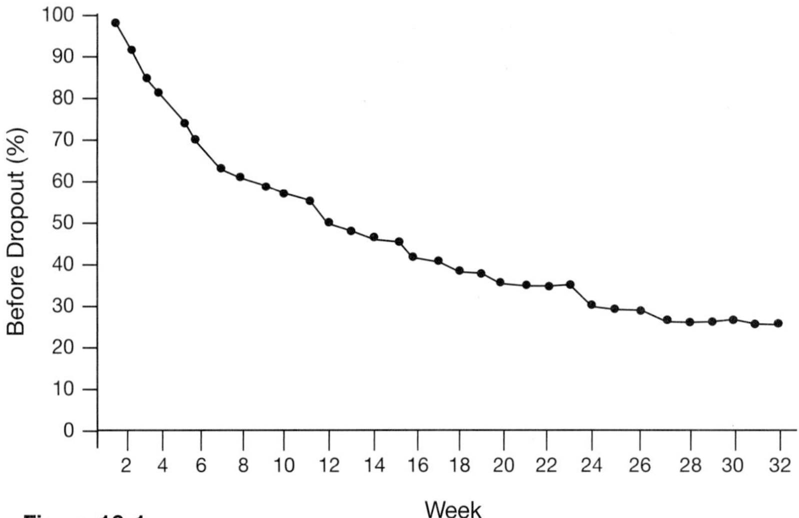

Figure 16-1
Observed drop-out of new and returning exercise-program participants over eight months, within a fitness center setting.

Adapted from: Annesi, J.J. (1998). Effects of computer feedback on adherence to exercise. *Perceptual and Motor Skills*, 87, 723–730.

Along with the observed attrition rates from exercise programs, rates of long-term success with nutritionally based weight-control efforts are similarly problematic (Miller, Koceja, & Hamilton, 1997). As with exercise, drop-out rates during the initial months of weight-management programs is found to be 50% or more (Graffagnino et al., 2006; Wadden et al., 1992). Indications are that less than 2% of individuals who attained significant weight loss in their twenties maintain even 10% of their original loss through their forties. Only 10 to 20% will keep their original weight lost off for even one full year. Between 75 and 85% of individuals have, over the past several years, used decreased fat intake, reduced amounts of food, reduced calories, and increased exercise to lose weight. However, none of these methods were practiced more than 20% of the time.

By any measure, it is clear that individuals' initial weight loss is not regularly maintained, and behaviors associated with weight loss are difficult to adhere to. In fact, the natural history of weight loss is extremely consistent regardless of a participant's gender and age, assigned caloric intake, or initial amount of weight loss. Maximum weight loss is typically reached about six months after initiating a program. Much of this weight loss is regained soon after treatment or intervention ends, and there is a more gradual weight increase over the next several years, often ending with greater weight than at the program's start (Jeffery et al., 2000). A study of working-age adults found that dieting used to reduce weight was actually associated with weight gain, not loss, over two years for the typical participant. In a position stand by the American Psychological Association (Mann et al., 2007), the use of diets, without strong and sustained behavioral support for both eating and physical activity, were deemed ineffective for improving health. They state, "It appears that dieters who manage to sustain a weight loss are the rare exception, rather than the rule. Dieters who gain back more weight than they lost may very well be the norm rather than the unlucky minority" (p. 230). They go on to state their concern for the potential health damages of frequent losses and gains of weight. Without fresh approaches to enable people to stick with behaviors associated with weight loss, numerous health-risk factors will continue to be adversely affected, and the United States' healthcare system may soon become overloaded. Clearly, if current trends continue, they will take a toll on many people's longevity and quality of life (Mokdad et al., 2001).

Although the universal prescription for weight loss is eating less and exercising more, these behaviors are not typically well-assimilated. Individuals' acknowledgement of the absolute need, the accrued health benefits, and the risks of not acting on behalf of their own health is, unfortunately, not a predictor of *maintenance* of health-related behaviors. This has been demonstrated over the past several decades by the disappointing outcomes of the increased social marketing of people's need to be more physically active and eat better. Based on reported trends, these public education-based efforts may actually be associated with less exercise, more obesity, and increased health risks over time.

Because approaches for providing information on the need to be more physically active and incorporate better eating appear ineffective at sustaining change, and teaching individuals how to properly exercise and diet have worked for only a select few, improvements in traditional methods are required. Rather than maintaining a primarily educational focus (and blaming individuals for not having enough "motivation" or "commitment" when they fail), LWMCs should seek alternate routes. They should attempt to systematically *nurture* healthy habits using what is presently known, as the result of research, about fostering sustained health-behavior changes. Hopefully, as the field of weight management moves from the status quo to the science of systematic behavior change, methods will become more focused, refined, and effective. As a result, individuals will be more readily empowered to effectively counter the many personal, social, and environmental barriers to maintaining weight-loss and exercise programs. Although the health-behavior change methods covered in this chapter are not new, they have failed to gain widespread usage within fields related to exercise, nutrition, and weight loss. The predominant approach is still to inform individuals on what should be done to lose weight and complete sufficient amounts of physical activity—and "hope for the best" regarding continuity of these obviously difficult sets of behaviors.

This chapter covers much of what LWMCs must understand to reliably affect *sustained* changes in critical health behaviors. These reviews begin with some of the theories of health-behavior change. This is not just an academic exercise, however. The focus is on how sound theories may be used to induce sustainable changes in eating and exercise behaviors. After a review of theories in this practical manner, an overview of the **correlates** of, or the variables associated with, physical activity and weight-loss behaviors is presented. Only when methods "hit at the heart" of factors known to reliably affect long-term success can practitioners promote replicability of results and improve the lives of many, rather than just a select few.

A review of a number of specific techniques that have been shown to be effective at enabling participants to maximize their success with newly adopted health behaviors is then given. Based on existing research, many of these interventions focus on improving individuals' self-management and self-regulatory abilities, but also consider their expectations, daily demands, personalities, and available social-support structures. Some behavior-change techniques have had increased success when delivered as a part of a multi-modal "treatment package." A sample of these packages is also overviewed, exemplifying movement from the science to the practice of effectively empowering individuals toward a path to improved health. How LWMCs may provide the best service to clients is also related to their ability to reliably deliver evidence-based treatments using effective counseling techniques. Thus, a brief review of some salient elements of the counseling process will be presented.

Without a high degree of ability to promote adherence, success at facilitating exercise and weight loss will be limited to those with the most internal volition, which in actuality is the group that needs the *least* help. An individual with a more typical profile—that is, the average person—will continue to demonstrate the familiar start-and-stop cycles. However, with appropriate use of research-driven adherence methods, widespread assimilation of improved health behaviors becomes possible. Sustained, favorable results can then become the norm, rather than the exception. Understanding the theoretical rationale of health-behavior-change treatments—the results of methods that are an outgrowth of systematic scientific scrutiny—along with optimal techniques for direct practical application of the best evidence-based practices, will enable LWMCs to make meaningful contributions to their clients. Although many individuals in health-related professions are novices at reliably fostering health-behavior changes, they too can reap the rewards if they pay close attention to what is presently understood through the behavioral sciences.

Theories of Motivated Behavior Change

Theoretical models provide high-level, testable hypotheses of factors that may predict behavior, how these factors interact to affect behaviors in a specific manner, and, in many cases, what may be done to affect positive change (Baranowski, 2006; Culos-Reed, Gyurcsik, & Brawley, 2001; Rejeski, 1992). Although many such theories are somewhat abstract and include variables that may not be readily changeable, this chapter focuses on models with implications for helping clients and avoids an exclusively explanatory focus. Some constructs are similar across theories. There has been some criticism of theories that attempt to be all-encompassing. For example, some researchers feel that *initiation* of health behaviors is a very different situation than *maintenance* of the behaviors (Rothman, 2002). Research suggests that what works to get people to begin exercising or modifying their eating program may not be related to maintenance. Although this debate is not covered in full, this chapter emphasizes the contribution that the selected theories make on the practice of promoting adherence to newly adopted health behaviors.

Decision-making Theories

The theory of reasoned action suggests that individuals usually act based on the information available to them. It also assumes that people consider in great depth the implications of their actions before undertaking them, and that the "intentions" that follow are the primary determinants of the attempted health behaviors. The bases of the intentions are, first, the attitude that completing the behaviors will lead to desired outcomes and, second, the social norms influencing the person (e.g., influences from family and friends). These two factors are weighed against any constraints a person may have (e.g., perceived lack of time, dislike of feelings associated with physical exertion) (Godin, 1994). The theory of reasoned action was subsequently extended and renamed the theory of planned behavior. This theory additionally accounts for a construct called "perceived behavioral control," or one's perception of how easy or difficult maintenance of the behavior is likely to be. This is similar to the concept of **self-efficacy** in the self-efficacy theory (reviewed later in this chapter), although not as much emphasis is placed upon this aspect in this context.

While these two theories point LWMCs in some general directions for helping methods, such as emphasizing progress toward goals, setting up social situations that are supportive, and emphasizing "mastery" over the processes that lead to reduced weight and better health, more specific directives for methodologies are lacking. Although there is a high dependence on intentions, it must be acknowledged that this is not a static concept; it may change as a person's persistence is challenged by slow progress, competing personal demands, and boredom.

Health-risk-reduction Theories

The following two theories are included in this chapter not because of their contribution to treatment research, but rather to illustrate how "common sense" does not always work when dealing with individuals' persistence with health behaviors. Both are focused on the association between the perceived need for improved health behaviors and the amount of behavior change that a person actually accomplishes. In actuality, neither model has had much success at predicting *sustained* health-behavior changes. To illustrate, research has found that approximately 90% of people could name multiple benefits of regular exercise, as well as articulate a high need for sufficient physical activity in their own lives (Kearny et al., 1999). However, only a small fraction of those people actually completed the recommended amounts. There has not been a strong association between perceived need and sustained health behaviors.

The **health belief model** hypothesizes that the likelihood of initiating and staying with a health behavior is linked directly to the perception of a personal health threat, and the belief that the recommended actions will reduce that threat. It is proposed that individuals will weigh the perceived benefits against the perceived barriers to initiation or continuance of the advised behaviors (Godin, 1994). Similarly, the **protection motivation theory** emphasizes action based on the severity of a threatened event (e.g., a heart attack). To strengthen the protection motivation theory, concepts were added that related to the level of confidence one has regarding the effectiveness of the recommended behaviors (i.e., response efficacy) and the level of confidence one has in his or her ability to successfully complete the recommended behaviors (i.e., personal efficacy).

Although individuals are more ready to start or restart weight-loss and exercise regimens when they perceive an acute need, the same does not hold true for adherence. In reality, this concept supports the suggestion mentioned at the start of this section that separate theories may be required to best deal with scenarios related to initiating vs. maintaining health behaviors. This also suggests that interventions should be specifically tailored based on an individual's readiness for change, as is reviewed in the later section on the **transtheoretical model.**

Behavioral Theory

Although it is often criticized for being simplistic or reductionist, **behavioral theory** (sometimes referred to as **operant conditioning** or **learning theory**) is one of the most (if not *the* most) clearly supported paradigms in the behavioral sciences. It posits that the internal processes (e.g., intentions, perceived need) that individuals go through are of minimal concern when attempting to predict, explain, and affect behavior change. It is proposed that whether one continues a health behavior or not is directly related to the reinforcers (vs. punishers) associated with the behavior (Knapp, 1988) (Figure 16-2). Thus, although many events may prompt a positive behavior, such as eating a salad (instead of, say, a cheeseburger), or spending 30 minutes on a treadmill (rather than spending time with friends at the pub after work), their consequences are the primary determinants of maintaining or terminating such a behavior over time (under similar conditions). Followers of behavioral theory focus their attention on what occurs directly following a behavior that may serve as a reinforcer (i.e., something perceived as positive), negative reinforcer (i.e., removing something perceived as negative), or punisher (i.e., something perceived as negative). The systematic use or manipulation of reinforcers and punishers can purposefully "shape" behaviors and aid in forming habits. The practical application of behavioral theory is strong, because people can directly observe resultant behaviors (which they cannot do with the internal processes often depended upon by other theories).

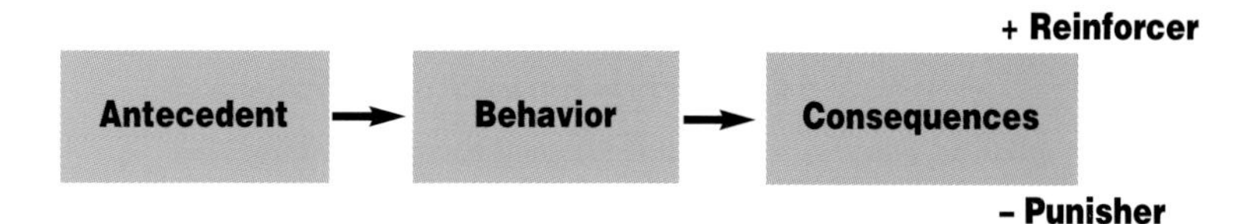

Figure 16-2
Primary tenet of behavioral theory

When considering the descriptions of interventions intended to promote health-behavior change, the implications of behavioral theory become evident. For example, methods are described to adjust exercise intensities and durations to reduce unpleasant sensations (e.g., fatigue, exhaustion) that may serve as punishers and reduce the chance of adherence over time, and maximize reinforcing effects such as feeling reenergized for further activities that day. Behavioral theory acknowledges that consequences may affect individuals differently. For example, experienced exercisers may perceive the "lactic-acid burn" as reinforcing because of its association with physiological progress, while the same feeling may lead novice exercisers to rapidly terminate the behavior. It becomes the domain of LWMCs to identify reinforcers and punishers for every individual so that they can organize a process for continuity of desired behaviors. Behavioral theory assumes (and has proven) great possibilities for purposely deriving situations that enable the systematic establishment of desirable habits.

Cognitive-behavioral Theories

The self-efficacy theory is a powerful explanatory model for predicting initiation and maintenance of health behaviors. This model hypothesizes that *all* sustained changes in behaviors are mediated by the common mechanism of self-efficacy, or the belief that one can successfully deal with barriers and competently perform desired behaviors (Bandura, 1997). The degree of situation-specific self-efficacy can determine the following:

- Whether a health behavior is attempted in the first place
- The degree of persistence when encountering difficulties
- Actual success of the resulting behaviors

Research strongly suggests that self-efficacy and related constructs predict adherence to exercise and weight-loss behaviors, and that self-efficacy is advanced through perceived incremental successes (Strecher et al., 1986) (Figure 16-3).

There are a number of methods that seek to improve self-efficacy to help foster persistence. The individual methods are covered in some detail later in the chapter. Each focuses on demonstrating how a person is competent and able to make adequate progress as a result of being persistent. For example, when a client sets a short-term goal and commits to (preferably in writing) the attainment of what is perceived to be a worthwhile short-term goal (e.g., increasing total cardiovascular exercise output by 20 minutes per week, or eating one fast-food meal per week instead of five) and achieves it, a sense of accomplishment and competence to persist (i.e., self-efficacy) may be derived. This may serve to counter another common scenario in which self-efficacy is diminished, such as when a client sets a lofty goal [e.g., to lose 45 pounds (20 kg) as soon as possible] and fails to achieve the desired result (e.g., perceived slow progress and incompetence is associated with weighing one's self each morning and seeing little or no positive change). Thus, self-efficacy is both a predictor and a result of perceived success with specific health behaviors. It also has great possibilities for interventions to benefit clients' persistence.

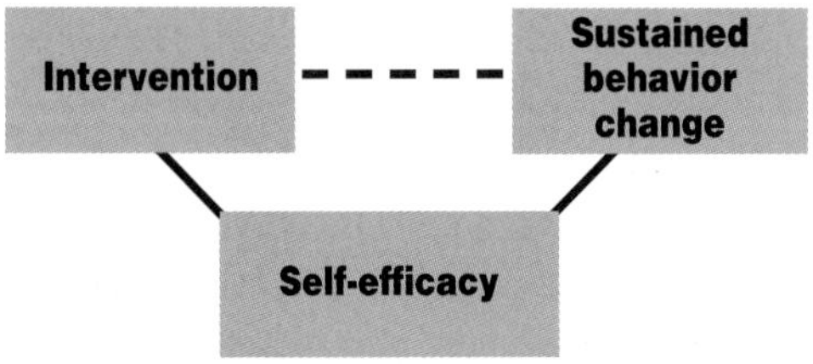

Figure 16-3
Proposed mediating effects of self-efficacy

Intervention
Sustained behavior change
Self-efficacy

Self-efficacy has been extended by its developer, Albert Bandura, into a broader theory named **social-cognitive theory.** It should be noted that the development of this theory in no way diminishes the importance of the self-efficacy construct on its own. The central principle of social-cognitive theory is called triadic reciprocal causation. The components of the triad, which greatly influence each other, are as follows (Bandura, 1986):

- Cognitions (thoughts that allow individuals to consider present situations based on previous situations and expected outcomes)
- Behaviors (previous actions)
- Environment (social and physical situations in which people operate)

Social-cognitive theory posits that all health behaviors are goal-driven through anticipation of outcomes. Perceived capabilities (self-efficacy) interact with goals through the simultaneous influence that cognitions, behaviors, and the environment have on one another. An important tenet of social-cognitive theory, for the purposes of LWMCs, is that people are capable of self-regulating their actions, choosing situations that will positively influence their behaviors, and altering their environment to best promote desirable health behaviors. Individuals may also purposefully manipulate their incentives and use knowledge of others' experiences to guide their own actions. Social-cognitive theory views the person as an active participant in maintaining his or her own health behaviors. That is in contrast to behavioral theory, where behaviors are viewed as simply being acted upon, and their continuance or termination is largely determined by their consequences.

Stages-of-change Theory

In contrast to most of the theories just reviewed, the transtheoretical model is a straightforward theory with obvious applicability for health-promotion practice. In fact it has been the basis of a number of well-developed interventions for both the initiation and maintenance of exercise, weight loss, and many other health-behavior issues including smoking cessation and alcohol rehabilitation. The transtheoretical model suggests that individuals are in one of five "stages of change" at any given time. These stages are: **precontemplation, contemplation, preparation, action,** and **maintenance.** Cyclical movement through, and relapse back from, these stages is common (Reed, 1999). Specific mechanisms are hypothesized to help individuals move forward through the stages (or relapse).

Individuals in the precontemplation stage have no intention of altering their current unhealthy behavior, while those in the contemplation stage are considering adopting a target behavior within six months. The focus of intervention for people in these two stages is to prompt them to identify an urgency to act on their own behalf. People in the preparation stage accomplish their target health behavior only sporadically. While they generally have identified a need, they have not yet been able to incorporate a regular regimen of action. Approaches that highlight the pros and cons of a higher level of action are often helpful for these individuals, as are methods that enable them to clearly envision themselves as being successful.

People in the action stage have begun a regular routine, but have been participating for less than six months. These individuals are the most likely to relapse to an earlier stage (and often begin the desired behavior again another time). Because the personal resources needed to begin a health behavior differ greatly from those needed to maintain it, a focus on countering psychological, social, and environmental barriers is a great help for this group (Annesi, 1998; Dishman, 1988). Adequate use of self-management and self-regulatory skills predicts success for individuals in the action stage. Persons in the maintenance stage have persisted at the target health behavior for at least six months. Research in exercise adherence confirms a notable reduction in the propensity to drop out for this group. Because evidence exists that skills for persistence are at least somewhat established in individuals in the maintenance stage, they must be convinced that the effort being given has sufficient payoff for them to continue.

Although the transtheoretical model appears quite reasonable and has held up fairly well to scientific scrutiny, it does not yet predict with much certainty what specific variables are associated with people "moving up" in stages, what circumstances predict a relapse, or if people react differently after several starts and stops. Research suggests a significant association between how advanced an individual's stage of change is and the amount of self-efficacy possessed regarding completion of that health behavior (Marcus et al., 1992).

Adaptation-relapse Process Theory

Although the preceding theories are broad and explanatory in nature, each has at least some implication for the selection and use of methods to promote maintenance of health behaviors. Researchers have tested a model with the working title of **adaptation-relapse process model,** which was specifically designed around intervention to promote exercise adherence (Annesi, 2004a). A version of the model will also be tested for adjusting eating behaviors. The model borrows heavily from several of the theories previously reviewed in this chapter. After considerable investigation, it was determined that the following factors explained approximately 45% of the variance in exercise adherence for new and returning participants:

- Self-management/self-regulatory skills
- Ability to tolerate discomfort
- Social support

Although the research team could increase the *considerable* predictive accuracy of the model if variables that were not readily changeable were added, it did not make these additions so that effective intervention design could remain the primary focus.

By developing a brief survey that assesses the three aforementioned factors, helping methods based on individuals' needs, weaknesses, and propensity for early drop-out could be specified. For example, if a person had an especially low score on the "ability to tolerate discomfort" factor, physical-activity amounts that were associated with pleasant, rather than aversive, feelings were emphasized. When the "self-management/self-regulation" factor score was low, practitioners may use an array of self-management and self-regulatory skills to help clients overcome barriers. Participation in non-threatening, supportive group-exercise environments that help build social support and feelings of camaraderie was emphasized when the "social support" score was low. This model is only applicable to new and returning exercisers. It does not address prompts that will *initiate* a physical-activity regimen for presently sedentary people. It does, however, directly relate variables that predict adherence to corresponding interventions that are likely to be effective.

Correlates of Sustained Physical Activity and Weight-loss Behaviors

This section reviews personal variables associated with sustained physical activity and weight-loss behaviors. These variables are referred to as correlates or determinants. While theories often deal with the interaction of several variables dynamically, correlates allow researchers to refine their focus for selection and use of helping methods by isolating the effects of distinct factors. Many of these factors emanate from theoretical propositions.

A thorough review of approximately 350 studies examining potential correlates of physical activity accounts for variables that are both changeable through helping efforts, and quite stable and not subject to much change (Trost et al., 2002). Examples are as follows:

- Various demographic and biological factors (e.g., education level, marital status, genetic health risks)
- Social factors (e.g., past family influences, physician influences)
- Physical-environment factors (e.g., perceived and actual access to recreation facilities, presence of sidewalks, safe environment)
- History of physical activity (in both childhood and adulthood)

Although the corresponding research on correlates of eating behaviors is not as well developed as research addressing physical activity, and is based on far fewer studies, much can be gleaned from the currently available findings. The following sections cover correlates of exercise adherence first, and then move on to determinants of maintenance of weight-management behaviors that focus primarily on modification of eating patterns.

Correlates of Sustained Physical Activity

As could be anticipated based on the earlier review of theories, individuals' knowledge of health and exercise, the beliefs of their family and friends about physical activity, "attitudes" toward exercise, the perceived value of exercise outcomes, and susceptibility to illness *are not* correlates of ongoing physical activity. LWMCs promoting exercise maintenance may see little payoff when presenting information to clients that focuses on the need to incorporate physical activity into their lives to improve health and avoid future physical problems, as counterintuitive as that may seem.

Some psychological factors that have been proven to be reliable *negative* correlates of physical activity are the amount of perceived barriers, perceived lack of time, poor body image, and mood disturbance. Methods to attempt to counter these factors are warranted. It should be noted that while perceived lack of time is the single most cited reason for quitting exercise, there is little evidence that adherents have more discretionary time than dropouts. "Perceived" is the key word here.

Psychological factors that are known to be *positive* correlates of physical activity include the expected attainment of personal goals, self-efficacy, self-motivation, feelings of social support, seeing one's self as a competent exerciser, the ability to accommodate physical sensations associated with exertion, and enjoyment of physical activity. Additionally, possessing the skills to effectively cope with barriers to physical activity and the ability to perceive the "positives" related to physical activity as outweighing the "negatives" are positive correlates of maintained exercise. Specific interventions should be incorporated to effectively deal with these personal variables, as is discussed later in this chapter.

The quality of dietary habits is a correlate of ongoing exercise, a fact that was replicated in studies of multiple age groups, as are feelings of support from a spouse, family members, peers, and one's physician. With regard to physical-activity programs, as perceived effort, intensity, and duration increase, adherence is reduced. At the onset of a program, participants and practitioners often try to expedite the physiological effects of exercise through very challenging amounts of exercise. Due to a low tolerance for exercise-induced discomfort, this practice may be linked to drop-out well before much progress is made. Whether frequency of exercise is a correlate remains unknown. While seeking to accomplish at least *some* physical activity each day may lead to consistency, fewer bouts per week may be less taxing on finite abilities to self-manage.

Correlates of Sustained Weight-loss Behaviors

As mentioned earlier, correlates of weight loss have not been studied as extensively as correlates of physical activity (Foreyt et al., 1995). Thus, the following review is based on the limited research available. Factors that appear *not* to be related to maintaining weight-loss behaviors include motives for losing weight (e.g., health, physical appearance, payment for weight loss), type of diet (e.g., proportions of macronutrients), degree of caloric restriction, and length of treatment (unless long-term continuance of treatment is classified as maintenance). In reality, *whenever* treatment is terminated, a gradual regain of weight is predicted. While the evidence is not completely clear, low mood and mood disturbance are thought to be negatively associated with maintaining weight-loss behaviors, as are loss of self-motivation and competing social pressures. Every effort should be made to reduce the chance of a client's low mood prompting a relapse into previous poor eating behaviors. Fortunately, the completion of even moderate amounts of physical activity positively affects mood for most individuals. This may be leveraged early in the treatment process to improve resilience. The importance of the proportion of fat, carbohydrates, and protein in the diet remains highly debated and unresolved with regards to maintenance of weight loss. Adjustments of macronutrient proportions may promote early, but unsustained, weight loss.

Social support is a correlate of maintaining appropriate eating patterns, along with self-efficacy. Clearly, the type of social environment present can have an effect on maintenance of weight loss, so LWMCs should make an effort to collaborate with clients on managing this important variable. Improvement in body image and body satisfaction tends to be associated with increased self-efficacy. The *best* predictor of weight-loss maintenance is physical activity. Apparently, there are still-unknown mechanisms at work with regular exercise that help an individual maintain weight loss that go well beyond what may be explained through caloric expenditure alone. Although compliance can be difficult, ongoing self-monitoring of caloric or fat intake is clearly a correlate of weight-loss maintenance. Some researchers advocate that practitioners spend considerable energies enabling individuals to become proficient and consistent at tracking food consumption.

Some behavioral correlates of weight-loss maintenance are suggested through findings from the National Weight Control Registry (Klem et al., 1997; National Weight Control Registry, 2006). This is a database of approximately 5000 adults who, on average, lost more than 60 pounds and maintained it for more than five years. Clearly, these persons are unusually successful. These individuals tend to monitor their weight regularly and act when they observe even small gains. Members of the Registry also tend to eat breakfast every day, eat four to five times per day, and limit fast foods to one time per week. This group also engages in amounts of physical activity that go beyond governmental recommendations, completing 60 to 90 minutes of moderate-intensity physical activity on a daily basis. This activity converts to approximately six miles of walking (their most frequent form of physical activity). Weekly caloric expenditure approximates 3300 calories for men and 2500 calories for women. Fewer than 10% of Registry participants were successful at keeping their weight off without engaging in regular exercise.

Methods to Improve Adherence to Exercise and Maintenance of Weight Loss

Specific methods to improve exercise and eating behavior follow from theories of health-behavior change and known correlates, many of which were reviewed earlier in this chapter. Ideally, treatments will be grounded in one or more tenet of a theory, be tested for their intended effect on the desired behavior, and, finally, be analyzed to determine if the expected mechanisms were associated with the observed changes in behavior (Baranowski, Anderson, & Carmack, 1998). In that manner, refinement of helping methods may proceed in a systematic manner. For example, it may be assumed that the use of short-term goal-setting and feedback that emphasizes small but consistent gains will improve maintenance of exercise by fostering improved exercise-related self-efficacy—a known correlate of adherence and a central element of both the social-cognitive theory and the self-efficacy theory. If ongoing study confirms that self-efficacy improves as a result of treatment, then goal-setting methods and progress feedback facilitators may be refined to address the associated feelings of competence and mastery. What should follow then is improvement in the consistency of the desired behavior changes, which is likely to benefit more people more often. It is essential for LWMCs to study the latest research, so they can understand the scientific progress being made in facilitating ongoing health-behavior changes with clients. This process is constantly evolving.

Within this section, a number of specific treatments, methods, and interventions are reviewed. Although this review is not exhaustive, treatments with good empirical foundations were chosen. After an explanation of each treatment, its rationale—or the expected reason why it may serve to help improve consistency of clients' long-term health behaviors—will be reviewed. Its application in the formation of both favorable exercise and eating habits is then covered. Some weight-loss and exercise-adherence programs have had success when interventions were delivered as a treatment package. A brief review of these programs is included. It is expected that clients will have preferences and respond differently to techniques based on their own personal makeup.

Assessment of Risk for Dropping Out

Researchers and practitioners who use the transtheoretical model base their interventions on individuals' stage of readiness to change. Because a person's stage is easily assessed through self-report, an appraisal of which methods may be most suited for which individual is readily available (Marcus & Forsyth, 2003). For example, individuals classified as being in the action stage (started the target health behavior less than six months ago) may require thorough attention when building the self-management skills needed to effectively address issues such as barriers to eating appropriately while "eating on the run" or when work or travel interrupts the exercise routine. Individuals in the maintenance stage may, however, be best served through activities that provide a variety of exercise routines to counter boredom, as well as acknowledgment of the importance of *maintaining* weight after a number of months of losing weight.

Because self-efficacy is such a strong correlate of sustained exercise, a number of measurement tools have been developed to assess "exercise barriers self-efficacy," or the ability to effectively deal with the many social, personal, and environmental barriers to maintaining exercise (McAuley & Mihalko, 1998). These surveys tend to evaluate the confidence one has for overcoming potential barriers (e.g., social demands on one's time, feeling "out of place," unfavorable weather) and remaining consistent. This method brings to light a practical picture of what it may take to enable different individuals to persist. Counselors may thereby refine their focus on individualized needs, and choose methods that are especially well-suited. Versions of this approach have also been used to identify vulnerable situations with regard to maintaining appropriate eating behaviors.

Self-motivation has been effectively measured in both research and practice settings. Because it has a demonstrated association with persistence (Buckworth & Dishman, 2002), there has been some success at assessing self-motivation, or the ability to persevere in the absence of external reinforcement, and then tailoring interventions intended to foster adherence to exercise. Because self-motivation is viewed as a trait, or a stable aspect of one's personal makeup, efforts are not usually expended in trying to change it. Thus, "motivating" someone may be a misleading phrase. Implications for practice may be that when minimal self-motivation is identified, practitioners may work to avoid overstressing the system with demands (e.g., immediately reducing caloric intake from 2700 per day to 1200 per day; rapidly progressing from little or no planned physical activity to a full hour of moderate-to-vigorous cardiovascular exercise each day). It may also be a good practice to empower clients with specific behavioral skills to counter effects of minimal self-motivation (e.g., positive self-talk, seeking energizing surroundings). With regard to sustaining an exercise program, research indicates that individuals with self-motivation scores even somewhat above average are still vulnerable to early drop-out if their lack of ability to overcome perceived barriers is not effectively addressed.

Consistent with the adaptation-relapse process model, researchers have developed a brief self-report inventory, called the "resources for exercise maintenance scale" (REMS) (Annesi, 2004a). Through use of the REMS, new and returning exercisers are assessed on their propensity for early drop-out based on their responses to nine items that correspond to the factors described earlier in this chapter (1 = strongly disagree to 5 = strongly agree):

- Ability to tolerate discomfort (e.g., "I can persist when a task is tiring, uncomfortable, and/or painful.")
- Self-management/self-regulatory skills (e.g., "I find it difficult using 'self control' to keep myself successful.")
- Social support (e.g., "I don't have people around who support my interests and efforts.")

By using a triage approach, counseling attention is prioritized and specific treatment emphases are suggested. For example, an individual scoring in the thirtieth percentile on REMS, with low scores on the "ability to tolerate discomfort" and "self-management/self-regulatory skills" subscales, may be assigned to frequent counseling that focuses on methods that address making the exercise regimen associated with pleasant, rather than exhausting, feelings. Considerable attention would also be given to teaching specific self-management and self-regulatory skills. Conversely, individuals scoring in the eighty-fifth percentile may initially be successful with less frequent appointments and more intense exercise plans. Their current abilities may already adequately address the demands of a fairly challenging exercise program.

Self-management/ Self-regulatory Skills

Goal-setting/Progress Feedback

Goals serve to direct participants' attention and action by mobilizing energy and prolonging effort (Locke & Latham, 1985). Goals also facilitate individuals' interest in developing relevant self-management strategies for sustained progress. Research suggests that optimal methods of setting goals for health behaviors should have the following traits (see Chapter 13):

- Goals should be specific (e.g., "do your best" goals may be the least effective).
- Ultimate goals should be broken down into incremental, short-term (e.g., one- to two-month) goals.
- Goals should be time-based.
- Goals should be accepted by the participant. LWMCs should play an active role in helping adjust goals so that they are reasonably attainable.
- A formal method of tracking progress is required.
- A formal plan of action (e.g., exercise plan, eating plan) is needed to facilitate goals.
- Goals should be prioritized.

Based on the preceding information, LWMCs should regularly cross-check their goal-setting methods with clients to ensure that they include the following principles:

- Long-term (six months or longer) goals are broken down into manageable short-term (e.g., one- to two-month) goals.
- A challenging, but reasonable, plan of action is established.
- There are processes for clients to gain relevant progress feedback (Figure 16-4).

Tailoring progress feedback is important because clients may rely only on readily available measures such as body weight, while incremental feedback in areas such as accumulated minutes of cardiovascular exercise per week and number of fruits and vegetables consumed per day may be more important for highlighting small gains and facilitating persistence. It should be noted that focusing only on obvious outcome measures (e.g., pounds or kilograms lost) may promote clients' frustration when progress is slower than desired. Because mood improvements are typically associated with moderate amounts of newly initiated exercise (Annesi, 2004b), LWMCs should measure, graph, and highlight positive changes such as levels of stress, depression, energy, and fatigue for their clients' inspection. Ongoing use of standardized surveys for mood changes have, when used in this manner, been associated with improvements in adherence to exercise programs (Annesi, 2004b). Participants are able to see progress in psychological areas that may be considerably meaningful for them.

Research indicates positive results when short-term goals are process-focused rather than outcome-focused. For this to successfully occur, there must be an adequate plan for the provision of feedback for these process goals (e.g., steps walked per day, calories consumed per day). For example, LWMCs could emphasize a one-month goal of increasing caloric expenditure through exercise from 500 to 1000 per week (a process goal), rather than a weight loss of 1.5 pounds (0.7 kg) per week, or 6 pounds (2.7 kg) in a month (an outcome goal).

Some researchers advocate attempting to adjust clients' long-term goals so that they will be more easily met (Foster et al., 1997).

Figure 16-4
Essential components of the goal-setting process

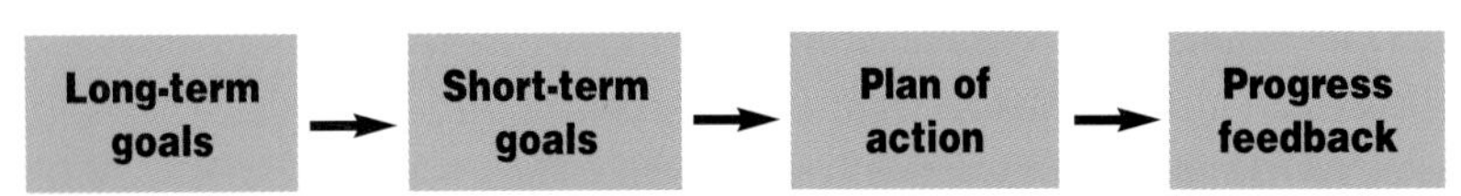

For example, a woman who is overweight by 85 pounds (39 kg) and wants to get down to 120 pounds (54 kg) because she feels that her social life will greatly improve, may be counseled to establish a (more realistic) goal weight that is the highest acceptable weight for her. Desires (possibly unreasonable ones), such as weight loss being associated with greatly increased amounts of attention and popularity, may be addressed as well. While this is a reasonable strategy, others have had success at maintaining exercise and weight-loss behaviors when ultimate goals were given relatively little attention initially, and when most of the early session-to-session focus was placed on the attainment of short-term goals (which were established in consultation with the LWMC). This technique prevents direct confrontation with the always-present social pressures (especially for females) to attain a certain body type, while maintaining a clear focus on adherence to the target behaviors through use of a more proximal goal. It was thought that habit formation, not rapid change, should remain the priority. This approach purposefully avoids confronting social pressures for thinness.

Clients are often able to articulate their desires when setting goals for both weight loss and physical activity. LWMCs should focus on aiding in the establishment, evaluation, and resetting of short-term goals. Attainment of agreed-upon short-term goals greatly contributes to increased self-efficacy and provides tangible evidence for clients that they can negotiate the system and be successful. Goal-setting and progress feedback are, therefore, essential strategies for LWMCs.

Self-monitoring

Self-monitoring is the organized recording of relevant behaviors. It may include manual recording of calories or fat for each food consumed, the review of an electronic compilation of completed cardiovascular exercise, or writing down each set and repetition of completed resistance exercise. Although self-monitoring methods may provide the information required to indicate when adjustments in eating or exercising are required, simply the act of self-monitoring may promote persistence. Often, it is an acknowledgement of incremental progress made (Knapp, 1988).

There is evidence of the benefits of self-monitoring for both exercise and reduced food intake. Some researchers believe that it is the single most important self-management tool for weight loss. In fact, some specialists suggest that an array of self-management skills should be learned so that the client becomes more proficient and consistent at self-monitoring calories or fat. Although it can be difficult to get compliance with comprehensive food tracking over time, the evidence for the efficacy of its continued use is compelling (Boutelle & Kirschenbaum, 1998). Methods have also sometimes required the recording of corresponding mood states, physical settings, and whether the food consumed was part of a scheduled eating time or not. This information may be used to identify prompts to eating, which may be acted upon as needed in consultation with a client. Some intervention packages have required self-monitoring for clients' weight-loss phase (typically around the initial six months), but not for their weight-maintenance phase. Some programs resume self-monitoring with evidence of non-adherence. Self-monitoring is usually complementary to goal-setting processes. Its use has been strongly related to weight-loss maintenance.

Cognitive Restructuring

Cognitive restructuring focuses on clients' purposeful use of internal processes to counter what may be harmful antecedents, or prompts, to health behaviors (Wing, Gorin, & Tate, 2001). With cognitive restructuring, a person is trained to first recognize an unproductive self-statement, then change or reframe it to be more productive. The cognitive-behavioral technique of "thought stopping" may also be incorporated to purposefully terminate problematic self-talk the moment it is recognized. At that point, another self-statement (which may be prepared beforehand with the LWMC) may be substituted. Done properly, cognitive restructuring can help individuals gain control of ruminations and self-talk, that, if left unchecked, can undermine individual occurrences of desired behaviors and their maintenance.

Cognitive restructuring is a useful technique when applied to both exercise and eating behaviors. For exercise, self-statements such as, "I can't believe I'm supposed to exercise after work today. I feel exhausted. Because it has been such a hard week, maybe I will skip it and just try to do more next week," could be stopped, and be substituted with more positive (but realistic) statements. For example, "Once I get going I will feel fine. Exercise is one of the best things that I can do for myself. It's important that I stay consistent." For eating, statements such as, "It is okay to have that (high-calorie) dessert today. It's been a bad week and I deserve it," could be stopped (hopefully, after only the first few words), and be substituted with such statements as, "It's not worth it, given all the hard work I have already put in. Progress has been good, and I don't want to regress."

Relapse Prevention

Relapse prevention is a well-developed, multiple-component treatment model that has previously addressed health behaviors, including tobacco and alcohol use (Marlatt & Gordon, 1985) (Figure 16-5). Its contribution to maintenance of physical activity and appropriate eating comes basically in two forms. The first is problem-solving related to identification of personal high-risk situations that are likely to cause a disruption in one's routine if they are not sufficiently dealt with. The other is developing awareness that the formation of healthful habits is not always a clean, linear process. In reality, it is almost inevitable that some disruptions, or "violations," will occur. The focus of treatment must therefore include both the development of behavioral skills needed for countering problems when they occur and the addressing of feelings of guilt, frustration, and incompetence often associated with a lapse in an established routine.

Research on relapse prevention suggests that clients should receive training in the following areas:

- Identifying situations that present a high risk for lapse of the desired behavior
- Improving the ability to either avoid or effectively cope with such high-risk situations
- Emphasizing the positives related to completed health behaviors rather than dwelling on minor violations
- Planning for inevitable slips in desired behaviors
- Setting rules for the behaviors that have some degree of flexibility
- Choosing enjoyable foods, physical activities, and environments associated with both of these components

Figure 16-5
Proposed model of the relapse process

Adapted from: Marlatt, G.A. (1985). Relapse prevention: Theoretical rationale and overview of the model. In: Marlatt, G.A. & Gordon, J.R. (Eds.) *Relapse Prevention* (p. 38). New York: Guilford.

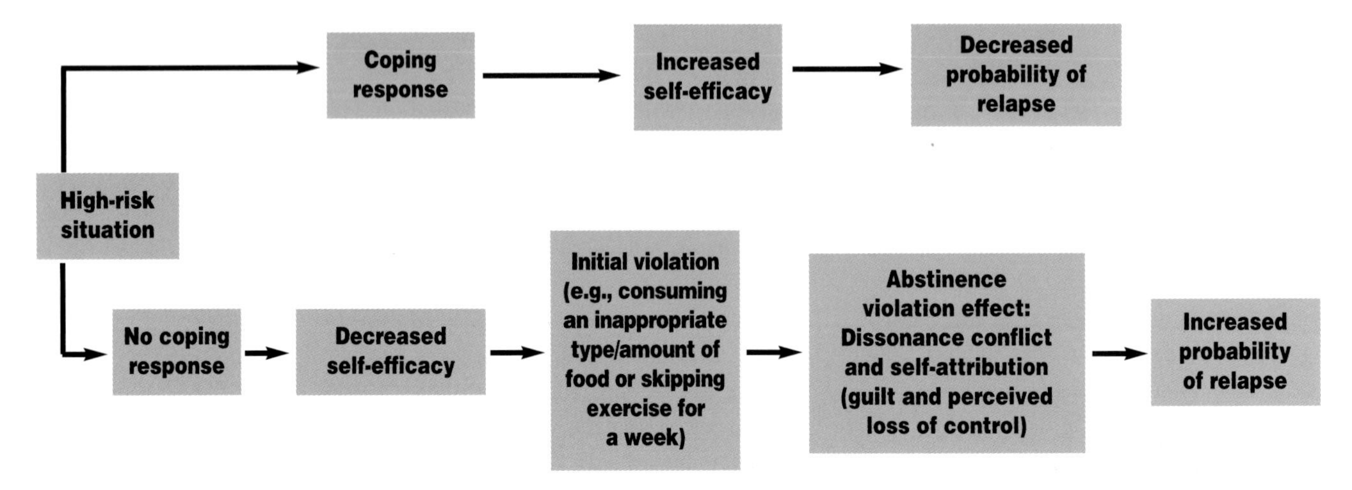

Although it may seem inappropriate, or unduly negative, to address relapse with a client when an exercise or eating plan is going well, the future rewards could be great. For example, if fast-food consumption is a risk when the client is rushed or is traveling for business, coping strategies may be devised before the problem is encountered. When a week of exercise is missed because a family emergency is being addressed, efforts can be made toward an enhanced capability to resume the routine as early as possible, rather than "trying to start fresh at the beginning of next month." The guilt and frustration of minor slips may be appropriately assimilated into the "big picture" of building healthful, long-term habits. LWMCs may also effectively address the "black-and-white thinking" of either being *on* or *off* the diet. Clients may also acknowledge that there is no absolute "gold standard" amount of exercise to either completely maintain or completely fail with—instead, any physical activity is productive.

When counseling for health-behavior change, relapse prevention is of great use. Although there are a number of possible variations for the effective delivery of this important cognitive-behavioral method, the following aspects should be included:

- Identification of high-risk situations
- The design of actions to counter the identified risky situations
- Preparation for feelings associated with minor breaks in routine

Dissociation

Dissociation, also referred to as cognitive dissociation or distraction, is a method by which a person's attentional focus is purposefully diverted away from unpleasant sensations (Annesi, 2001). In behavioral theory, it is an attempt to neutralize sensations that may be distasteful (e.g., hunger, fatigue) and therefore yield negative effects on the desired behavior. Left unchecked, undesirable sensations being "paired" with avoidance of food or completion of a physical activity will greatly diminish a person's chances for adherence. Although some researchers have questioned the usefulness of distancing one's self from physical sensations related to exercise—as such feedback has enhanced performance outputs—research is quite clear regarding the benefits of dissociation for the *typical* participant who struggles with both exercise-induced discomfort and consistency.

Methods used for dissociation with exercise include the use of television, reading, conversation, music, interesting surroundings, and participation in new or absorbing tasks (e.g., a new sport). Even the use of video games attached to exercise apparatus has been tested successfully. Methods to dissociate from feelings of hunger are usually based around initiating a task so that the person's attention will be redirected. Because exercising is incompatible with eating, and is productive for both weight loss and mood improvement, sometimes it may be suggested as an alternate activity. Dissociation is most productive when counselors discuss it early in the behavior-change process. Clients' successful resolution of challenging situations is likely to lead to feelings of increased self-efficacy, and thus improved maintenance of the desired behaviors.

Behavioral Contracting

Behavioral contracting, sometimes referred to as **contingency contracting,** is a method for outlining an agreement to fulfill a specific set of behaviors within a specified timeframe. Researchers state that aspects of contracting that promote health-behavior maintenance are as follows:

- Clarity
- Direct involvement with each participant's commitment
- A public, rather than private, commitment (promotes accountability)
- Ability to serve as support for a reward system (i.e., a marker of success)

LWMCs should consult closely with clients in developing behavioral contracts for both eating and physical activity. Contracts should reflect previously set goals and be newly generated as short-term goals are revised. A clear method of feedback is required to determine if the behavioral contract has been met. An example of a contract for revised eating may include a commitment to keep caloric intake between 1200 and 1600 per day, or limit fat intake to 25 grams each day. Examples for physical activity may be to complete four 30- to 40-minute sessions of moderate-to-vigorous cardiovascular exercise each week, or to complete a prearranged resistance-training program twice a week. There is an obvious need for LWMCs to provide empirical measurement tools to evaluate compliance. Behavioral contracts should be framed as serious commitments between the client and LWMC, and the client and himself or herself. Expected behaviors should be clearly defined, and the agreement should be formalized in writing and signed by all involved.

Decisional Balance Sheet

While decisional balance is a process suggested within the transtheoretical model for *adopting* regular health behaviors, it is also useful for *maintenance* of desired behaviors. It is a cognitive technique that seeks to clearly define both the benefits (pros) and costs (cons) related to a target behavior. Participants must perceive the "payoffs" from a health behavior to be greater than the costs if there is to be adherence. Decisional balance is an attempt to organize this information for individuals and tailor it to their specific circumstances (Marcus & Forsyth, 2003).

LWMCs may utilize a prepared set of possible benefits and costs to which clients can respond, or clients may create a new balance sheet based on their specific circumstances and perceptions. Because the perceived costs of maintaining a modified eating pattern and regular exercise may be great, time is well spent on this rational approach for highlighting the benefits of behavioral maintenance. For example, it is hoped that discomfort and time demands, which are often perceived to be associated with regular physical activity, may be countered by the improved mood, energy level, strength, stamina, and feelings of productivity and mastery that the completion of these important behaviors may bring. The sacrifice of significantly reducing portion sizes, limiting fast-food consumption, and restricting high-calorie desserts may be countered by the feelings associated with being more fit and maintaining an improved body shape.

Stimulus Control

Although much of what has been discussed in this chapter regarding behavioral theory focused on consequences, **antecedents**—those things that may prompt occurrence of a desired health behavior—are also critical. It is quite possible for clients to gain substantial control of environmental aspects that reliably induce health behaviors. Purposefully setting up or modifying one's environment and perceptions to prompt desired behaviors can be an important asset in the formation of appropriate eating and physical-activity habits (Knapp, 1988). Stimulus-control methods for appropriate eating include an increased awareness of hunger cues, a prominent location for fruits and vegetables, and a requirement to eat only at designated locations (to avoid having eating become associated with other activities, such as watching television or reading). Stimulus control may also work in reverse, such as removing salt shakers and keeping high-fat snacks out of sight.

Adverse psychological states such as low mood (e.g., transient mild depression) may prompt a relapse into former problematic eating patterns. Physical activity may be useful as a response because of its acute mood-improving effects. Physical activity very early in programming (or even *prior* to imposing a caloric restriction), may also be useful to bolster a client's "psychological profile," thereby enabling more resilience to mood-related relapses. Along these lines, Baker and Brownell (2000) proposed a model of the relationship between physical activity, changes in various psychological factors, and adherence to diet and exercise regimens (Figure 16-6).

Methods for prompting exercise sessions may include formally scheduling workouts (e.g., in a daily planner), blocking the home exit door with an exercise bag, and confirming an exercise appointment with a friend. Participants have even reported sleeping in their exercise clothes (and athletic shoes) to prompt adherence. The goal of stimulus control is, therefore, to set up situations that reliably **trigger** desired behaviors (and minimize triggers to competing behaviors) as habits become more completely formed.

Self-reward

A self-reward can serve as a well-deserved marker of completing what was agreed upon in a contract or reaching a short-term goal. The acknowledgement of an incremental success serves to reinforce ongoing persistence. Examples of self-rewards can include relaxation time in a whirlpool after a challenging workout, dinner out after a week of adhering to an exercise plan, or buying that desired piece of clothing after reaching a short-term process goal with a new eating plan. Clients should take time to reflect on recent successes, as well as look to forward to the next wave of efforts.

Program Aspects

Programming for Weight-loss Maintenance

Although many people who are seeking weight loss will evaluate their degree of success based on how quickly and extensively weight is lost, this section reviews various program components associated with the *maintenance* of weight loss. Obviously, for health-risk reduction, long-term maintenance is a precondition. Fewer analyses have been completed on this topic. Often, when long-term follow-ups of weight-loss interventions are attempted, there are considerable data missing, because individuals are hard to track over long periods of time. Those with the poorest results are often unwilling to be subjected to ongoing assessment. Also, many studies rely on self-reported weight, which is often inaccurate. With these confounds in mind, the following review should be considered somewhat limited.

Although diets advocating low carbohydrate consumption, as compared to fat and protein consumption, tend to produce greater initial weight loss, they are no better than others over time. Research suggests little association between macronutrient proportions and maintenance of weight loss [American College of Sports Medicine (ACSM), 2001]. Although diets requiring a lower

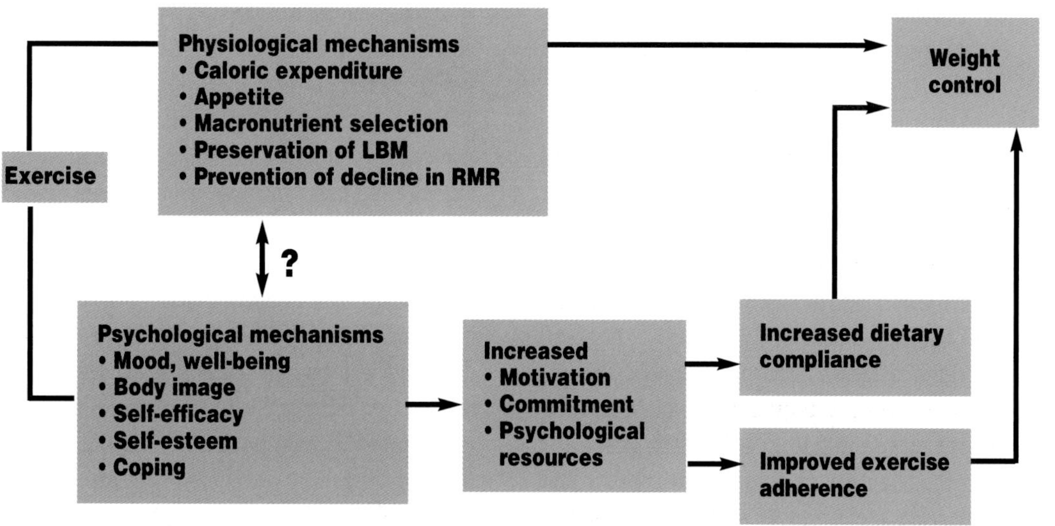

Figure 16-6
Proposed pathways linking exercise, psychological change, dietary compliance, and weight control

Adapted, with permission, from W.W. Baker and K.D. Brownell, 2000, Physical activity and maintenance of weight loss: physiological and psychological mechanisms. In *Physical activity and obesity*, edited by C. Bouchard. (Champaign, IL: Human Kinetics), 315.

caloric intake produce greater initial losses, weight gain is greater after treatment is terminated. Therefore, assigned caloric intake is also not associated with maintenance of weight loss. Treatment length is not related to weight-loss maintenance unless treatment is ongoing. Whether treatment length was 12, 20, or 40 weeks, there was a clear pattern of weight regain after treatment stopped (Jeffery et al., 2000).

When food was provided for six months, weight loss was better maintained at 18 months. After that point, however, maintenance of weight lost compared to individuals who did not have food provided was similar. Preliminary research also indicates that payment or other compensation for maintaining weight loss is ineffective. However, extensions of this approach are being planned in which financial incentives for maintaining an appropriate weight are given through health-insurance cost adjustments.

Based on cross-sectional findings from the National Weight Control Registry (2006), the following aspects, based on self-report, appear to have had a positive effect on weight-loss maintenance:

- A low-fat (23 to 24%), low-calorie (1300 to 1500 calorie) diet
- Regularly eating breakfast
- High amounts of physical activity (60 to 90 minutes per day)
- Regular weighing (at least once per week)

Although some practitioners do not advocate frequent weighing, findings from the Registry were contrary. For successful weight-loss maintainers, it seemed that the feedback from weighing prompted them to make rapid caloric-intake adjustments when observing a short-term weight gain. Although physical activity is the strongest predictor of weight-loss maintenance, many programs either do not emphasize its importance or, because of its association with weight-loss maintenance rather than initial loss, phase it in after months of actively losing weight through diet changes alone. Often, the rationale is that it may be a disadvantage to attempt too many challenging tasks simultaneously. Deferred inclusion of a physical-activity program may be problematic, however, because most individuals need time to establish a habit of regular exercise. It also may be possible to leverage common self-management and self-regulatory skills (e.g., cognitive restructuring, relapse prevention), and benefit from associated mood improvements.

Based on limited evidence, LWMCs should start planning for the maintenance of weight loss soon after establishing a modified eating plan for a client with the assistance of a properly credentialed nutrition professional (Wing, Gorin, & Tate, 2001). These efforts should anticipate the typical pattern of achieving substantial weight loss over several months of treatment, followed by a gradual, but steady, return to baseline weight (and sometimes beyond) beginning soon after active treatment is completed. New approaches under consideration are based on the understanding that treatment termination predicts weight gain. For example, ongoing periodic follow-up through economical methodologies such as phone, email, and the Internet are being tested. Elongation of treatment is also common, and may be the primary reason for the minor improvements observed over the past several decades.

Programming for Exercise Adherence

The research related to program factors associated with maintaining exercise is better developed than that for weight-loss maintenance. Several researchers are testing "lifestyle" activities (e.g., gardening, walking the dog), as opposed to more structured exercise regimens, for their effectiveness. Although both seem to have similar short-term adherence effects, the former may be more acceptable to some individuals. Multiple brief bouts of physical activity throughout the day have also been shown to have comparable effects to a more traditional exercise session of 30 minutes to an hour. Many clients may maintain regimens best when they are offered a "mix-and-match" programming strategy. An example may be one day per week of a sport, two days walking in the neighborhood, one group exercise class, and two days in the gym using resistance machines. Clearly, clients' preferences should be considered, because their inclusion in choosing elements of programming is positively associated with adherence (vs. exercise assigned without choice). Modality of exercise (e.g., walking, running, swimming) does not appear to be directly related to adherence. Again, LWMCs should actively seek participants' preferences when suggesting and revising exercise plans.

The length and intensity of exercise sessions are inversely related to adherence in novice participants. Generally, the more demands placed on individuals' ability to tolerate exercise-induced feelings, the more their existing self-management and self-regulation skills will be tested. The typical individual may often have programmed exercise amounts, or even amounts that they choose themselves, inadvertently paired with unacceptable physical sensations—thus prompting early drop-out. Researchers are testing methods by which feeling states that occur either during an exercise session or as a result of completing a session (i.e., changes in feelings from before to after exercise), may be accurately measured and evaluated for their adherence implications (Annesi, 2002). These methods allow assessment of the adequacy of an exercise program and whether the associated feelings are acceptable or unacceptable to the participant—on an individual basis.

Researchers have yet to clearly identify the relationship between exercise frequency and adherence. Some researchers suggest that the avoidance of "overtaxing" the system with more than three or four sessions per week is preferable. Others suggest that each day should include some physical activity so that a routine is more easily established. Until further research is available, clients' preferences regarding frequency should be the guideline. Further research is also required to determine the adherence effects of very convenient physical-activity programming, such as neighborhood walking paths and recreation areas. It also will be interesting to see an evaluation of the long-term maintenance implications of lifestyle physical activities vs. more structured approaches such as exercising at a fitness center or a YMCA.

Based on the available evidence, LWMCs should suggest exercise modalities based on clients' preferences, and exercise amounts based on associated feelings (Parfitt & Gledhill, 2004). LWMCs should strive to develop enjoyable experiences that clients can easily maintain (Wankel, 1993). For most individuals, too much emphasis on early physiological gains is likely to associate exercise with feelings of discomfort, dread, and early drop-out. LWMCs should allow for variety and choice in exercise programming, and make certain that suggested amounts yield feelings of being energized and having accomplished something productive. Although many experts suggest that programs should include enough cardiovascular, strength, and flexibility activities to make sufficient physiological gains, LWMCs should tailor regimens to ensure conditions that promote long-term adherence (Willis & Campbell, 1992).

Social Support

Social support has strong positive possibilities for maintaining physical activity and weight-control programs (Carron, Hausenblas, & Mack, 1996; Wing, Gorin, & Tate, 2001). Participants in group programs reported advantages related to enjoyment, support, camaraderie, and an increased sense of personal commitment to continue. Social support may be provided by a spouse, friend, coworker, or by either a spontaneously occurring or assigned group. Generally speaking, the social aspects of diet and exercise programming fall on a negative to positive continuum from feelings of social threat [e.g., social physique anxiety occurring when a person's (perceived) deconditioned body is being compared to more fit and attractive ones] to feelings of high social cohesion (e.g., a sense of bonding and camaraderie within the group, and of a shared goal).

Regarding physical activity, a full 90% of participants report a preference for exercising either in a group or with a friend. A series of studies evaluated the impact of regular "team building" and supervision (three to four times per week) on groups of novice exercisers. An increase in social cohesion was found, and greater cohesion was related to better adherence. The results were similar even when counselors had a much less active role in facilitating social support (Annesi, 1999). In fact, it seemed that little more than a setting where those with similar goals (e.g., weight loss, diabetes management) were gathered in nonthreatening surroundings with others of similar characteristics (e.g., at least somewhat overweight, a novice exerciser) was required to facilitate feelings of cohesion. Beneficial socialization between group members appeared to occur spontaneously.

Based on that evidence, LWMCs should endorse clients' participation in group physical activities in nonthreatening formats (e.g., walking groups). It should be noted, however, that a minority of clients will prefer to exercise alone. Participation in many types of sports may also provide moderate-to-vigorous forms of cardiovascular exercise within supportive social settings. As with group exercise, the possibility should be considered that clients may feel overwhelmed, embarrassed, or threatened. Social-support interventions may also beneficially interact with other adherence techniques, such as dissociation (e.g., through having a conversation while walking together), enhanced self-efficacy (e.g., through receiving compliments from others), and stimulus control (e.g., through reminders to attend a scheduled session).

Although group sessions are popular in commercial weight-loss programs, data are sparse regarding their effects on the maintenance of weight loss. A number of studies have attempted to include the spouse in either losing weight with the participant or providing support. Across these investigations, a small positive effect on maintained weight loss was found compared to methods that did not include the spouse. Interestingly, women who received spousal support had better results than men. Another somewhat successful method included incorporating friends into the program. Maintenance-support strategies were taught, and weight loss at six-month follow-ups was improved with this method. Also, group-based contests for weight loss tended to be associated with greater success at follow-up, compared to when the individual's maintained weight loss was the measure used.

Providing social support for maintenance of weight loss and recruiting the help of a spouse may be beneficial, especially for women clients. Social support derived from other groups (e.g., friends, coworkers) may also be beneficial. It is not clear, however, whether weight-loss interventions in large groups, small groups, or individual-counseling formats help to better maintain weight loss.

Treatment Packages

Although LWMCs should use specific interventions as they deem appropriate for individual clients, there are also a number of structured treatment packages that aim to increase and maintain regular exercise while reducing and maintaining each individual's weight. These packages tend to be based on predominant health-behavior-change theories. They incorporate several of the individual treatments already described in this chapter, and are evaluated based on their effect as a unified system or protocol. Thus, there is less choice for LWMCs regarding administration of specific methods. Although this is certainly preferable when large-scale, replicable efforts are required, many health-behavior-change specialists advocate using at least partially structured behavior-change methodologies for virtually all clients. While acknowledging the individual differences among clients, they emphasize that most people who look for help to achieve similar goals have enough in common to justify using a fairly defined (but individually adaptable) system. This section provides an overview of selected protocols. Only systems with their bases grounded in behavioral science should be considered for use by LWMCs.

For adoption of, and adherence to, physical activity, Marcus and Forsyth (2003) describe a system based on the transtheoretical model. There are specific treatment components tailored to each stage of readiness in which an individual may presently be. This system allows LWMCs to systematically advance individuals through the stages and react purposefully when they relapse into an earlier stage. With regard to adherence to exercise in Marcus and Forsyth's "Stage 5: Making Physical Activity a Habit," it is suggested that clients:

- Review successful behavior-change skills that have worked for them in the past for other behaviors, and resolve methods that have not previously worked
- Utilize a balance-sheet method to derive benefits gained from being physically active, and address costs and barriers
- Explore options for making exercise more enjoyable
- Review short-term progress toward goals
- Review new and revised goals
- Enlist social support
- Engage in self-reward for recently attained accomplishments
- Ensure that there are means to continue to track progress

A list of treatment tasks are annotated for each stage of readiness. Timeframes for application of specific treatments are based on the assessment of individuals' present stage. Within this system, informal self-report forms support the administration of many of the aforementioned processes.

Another treatment package, which is specifically designed to help new and returning exercisers assimilate regular exercise into their lives, is based on tenets of social-cognitive theory and the adaptation-relapse process model (Annesi, 2003). Because this protocol has been delivered by counselors within community-wellness-center settings (e.g., YMCAs) and must accommodate hundreds of individuals each month, a highly structured approach is taken. A specifically developed computer program directs treatment selections for six individual counseling sessions over six months (four in the first three months, two from the fourth month to the sixth month), based on the validated REMS survey described earlier in this chapter. In one-on-one meetings, counselors are directed through the delivery of an array of cognitive-behavioral methods, including the following:

- Long- and short-term goal-setting
- Provision of progress feedback
- Assessment of mood-state changes
- Assessment of feeling-state changes associated with suggested exercise amounts
- Instruction on a number of self-management and self-regulatory skills (e.g., relapse prevention, cognitive restructuring, dissociation)
- Recruiting social support
- Behavioral contracting

Each appointment somewhat differs based on when it occurs and the client's individual progress to date. All of the behavioral methods focus on assessed factors of clients' ability to tolerate exercise-induced discomfort, their self-management and self-regulatory abilities, and their available social-support systems. Ongoing results of goal-setting forms, surveys of psychological factors, progress reports, and behavioral contracts are incorporated into algorithms that yield directives on how counselors should proceed based on individual variables accounted for within the supporting computer application. This protocol is an example of a theoretically based intervention package intended for large-scale dissemination. Given the lack of success with informational and social-marketing approaches to assimilate regular physical activity, this program attempts to administer evidence-based, cognitive-behavioral interventions through time-limited, individual contacts with counselors.

Cooper, Fairburn, and Hawker (2003) outlined a protocol for weight reduction that has a much greater emphasis on the maintenance of weight loss than many other programs. Although designed to be administered through individual counseling sessions, it may be adapted to group settings as well. The 44-week protocol consists of nine structured "modules" that have a range of time for administration. Early in the protocol, calorie counting (typically 1200 to 1500 calories per day) and recording are instituted, and barriers to weight loss are addressed. It is intended that clients become highly proficient at self-monitoring food intake, as well as associated factors such as location, time of consumption, whether the food was part of a meal or not, and feelings associated with specific periods of eating (e.g., feelings of guilt, social pressure to eat). Barriers to appropriate eating, and potential remedies, are prompted through a standardized form. After approximately five months of treatment, physical activity is formally incorporated as a component. Issues around body image, periodic weight fluctuations, and "primary goals" (e.g., client-perceived desirable effects of weight loss, such as receiving admiration from others and a much-improved social life) are addressed as well. Clients are encouraged to accept manageable amounts of weight loss as a success.

At around the seventh month, weight-loss maintenance is specifically addressed. Within this module, clients formally adopt a goal of maintaining weight rather than losing more weight. LWMCs must review previous modules for methods that may be adapted to this new focus. Clients are prepared on how to react when they gain weight beyond what may be expected from natural fluctuations. Results of weekly weighings are graphed to provide enhanced feedback. A number of self-management skills are reviewed specifically in the revised context of weight-loss maintenance. Self-monitoring of food intake is also phased out around the seventh month through a step-by-step process. Finally, suggestions are given to address the following topics, guided by a standardized form:

- Reasons that the client does not want to gain weight
- Goal weight range
- Eating habits
- Physical-activity habits
- Danger areas
- Weight monitoring and reviewing
- When to act
- Devising a plan for dealing with a change in weight
- Dealing with the cause of weight gain

At treatment termination (after approximately 44 weeks), LWMCs should offer several follow-up sessions at two-month intervals.

This protocol is an example of a modular approach, in which counselors are provided specific treatment components to be completed at specified times. There is, however, a great amount of flexibility given based on clients' differences and goals. Unlike most systems, this protocol places specific attention on maintaining the weight that was lost.

Considerations for Professional Practice

Skills for Counseling

Being an effective practitioner of health-behavior change requires more than just technical knowledge of current theories and methods (although this knowledge is generally a precondition for success). Most interventions are delivered on a face-to-face basis. Thus, a level of trust and partnership with clients is required. Systems in which clients were provided behavioral guidelines and skills through audio or written materials, and then left to their own devices to self-administer them, have had minimal effect to date. The most productive LWMCs will have the interpersonal skills required to effectively facilitate a wide array of treatments for many types of clients.

The field of counseling has identified a number of skills thought to be essential for effective individualized delivery of behavior-change treatments. Especially when adherence is a concern, it is essential that clients have an ongoing relationship with LWMCs and trust that they will support their endeavor of developing resilient health habits over the long haul. Practitioners' innate abilities in terms of counseling skills vary greatly. Through role play, observation, and seeking constructive feedback, LWMCs may make improvements and maximize their professional effectiveness.

Communication Skills

Attending—This skill requires centering one's energy, focus, and thoughts on the client. Nonverbal behaviors that are part of attending include:

- Squaring—turning the body to fully face the client
- Posture—conscientiously giving bodily signals and showing genuine interest
- Eye contact—providing direct eye contact at all times
- Energy level—signaling and maintaining high energy and enthusiasm

Listening—Effective listening is an active process. LWMCs should identify possible incongruities and clarify them with clients. For example, when initiating an exercise regimen, clients will often say that they do not have "enough time" to exercise and offer a long list of time-consuming activities that seem to take priority over the target health behaviors (which will ultimately have a much greater impact on their health, longevity, and quality of life). Also, summarizing clients' statements for clarification signals that LWMCs pay attention.

Content—Many clients are talkative during meetings, but it is up to LWMCs to select relevant aspects to enhance behavioral support. Hence, LWMCs should become proficient at separating meaningful content from superfluous talk. Although rapport-building is essential, LWMCs should focus on health-behavior change.

Affect—Counselors should be aware of the emotional patterns of clients, especially as they are associated with specific content areas. This may serve as a reference for how to approach a topic in the future. For example, weight and body-esteem are often emotionally charged areas. When this is the case, LWMCs should be sensitive in their approach to corresponding measurements. Nonverbal signals of clients' frustration with slow progress also require identification and appropriate communication.

Empathy—Empathy is the ability to understand another's situation from his or her frame of reference. It is important for building rapport, especially when a client is considerably more overweight and less fit than the LWMC. An understanding of nonverbal expressions and verbal intonations may help LWMCs better absorb the frame of reference that is unique for each client.

Personal Characteristics

Self-awareness—This involves being open to clients' feedback, as well as being self-reflective regarding one's own effectiveness at promoting sustained health-behavior changes.

Good Will— LWMCs must, at all times, work on behalf of their clients in a positive and trustworthy manner.

Support—Effective LWMCs encourage their clients to become self-reliant. Although they play an important role in providing support, they should not purposefully create relationships that foster dependency.

Flexibility—Effective management of clients requires self-management and other techniques that may need to be adjusted to accommodate individual needs.

Energy—It is important for LWMCs to be highly energetic and enthusiastic with clients.

Intellectual Competence—LWMCs should have a superior working knowledge of the theory and practice of health-behavior change and, specifically, sustaining changes. They should continually seek to improve and increase their knowledge through the newest evidence-based material.

Trustworthiness—LWMCs should respect confidentiality, be considerate, and try to be understanding with clients.

Ethics

LWMCs should use good judgment when referring clients to use other professionals' services. They should keep a referral list of properly credentialed dieticians (R.D.); psychotherapists, psychologists, and psychiatrists (M.S.W., Ph.D., Psy.D., M.D.); and physicians (M.D., D.O.). It is paramount for LWMCs to understand their own professional qualifications and the limitations of their professional conduct. For example, counseling clients on psychological and interpersonal issues, special dietary requirements, and specific physical pathologies clearly falls outside of the professional scope of practice of most LWMCs. Appendix A presents the ACE Code of Ethics.

Behavioral Measurement

Although often thought to be the domain of researchers, a wide assortment of validated measurement instruments is available for LWMCs' use. A number of factors that may be readily measured focus on the following:

- Outcomes (e.g., mood, energy level)
- Delivery of treatments (e.g., changes in exercise-induced feelings, assimilation of self-management skills)
- Possible mediators and moderators of the health-behavior-change process (e.g., body image, self-efficacy).

Ostrow (1996) and Duda (1998) present comprehensive reviews, sources, and suggestions for application of easily administered and scored surveys that are relevant to the development of appropriate exercise and weight-loss behaviors. Practitioners are encouraged to make use of these assessments to evaluate both the processes and outcomes of their work. Appropriate use of such survey instruments is suggested by Kimiecik and Blissmer (1998).

Interventions often seek to induce ongoing changes in specific behavioral and psychological factors. Thus, their relationship with exercise adherence and weight-loss measures is an important one. Empirical scrutiny of changes in such variables may be time well spent for assessing a treatment's effect on an individual client and the treatment's propensity for favorable effects across most individuals with similar needs. Table 16-1 outlines relevant categories of self-report surveys that are presently available.

Table 16-1
Relevant Categories of Validated Self-report Measurement Instruments

- Self-concept and body image
- Stage of change
- Self-efficacy and self-confidence
- Locus of control
- Mood
- Energy level
- Perceived exertion
- Group dynamics and social cohesion
- Perceived barriers
- Self-motivation
- Personal incentives
- Attentional focus
- Decisional balance

Summary

Most people have a problem with maintaining physical-activity and weight-management programs. High amounts of attrition from exercise and weight-loss regimens have been prevalent, and regain of lost weight is nearly a certainty for most individuals. Behavioral science yields important suggestions on how LWMCs may proceed to sustain positive changes in health behaviors. A number of theoretical models provide perspectives on what may enable individuals to successfully adapt to exercise and appropriate eating. Some are focused on participants' thought systems, while others view environmental conditions as primary factors. Each posits an interaction of variables, some of which may be purposefully adjusted for the benefit of clients. A number of individual factors are also associated with changes in health behaviors. Again, the astute LWMC benefits from knowledge of these correlates of maintained physical activity and weight loss in their helping efforts. Individual interventions have been developed and tested based on theoretical models and determinants of health behaviors. They present a diverse array of evidence-driven methodologies that LWMCs may incorporate. With a thorough grasp of the theory and research behind health-behavior-change processes and methods, LWMCs are in an advantageous position to improve and sustain the health and quality-of-life of their clients.

References

American College of Sports Medicine (2001). Appropriate intervention strategies for weight loss and prevention of weight regain for adults. *Medicine & Science in Sports & Exercise,* 33, 2145–2156.

Annesi, J.J. (2004a) Relationship of social cognitive theory factors to exercise maintenance in adults. *Psychological Reports,* 99, 142–148.

Annesi, J.J. (2004b). Psychological improvement is associated with exercise session attendance over 10 weeks in formerly sedentary adults. *European Journal of Sport Science*, 4, 2, 1–10.

Annesi, J.J. (2003). Effects of a cognitive behavioral treatment package on exercise attendance and drop out. *European Journal of Sport Science,* 3, 2, 1–16.

Annesi, J.J. (2002). Relationship between changes in acute exercise-induced feeling states, self-motivation, and adults' adherence to moderate aerobic exercise. *Perceptual and Motor Skills,* 94, 425–439.

Annesi, J.J. (2001). Effects of music, television, and a combination entertainment system on distraction, exercise adherence, and physical outputs in adults. *Canadian Journal of Behavioural Science,* 33, 193–202.

Annesi, J.J. (1998). Effects of minimal group promotion on cohesion and exercise adherence. *Small Group Research,* 30, 542–557.

Annesi, J.J. & Unruh, J.L. (2007). Effects of THE COACH APPROACH® intervention on drop out rates among adults initiating exercise programs at nine YMCAs over three years. *Perceptual and Motor Skills,* 104, 459–466.

Baker, C.W. & Brownell, K.D. (2000). Physical activity and maintenance of weight loss: Physiological and psychological mechanisms. In: Bouchard, C. (Ed.) *Physical Activity and Obesity* (pp. 311–328). Champaign, Ill.: Human Kinetics.

Bandura, A. (1997). *Self-Efficacy: The Exercise of Control.* New York: Freeman.

Bandura, A. (1986). *Social Foundations of Thought and Action: A Social Cognitive Theory.* Englewood Cliffs, N.J.: Prentice Hall.

Baranowski, T. (2006). Advances in basic behavioral research will make the most important contributions to effective dietary change programs at this time. *Journal of the American Dietetic Association*, 106, 808–811.

Baranowski, T., Anderson, C., & Carmack, C. (1998). Mediating variable framework in physical activity interventions. How are we doing? How might we do better? *American Journal of Preventive Medicine,* 15, 266–297.

Boutelle, K.N. & Kirschenbaum, D.S. (1998). Further support for consistent self-monitoring as a vital component of successful weight control. *Obesity Research,* 6, 219–224.

Buckworth, J. & Dishman, R. K. (2002). *Exercise Psychology.* Champaign, Ill.: Human Kinetics.

Carron, A.V., Hausenblas, H.A., & Mack, D. (1996). Social influences and exercise: A meta-analysis. *Journal of Sport and Exercise Psychology,* 18, 1–16.

Cooper, Z., Fairburn, C.G., & Hawker, D.M. (2003). *Cognitive-Behavioral Treatment of Obesity: A Clinician's Guide.* New York: Guilford.

Culos-Reed, S.N., Gyurcsik, N.C., & Brawley, L.R. (2001). Using theories of motivated behavior to understand physical activity. In: Singer, R.N., Hausenblas, H.A., & Jannelle, C.M. (Eds.) *Handbook of Sport Psychology* (2nd ed., pp. 695–717). New York: Wiley.

Dishman, R.K. (1988). Overview. In: Dishman, R.K. (Ed.) *Exercise Adherence: Its Impact on Public Health* (pp. 1–9). Champaign Ill.: Human Kinetics.

Duda, J.L. (Ed.) (1998). *Advances in Sport and Exercise Psychology Measurement.* Morgantown, W.V.: Fitness Information Technology.

Foreyt, J.P. et al. (1995). Psychological correlates of weight fluctuation. *International Journal of Eating Disorders,* 17, 263–275.

Foster, G.D. et al. (1997). What is a reasonable weight loss? Patients' expectations and evaluations of obesity treatment outcomes. *Journal of Consulting and Clinical Psychology,* 65, 79–85.

Godin, G. (1994). Social-cognitive models. In: Dishman, R.K. (Ed.) *Advances in Exercise Adherence* (pp. 113–136), Champaign, Ill.: Human Kinetics.

Graffagnino, C.L. et al. (2006). Effect of a community-based weight management program on weight loss and cardiovascular disease risk factors. *Obesity,* 14, 280–288.

Jeffery, R.W. et al. (2000). Long-term maintenance of weight loss: Current status. *Health Psychology,* 19 (Suppl.), 5–16.

Kearney, J.M. et al. (1999). Stages of change toward physical activity in a nationally representative sample in the European Union. *Public Health Nutrition,* 2, 115-124.

Kimiecik, J.C. & Blissmer, B. (1998). Applied exercise psychology: Measurement issues. In: Duda, J.L. (Ed.). *Advances in Sport and Exercise Psychology Measurement* (pp. 447–460). Morgantown, W.V.: Fitness Information Technology.

Klem, M.L. et al. (1997). A descriptive study of individuals successful at long-term maintenance of substantial weight loss. *American Journal of Clinical Nutrition,* 66, 239–246.

Knapp, D.N. (1988). Behavioral management techniques and exercise promotion. In: Dishman, R.K. (Ed.) *Exercise Adherence* (pp. 203–235). Champaign, Ill.: Human Kinetics.

Locke, E.A. & Latham, G.P. (1985). The application of goal setting to sports. *Journal of Sport Psychology,* 7, 205–222.

Mann, T. et al. (2007). Medicare's search for effective obesity treatments: Diets are not the answer. *American Psychologist,* 62, 220–233.

Marcus, B.H. & Forsyth, L.H. (2003). *Motivating People to Be Physically Active.* Champaign, Ill.: Human Kinetics.

Marcus, B.H. et al. (1992). Self-efficacy and the stages of exercise behavior change. *Research Quarterly for Exercise and Sport,* 63, 60–66.

Marlatt, G.A. & Gordon, J.R. (Eds.) (1985). *Relapse Prevention.* New York: Guilford.

McAuley, E. & Mihalko, S.L. (1998). Measuring exercise-related self-efficacy. In: Duda, J.L. (Ed.) *Advances in Sport and Exercise Psychology Measurement* (pp. 371–390). Morgantown, W.V.: Fitness Information Technology.

Miller, W.C., Koceja, D.M., & Hamilton, E.J. (1997). A meta-analysis of the past 25 years of weight loss research using diet, exercise, or diet plus exercise intervention. *International Journal of Obesity,* 21, 941–947.

Mokdad, A.H. et al. (2001). The continuing epidemic of obesity in the United States. *Journal of the American Medical Association,* 286, 1195–2000.

National Weight Control Registry (2006). *The National Weight Control Registry: Research Findings.* http://www.nwcr.ws/Research/default.htm.

Ostrow, A.C. (Ed.) (1996). *Directory of Psychological Tests in the Sport and Exercise Sciences* (2nd ed.). Morgantown, W.V.: Fitness Information Technology.

Parfitt, G. & Gledhill, C. (2004). The effect of choice of exercise mode on psychological responses. *Psychology of Sport and Exercise,* 5, 111–117.

Reed, G.R. (1999). Adherence to exercise and the transtheoretical model of behavior change. In: Bull, S.J. (Ed.) *Adherence Issues in Sport and Exercise* (pp. 19–45). New York: Wiley.

Rejeski, W.J. (1992). Motivation for exercise behavior: A critique of theoretical directions. In: Roberts, G.C. (Ed.) *Motivation in Sport and Exercise* (pp. 129–157). Champaign, Ill.: Human Kinetics.

Rothman, A.J. (2002). Toward a theory-based analysis of behavioral maintenance. *Health Psychology,* 19 (Suppl.), 64–69.

Strecher, V.J. et al. (1986). The role of self-efficacy in achieving health-behavior change. *Health Education Quarterly,* 13, 73–91.

Trost, S.G. et al. (2002). Correlates of adults' participation in physical activity: Review and update. *Medicine & Science in Sports & Exercise,* 34, 1996–2001.

Wadden, T.A. et al. (1992). A multicenter evaluation of a proprietary weight reduction program for the treatment of marked obesity. *Archives of Internal Medicine,* 152, 961–966.

Wankel, L.M. (1993). The importance of enjoyment to adherence and psychological benefits from physical activity. *International Journal of Sport Psychology,* 24, 151–169.

Willis, J.D. & Campbell, L.F. (1992). *Exercise Psychology*. Champaign, Ill.: Human Kinetics.

Wing, R.R., Gorin, A., & Tate, D. (2001). Strategies for changing eating and exercise behavior. In: Bowman, B.B. & Russell, R.M. (Eds.) *Present Knowledge in Nutrition* (8th ed.). Washington, DC: International Life Sciences Institute.

Suggested Reading

Annesi, J.J. (1996). *Enhancing Exercise Motivation.* Los Angeles, Calif.: Leisure Publications.

Bray, G.A., Bouchard, C., & James, W.P.T. (Eds.) (1998). *Handbook of Obesity*. New York: Dekker.

Dishman, R.K. (Ed.) (1994) *Advances in Exercise Adherence.* Champaign, Ill.: Human Kinetics.

Dishman, R.K. & Buckworth, J. (1996). Increasing physical activity: A quantitative synthesis. *Medicine & Science in Sports & Exercise,* 28, 706–719.

Ekkekakis, P. & Lind, E. (2006). Exercise does not feel the same when you are overweight: The impact of self-selected and imposed intensity on affect and exertion. *International Journal of Obesity,* 30, 652–660.

Fairburn, C.G. & Brownell, K.D. (Eds.) (2002). *Eating Disorders and Obesity: A Comprehensive Handbook* (2nd ed.). New York: Guilford.

Flegal, K.M. et al. (2002). Prevalence and trends in obesity among U.S. adults, 1999–2000. *Journal of the American Medical Association,* 288, 1723–1727.

Kahn, E.B. et al. (2002). The effectiveness of interventions to increase physical activity: A systematic review. *American Journal of Preventive Medicine,* 22, 73–107.

Prochaska, J.O., Norcross, J.C., & DiClemente, C.C. (1994). *Changing for Good.* New York: Avon.

U.S. Department of Health and Human Services (1996). *Physical Activity and Health: A Report of the Surgeon General.* Atlanta, Ga.: U.S. Department of Health and Human Services, Centers for Disease Control and Prevention, National Center for Chronic Disease Prevention and Health Promotion.

U.S. Department of Health and Human Services (1999). *Promoting Physical Activity: A Guide for Community Action.* Champaign, Ill.: Human Kinetics.

Wadden, T.A. & Stunkard, A.J. (2002). *Handbook of Obesity Treatment.* New York: Guilford.

Wing, R.R. (2003). Behavioral interventions for obesity: Recognizing our progress and future challenges. *Obesity Research,* 11(Suppl.), 3–6.

Part VI

Special Considerations

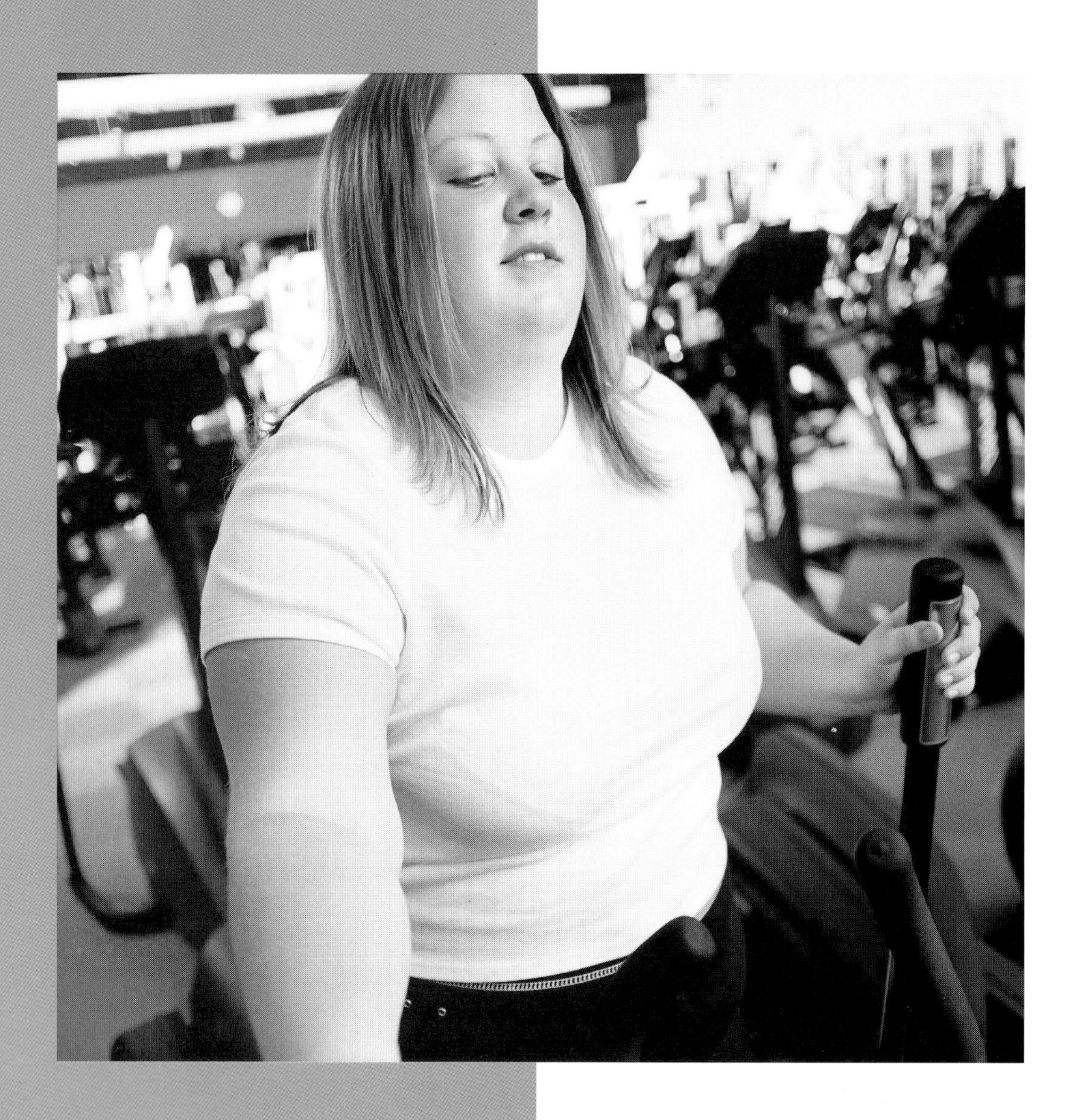

Kara A. Witzke

Kara A. Witzke, Ph.D., is an associate professor and department chair of kinesiology at California State University San Marcos in San Diego County. She has worked in industry and various wellness venues around the country and has promoted wellness and lifestyle management to children and adults of all ages through education, research, and community involvement. She is active in the ACE exam development process and is an ACE media spokesperson. Her current research focuses on the effects of exercise on both diabetes and bone health.

Chapter 17

Physiology of Obesity

Prevalence of Overweight and Obesity

The **obesity** epidemic is recognized as a complex problem that affects people around the world, regardless of gender, socioeconomic status, race, or ethnicity. One of the goals of the U.S. initiative entitled Healthy People 2010 is to reduce the percentage of obese adults to less than 15% and to develop strategies to prevent **overweight** and obesity. However, this goal is far from being attained. According to the National Health and Nutrition Examination Surveys (NHANES) I and II (1960–1980), the prevalence of overweight (BMI = 25–29.9) and obesity (BMI ≥30) among adults and children was relatively stable in the U.S (Engel et al., 1978; McDowell et al., 1984). However, the NHANES III survey (1988–1994), for the first time in the nation's history, showed an alarming statistic: The prevalence of obesity among adults had increased a full 8% since the previous survey (Crespo & Wright, 1995; Executive Summary, 1994). In fact, between 1980 and 2002, the number of obese adults age 20 and older has doubled, and the incidence of overweight children and adolescents has tripled. The newest estimates still reveal an upward trend in the prevalence of overweight and obesity in children, adolescents, and adults (Flegal, 2005) (Table 17-1).

The chance of having a **body mass index (BMI)** greater than 25 starts to rise around age 35 and declines around age 75 in

IN THIS CHAPTER:

Table 17-1
Prevalence of Overweight and Obesity Among Children, Adolescents, and Adults in the U.S. From 1960 to 2004

Survey Year	Children 6–11 Overweight (%)	Adolescents 12–19 Overweight (%)	Adults 20–74 Overweight or Obese (%)	Adults 20–74 Overweight (%)	Adults 20–74 Obese (%)
1960–1962	–	–	44.8	31.5	13.3
1963–1965	4.2	–	–	–	–
1966–1970	–	4.6	–	–	–
1971–1974	4.0	6.1	47.7	33.1	14.6
1976–1980	6.5	5.0	47.4	32.3	15.1
1988–1994	11.3	10.5	56.0	32.7	23.3
1999–2002	15.8	16.1	65.2	34.1	31.1
2003–2004	18.8	17.4	66.3	34.1	32.2

Sources: Flegal, K.M. (2005). Epidemiologic aspects of overweight and obesity in the United States. *Physiology and Behavior*, 86, 5, 599–602; Ogden, C.L. et al. (2006). Prevalence of overweight and obesity in the United States, 1999–2004. *Journal of the American Medical Association*, 295, 13, 1549–1555.

both men and women. However, women are still more likely to be obese at all ages.

Not surprisingly, these trends are similar in other countries throughout the world. In Great Britain, the prevalence of obesity among adults has also tripled since 1980, and among preschool children in China, the obesity rate increased from 1.5% in 1989 to 12.6% in 1997, a greater than eightfold increase in just eight years.

There are also differences in overweight and obesity prevalence by racial/ethnic group. It is estimated that 54% of non-Hispanic black women are obese, compared with 32% of Mexican-American women and 30% of non-Hispanic white women of the same age. Among males, 34% of black males are obese, compared to 31% of white males and 32% of Mexican-American males (Ogden et al., 2006). These racial differences may be explained by a combination of genetics, food, and exercise habits, as well as cultural attitudes toward body weight. On average, non-Hispanic black women burn approximately 100 fewer calories each day during rest than white women, which translates into nearly 1 pound (0.45 kg) of body fat gained each month (Carpenter et al., 1998). These women also tend to experience a more dramatic lowering of resting metabolic rate during dieting than non-Hispanic white women, which may also explain why they tend to have greater difficulty in achieving a goal body weight than overweight white women (Foster et al., 1999). Again, however, the trend toward increasing overweight and obesity continues to increase among all racial/ethnic and socioeconomic groups.

Overweight vs. Obesity

There is some confusion around the precise meaning of the terms overweight, overfat, and obesity as they pertain to body composition and risk for health problems. In proper context, the term "overweight" simply refers to a body weight that exceeds some predetermined average for a specific height. A person who is overweight has usually experienced an increase in body fat, but not always, as in the case of muscular athletes. The term "obesity" refers to the overfat condition that accompanies a host of comorbidities, including components of the metabolic syndrome: **glucose** intolerance, **insulin** resistance, **dyslipidemia, type 2 diabetes, hypertension,** elevated plasma **leptin** concentrations, increased **visceral fat** tissue, and increased risk of **coronary heart disease** and cancer. Available research indicates a much clearer relationship between these conditions and increased body fat, rather than merely an increase in body weight. It is certainly possible for an individual to be overweight or overfat, but not exhibit components of the obesity syndrome described here. In most medical literature, the term "overweight" is used to describe an "overfat" condition, even in the absence of accompanying body-fat measures. In this context, obesity then refers to individuals at the extreme end of the overweight continuum. This is the framework used to determine BMI, which is the most common technique for estimating healthy bodyweight levels.

Determination of Body Fatness Using BMI

BMI is calculated as a ratio of one's weight to height:

$$BMI = weight (kg)/height^2 (m)$$

Example:

Male, height 5'9", 214 lb

5'9" = 69 in 69 in x 0.0254 m/in = 1.753 m

214 lb 214 lb ÷ 2.2 kg/lb = 97.3 kg

$BMI = 97.3 \div (1.753)^2 = 31.7 \text{ kg/m}^2$

Table 17-2 provides an easy way to determine BMI by intersecting a client's height and weight in standard units. Easy-to-use BMI calculators also are available online. In 1997, the World Health Organization published guidelines that classified people with BMIs greater than 25 as overweight and those with BMIs greater than or equal to 30 as obese. Individuals who display BMIs greater than or equal to 40 are considered morbidly, or extremely, obese. These individuals clearly have a higher risk of death and disability due to their weight (Table 17-3). These revised standards place 97 million Americans in the overweight and obese categories, up from 72 million people using the previous standards.

Limitations of BMI

Similar to height-weight tables, the BMI also fails to consider the body's proportional distribution of body fat and the composition of overall body weight. The possibility of

Table 17-2
Body Mass Index

	19	20	21	22	23	24	25	26	27	28	29	30	35	40
Height (inches)							**Weight (pounds)**							
58	91	95	100	105	110	115	119	124	129	134	138	143	167	191
59	94	99	104	109	114	119	124	128	133	138	143	148	173	198
60	97	102	107	112	118	123	128	133	138	143	148	153	179	204
61	100	106	111	116	121	127	132	137	143	148	153	158	185	211
62	104	109	115	120	125	131	136	142	147	153	158	164	191	218
63	107	113	118	124	130	135	141	146	152	158	163	169	197	225
64	110	116	122	128	134	140	145	151	157	163	169	174	203	233
65	114	120	126	132	138	144	150	156	162	168	174	180	210	240
66	117	124	130	136	142	148	155	161	167	173	179	185	216	247
67	121	127	134	140	147	153	159	166	172	178	185	191	223	255
68	125	131	138	144	151	158	164	171	177	184	190	197	230	263
69	128	135	142	149	155	162	169	176	182	189	196	203	237	270
70	132	139	146	153	160	167	174	181	188	195	202	209	243	278
71	136	143	150	157	165	172	179	186	193	200	207	215	250	286
72	140	147	155	162	169	177	184	191	199	206	213	221	258	294
73	144	151	159	166	174	182	189	197	204	212	219	227	265	303
74	148	155	163	171	179	187	194	202	210	218	225	233	272	311
75	152	160	168	176	184	192	200	208	216	224	232	240	279	319
76	156	164	172	180	189	197	205	213	221	230	238	246	287	328

Note: Find the client's height in the far left column and move across the row to the weight that is closest to the client's weight. His or her body mass index will be at the top of that column.

Table 17-3
BMI Reference Chart

Weight Category	BMI Range
Underweight	<18.5
Normal weight	18.5–24.9
Overweight	25.0–29.9
Grade I Obesity	30.0–34.9
Grade II Obesity	35.0–39.9
Grade III Obesity	≥40

misclassifying someone as overweight using BMI standards applies particularly to shot putters, bodybuilders, heavier wrestlers, and football players. Although there are inherent problems with assessing fatness of an individual using this method, it remains the method of choice for large-scale epidemiological studies due to the ease of obtaining the two measurements required and its acceptable correlation with more technical measures (e.g. hydrostatic weighing, skinfolds). It should be emphasized, however, that the number obtained using BMI is not a measure of body composition per se, but merely a calculated ratio using height and weight.

Fat Cell Size and Number: Hypertrophy vs. Hyperplasia

Obesity can also be classified by fat cell size and number.

Fat cell **hypertrophy:** Existing fat cells enlarge or fill with fat

Fat cell **hyperplasia:** Total **adipocyte** number increases

One technique for studying body fatness involves extracting small fragments of tissue through a syringe needle inserted directly into a fatty area on the body. Chemical treatment of the sample isolates the individual fat cells for counting. Dividing fat mass in the sample by fat cell number determines the average quantity of fat per cell.

Obesity that occurs early in life (before age one) or during the adolescent growth spurt (ages nine through 13), with a BMI >40, can cause an increase in the number of adipocytes (fat cells), called hypercellular or hyperplastic obesity. This type of obesity can easily predispose an individual to obesity throughout adulthood, merely due to the increased numbers of adipose cells available to store and metabolize fat. In fact, children who are obese between the ages of six and nine have a 55% chance of becoming obese adults, which is 10 times the risk of children of normal weight. A child does not generally "outgrow" obesity. In fact, once established, the number of fat cells remains constant in spite of weight gain or loss. Reducing body fatness is especially difficult, though not impossible, for those with a high number of fat cells. Individuals with hyperplastic obesity are not easily treated with ordinary dietary and exercise regimens. When treated with a conventional low-energy diet, they seem to fail to lose weight after reaching a certain fat-cell size. Obese people who have lost weight by restricting energy intake are very prone to weight regain. Unfortunately for these individuals, no amount of dietary restriction or exercise can reduce fat-cell *number* (Vinten & Galbo, 1983). Therefore, lifestyle-modification plans that strive to reduce overall body fat will only reduce the *amount* of fat in each existing cell, which means that it will be more difficult to reduce body-fat percentage, and then to maintain any fat loss.

Obesity that occurs later in life, called hypertrophic obesity, is associated with an enlargement of the existing fat cells, but a normal fat-cell number. This pattern is correlated with truncal fat distribution (an apple-shape) and health consequences later in life (McArdle, Katch, & Katch, 2001). Men, on average, gain between 0.4 and 1.8 pounds (0.2 and 0.8 kg) of fat each year until their 60s, despite a gradual decrease in food consumption. Approximately 14% of women gain more than 30 pounds (13.6 kg) between the ages of 25 and 34. Women in general have more fat cells than men (McArdle, Katch, & Katch, 2001).

Health Consequences of Obesity

Obesity is an independent risk factor for coronary heart disease, even when adjusted for the influences of other risk factors such as age, cholesterol, systolic blood pressure, smoking, left ventricular hypertrophy, and glucose intolerance (Hubert et al., 1983). Obesity is the second leading cause of preventable death in America, with smoking being the first (Allison et al., 1999). Obese individuals have an overall mortality rate almost twice that of normal-weight individuals, and even moderate overweight is associated with a significant increase in the risk of premature death. Obesity reduces life expectancy by 10 to 20 years, causing 280,000 to 325,000 premature deaths in the U.S. each year (Allison et al., 1999), at a cost of more than $100 billion annually.

Obesity is associated with cardiovascular disease, hypertension, elevated total cholesterol and low HDL cholesterol, impaired heart function, postmenopausal breast cancer, impaired immune function, gallbladder and kidney diseases, skin problems, sleep and breathing disorders, impotence, pregnancy complications, back pain, arthritis, and other bone and joint disorders. Of special importance is the strong association between excess body fat and diabetes. Obesity increases the risk of developing this debilitating disease by more than three times.

Excessive fatness in childhood and adolescence predicts poor health outcomes in adulthood. Children who gain more weight than their peers tend to become overweight adults with increased risk of hypertension, elevated insulin, **hypercholesterolemia,** and heart disease (Sinaiko et al., 1999). Therefore, being overweight is associated with adverse health effects 55 years later. The Harvard Growth Study from 1922 to 1935 evaluated 3000 school children annually throughout high school and up until eight years later. The overweight children showed an overall greater risk of mortality from all causes and a twofold higher coronary heart disease risk as adults (Dearborn, 1938).

Specific Risks

Excessive body fat is associated with various specific health risks (Table 17-4). It is also closely related to the explosion of type 2 diabetes diagnosed in children. Approximately 66% of adults are overweight and 32% are classified as obese. According to the National Institutes of Health (NIH), obesity represents a chronic, degenerative disease, even at low levels of excessive body fat. A moderate 4 to 10% increase in body weight after the age of 20 correlates with a 50% greater risk of death from coronary artery disease and nonfatal heart attack (Rosengren, Wedel, & Wilhelmsen, 1999). Even long-term body weight at the high end of the normal range increases heart disease and cancer risk (Manson et al., 1995). In the Nurses Health Study, even nurses of average weight experienced 30% more heart attacks compared to their thinnest counterparts, and the risk for a moderately overweight nurse was 80% higher. This means that a woman who gains only 20 pounds (9 kg) from her late teens to middle age doubles her risk of having a heart attack. Research has established obesity as

Table 17-4
Specific Health Risks of Excessive Body Fat

- Impaired cardiac function due to increased workload on the heart
- Hypertension
- Stroke
- Deep-vein thrombosis
- Increased insulin resistance in children and adults
- Renal disease
- Sleep apnea and pulmonary disease
- Problems receiving anesthesia during surgery
- Osteoarthritis, degenerative joint disease, and gout
- Endometrial, breast, prostate, and colon cancers
- Abnormal plasma lipid and cholesterol levels
- Menstrual irregularities
- Gallbladder disease
- Psychological distress, social stigma, and discrimination

Source: Adapted from McArdle, W.D., Katch, F.I., & Katch, V.L. (2001). Overweight, obesity, and weight control. In *Exercise Physiology: Energy, Nutrition, and Human Performance* (5th ed., pp. 820-863). Philadelphia: Lippincott Williams & Wilkins.

an independent heart-disease risk, similar in nature to cigarette smoking, high cholesterol, and hypertension. It also appears to correspond to higher levels of arterial inflammation that slowly and progressively increases heart attack and stroke risk over many years.

The Importance of Body-fat Distribution Pattern

Where a person tends to store body fat is also an important determinant of future health. Studies suggest that weight gain in the abdominal area (apple shape), or **android obesity,** doubles the risk for coronary heart disease, high blood pressure, diabetes, and **stroke,** compared to individuals of the same overall body fat who tend to store fat in the **gynoid** pattern, namely in the hips, buttocks, and thighs (pear shape). The reason for this difference seems to be that fat in the abdomen is more easily mobilized and sent into the bloodstream, increasing the disease-related blood fat levels. In general, men tend to gain weight in the android pattern, while women tend to store in the gynoid pattern, although any person with android obesity carries the increased health risks. To determine body-fat distribution pattern, a simple waist-to-hip ratio can be performed, whereby the girth of the waist at the smallest point at or near the navel is divided by the girth of the hips, at the largest point around the buttocks (see Chapter 10 for a more detailed discussion of waist-to-hip ratio). If the ratio exceeds 0.86 for women and 0.95 for men, there is a tendency to store fat in the android pattern, and therefore, also a higher risk of death. Central body-fat distribution (android) is associated with higher blood **cholesterol, triglycerides,** higher insulin levels, and lower HDL cholesterol, in addition to higher blood pressure and increased left ventricular wall thickness (Freedman et al., 1999).

Some clinicians use waist girth as a simple gauge of abdominal obesity and to complement measures of body fat for normal-weight individuals. Waist girth alone has been shown to relate more strongly to direct measures of abdominal visceral fat accumulation and other heart-disease risks than waist-to-hip ratio. Specifically, women with waist measurements higher than 30 inches (76 cm) display heart disease twice as frequently as slimmer women. In general, men with waist circumferences above 40 inches (102 cm) and women with waist circumferences above 35 inches (88 cm) display elevated cardiovascular risk profiles (Executive Summary, 1998).

Theories of Obesity

The exact cause of obesity remains a mystery. If obesity was a simple disorder caused by gluttony and overindulgence, then reducing food intake would cause permanent weight loss and improved health. Unfortunately, obesity involves a complex interaction of many factors involving psychological, environmental, evolutionary, biologic, and genetic causes. Individual differences in factors that predispose humans to excessive weight gain include eating patterns and eating environment; food packaging; body image; variations related to resting metabolic rate; diet-induced thermogenesis; level of spontaneous physical activity (e.g., fidgeting); basal body temperature; susceptibility to viral infections; levels of cellular **adenosine triphosphate (ATP)** and metabolic enzymes; and metabolically active brown adipose tissue. Interestingly, while the cause of obesity is usually not related to hormonal problems, obesity often triggers a cascade of abnormal hormonal responses. This section reviews some of the prevalent historical theories of obesity that incorporate the complex interaction of these factors.

Set Point

Permanent weight loss remains elusive for most people. It is estimated that as many as 85% of dieters regain lost body weight within five years (Miller & Groziak, 1997). These observations have raised suspicion that metabolic factors are important in the regulation of body weight. The set-point theory maintains that the body has a homeostatic control system for regulating its fat stores, and that the body's efficiency (resting metabolism) changes based on the amount of energy coming in, in an attempt to maintain fixed fat stores and body weight.

This theory was developed after early studies reported that weight loss and weight gain result in adaptive changes in **resting metabolic rate (RMR)** that attempt to return the individual back to his or her previous body weight (Bennett, 1995). Reductions in **thyroid hormones** were also shown to accompany slower RMR. However, studies conducted in metabolic wards, where energy input and energy output are carefully controlled and monitored and include long-term follow-up, do not support the theory that obese individuals in a weight-reduced state are more energy conservative than they were before weight loss. In fact, it appears that obese individuals who have lost weight have the same RMRs as individuals of the same body size and composition who have never been obese. These more carefully controlled studies conclude that the weight-gain tendency of obesity-prone persons is caused by factors other than variations in metabolic rate (e.g., physical inactivity), and therefore do not support the set-point theory of weight loss and weight gain (Weinsier et al., 2000).

It is interesting to note, however, that ethnic differences in metabolic rate do seem to exist. In general, black women have RMRs approximately 12% *lower* than white women. This difference appears to be genetically determined and may be explained by their lower metabolically active organ mass relative to muscle mass (Weinsier et al., 2001).

Mutant Gene (Leptin)

Leptin was discovered in 1994, quite by accident, when researchers found a strain of hybrid mice that ballooned up to five times the girth of normal mice due to their uncontrollable urge to eat. These mice were predestined to become obese due to a mutation of the gene called *obese,* or *ob.* It was believed that mice with the *ob* gene had low levels of the appetite-controlling hormone leptin. There was initially considerable excitement among obesity researchers, who thought that perhaps they had found the gene that controlled obesity. It has since been shown, however, that most obese individuals actually have *elevated* plasma leptin levels (Arch, 2005).

Leptin is a cytokine hormone released from adipocytes (fat cells), especially fat-filled adipocytes. It is secreted by adipose tissue in direct proportion to the total amount of body fat. Leptin has been called a regulator of appetite, but more specifically, it is a hormone that acts on the hypothalamus in the brain to regulate energy intake (Arch, 2005). Since it is a hormone, it also plays an important role in a negative-feedback loop whereby the fat cells communicate with the brain. In a normal situation, increases in triglyceride deposits into the adipocyte causes a release of leptin from the adipocyte, which in turn tells the hypothalamus to reduce appetite and the drive to eat. Fasting induces a decrease in leptin produced in adipose tissue and a subsequent decrease in serum leptin levels, which stimulate hunger (Arch, 2005).

The hormone-hypothalamic control mechanism fits well with the set-point theory of body-fat accumulation. It also helps explain the extreme difficulty that many obese individuals experience in sustaining significant fat loss. In obese children and adults, plasma leptin circulates in direct proportion to adipose tissue mass when weight is stable, in amounts four times higher than in lean individuals (Gutin et al., 1999). It is thought that obese individuals might be "leptin resistant," similar to the phenomenon of insulin resistance that also often accompanies obesity. This theory is supported by the observation that leptin transport across the blood-brain barrier is impaired in obese individuals. Research continues with regard to leptin resistance, and its apparent close parallel with insulin resistance in obese individuals.

Weight loss reduces serum leptin levels and weight gain increases circulating levels. Even without significant weight loss, a prolonged state of negative caloric balance decreases circulating leptin concentrations and increases hunger sensations. Interestingly, neither short- nor long-term exercise significantly affects leptin independently of the effects of exercise on total body-fat loss. Injections of leptin in both lean and obese subjects do produce a dose-dependent response with body-fat loss, suggesting a potential role for leptin and related hormones in treating obesity.

Leptin alone does not determine whether a person becomes obese, nor does it explain why some people can eat without restriction and maintain a stable body weight while others become overfat with the same caloric intake. It may, however, be a very important regulatory component of the obesity puzzle. Researchers are already designing compounds such as ob-protein, a natural body protein, that may reduce appetite and accelerate fat metabolism, and ob-receptor stimulator, a drug that suppresses appetite when the ob protein binds to its receptor in the brain and therefore causes leptin receptors to work more effectively.

Hormonal Factors

Probably the single greatest advance in the understanding of obesity has been the identification of hormones involved in appetite regulation. Besides leptin, adipocytes (fat cells) have also been shown to secrete other substances involved in the regulation of food intake and energy homeostasis. Adipocyte-derived factors have been identified, including adipsin, agouti, adiponectin, resistin, tumor necrosis factor (TNF), and secreted protein that is acidic and rich in cysteine (SPARC).

Other organs in the body, apart from but related to adipocyctes, also serve to regulate appetite and, therefore, energy intake. Certainly the gland with the most control over appetite regulation is the hypothalamus. Neuroendocrine activity is centered in the arcuate nucleus, a group of cells in the hypothalamus, and is mediated by two types of neurons, the appetite-inhibiting melanocortin (MC), which is derived from pro-opiomelanocortin (POMC), and the appetite-stimulating neuropeptide Y (NPY). These neurons relay feedback signals to the hypothalamus via the **central nervous system,** the digestive tract, thyroid gland, adrenal glands, and the pancreas to signal the individual to either start or stop eating. The following hormones are important in relaying feedback information to the hypothalamus via the neurons, POMC, and NPY (Orr & Davy, 2005):

- Thyroid hormones are involved in regulating resting metabolic rate, which comprises approximately 60 to 70% of the total calories the body burns every day. Genetics determine approximately 41% of the variability in thyroid levels. Thyroid hormones also have an inverse relationship with leptin secretion, such that increases in thyroid secretion and metabolic rate inhibit leptin secretion, which in turn stimulates appetite.
- Cholecystokinin (CCK) is a peptide hormone secreted in the duodenum and jejunum of the small intestine in response to digestive enzymes. It slows emptying of the stomach and sends **satiety** signals to the hypothalamus, which should inhibit food consumption. While its role in obesity is not known, there are currently drugs in development called CCK-A promoters that enhance the effects of CCK-A, an intestinal hormone that may inhibit appetite.
- Peptide YY (PYY) is a hormone rapidly released from the descending colon and rectum in proportion to the amount of calories consumed. PYY acts on the hypothalamus to suppress appetite, on the pancreas to increase its exocrine secretion of digestive juices, and on the gallbladder to stimulate the release of bile. The appetite suppression mediated by PYY works more slowly than that of cholecystokinin and more rapidly than that of leptin. Subjects given PYY were less hungry and ate less food over the next 12 hours than those who received a placebo (Batterham et al., 2003). In obese individuals, circulating levels of PYY are decreased and the release of PYY following a meal is lower than in normal-weight individuals (Daniels, 2006).

- **Cortisol,** a **glucocorticoid,** is released from the adrenal glands in response to corticotrophin-releasing hormone. It functions to raise blood glucose levels by facilitating **gluconeogenesis,** stimulating NPY, and promoting **lipolysis** (release of triglyceride from fat cells). Cortisol also stimulates the storage of fat, especially in the central and visceral areas. Levels of cortisol are most notably higher during times of stress, which is why eating in response to stress may be linked to increased or altered cortisol production and abdominal fat deposition.
- Insulin is a peptide hormone produced by the pancreas and secreted in response to elevated blood glucose levels. Circulating levels of insulin are directly proportional to adipose level and rise rapidly after eating. Insulin suppresses NPY and stimulates POMC. Fat cells themselves produce peptides that elicit insulin resistance, and high-fat diets inhibit insulin communication with the hypothalamus to reduce appetite and food intake.
- **Ghrelin,** a hormone discovered in 1999, is produced mainly in the stomach. It is responsible for stimulating appetite via stimulation of the NPY receptors and by stimulating the adrenal glands to release **adrenocortiocotrophic hormone (ACTH),** which ultimately stimulates the release of cortisol. Ghrelin levels in the blood are inversely correlated with weight, meaning that high ghrelin levels are associated with low body weight. Circulating blood levels of ghrelin increase shortly before eating and decrease quickly after eating.
- Obestatin is the newest hormone discovery in obesity research. Found in 2005 on the same gene as ghrelin, and only studied in animals thus far, obestatin decreases food ingestion, unlike ghrelin, which increases the feeding response. Scientists have not yet determined whether obestatin acts mainly on the hypothalamus, thereby reducing appetite, or in the other regions of the brain, causing taste aversion.

High Energy Intake

Probably the most obvious, but most misunderstood, theory of why individuals become obese is that they simply consume too many calories. Short-term overeating is a common habit that does little to adversely affect health, whereas overeating over long periods can become a health risk. Overeating can be either active or passive and can be induced by a number of conditions. Active overeating can be caused by a cognitive drive to consume too many calories (driven by internal or external cues), a physical defect in appetite and/or satiety regulation, or an inappropriate psychological response to stress. Passive overeating is a different phenomenon, in which the consumption of what would otherwise be a "normal" amount of food becomes excessive due to a sedentary, inactive lifestyle.

Active Overeating

One of the clearest examples of active overeating is illustrated by what happens to laboratory rats when their normal, bland chow is replaced by chocolate chip cookies and other high-calorie foods. This substitution disrupts energy balance, which normally defends the body's current weight, and replaces it with a fourfold fat gain in these animals (Jequier, 2002).

Active overeating in humans can occur due to cultural norms that favor fatness and regard high body weight (in women in particular) as a symbol of affluence and attractiveness. In Western society, however, active overeating is mostly driven by marketing. Huge portion sizes and fast-food "combo" meals that are less expensive than the *a la carte* option, and generally more convenient to order, provide an excessive amount of calories that bear no relationship to the single-meal energy requirement of most individuals. Barbara Rolls calls this phenomenon "volumetrics." In one study, 23 normal-weight men and women were provided with standard-portion meals for 11 consecutive days, and large-portion meals (additional 50%) for 11 days. When presented with the large-portion meals, subjects still voluntarily consumed all of the additional food, which contained approximately 423 extra calories per day. They did not compensate for the additional calories by decreasing intake during the study period. Therefore, increased portions contributed to energy overconsumption and excess body-weight gain (Rolls, Roe, & Meengs, 2007). However, evidence suggests that active overeating contributes to the obesity epidemic to a lesser degree in the general population than does passive overeating.

Passive Overeating

It is easy to demonstrate how increases in energy intake lead to positive energy balance and weight gain. In contrast, there is strong evidence to suggest that the modern sedentary lifestyle, and the resultant low levels of energy expenditure, is the driving force behind the obesity epidemic. In fact, evidence suggests that reduced energy expenditure increases a person's vulnerability to overeating, primarily due to the fat content of foods that provide excessive amounts of calories even though overall "portions" of these high-fat foods may be quite normal.

In an interesting study of this phenomenon, men were allowed to eat freely from seemingly identical diets that had been secretly manipulated to contain 20%, 40%, or 60% energy from fat. Regardless of the fat content of their diets, each group of men ate the same bulk of food. Therefore, the energy overload provided in the 60% fat diet was an "accidental" phenomenon (hence the term "passive overeating") (Stubbs et al., 1995). Independent of fat content, low-energy-dense diets generate greater satiety than high-energy-dense diets, suggesting that an important regulatory signal may be the weight or volume of food consumed rather than the actual caloric content of the food (Poppitt & Prentice, 1996). Therefore, high-fat foods do not decrease consumption, but rather only serve as a source of unnecessary excessive calories.

Low Energy Expenditure

Many people believe that excessive caloric consumption is the sole cause of obesity. If this were true, then some form of caloric restriction by dieting would become the number-one recommended approach to weight loss. Studies have shown, however, that this strategy is very ineffective at promoting long-term weight loss. It is true, however, that weight gain often parallels a reduction in physical activity rather than an increase in caloric intake. In fact, it could be argued that the "creeping obesity" common during middle-age is more a function of reductions in physical activity, because most people tend to eat the same relative number of calories throughout adulthood. Physically active individuals are usually the ones who consume the most calories, yet weigh the least.

It is interesting to note that the per capita caloric intake in the U.S. has decreased by approximately 400 kcal per day over the last 100 years, but body weight and body fat have increased steadily. From 1977 to 1987, average caloric intake decreased by 4%, yet the number of overweight people increased by 8%. If caloric intake alone were responsible, then reductions in caloric intake would equal reductions in body weight.

Individuals who maintain a physically active lifestyle do not exhibit the "normal" pattern of weight gain in adulthood. This is also true in young, growing children. From age three months to one year, the total energy expenditure of infants who later became overweight is 21% lower than infants with normal body weights. Children age four to six years are an average of 25% below energy-expenditure recommendations for their energy-intake levels. As many as 50% of boys and 75% of girls in the U.S. fail to engage in moderate physical activity three or more times per week, and overweight elementary-school children are considerably less active than normal-weight children, despite lower caloric intake.

The observation that overweight children often eat the same or less than their normal-weight peers also corresponds to less physically active adults who slowly, progressively gain weight. Overweight individuals do not typically eat more than persons of normal weight, which partially explains why dieting alone, without exercise, is often ineffective for long-term weight loss.

Influence of Genetics vs. Environment

Research indicates that genetic factors that affect metabolism and appetite determine approximately 25% of the variation in body fatness, and a larger percentage is explained by environmental influences. The epidemic of obesity, which began 20 years ago, has occurred within a gene pool that has not changed in 100 years or more. Nonetheless, it is clear that genetic factors play an important role in a person's susceptibility to becoming obese in an obesity-promoting environment (Snyder et al., 2004), which is rich with sedentary and stressful activities, and ready access to inexpensive, large-portion, high-calorie, good-tasting food (Bouchard, 1997). Genetics contributes to the development of obesity in two ways:

- Single rare mutations in certain genes wholly explain the development of obesity (monogenic obesity). These forms are rare, very severe, and generally begin in childhood (e.g., lacking the gene that produces leptin).
- Several genetic variants interact with an "at-risk" environment (polygenetic obesity). In this case, each gene, taken individually, would only contribute to body weight in a small way, and the cumulative effect of these genes would only become significant when there is an interaction with environmental factors that cause their expression (e.g., overeating, sedentary lifestyle). This form is common and is the form that is emphasized in this discussion (Pritchard, 2001).

The unique interaction between an individual's genetic composition and the environment in which their genes have an opportunity to express themselves makes it difficult to quantify the role of each in the development of obesity. While a person's genes do not necessarily cause obesity, they may lower the threshold for its expression. Researchers are just now starting to identify key genes and specific DNA sequences that relate to the causes of appetite regulation and predispose a person to obesity. To date, more than 50 genes and polymorphisms have been tested and implicated in controlling food intake, energy expenditure, and fat and carbohydrate metabolism. While no conclusive role in obesity development has been established for these genes, certain variants are associated with different aspects of obesity, such as time to onset, aggravation with time, metabolic and cardiovascular complications, appetite, and the interaction between excess body weight and physical activity (Clement, 2005). This area of research, however, is extremely complex, and progress in the knowledge of the human genome and the development of computing tools and new analysis strategies that can handle several hundreds of items of genetic and environmental information at once will be necessary to tackle these questions (Clement, 2005).

Genetic Factors

Insightful information about the causes of obesity has come from the cloning of obesity genes in animals. Molecular and reverse genetic studies (using mouse "**knockouts**") have also helped to establish important pathways that regulate body fat and food intake. Leptin deficiency, produced by a single gene mutation as described earlier in this chapter, has shown that true metabolic-gene pathways do exist. Similar deficiencies in food intake have been found, where changes to the amino-acid sequence of a key regulator of food intake, melanocortin-4 receptor, causes uncontrolled food intake similar to that seen in leptin deficiency. These insights into biology have shown that body-fat regulation may be independent of willpower.

In a landmark study by Bouchard et al. (1990), the importance of genetics in body-weight regulation was clearly shown. Researchers intentionally overfed 12 pairs of male identical twins for 100 days (total overfeeding of 84,000 kcal) to observe differences within and between twin pairs. What they found was a striking similarity in the amount of weight gain, skinfold changes, and changes in BMI within the twin pairs, but three times more variance between twin pairs for these same variables. The within-pair similarity was particularly evident with respect to the changes in regional fat distribution and amount of abdominal visceral fat, with approximately six times as much variance between pairs as within pairs. They concluded that the most likely explanation for the similarity within a pair of twins in the adaptation to long-term overfeeding, while the explanation for the large variations in weight changes and body-fat distribution between pairs of twins is that genetic factors were involved. These genetic factors may regulate a person's tendency to store extra calories as either fat or lean tissue and alter resting metabolism accordingly.

Genetic researchers have identified a specific gene, the uncoupling protein-2 gene (UCP2), as another important link in the obesity puzzle. High activity of this gene, which is present in all human tissue, activates a protein that burns extra calories as heat (Fleury et al., 1997). This type of metabolism blunts excess fat storage and may help to explain why some people store extra calories as fat while others do not, as was previously shown in the work of Bouchard et al. (1990). Finding a drug that turns on the UCP2 gene could prove to be an obesity-treatment breakthrough.

Environmental Factors

Higher rates of obesity are found in people with the lowest incomes and the least education, especially among women and certain ethnic groups. This association may be partially explained by the relatively low cost of energy-dense, high-fat food, and the association of lower incomes with the unavailability of fresh fruits and vegetables (Turrell et al., 2002). Observational studies in many different countries confirm that dietary patterns and obesity rates vary between neighborhoods, where living in a low-income neighborhood is independently associated with obesity and a poor diet (Cummins & Macintyre, 2006). These environmental influences on diet involve two pathways: access to foods for home consumption from supermarkets and grocery stores, and access to ready-made food (e.g., fast food, restaurants).

Studies consistently show that the presence of supermarkets is associated with a lower prevalence of obesity. In the U.S. and Canada, "healthier" and more expensive foods are less available in poorer communities, and access to supermarkets is more difficult in low-income neighborhoods, where independent stores dominate and tend to charge higher prices. Foods purchased from fast-food and other restaurants are becoming an increasingly important part of people's diets, especially in the U.S. These foods, which can be up to 65% more energy dense than those found in the average diet, provide fewer nutrients and higher amounts of fat and tend to be larger in portion size than foods consumed at home (Prentice & Jebb, 2003; Rolls, 2003).

Several components of the American food supply and food "environment" may be important determinants of obesity. Research on portion sizes, packages, and servings clearly indicates that when more food is provided, more food is eaten (Diliberti et al., 2004). Portion sizes have increased dramatically in the past 40 years, and while containers do state that a particular package may contain more than one serving, it is common to consume food by the package and not by the serving size.

Modifying Body Fat Early in Life

Behavior is an important determinant of body fatness, even at a very young age. Maternal nutrition during pregnancy has an effect on the developing fetus. Mothers who gain more than 40 pounds (18 kg) during pregnancy generally have babies with larger skinfold thicknesses than babies of mothers who gained less weight during pregnancy (Udal et al., 1978). Bottle-feeding and the introduction of solid foods too early have also been associated with childhood obesity, whereas breastfeeding, which allows the infant's natural appetite to set limits on food intake, may prevent overfeeding and the development of obesity (Kramer, 1981). Certainly, moderate food intake and regular physical activity during growth has the potential to attenuate an increase in fat-cell number and fat-cell size, whereas these positive choices only have the potential to reduce fat-cell size if done later in life. Early prevention of obesity through proper diet and exercise offers the greatest potential for reducing the prevalence of obesity in all individuals.

Summary

Obesity is a multifaceted disorder with a common final outcome, whereby energy intake exceeds expenditure, leading to an excess accumulation of body fat. The average body weight of American adults has increased by 8 pounds (3.6 kg) over the past 20 years, and today approximately 66% of Americans are classified as either overweight or obese. Excessive body fat is the second leading cause of preventable death in the United States, behind only smoking. Obesity increases a person's risk for **hypertension, hyperglycemia,** breast cancer, and hypercholesterolemia. The location of body-fat accumulation, namely around the trunk and abdomen, is also an important determinant of risk for cardiovascular disease. Hormones such as leptin and adipocyte-derived factors play an important role in regulating appetite, and therefore, energy intake. While genetic factors account for 25 to 30% of excess body-fat accumulation, environmental factors such as an abundance of low-cost, energy-dense, high-fat foods and a society that favors inactivity provide the optimal condition for obesity to express itself.

References

Allison, D.B. et al. (1999). Annual deaths attributable to obesity in the United States. *Journal of the American Medical Association*, 282, 16, 1530–1538.

Arch, J.R. (2005). Central regulation of energy balance: Inputs, outputs and leptin resistance. *Proceedings of the Nutrition Society,* 64, 1, 39–46.

Batterham, R.L. et al. (2003). Inhibition of food intake in obese subjects by peptide YY3-36. *New England Journal of Medicine,* 349, 10, 941–948.

Bennett, W.I. (1995). Beyond overeating. *New England Journal of Medicine,* 32, 10, 673–674.

Bouchard, C. (1997). Human variation in body mass: Evidence for a role of the genes. *Nutrition Review,* 55, 1, S21–27; discussion S27–30.

Bouchard, C. et al. (1990). The response to long-term overfeeding in identical twins. *New England Journal of Medicine*, 322, 21, 1477–1482.

Carpenter, W.H. et al. (1998). Total daily energy expenditure in free-living older African-Americans and Caucasians. *American Journal of Physiology,* 274, 1, E96–101.

Clement, K. (2005). Genetics of human obesity. *Proceedings of the Nutrition Society,* 64, 2, 133–142.

Crespo, C.J. & Wright, J.D. (1995). Prevalence of overweight among active and inactive U.S. adults from the Third National Health and Nutrition Examination Survey. *Medicine & Science in Sports & Exercise,* 27, S73.

Cummins, S. & Macintyre, S. (2006). Food environments and obesity—neighbourhood or nation? *International Journal of Epidemiology,* 35, 1, 100–104.

Daniels, J. (2006). Obesity: America's epidemic. *American Journal of Nursing,* 106, 1, 40–49.

Dearborn, W. et al. (1938). Data on the growth of public school children (from the materials of the Harvard Growth Study). *Monographs of the Society for Research in Child Development*, 1.

Diliberti, N. et al. (2004). Increased portion size leads to increased energy intake in a restaurant meal. *Obesity Research,* 12, 3, 562–568.

Engel, A. et al. (1978). Plan and operation of the HANES I augmentation survey of adults 25–74 years: United States, 1974-1975. *Vital Health Statistics,* 1, 14, 1–110.

Executive Summary (1994). Plan and operation of the Third National Health and Nutrition Examination Survey, 1988-94. Series 1: programs and collection procedures. *Vital Health Statistics,* 1, 32, 1–407.

Executive Summary (1998). Executive summary of the clinical guidelines of the identification, evaluation, and treatment of overweight and obesity in adults. *Archives of Internal Medicine,* 158, 1855.

Flegal, K.M. (2005). Epidemiologic aspects of overweight and obesity in the United States. *Physiology and Behavior,* 86, 5, 599–602.

Fleury, C. et al. (1997). Uncoupling protein-2: A novel gene linked to obesity and hyperinsulinemia. *Nature Genetics,* 15, 3, 269–272.

Foster, G.D. et al. (1999). Changes in resting energy expenditure after weight loss in obese African American and white women. *American Journal of Clinical Nutrition,* 69, 1, 13–17.

Freedman, D.S. et al. (1999). The relation of overweight to cardiovascular risk factors among children and adolescents: The Bogalusa Heart Study. *Pediatrics,* 103, 6, 1175–1182.

Gutin, B. et al. (1999). Plasma leptin concentrations in obese children: Changes during 4-month periods with and without physical training. *America Journal of Clinical Nutrition,* 69, 3, 388–394.

Hubert, H.B. et al. (1983). Obesity as an independent risk factor for cardiovascular disease: A 26-year follow-up of participants in the Framingham Heart Study. *Circulation,* 67, 5, 968–977.

Jequier, E. (2002). Pathways to obesity. *International Journal of Obesity-related Metabolic Disorders,* 26, Supplement 2, S12–17.

Kramer, M.S. (1981). Do breast-feeding and delayed introduction of solid foods protect against subsequent obesity? *Journal of Pediatrics,* 98, 6, 883–887.

Manson, J.E. et al. (1995). Body weight and mortality among women. *New England Journal of Medicine,* 333, 11, 677–685.

McArdle, W.D., Katch, F.I., & Katch, V.L. (2001). Overweight, obesity, and weight control. In: *Exercise Physiology: Energy, Nutrition, and Human Performance* (5th ed., pp. 820–863). Philadelphia: Lippincott Williams & Wilkins.

McDowell, A. et al. (1981). Plan and operation of the Second National Health and Nutrition Examination Survey, 1976–1980. *Vital Health Statistic,* 1, 15, 1–144.

Miller, G.D. & Groziak, S.M. (1997). Diet and gene interaction. *Journal of the American College of Nutrition,* 16, 4, 293–295.

Ogden, C.L. et al. (2006). Prevalence of overweight and obesity in the United States, 1999–2004. *Journal of the American Medical Association,* 295, 13, 1549–1555.

Orr, J. & Davy, B. (2005). Dietary Influences on peripheral hormones regulating energy intake: Potential applications for weight management. *Journal of the American Dietetic Association,* 105, 1115–1124.

Poppitt, S.D. & Prentice, A.M. (1996). Energy density and its role in the control of food intake: Evidence from metabolic and community studies. *Appetite,* 26, 2, 153–174.

Prentice, A.M. & Jebb, S.A. (2003). Fast foods, energy density and obesity: A possible mechanistic link. *Obesity Review,* 4, 4, 187–194.

Pritchard, J.K. (2001). Are rare variants responsible for susceptibility to complex diseases? *American Journal of Human Genetics*, 69, 1, 124–137.

Rolls, B.J. (2003). The supersizing of America: Portion size and the obesity epidemic. *Nutrition Today,* 38, 2, 42–53.

Rolls, B.J., Roe, L.S., & Meengs, J.S. (2007). The effect of large portion sizes on energy intake is sustained for 11 days. *Obesity* (Silver Spring), 15, 6, 1535-1543.

Rosengren, A., Wedel, H., & Wilhelmsen, L. (1999). Body weight and weight gain during adult life in men in relation to coronary heart disease and mortality: A prospective population study. *European Heart Journal,* 20, 4, 269–277.

Sinaiko, A.R. et al. (1999). Relation of weight and rate of increase in weight during childhood and adolescence to body size, blood pressure, fasting insulin, and lipids in young adults: The Minneapolis Children's Blood Pressure Study. *Circulation,* 99, 11, 1471–1476.

Snyder, E.E. et al. (2004). The human obesity gene map: The 2003 update. *Obesity Research,* 12, 3, 369–439.

Stubbs, R.J. et al. (1995). Covert manipulation of dietary fat and energy density: Effect on substrate flux and food intake in men eating ad libitum. *American Journal of Clinical Nutrition,* 62, 316–329.

Turrell, G. et al. (2002). Socioeconomic differences in food purchasing behaviour and suggested implications for diet-related health promotion. *Journal of Human Nutrition and Dietetics,* 15, 5, 355–364.

Udal, J.N. et al. (1978). Interaction of maternal and neonatal obesity. *Pediatrics,* 62, 1, 17–21.

Vinten, J. & Galbo, H. (1983). Effect of physical training on transport and metabolism of glucose in adipocytes. *American Journal of Physiology,* 244, 2, E129–134.

Weinsier, R.L. et al. (2001). Body fat distribution in white and black women: Different patterns of intraabdominal and subcutaneous abdominal adipose tissue utilization with weight loss. *American Journal of Clinical Nutrition,* 74, 5, 631–636.

Weinsier, R.L. et al. (2000). Do adaptive changes in metabolic rate favor weight regain in weight-reduced individuals? An examination of the set-point theory. *American Journal of Clinical Nutrition,* 72, 5, 1088–1094.

Suggested Reading

Allison, D.B. & Saunders, S.E. (2000). Obesity in North America: An overview. *Medical Clinics of North America,* 84, 2, 305–332, v.

American College of Sports Medicine (2001). Position stand: Appropriate intervention strategies for weight loss and prevention of weight regain for adults. http://www.acsmmsse.org/pt/re/msse/positionstandards.htm

Bachman, C.M. et al. (2006). Is there an association between sweetened beverages and adiposity? *Nutrition Review,* 64, 4, 153–174.

Lissner, L. et al. (1987). Dietary fat and the regulation of energy intake in human subjects. *American Journal of Clinical Nutrition,* 46, 6, 886–892.

Prentice, A.M. (2001). Overeating: The health risks. *Obesity Research,* 9, Supplement 4, 234S–238S.

Wyatt, S.B., Winters, K.P., & Dubbert, P.M. (2006). Overweight and obesity: Prevalence, consequences, and causes of a growing public health problem. *American Journal of the Medical Sciences,* 331, 4, 166–74.

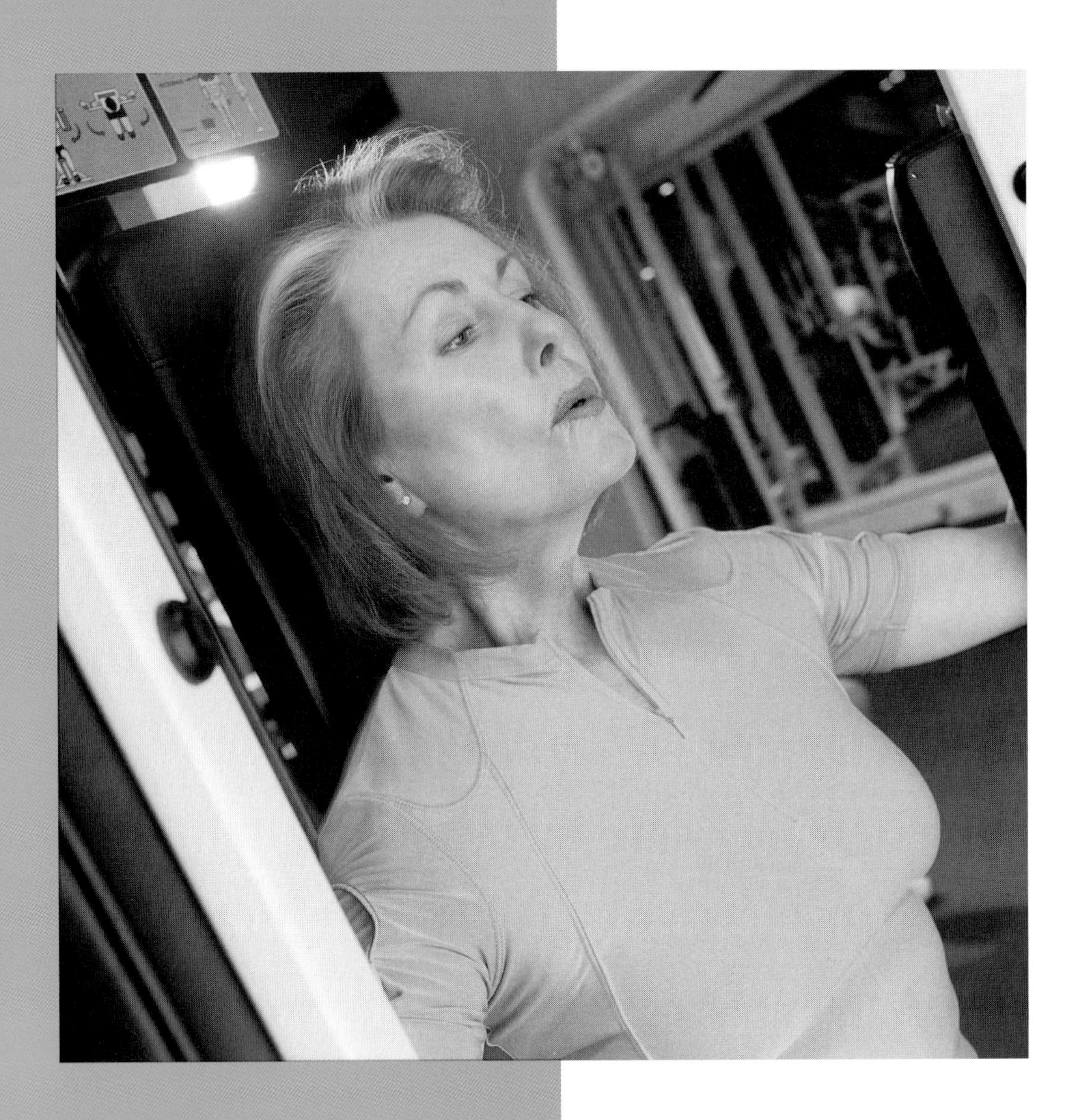

Scott Roberts

Scott Roberts, Ph.D., is an associate professor and program coordinator for the Exercise Physiology Program at California State University, Chico. He is a fellow of both the American College of Sports Medicine and the American Association of Cardiovascular and Pulmonary Rehabilitation. He is a widely published author and coauthor and an editor for several publications. Dr. Roberts authored the chapter "Exercise Guidelines for Individuals with Pacemakers and AICDs" and served as the section editor for cardiovascular disease chapters in ACSM's Exercise Management for Persons With Chronic Diseases and Disabilities, *2nd edition. He also coauthored* Clinical Exercise Testing and Prescription: Theory and Application.

Chapter 18

Exercise for Individuals With Medical or Health Limitations

IN THIS CHAPTER:

Fitness professionals frequently encounter clients with special needs and health concerns. For those who work with clients of middle age or older, this will be a regular event. It is important for Lifestyle & Weight Management Consultants (LWMCs) to identify health conditions that will influence the development of lifestyle-modification programs in the initial screening portion of the client–LWMC interaction. LWMCs should regularly update their client screening records to identify and effectively address changes in health status as they occur. Once an LWMC has identified that a client has a medical and/or health condition, he or she must obtain physician approval before proceeding with exercise-program development, testing, or training. Along with physician approval, LWMCs also should request exercise guidelines and limitations from the client's physician. In many cases, a physician will appoint another health professional to assist in providing exercise guidelines. This may be, for example, a nurse, physical therapist, clinical exercise physiologist, or a diabetes educator, depending on the clinical status of the client. It is important to obtain and follow the guidelines given and to maintain close contact with the appropriate health professional to have all questions answered and to provide status reports at predetermined intervals. An ACE-certified LWMC should not work with clients with health challenges until they have received medical clearance. This chapter addresses basic guidelines for working with clients with the following health conditions and/or special needs:

- Coronary artery disease
- Hypertension
- Peripheral vascular disease
- Diabetes
- Asthma
- Osteoporosis
- Low-back pain
- Arthritis
- Older adults
- Children
- Pregnancy

As a rule of thumb, if clients have been released to take part in independent **activities of daily living (ADL)** (including a limited exercise program), they will probably be cleared to work with an LWMC who can then provide guidance and motivation.

Generally speaking, clients with one or more of the previously listed characteristics should follow a low- or non-impact, low-intensity exercise program that progresses gradually. In many cases, there are specific exercises or modifications to exercises that will enhance the safety and effectiveness of the exercise program. If an LWMC works with clients with special needs, it is the LWMC's responsibility to enhance his or her knowledge and skills in this area through continuing education opportunities.

Cardiovascular Disorders

Cardiovascular disease is the leading cause of death in the Western world, and the majority of cases are attributed to **coronary artery disease (CAD)**. CAD results from **atherosclerosis,** which is caused by a narrowing of the coronary arteries that supply the heart muscle with blood and oxygen. The narrowing may result from an initial injury to the inner lining of the arteries (due to high blood pressures, high levels of **low-density lipoproteins,** elevated blood **glucose,** or other chemical agents, such as those from cigarettes). Once the inner lining has been damaged, the accumulation of plaque (consisting of calcified cholesterol and fat deposits) reduces the diameter of the coronary artery.

Atherosclerosis also is the underlying cause of cerebral and **peripheral vascular diseases.** Manifestations of these diseases include heart attack, **angina, stroke,** and intermittent **claudication.**

Exercise and Coronary Artery Disease

Regular physical activity reduces the risk of CAD, but how effective is exercise in treating it? In the early 1960s, physicians began experimenting with getting patients up and out of bed soon after a cardiac event, and the results were favorable. Unlike those who were advised to stay in bed, cardiac patients who stayed mobile experienced fewer clinical complications, a faster recovery, and fewer complications related to bed rest. In almost all cases, individuals recovering from a **myocardial infarction,** cardiac surgery, or other cardiac procedure, can benefit from a supervised cardiac rehabilitation program (Wenger et al., 1995).

Exercise Guidelines for CAD

It is best if clients with a history of coronary artery disease first complete a supervised cardiac rehabilitation program before starting an exercise program. Most clients who have been released to take part in ADL will have been given a home exercise program and some basic activity guidelines. It is appropriate for LWMCs to inform prospective clients that cardiac rehabilitation programs are available and that they should ask their physician if participation is recommended. Exercise and activity guidelines are based on the clinical status of the client. A cardiologist or other designated health professional should provide an upper-limit heart rate, as well as guidelines and limitations to physical activity.

- Low-risk cardiac clients should have stable cardiovascular and physiological responses to exercise. The term low-risk is generally applied to those clients who have all of the following: (1) an uncomplicated clinical course in the hospital; (2) no evidence of resting or exercise-induced **ischemia;** (3) functional capacity greater than 7 **METs** or 24.5 ml/kg/min three weeks following any medical event or treatment that required hospitalization, such as a heart attack, episode of angina, or open heart surgery; (4) normal ventricular function greater than 50% ejection fraction (percent of blood pumped out of the heart with each beat); and (5) no significant resting or exercise-induced arrhythmias (abnormal heart rhythms identified by an electrocardiogram).

- Clients or potential clients who have two or more cardiac risk factors or a history of cardiac disease must have a physician release and referral to exercise (see Chapter 9).
- All clients with documented CAD should undergo a maximal graded exercise test administered by a physician or appropriately trained professional to determine their functional capacity and cardiovascular status to establish a safe exercise level.
- LWMCs should design all clients' exercise programs according to the guidelines given by their personal physicians. These guidelines will usually be based on exercise test results, medical history, clinical status, and symptoms. There are published guidelines available to assist LWMCs in working with these clients and interacting with their healthcare team [American College of Sports Medicine (ACSM), 2006; American Association of Cardiovascular and Pulmonary Rehabilitation (AACPR), 1999].
- Exercise should not continue if any abnormal signs or symptoms are observed before, during, or immediately following exercise. If symptoms persist, activate the emergency medical system.

Sample Exercise Recommendation

Mode. Low-intensity endurance exercise, such as low-impact aerobics, walking, swimming, or stationary cycling, should be the primary exercise mode. Avoid **isometric** exercises, as they can dramatically raise blood pressure and the workload or stress on the heart. Develop a weight-training program that features low resistance and a high number of repetitions.

Note: Any client who has had a cardiovascular event within the last month should, as appropriate, follow the exercise guidelines outlined below. If a low-risk client has been stable for at least six months, LWMCs should follow the exercise guidelines for sedentary, healthy adults.

Intensity. **Rating of perceived exertion (RPE)** of 9 to 14 (on the 6 to 20 scale); heart rate can be as low as 20 to 30 beats over resting heart rate and up to 40 to 75% of maximal **heart-rate reserve** (Karvonen formula).

Duration. The total duration should be gradually increased to 20 to 30 minutes of continuous or **interval training,** plus additional time for warm-up and cool-down activities.

Frequency. Three to five days per week.

Hypertension

Hypertension is one of the most prevalent **chronic diseases** in the United States. According to the Centers for Disease Control and Prevention (CDC), approximately one in three U.S. adults has chronically elevated blood pressure, or is taking antihypertensive medication. Unfortunately, nearly one-third of people in the U.S. living with hypertension don't know they have it and more than 40% of people with high blood pressure aren't receiving treatment. Hypertension is related to the development of CAD, increased severity of atherosclerosis, stroke, congestive heart failure, left ventricular hypertrophy, aortic aneurysms, and peripheral vascular disease. Hypertensive individuals are at three to four times the risk of developing coronary artery disease, and up to seven times the risk of having a stroke.

Exercise and Hypertension

Exercise is recognized as an important part of therapy for controlling hypertension. While it is known that regular aerobic exercise reduces both **systolic** and **diastolic blood pressure** by an average of 10 mmHg, how it does this is not completely understood. It appears that regular physical activity reduces both **cardiac output** and total peripheral resistance when the body is at rest, in addition to reducing sympathetic activity.

Exercise Guidelines for Hypertension

Since many hypertensive individuals are obese and have CAD risk factors, non-drug therapy is usually the first line of treatment. This therapy will usually include weight reduction, salt restriction, and increased physical activity. Consider the following factors when recommending exercise for hypertensive clients: (1) medical/clinical status; (2) current medications; (3) the frequency, duration, intensity, and mode of exercise the individual is currently participating in; and (4) how well the individual manages his or her hypertension.

- Do not allow hypertensive clients to hold their breath or strain during exercise **(Valsalva maneuver);** instead, cue them to exhale on the exertion.
- Weight training should supplement endurance training. Utilize **circuit training** rather than heavy weight lifting and keep resistance low and the number of repetitions high.
- Use the RPE scale to monitor exercise intensity, because some medications (e.g., **beta blockers**) can alter the accuracy of the training heart rate during exercise.
- Be aware of any changes in medications, which should come with written guidelines from the client's physician. Not all medication changes will require a change in the exercise program, but this should be communicated to the LWMC by the client's physician. See Appendix D for a listing of generic and brand names of common antihypertensive medications by class.
- Exercise should not continue if any abnormal signs or symptoms are observed before, during, or immediately following exercise. If symptoms persist, activate the emergency medical system. If symptoms stop, discontinue the exercise program until the client's physician gives clearance.
- Physicians may instruct their hypertensive patients to record their blood pressures before and after exercise.
- Instruct hypertensive clients to move slowly when getting up from the floor, because they are more susceptible to **orthostatic hypotension** when taking antihypertensive medication.
- Both hypertensive and hypotensive responses are possible during and after exercise for individuals with hypertension. Either of these responses should be reported, and additional exercise guidelines given as a result.
- Carefully monitor each hypertensive client's blood pressure during exercise initially, and possibly long-term. Blood pressure can be most accurately measured during lower-body aerobic activity (e.g., stationary cycling) and resistance training (e.g., leg extensions). Clients with more severe hypertension will likely be taking one or more hypertensive medications that may affect their responses to exercise.
- Individuals with hypertension may have multiple CAD risk factors, which should be considered when developing their exercise programs.

Sample Exercise Recommendation

Mode. The overall exercise-training recommendations for individuals with mild-to-moderate hypertension are basically the same as those for apparently healthy individuals. Endurance exercise such as low-impact aerobics, walking, and swimming should be the primary exercise mode. Exercises with a significant isometric component should be avoided. Weight training should feature low resistance and a high number of repetitions (initially, 12 to 20).

Intensity. The exercise-intensity level should be near the lower end of the heart-rate range (40 to 65% heart-rate reserve).

Frequency. Encourage hypertensive clients to exercise at least four times per week. Elderly clients or those with an initially low functional capacity may exercise daily for shorter durations.

Duration. Gradual warm-ups and cool-downs lasting longer than five minutes are recommended. Gradually increase total exercise duration to as much as 30 to 60 minutes per session, depending on the medical history and clinical status of the individual.

Peripheral Vascular Disease

Peripheral vascular disease (PVD) is caused by atherosclerotic lesions in one or more peripheral arterial and/or venous blood vessels (usually in the legs). Common sites for atherosclerotic lesions include the iliac, femoral, and popliteal arteries (see Figure 1-2a, page 4). Most people with PVD are older and have long-established CAD risk factors; PVD also is 20 times more common in diabetics than in non-diabetic individuals. The treatment for PVD usually involves a combination of medication (to increase dilation of the arteries and veins), exercise (to improve blood flow and functional capacity), medical procedures (to clean out the blockages), and surgery (artery bypass).

PVD is a painful and often debilitating disease, characterized by muscular pain caused by ischemia (reduced blood flow) to the working muscles. This ischemic pain is usually the result of spasms or blockages, referred to as claudication. Some people experience chronic claudication and pain even at rest. For others, activities such as walking, cycling, or stair climbing can cause painful, intermittent claudication that is usually relieved by immediate rest. Most people with PVD describe claudication as a dull, aching, cramping pain. The claudication pain scale is a subjective rating of discomfort that can be used to regulate exercise intensity, duration, and frequency (Table 18-1).

Table 18-1
Subjective Grading Scale for Peripheral Vascular Disease

Grade I –	Definite discomfort or pain, but only of initial or modest levels
Grade II –	Moderate discomfort or pain from which the client's attention can be diverted, by conversation, for example
Grade III –	Intense pain (short of Grade IV) from which the client's attention cannot be diverted
Grade IV –	Excruciating and unbearable pain

Exercise and Peripheral Vascular Disease

One of the primary benefits of exercise for individuals with PVD is that it helps to lower overall CAD risk (e.g., hypertension, **hypercholesterolemia**), as well as improve blood flow and overall cardiovascular endurance. Studies have shown that people with PVD can improve their peak work capacity with regular exercise (Regensteiner & Hiatt, 1995).

Exercise Guidelines for Peripheral Vascular Disease

Individuals with PVD should undergo a complete medical evaluation before embarking on an exercise program. Initially, the focus should be on low-intensity, non-weightbearing activities. Because of their chronic pain, individuals with PVD often have a high anxiety level when starting out. Gradual progression can build confidence, and additional activities may be added to the program. Individuals with PVD probably do not have ambitions to run a marathon; they simply want to be able to go shopping, climb stairs, and go for a walk without a great deal of pain. In addition to exercise, other lifestyle modifications, such as diet modifications and weight management, should be encouraged in an effort to lower overall CAD risk.

- Encourage daily exercise with frequent rest periods to allow for maximal exercise tolerance.
- Initially, recommend low-impact, non-weightbearing activities such as swimming, rowing, and cycling. Add weightbearing activities as exercise tolerance improves.
- Avoid exercising in cold air or water to reduce the risk of **vasoconstriction.**
- Interval training, which may involve five- to 10-minute exercise bouts, one to three times per day, may initially be appropriate for some PVD clients.
- Because many PVD clients also are diabetic, they need to take excellent care of their feet to avoid blisters and other injuries that could lead to infection.
- Ideally, individuals with PVD should be closely supervised, such as in a cardiac rehabilitation program.
- Gradually increase the time, duration, and intensity of PVD clients' programs. The degree of progress (absence or reduction of pain) will dictate how often and how much to increase these variables. As a client's functional capacity improves, increase these factors accordingly.
- Encourage PVD clients to walk as much and as often as they can tolerate.

Sample Exercise Recommendation

Mode. Non-impact endurance exercise, such as swimming and cycling, may allow for longer-duration and higher-intensity exercise. Recommend weightbearing activities that are shorter in duration and lower in intensity, with more frequent rest periods.

Intensity. Choose low-intensity exercises rather than high-intensity, high-impact exercises. PVD clients should exercise to the point of moderate to intense pain (Grade II to Grade III on the claudication pain scale; see Table 18-1). As functional capacity improves, gradually increase intensity.

Frequency. Daily exercise is recommended initially. As functional capacity improves, frequency can be reduced to four to six days per week.

Duration. A longer and more gradual warm-up and cool-down (longer than 10 minutes) is recommended. Gradually increase total exercise duration to 30 to 40 minutes.

Diabetes

Diabetes is characterized by reduced **insulin** secretion by the pancreatic beta cells and/or reduced sensitivity to insulin. Diabetes causes abnormalities in the metabolism of **carbohydrates, protein,** and **fat** and, if left untreated, can be deadly. This is of particular concern since the symptoms of diabetes are not always evident in the early stages.

People with diabetes are at greater risk for numerous health problems, including kidney failure, nerve disorders, eye problems, and heart disease, and are two to four times as likely to develop cardiovascular disease. Prolonged and frequent elevation of blood sugar can damage the capillaries, a condition called microangiopathy that leads to poor circulation. In addition, people with diabetes are at greater risk for permanent nerve damage.

There are two main types of diabetes. **Type 1 diabetes** is caused by the destruction of the insulin-producing beta cells in the pancreas, which leads to little or no insulin secretion. Type 1 diabetes generally occurs in childhood and regular insulin injections are required to regulate blood glucose levels.

The typical symptoms of type 1 diabetes are excessive thirst and hunger, frequent urination, weight loss, blurred vision, and recurrent infections. During periods of insulin deficiency, a higher-than-normal level of glucose remains in the blood because of reduced uptake and storage. A chronically elevated blood glucose level is a condition known as **hyperglycemia.**

Type 2 diabetes is the most common form of diabetes, affecting 90% of all diabetic patients. It typically occurs in adults who are overweight and is characterized by a reduced sensitivity of insulin target cells to available insulin, a condition called insulin resistance. Insulin resistance—in which the body is unable to use its own insulin efficiently—affects approximately 60 million people in the United States, one in four of whom will develop type 2 diabetes. Unfortunately, increasing numbers of children are being diagnosed with type 2 diabetes, making the term "adult-onset diabetes" obsolete. Some people with type 2 diabetes never exhibit any of the classic symptoms of diabetes. Treatment usually includes diet modification, medication, and exercise therapy.

Type 2 diabetes also is characterized by frequent states of hyperglycemia, but without the increased catabolism of fats and protein. Because 75% of individuals with type 2 diabetes are obese or have a history of **obesity,** it is important to note that this condition is often reversible with permanent weight loss.

Effective Diabetes Control

Long-term regulation of blood glucose levels is necessary to effectively control diabetes. In type 1 diabetes, glucose regulation is achieved through regular glucose assessment, proper diet, exercise, and appropriate insulin medication. For type 2 diabetes, it is achieved through lifestyle changes centered around proper diet, weight management, exercise, and insulin or oral agents if needed. A combined diet and exercise regimen results in weight loss and weight control, improved circulation and cardiorespiratory fitness, a reduced need for insulin, improved self-image, and an improved ability to deal with stress.

Exercise and Type 1 Diabetes

The role of exercise in controlling glucose levels has not been well demonstrated. Even so, individuals with type 1 diabetes can improve their functional capacity, reduce their risk for CAD, and improve insulin receptor sensitivity and number with a program of regular physical activity.

Exercise and Type 2 Diabetes

Exercise plays an important role in controlling type 2 diabetes, because it reduces both cholesterol levels and weight. With excessive blood glucose elevation, blood fats rise to become the primary energy source for the body. Higher-than-normal blood-fat levels put diabetics at greater risk for heart disease.

Exercise Guidelines for Diabetes

Before beginning an exercise program, clients with diabetes should speak with a physician or diabetes educator to develop a program of diet, exercise, and medication. The primary goal of exercise for type 1 diabetes is better glucose regulation and reduced heart disease risk. The timing of exercise, the amount of insulin injected, and the injection site are important to consider before exercising. Exercise should be performed consistently so that a regular pattern of diet and insulin dosage can be maintained. Ideally, the diabetic client should perform a similar exercise routine every day, within one to two hours of consuming a meal or snack.

The primary goal of exercise for individuals with type 2 diabetes is weight loss and control, as 80% of people with this condition are overweight. By losing weight through diet and exercise, they may be able to reduce the amount of oral insulin medication needed. The primary objective during exercise for those with type 2 diabetes is caloric expenditure, which is best achieved by long-duration exercise. Since the duration of exercise is often high, the intensity of exercise should be kept lower.

- Clients with diabetes should check their blood glucose levels frequently and work closely with their physicians to determine the right insulin dosage.
- People with diabetes should always carry a rapid-acting carbohydrate (such

as juice or candy) in case they develop **hypoglycemia.**

- Diabetic clients should not inject insulin into the primary muscle groups that will be used during exercise, because it will be absorbed too quickly, resulting in hypoglycemia.
- Encourage clients with diabetes to exercise at the same time each day for better control.
- People with diabetes should avoid exercise during periods of peak insulin activity.
- A carbohydrate snack should be consumed before and during prolonged exercise.
- People with diabetes need to take very good care of their feet, which should be regularly checked for any cuts, blisters, or signs of infection. High-quality exercise shoes also are very important.
- Physicians will usually instruct their patients to check their blood glucose level before and after exercise. Exercise should be curtailed if preexercise blood glucose is below 100 mg/dL. With additional carbohydrate consumption, exercise may be allowed to take place. Exercise should also be curtailed if preexercise blood glucose is greater than 300 mg/dL or greater than 240 mg/dL with urinary ketone bodies. In the latter scenario, exercise would need to be postponed until the client's blood sugar is under control. Clients with diabetes should have specific guidelines to follow in these situations. These guidelines will depend upon a client's clinical status and medical history with respect to blood glucose control.

Sample Exercise Recommendation

Mode. Endurance activities, such as walking, swimming, and cycling are a good choice for people with diabetes.

Intensity. Start at 50 to 60% of **cardiac reserve,** gradually progressing to 60 to 70%.

Frequency. Four to seven days/week. Some clients may need to start out with several shorter daily sessions.

Duration. Individuals with type 1 diabetes should gradually work up to 20 to 30 minutes per session. For individuals with type 2 diabetes, 40 to 60 minutes is recommended.

Special Precautions for Exercise and Diabetes

Individuals with type 1 diabetes face two potential problems during or following exercise: lack of insulin, which may cause a hyperglycemic effect; and rapid mobilization of insulin, which dangerously lowers blood glucose levels. Low blood glucose is referred to as hypoglycemia. One of the first rules for those with type 1 diabetes is to either reduce insulin intake or increase carbohydrate intake before exercise. If pre-exercise blood glucose is below 100 mg/dL in clients taking insulin, it is recommended that they consume 20 to 30 grams of additional carbohydrate before exercise. Individuals with either type of diabetes should exercise one to two hours after a meal and before peak insulin activity. Because exercise has an insulin-like effect, insulin dosages generally should be lowered prior to exercise. Clients with diabetes should check blood glucose levels frequently when starting an exercise program and be aware of any unusual symptoms prior to, during, or after exercise.

Other potential problems associated with exercise and diabetes include autonomic neuropathy (which may blunt the HR response to exercise); peripheral neuropathy (which may cause numbness in the extremities); microvascular complication (which may cause vision or kidney problems); and peripheral vascular disease (which may cause claudication).

Asthma

Asthma is a reactive airway disease characterized by shortness of breath, coughing, and wheezing. It is due to (1) constriction of the smooth muscle around the airways, (2) a swelling of the mucosal cells, and/or (3) increased secretion of mucous. Asthma can be caused by an allergic reaction, exercise, infections, stress, or other environmental irritants, such as pollens, inhalants, cigarette smoke, and air pollution. Asthma is one of the most common respiratory disorders affecting both adults and children.

Approximately 80% of people with asthma experience **exercise-induced asthma (EIA)**, which is characterized by moderate obstruction and is not life-threatening. The severity of an EIA attack is related to the intensity of exercise and the ventilatory requirement of the task, as well as the environmental conditions. Inhaling cold, dry air versus warm, moist air seems to cause greater airway obstruction.

The exact cause of EIA is not well understood, but it is believed to be caused when the airways become dry as moisture is absorbed from the air as it passes from the nose to the lower part of the lungs. While asthma is not a contraindication to exercise, people with asthma should work with their physicians to develop appropriate exercise programs.

Exercise and Asthma

Most individuals with controlled asthma will benefit from regular exercise, which helps to reduce the ventilatory requirement for various tasks, making it easier for them to participate in normal daily activities with less shortness of breath and fewer asthma attacks. Several studies have shown that regular exercise also can reduce the number and severity of EIA attacks (ACSM, 2001).

Exercise Guidelines for Asthma

- Before beginning an exercise program, individuals with asthma must have a medication/treatment plan to prevent EIA attacks.
- Clients with asthma should have a bronchodilating inhaler with them at all times and be instructed to use it at the first sign of wheezing.
- Keep the exercise intensity low initially and gradually increase it over time, since exercise intensity is directly linked to the severity and frequency of EIA.
- Reduce the intensity if asthma symptoms occur.
- Using an inhaler several minutes before exercise may reduce the possibility of EIA attacks.
- Use the results of pulmonary exercise testing to design an appropriate exercise program.
- Encourage clients with asthma to drink plenty of fluids before and during exercise.
- Individuals with asthma should extend their warm-up and cool-down periods.
- Individuals with respiratory disorders will often experience more symptoms of respiratory distress when exercising in extreme environmental conditions (high or low temperature, high pollen count, and heavy air pollution).
- Wearing a face mask during exercise helps keep inhaled air warmer and moister, and may minimize asthmatic responses during exercise.
- Individuals with respiratory disorders need to be carefully followed by their physician.
- Only people with stable asthma should exercise.
- If an asthma attack is not relieved by medication, activate the emergency medical system.
- Individuals with asthma often respond best to exercise in mid-to-late morning.
- Clients with asthma should avoid extremes in temperature and humidity.

Sample Exercise Recommendation

Mode. Walking, cycling, and swimming are good choices for clients with asthma. Upper-body exercises such as arm cranking, rowing, and cross-country skiing may not be appropriate because of the higher ventilation demands. Swimming may be particularly beneficial because it allows people with asthma to inhale the moist air just above the surface of the water.

Intensity. Recommend low-intensity dynamic exercise based on the client's fitness status and limitations.

Frequency. Encourage clients with asthma to exercise at least three to four times per week. Individuals with low functional capacities or those who experience shortness of breath during prolonged exercise may benefit from intermittent exercise (two 10-minute sessions).

Duration. Encourage a longer, more gradual warm-up and cool-down (longer than 10 minutes). Gradually increase total exercise duration to 20 to 45 minutes.

Osteoporosis

Osteoporosis is a major public health threat for an estimated 44 million Americans. In the U.S., 10 million individuals are estimated to already have the disease and almost 34 million are at an increased risk for osteoporosis. Of the 10 million estimated to have osteoporosis, 8 million are women and 2 million are men (National Osteoporosis Foundation, 2002).

After reaching its peak, bone mass declines throughout life because of an imbalance of "remodeling" of the bone. Remodeling, which refers to the replacement of old bone with new bone, keeps the skeletal system in peak form and helps maintain calcium homeostasis.

Exercise and Osteoporosis

The treatment of osteoporosis is aimed at preventing or retarding bone mineral loss. **Estrogen** replacement therapy is highly effective in maintaining bone mass and preventing osteoporosis in women by reducing bone reabsorption and retarding or halting **postmenopausal** bone loss. **Premenopausal** women should consume 1,000 to 1,500 mg of calcium per day, which appears to suppress age-related bone loss. While the role of exercise in the prevention and treatment of osteoporosis is not completely understood, it is known that physical stress determines the strength of bone. Physical inactivity is a known risk factor for osteoporosis, and exercise is recommended for its prevention and treatment because weightbearing exercise either retards the loss of, or increases, bone mass. Even individuals who have led **sedentary** lives can increase bone mass by becoming more active.

Exercise Guidelines for Osteoporosis

The greater the physical stress and compression on a bone, the greater the rate of bone deposition (this is why weightbearing exercise is recommended). Since most individuals who suffer from osteoporosis are elderly, LWMCs should refer to the exercise guidelines and recommendations for older adults that begin on page 406. Resistance training also is an important component in the prevention of osteoporosis. Individuals should initially use resistance levels that permit them to properly perform 15 to 20 repetitions, and then progress to eight to 12 repetitions to promote strength and bone development. Additionally, individuals with osteoporosis may need to avoid the following:

- Jumping, high-impact aerobics, jogging, and running
- Spinal flexion, crunches, and rowing machines
- Trampolines and step aerobics
- Wooden gym floors that may become slippery from sweat drops
- Abducting or adducting the legs against resistance (particularly machines)
- Moving the legs sideways or across the body
- Pulling on the neck with hands behind the head

Low-back Pain

Back injuries, including sprains and strains, are the number-one disability for people under age 45. It is estimated that 80% of the population will experience an episode of low-back pain (LBP) some time in their lives. Of these, 5% will go on to develop chronic LBP, which accounts for 10% of all chronic health conditions in the U.S. and 25% of days lost from work. LBP has been labeled the most expensive benign health condition in America.

Back injuries translate into millions of lost work days every year and cost billions for medical care, disability payments, and legal payments. Reducing back-injury rates is a top priority for all employers. In fact, the most common type of workers' compensation claim is a back strain/sprain, which accounts for up to 25% of all claims, representing annual payments of $2.5 to $7 billion, including one-half of all disability compensation payments annually.

While the cause of LBP is often elusive, four common causes have been identified: a **herniated disc** (rupture of the outer layers of fibers that surround the gelatinous portion of the disc); **spondylolisthesis** (forward sliding of the body of one vertebra on the vertebra below it); a trauma to the back (accident); and degenerative disc disease (progressive structural degeneration of the intervertebral disc). Lower-back problems are often associated with an imbalance of strength and flexibility of the lower back and abdominal muscle groups. Poor flexibility in the hamstrings and hip flexor muscles also has been linked to LBP.

Exercise and Low-back Pain

Appropriate exercise design for the low back must be individualized. According to McGill (2007), some people with a history of back troubles desire pain relief and spine stability (a health objective), while others may seek a performance objective (which may be counterproductive to optimal back health). Some people need more stability, while others may need more mobility. Some exercises will exacerbate the back troubles of some people, but may help others.

It is widely believed that stretching the back and increasing the **range of motion** is beneficial and reduces back problems. However, available scientific evidence shows that, on average, those who have more range of motion in their backs have a greater risk of future troubles. Clearly there is a tradeoff between mobility and stability; the optimal balance is a very personal and individual variable. Indeed, the "stability/mobility balance" may shift during a progressive exercise program as symptoms resolve, with advancing age, or as rehab/training objectives change.

Another generally perceived goal of training the back is to increase strength. Strength has little association with low-back health. In fact, many people hurt their backs in an attempt to increase strength. It could be argued that this is an artifact, in that some exercise programs intended to enhance strength contained poorly chosen exercises such as sit-ups. Performing sit-ups both replicates a potent injury mechanism (specifically posterior disc herniation) and results in high loads on the spine. On the other hand, muscle endurance, as opposed to strength, has been shown to be protective against future back troubles. Further, for many people, it is better to train for stability rather than stretching to increase range of motion.

Two other concepts should be emphasized. First, training approaches intended to enhance athletic performance are often counterproductive to the approaches used when training for health. Too many patients are rehabilitated using athletic philosophies or, worse yet, "body-building" approaches designed primarily to isolate and **hypertrophy** specific muscles, and progress is thwarted. Many bad backs are created from using inappropriate performance philosophies. Identifying the training objectives is paramount. The emphasis must be on enhancing spine health—training for performance is another topic. Second, many of the training approaches that are used at joints such as the knee, hip, and shoulder are mistakenly applied to the back. The back is a very different and complex structure, involving a flexible column, with complex muscle and ligamentous support. The spine contains the spinal cord and lateral nerve roots, and musculature intimately involved in several other functions, including breathing mechanics. Many of the traditional approaches for training other joints in the body are not appropriate for the back—either they do not produce the desired result or they create new injuries.

Exercise Guidelines for Low-back Pain

Advise clients with low-back pain to keep the following guidelines in mind (McGill, 2007):

- While there is a common belief that exercise sessions should be performed at least three times per week, it appears that low-back exercises have the most beneficial effect when performed daily.
- The "no pain, no gain" axiom does not apply when exercising the low back in pained individuals, particularly when applied to weight training.
- General exercise programs that combine cardiovascular components (like walking) with specific low-back exercises have been shown to be more effective in both rehabilitation and for injury prevention.
- Diurnal variation in the fluid level of the intervertebral discs (discs are more hydrated early in the morning after rising from bed) changes the stresses on the discs throughout the day. Specifically, these stresses are highest following bed rest and diminish over the subsequent few hours. It would be very unwise to perform full-range spine motion while under load shortly after rising from bed.
- Low-back exercises performed for maintenance of health need not emphasize strength; rather, more repetitions of less-demanding exercises will assist in the enhancement of endurance and strength. There is no doubt that back injury can occur during seemingly low-level demands (such as picking up a pencil) and that an injury due to a motor-control error can occur. While it appears that the chance of motor-control errors, which can result in inappropriate muscle forces, increases with fatigue, there is also evidence documenting the changes in passive tissue loading with fatiguing lifting. Given that endurance has more

Daily Routine for Enhancing Low-back Health

The following exercises will spare the spine, enhance the muscle challenge, and enhance the motor control system to ensure that spine stability is maintained in all other activities. Keep in mind that these are only examples of well-designed exercises and may not be for everyone—the initial challenge may or may not be appropriate for every individual, nor will the graded progression be the same for all clients. These are simply examples to challenge the muscles of the torso.

Cat-Camel

The routine should begin with the cat-camel motion exercise (spine flexion-extension cycles) to reduce spine viscosity (internal resistance and friction) and "floss" the nerve roots as they outlet at each lumbar level. Note that the cat-camel is intended as a motion exercise—not a stretch—so the emphasis is on motion rather than "pushing" at the end ranges of flexion and extension. Five to eight cycles have shown to be sufficient to reduce most viscous-frictional stresses.

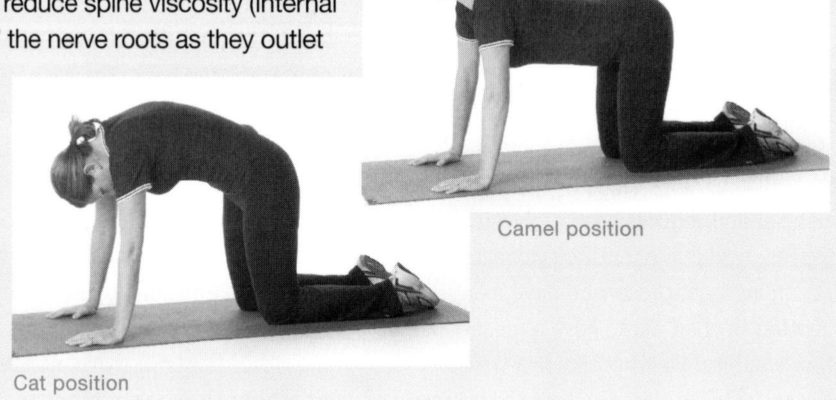

Camel position

Cat position

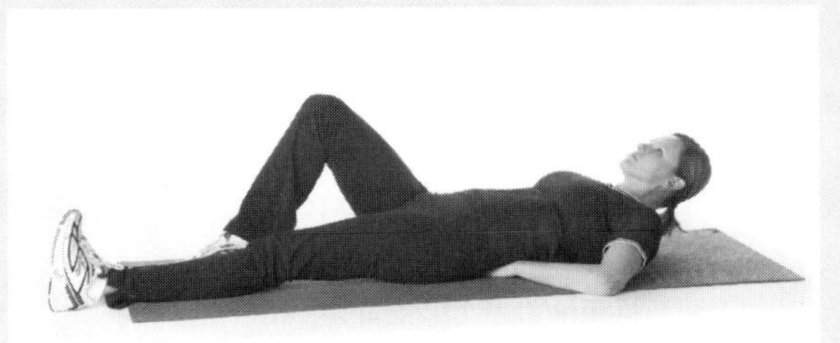

Curl-up

The cat-camel motion exercise is followed by anterior abdominal exercises, in this case the curl-up. The hands or a rolled towel are placed under the lumbar spine to preserve a neutral spine posture. Do not allow the client to flatten the back to the floor, as doing so flexes the lumbar spine, violates the neutral spine principle, and increases the loads on the discs and ligaments. One knee is flexed but the other leg is straight to lock the pelvis–lumbar spine and minimize the loss of a neutral lumbar posture. Have clients alternate the bent leg (right to left) midway through the repetitions.

Birddog

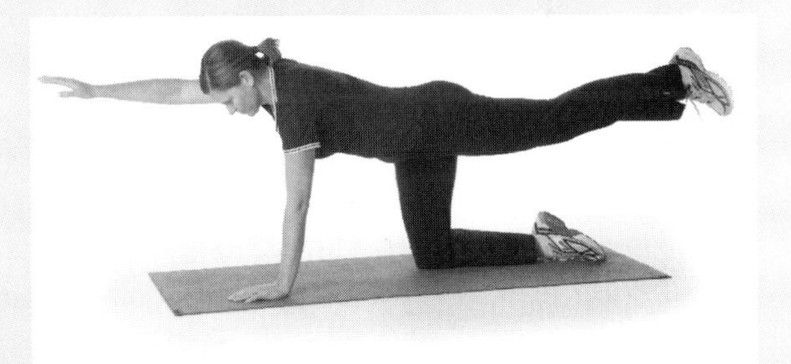

The extensor program consists of leg extensions and the "birddog." In general, these isometric holds should last no longer than seven to eight seconds given evidence from near infrared spectroscopy indicating rapid loss of available oxygen in the torso muscles when contracting at these levels; short relaxation of the muscle restores oxygen. The evidence supports building endurance with increased repetitions rather than extending "hold time."

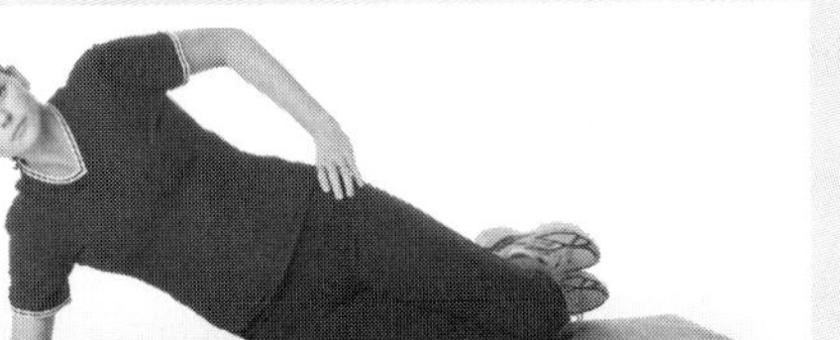

Side Bridge

The lateral muscles of the torso (i.e., quadratus lumborum and abdominal obliques) are important for optimal stability, and are targeted with the side bridge exercise. The beginner level of this exercise involves bridging the torso between the elbow and the knees. Once this is mastered and tolerated, the challenge is increased by bridging using the elbow and the feet. It is important when performing the side bridge exercise to maintin a neutral neck and spine position and not let the hips rotate forward.

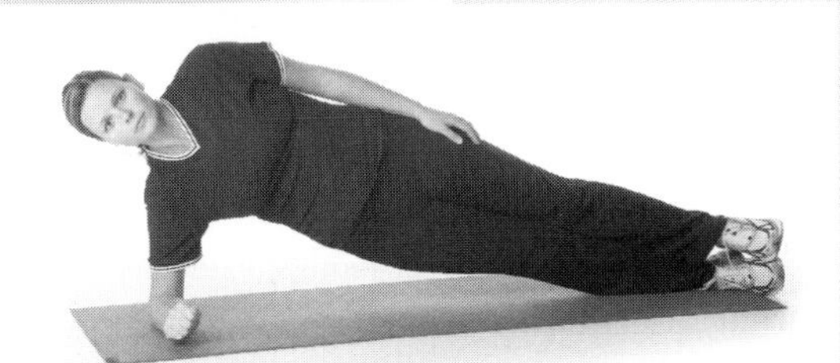

protective value than strength, strength gains should not be overemphasized at the expense of endurance.

- There is no such thing as an ideal set of exercises for all individuals. An individual's training objectives must be identified (e.g., rehabilitation specifically to reduce the risk of injury, optimize general health and fitness, or maximize athletic performance), and the most appropriate exercises chosen. While science cannot evaluate the optimal exercises for each situation, the combination of science and clinical experiential "wisdom" must be utilized to enhance low-back health.
- Encourage clients to be patient and stick with the program. Increased function and pain reduction may not occur for three months.

Arthritis

Arthritis means "joint inflammation," a general term that includes more than 100 kinds of rheumatoid disease. The most common forms of arthritis are **rheumatoid arthritis** and **osteoarthritis.** Osteoarthritis, also referred to as degenerative joint disease, is a degenerative process in which cartilage wears away, leaving two surfaces of bone in contact with each other. Rheumatoid arthritis is caused by an inflammation of the membrane surrounding the joint, and is often associated with pain and swelling in one or more joints. According to the CDC, more than 40 million people in the United States have some form of arthritis (one in every seven people). Osteoarthritis is a common and chronic condition affecting the joints in the elderly, aged 55 and above. More than 20 million people in the U.S. alone suffer from osteoarthritis. Most people over the age of 75 are affected with osteoarthritis in at least one joint, making this condition a leading cause of disability in the U.S. Rheumatoid arthritis, the most crippling and second most common form of arthritis, affects approximately 2.1 million Americans and two to three times more women than men. Further, the average onset for rheumatoid arthritis is between the ages of 20 and 45 years old.

The treatment of arthritis, which may involve medicine (corticosteroids), physical therapy, physiotherapy [transcutaneous electrical nerve stimulation (TENS) and hot packs], occupational therapy (to improve performance of ADL) and surgery (joint replacement), depends on the severity and the specific form of arthritis. Individuals with arthritis can be classified into four categories of functional capacity (Table 18-2) (Hochberg et al., 1992).

Table 18-2
American College of Rheumatology Revised Criteria for Classification of Functional Status in Rheumatoid Arthritis

Class I	Completely able to perform usual activities of daily living (self-care, vocational, and avocational)
Class II	Able to perform usual self-care and vocational activities, but limited in avocational activities
Class III	Able to perform usual self-care activities, but limited in vocational and avocational activities
Class IV	Limited in ability to perform usual self-care, vocational, and avocational activities

Note: Usual self-care activities include dressing, feeding, bathing, grooming, and toileting. Avocational activities (recreational and/or leisure) and vocational (work, school, homemaking) activities are patient-desired and age- and sex-specific.

Reprinted with permission from: Hochberg, M.C. et al. (1992). The American College of Rheumatology 1991 revised criteria for the classification of global functioning status in rheumatoid arthritis. *Arthritis and Rheumatism,* 35, 5, 498–502.

Individuals with arthritis should not be excluded from participating in a program of regular exercise. Stronger muscles and bones, improved cardiorespiratory fitness, and improved psychosocial well-being are some of the benefits they can gain from appropriate exercise. Exercise is contraindicated, however, during inflammatory periods, because it can aggravate or worsen the condition.

Exercise and Arthritis

Exercise is recommended for individuals with arthritis to help preserve muscle strength and joint mobility, improve functional capabilities, relieve pain and stiffness, prevent further deformities, improve overall physical conditioning, reestablish neuromuscular coordination, and mobilize stiff or contracted joints.

Fitness programs, which should be carefully designed in conjunction with a physician or physical therapist, must be based on the functional status of the individual. For example, someone in Functional Class I should be able to perform most activities that a typical healthy person can. For those in Class II, nonweightbearing activities, such as cycling, warm-water exercise, and walking, are recommended. Individuals in Class III should benefit from a cycling or warm-water aquatic program. Exercise should be avoided during acute arthritic flare-ups.

Clients with arthritis may complain of fatigue and some discomfort following exercise. Exercise programs need to achieve the proper balance of rest, immobilization of affected joints, and appropriate exercise to reduce the severity of the inflammatory joint disease.

Exercise Guidelines for Arthritis

- Encourage clients with arthritis to participate in low-impact activities such as stationary cycling, rowing, and aquatic-fitness classes.
- Begin with frequent low-intensity sessions.
- Reduce exercise intensity and duration during periods of inflammation or pain.
- Extend the warm-up and cool-down periods.
- Modify the intensity and duration of exercise according to how well the client responds, any changes in medication, and the level of pain.
- It is essential to put all joints through their full range of motion at least once a day to maintain mobility.
- Have the individual take a day or two of rest if he or she continues to complain about pain during or following an exercise session. If a client is still experiencing exercise-associated musculoskeletal pain or discomfort more than two hours after a workout, reduce the intensity of future bouts of exercise.
- Emphasize proper body alignment at all times. Poor posture and decreased joint mobility and strength disrupt the performance of efficient, controlled, and integrated movement. Misaligned body positions and awkward movements affect walking gait and increase fatigue. Special precautions should be taken for clients who have undergone a hip replacement (Table 18-3).

Table 18-3
Exercise Guidelines for Individuals With a Hip Replacement

- Lift the knee no higher than hip level or 90 degrees of flexion
- Toes straight ahead; no "pigeon toes"
- No adduction past midline
- Need leg/hip abduction and lateral movements and strengthening

- While pain is quite normal in people with arthritis, instruct clients to work just up to the point of pain, but not past it. Movements that are simple for healthy people can be quite painful for individuals with arthritis.
- Use isometric exercises, which strengthen the joint structures and surrounding muscles while placing the least amount of stress on the joint itself.
- If severe pain persists following exercise, clients should consult with their physician.
- Individuals with rheumatoid arthritis should not exercise during periods of inflammation, and regular rest periods should be stressed during exercise sessions.
- Keep in mind that clients with arthritis may be more limited by joint pain than by cardiovascular function.

Sample Exercise Recommendation

Mode. Non-weightbearing activities such as cycling, warm-water aquatic programs, and swimming are preferred because they reduce joint stress. Recommended water temperature is 83° F to 88° F (28° C to 31° C).

Intensity. Emphasize low-intensity, dynamic exercise rather than high-intensity, high-impact exercise. The exercise intensity should be based on the client's comfort level before, during, and after exercise.

Frequency. Encourage individuals with arthritis to exercise at least four to five times per week.

Duration. Encourage long, gradual warm-up and cool-down periods (longer than 10 minutes). Initial exercise sessions should last no longer than 10 to 15 minutes.

Older Adults

According to the CDC, the United States population is growing older. In fact, by the year 2030, more than 70 million Americans will be over the age of 65. The most rapid population increase over the next decade will be of those over 85 years of age. This is due, in large part, to modern medicine and health-promotion activities.

But what is the quality of these extended lives? One measure of the quality of life is an individual's ability to perform ADL, such as bathing, dressing, and eating. While these tasks may become more difficult as an individual grows older, it is possible to stay healthy and lead a long, satisfying life. The things that people must do to stay healthy (e.g., exercise, eat right, not smoke) become even more important as they age. Thus, while someone may be 65 years of age (chronological age), he or she may have a biological age of 45 based on fitness and health status. The importance of regular exercise and health promotion cannot be emphasized enough when looking at the association of chronological versus biological age.

Physiological Challenges of Aging

Aging is a normal biological process. The signs of progressive aging are familiar to most people and include loss of height, reduced lean body mass, gray hair, more wrinkles, changes in eyesight, and, to some extent, slightly less coordination. There are noticeable changes in the functioning of the cardiovascular, endocrine, respiratory, and musculoskeletal systems as well. To what extent these changes may be affected by exercise is not completely understood.

Heart Rate. Maximal heart rate declines with age, diminishing the accuracy of estimating training intensity based on heart rate. Other methods of monitoring exercise intensity, such as the RPE scale (sometimes in conjunction with heart rate), may be more effective. Even though exercise heart rate declines with age, **stroke volume** has been shown to increase or be maintained in healthy older subjects who exercise, thus overcoming the effect of a lowered heart rate.

Blood Pressure. Older individuals generally display higher blood pressure readings during submaximal and maximal exercise. In addition, they may have higher myocardial oxygen consumption requirements, which can result in higher blood pressures. Endurance training can significantly reduce the mean blood pressure and the systemic vascular resistance in older individuals.

Cardiac Output and Stroke Volume. Cardiac output is typically lower in older individuals, and resting cardiac output declines 1% per year upon reaching adulthood. Resting stroke volume declines approximately 30% between the ages of 25 and 85 and, when combined with the decrease in maximal heart rate, leads to a drop in cardiac output of 30 to 60%. This effect may be countered, however, by exercise.

Maximal Oxygen Uptake. With normal aging, **maximal oxygen uptake ($\dot{V}O_2$ max)** declines approximately 8 to 10% per decade after age 30. This decline is associated with a decrease in maximal heart rate and stroke volume, and a decrease in oxygen extraction by contracting muscles. It is clear, however, that aerobic capacity can be improved at any age.

Bones. With age, bones become more fragile and porous, and often debilitating fractures are common in the elderly. By the age of 90, as many as 32% of women and 17% of men will have sustained a hip fracture, and many will die of related complications. With age, the loss of calcium results in decreased bone mass, but weightbearing and resistance-training exercises are known to help maintain bone mass.

Skeletal Muscle. Muscle mass declines with age, resulting in decreased muscular strength and endurance. For each decade after the age of 25, 3 to 5% of muscle mass is lost. This is primarily attributed to changes in lifestyle and the decreased use of the neuromuscular system. Several studies, however, have reported significant strength gains in previously sedentary older adults following a program of regular exercise (Peterson & Franklin, 2005).

Body Composition. As lean body weight (muscle and bone) declines with age, body fat increases. The changes in body composition resulting from age are primarily due to a lack of physical activity and a decrease in muscle mass and **basal metabolic rate (BMR).** On average, there is a 10% reduction in BMR between early adulthood and retirement age, and a further 10% decrease after that. Regular physical activity, which preserves lean body mass, decreases fat stores, and stimulates protein synthesis, may reverse the adverse changes in body composition that are associated with growing older.

Exercise Guidelines for Older Adults

Before starting an exercise program, older adults should first see their physician. Although the principles of exercise design are similar to those for any group, special care should be given when setting up fitness programs for older participants. A pre-exercise evaluation may need to include a complete medical history, a physical, and a treadmill test. The exercise program should combine endurance, flexibility, and balance training, as well as muscle strengthening and joint mobilization. For most elderly patients, low-impact exercise is advisable. Older individuals should be encouraged to become more physically active in all of their daily activities (e.g., use the stairs, walk to the store), and to bend, move, and stretch to keep joints flexible.

Sample Exercise Recommendation

Mode. Endurance exercise, such as low-impact aerobics, walking, using cardiovascular equipment, and swimming, should be the primary exercise mode. Recommend a program of weight training that features low resistance and high repetitions.

Intensity. Keep the exercise intensity level near the lower end of the heart-rate range (40 to 65% heart-rate reserve).

Frequency. Encourage elderly clients to exercise at least four to five times per week. Daily exercise of shorter duration may be appropriate for certain individuals with an initial low functional capacity.

Duration. A longer and more gradual warm-up and cool-down period (greater than five minutes) is recommended. Gradually increase total exercise duration to 30 to 60 minutes per session, depending on the medical history and clinical status of the individual.

Special Precautions for Older Adults

Individuals with high blood pressure, heart disease, or arthritis should take particular care when performing weight-training exercises. LWMCs should incorporate an extended warm-up and cool-down period—approximately 10 to 15 minutes. LWMCs may find that older clients have a more difficult time exercising in extreme environmental conditions, which should be avoided. Some elderly individuals with arthritis or poor joint mobility should participate in non-weightbearing activities such as cycling, swimming, and chair and floor exercises.

Exercise and Children

Within the past 20 years, a great deal of research has focused on the effects of exercise in children and adolescents.

It appears that children respond to exercise in much the same way as adults. With little encouragement, most children in good health are willing to be physically active. Recent national attention on the health and fitness of American children has sparked a great deal of debate over topics such as (1) how much exercise should children and adolescents be getting; (2) who is responsible for making sure children get enough exercise; and (3) what kind of exercise is important, and at what age. Many of these issues have yet to be resolved.

Millions of youth in the United States are at risk for developing degenerative diseases in their adult years because they are not active enough. The percentage of overweight boys and girls has more than doubled during the past two decades (National Center for Health Statistics, 2000), and of youngsters ages five to 15 who are overweight, 61% have one or more cardiovascular disease risk factors, and 27% have two or more (Freedman et al., 1999). Results of the 1999 California Physical Fitness Test indicate that a staggering 80% of fifth-, seventh-, and ninth-graders tested were unable to meet minimum standards to be considered physically fit. In the United States, television viewing, "surfing" the Internet, and playing video games contribute substantially to the amount of time youth spend in sedentary pursuits. On average, young people between the ages of two and 18 spend an astounding four hours a day using electronic media (e.g., watching television, playing video games, or using a computer) (Kaiser Family Foundation, 1999). By high school graduation, it is likely that the average American teen will have spent more time in front of the television than in school (Strasburger, 1992).

The negative health consequences associated with childhood obesity and physical inactivity include hypertension, the development of atherosclerosis, and type 2 diabetes (formerly known as adult-onset diabetes) among children and teenagers. Furthermore, since both positive and negative behaviors established at a young age have a high probability of persisting into adulthood, it is likely that inactive kids will become inactive adults (Janz, Dawson, & Mahoney, 2000; Trudeau et al., 1999). As such, preventive health efforts that increase physical activity during childhood and adolescence will likely have favorable health benefits in later years. In the long run, health-promotion strategies that ensure healthy levels of physical activity among children and teenagers could help to maintain the progress that has been made over the past few decades in reducing deaths from cardiovascular disease. The Healthy People 2010 report includes participation in physical activity as one of the nation's 10 leading health indicators (U.S. Department of Health and Human Services, 2000).

Exercise Guidelines for Children

Sufficient evidence exists that children can physiologically adapt to endurance training. However, the amount of exercise required for optimal functional capacity and health at various ages has not been precisely defined. Until more definitive evidence is available, current recommendations are that children and youth accumulate 60 total minutes of exercise each day, 20 to 30 minutes of which is vigorous (Table 18-4).

Sample Exercise Recommendation

Mode. Encourage children to participate in sustained activities that use large muscle groups (e.g., swimming, jogging, aerobics). Incorporate other activities, such as recreational sports and fun activities that develop other components of fitness (speed, power, flexibility, muscular endurance, agility, and coordination) into a fitness program.

Intensity. Start with low-intensity exercise and progress gradually. There are currently no universal recommendations available for the use of training heart rate during exercise for children. Using the RPE scale is a more practical method of monitoring exercise intensity with children.

Frequency. Two to three days of endurance training will allow adequate time to partici-

Table 18-4
General Endurance Training Guidelines for Children

- Although children are generally quite active, most choose to participate in activities that consist of short-burst, high-energy exercise. Encourage children to participate in sustained activities that use large muscle groups.
- The type, intensity, and duration of exercise activities need to be based on the maturity of the child, medical status, and previous experiences with exercise.
- Regardless of age, the exercise intensity should start out low and progress gradually.
- Because of the difficulty in monitoring heart rates with children, the use of a perceived exertion scale is a more practical method of monitoring exercise intensity in children.
- Children are involved in a variety of activities throughout the day. Because of this, a specific time should be dedicated to sustained aerobic activities.
- The duration of the exercise session will vary depending on the age of the children, their previous exercise experience, and the intensity of the exercise session.
- Because it is often quite difficult to get children to respond to sustained periods of exercise, the session periods need to be creatively designed.

pate in other activities, and still be sufficient enough to cause a training effect.

Duration. Since children will be involved in a variety of activities during and after school, dedicate a specific amount of time to endurance training. Gradually increase endurance-exercise activities to 30 to 40 minutes per session. With younger children, it will be necessary to start out with less time.

Although there are fewer resistance-training studies involving children than adults, the evidence that demonstrates increases in strength following structured resistance training in children is mounting (ACSM, 2005). These studies indicate that strength increases in children are similar to those observed in older age groups. Furthermore, the safety and efficacy of resistance-training programs for prepubescent children has been well-documented.

The risk of injuries to children participating in resistance-training programs is low. However, injuries can occur in any sport or strenuous physical activity. To minimize the risk of injury during resistance training, adhere to the following guidelines:

- Obtain medical clearance or instructions regarding physical needs.
- Children should be properly supervised at all times.
- Do not allow children to exercise unless the weight-training facility is safe for them.
- Never have children perform single maximal lifts, sudden explosive movements, or try to compete with other children.
- Teach children how to breathe properly during exercise movements.
- Never allow children to use any equipment that is broken or damaged, or that they do not fit on properly.
- Children should rest for approximately one to two minutes between each exercise, and for longer if necessary. In addition, they should have scheduled rest days between each training day.
- Encourage children to drink plenty of fluids before, during, and after exercise.
- Tell children that they need to communicate with their coach, parent, or teacher when they feel tired or fatigued, or when they have been injured.

Exercise and Pregnancy

Numerous studies of the cardiovascular responses of pregnant women have demonstrated that women can maintain and even improve their cardiovascular, respiratory, and aerobic capacities during pregnancy (Sternfeld, 1997). Since exercise causes a redistribution of the blood flow to the working muscles, it was believed that a reduction of blood flow to the uterus might harm the fetus. However, several studies have shown that although there is a slight decrease in overall uterine blood flow during moderate exercise, blood flow to the placenta appears to be adequate.

Cardiac reserve, or the difference between resting and maximum cardiac function, is reduced in pregnant women. As pregnancy progresses, it seems the heart is less able to adapt to the increased demand, especially in the supine position, because the heart may already be working at a very high level due to the increased demands of pregnancy. This is why pregnant women should be discouraged from exercising at high levels or participating in activities that require sudden bursts of movement.

Many women are more flexible during pregnancy due to joint laxity. With the release of the hormone **relaxin,** joints become looser, increasing the risk for injury during exercise.

Pregnant exercisers must be aware of the ambient temperature prior to each workout. Exercise increases body temperature, which can be harmful to the fetus, particularly if the core body temperature exceeds 100° F (38° C). Pregnant women should be conservative when exercising in hot, humid environments, since body-temperature regulation is more difficult for them.

Exercise Guidelines for Pregnant Women

Most women should be able to continue exercising during their first trimester without much difficulty. While morning sickness, mild weight gain, and fatigue might sideline some, most women should be able to continue their normal exercise program. Exercise in the supine position should be performed with caution and possibly avoided after the first trimester. Some forms of exercise, such as running, may be difficult during the second and third trimesters due to increased body weight, **edema,** varicose veins, and increased joint mobility.

A woman should clearly understand the risks and potential benefits associated with exercising during pregnancy, and should make the decision to exercise in conjunction with her physician.

The conclusion of the American College of Obstetricians and Gynecologists (1994; 2002) that exercise during pregnancy is safe for most women is based on the recommendation that participants be carefully monitored by their physician, and that they understand and adhere to the following guidelines as appropriate:

- Exercise goals during pregnancy should be discussed with a physician.
- Do not begin a vigorous exercise program shortly before or during pregnancy.
- Gradually reduce the intensity, duration, and frequency of exercise during the second and third trimesters. For example, a woman who walks or runs an average of 4 miles per day might reduce her mileage to 3 miles per day during the first trimester; to 2 miles per day during the second trimester; and to 1 or 1.5 miles during the final trimester.
- Avoid exercise when the temperature and/or humidity is high.
- Try to run or walk on flat, even surfaces.
- Wear supportive shoes while walking or running during pregnancy.
- If running becomes uncomfortable during the second and third trimesters, try other forms of aerobic exercise, such as swimming, running in water, and bicycling.
- Extend warm-up and cool-down periods.
- Body temperature, which should not exceed 100° F (38° C), should be taken immediately after exercise. If body temperature exceeds 100° F (38° C), modifying intensity and duration, as well as exercising during the cooler part of the day, should help.
- Use the RPE scale rather than heart rate to monitor exercise intensity. Choose an intensity that is comfortable; a pounding heart rate, breathlessness, or dizziness are indicators that intensity should be reduced.

- Eat a small snack before exercise to help avoid hypoglycemia.
- Drink plenty of water before, during, and after exercise.
- Avoid overstretching or going beyond normal range of motion.
- Any unusual physical changes, such as vaginal bleeding, severe fatigue, joint pain, or irregular heartbeats, should immediately be reported to a physician.

For more detailed information regarding exercise and pregnancy, please refer to ACE's Fitness Guide, *Pre- and Post-Natal Fitness,* by Lenita Anthony.

Summary

Training clients with health concerns and special needs can be very gratifying. One of the keys to success is to maintain contact with each client's physician and health-care team. Always obtain written guidelines before proceeding with exercise training. LWMC must keep programs more conservative than they would for clients that are without health concerns. This can be an area of tremendous professional growth for LWMCs. LWMCs should investigate continuing education opportunities to maximize the safety and effectiveness of their services.

References

American Association of Cardiovascular and Pulmonary Rehabilitation (1999). *Guidelines for Cardiac Rehabilitation and Secondary Prevention Programs.* Champaign, Ill.: Human Kinetics.

American College of Obstetricians and Gynecologists (2002). *ACOG Committee Opinion: Exercise During Pregnancy and the Postpartum Period.* Washington, D.C.: American College of Obstetricians and Gynecologists.

American College of Obstetricians and Gynecologists (1994). *ACOG Technical Bulletin #189.* Washington D.C.: American College of Obstetricians and Gynecologists.

American College of Sports Medicine (2006). *ACSM's Guidelines for Exercise Testing and Prescription* (7th ed.). Philadelphia: Lippincott Williams & Wilkins.

American College of Sports Medicine (2005). *ACSM's Resource Manual for Exercise Testing and Prescription* (5th ed.). Philadelphia: Lippincott Williams & Wilkins.

Freedman, D. et al. (1999). The relationship of overweight to cardiovascular risk factors among children and adolescents: The Bogalusa heart study. *Pediatrics,* 103, 1175–1182.

Hochberg, M.C. et al. (1992). The American College of Rheumatology 1991 revised criteria for the classification of global functioning status in rheumatoid arthritis. *Arthritis and Rheumatism,* 35, 5, 498–502.

Janz, K., Dawson, J., & Mahoney, L. (2000). Tracking physical fitness and physical activity from childhood to adolescence: The Muscatine Study. *Medicine & Science in Sports & Exercise,* 32, 7, 1250–1257.

Kaiser Family Foundation (1999). *Kids & Media @ The New Millennium* [monograph]. Menlo Park, Calif.: Kaiser Family Foundation.

McGill, S.M. (2007). *Low Back Disorders* (2nd ed.). Champaign, Ill.: Human Kinetics.

National Center for Health Statistics (2000). *Health, United States. With adolescent health chartbook.* Online at: http://www.cdc.gov.nchs/products/pubs/pudshus/ tables/2000/updated/00hus69.pdf.

National Osteoporosis Foundation (2002). *America's Bone Health: The State of Osteoporosis and Low Bone Mass.* Washington, D.C.: National Osteoporosis Foundation.

Peterson, J.A. & Franklin, B.A. (2005). Basic strength-training guidelines for older adults. In: American Council on Exercise. *Exercise for Older Adults* (2nd ed.). San Diego, Calif.: American Council on Exercise.

Regensteiner, J.G. & Hiatt, W.R. (1995). Exercise rehabilitation for patients with peripheral arterial disease. *Exercise and Sports Science Reviews,* 23, 1–24.

Sternfeld, B. (1997). Physical activity and pregnancy outcome: Review and recommendations. *Sports Medicine,* 23, 33–47.

Strasburger, V. (1992). Children, adolescents and television. *Pediatrics Review,* 13, 144–151.

Trudeau, F. et al. (1999). Daily primary school physical education: Effects on physical activity during adult life. *Medicine & Science in Sports & Exercise,* 31, 1, 111–117.

U.S. Department of Health and Human Services (2000). *Healthy People 2010: Understanding and Improving Health.* Washington, D.C.: U.S. Department of Health and Human Services, Government Printing Office.

Wenger N.K. et al. (1995). *Cardiac rehabilitation: Clinical practice guidelines no. 17.* Rockville, Md.: US Department of Health and Human Services, Public Health Service Agency for Health Care policy and Research and the National Heart, Lung and Blood Institute, Agency for Health Care Policy and Research. Publication no. 96-0672.

Suggested Reading

American College of Sports Medicine (2003). *ACSM's Exercise Management for Persons with Chronic Diseases and Disabilities.* Champaign, Ill.: Human Kinetics.

American College of Sports Medicine (1993). Position stand: Physical activity, physical fitness and hypertension. *Medicine & Science in Sports & Exercise,* 25, 10, i–x.

American Council on Exercise (2007). *Clinical Exercise Specialist Manual.* San Diego, Calif.: American Council on Exercise.

American Diabetes Association (1993). *Standards of Medical Care for Patients with Diabetes Mellitus.* 1992–93 Clinical Practice Recommendations. Alexandria, Va.: American Diabetes Association.

Anthony, L. (2002). *Pre- and Post-Natal Fitness.* San Diego, Calif.: American Council on Exercise.

Bartram, H.P. & Wynder, E.L. (1989). Physical activity and colon cancer risk? Physiological considerations. *American Journal of Gastroenterology,* 84, 109.

Blair, S.N. et al. (1992). How much physical activity is good for health? *Annual Review of Public Health,* 13, 99.

Bonnick, S.L. (2001). *The Osteoporosis Handbook: Every Woman's Guide to Prevention and Treatment* (3rd ed.). Dallas: Taylor Publishing Company.

Brownell, K.D. & Foreyt, J.P. (Eds.) (1986). *Handbook of Eating Disorders: Physiology, Psychology and Treatment of Obesity, Anorexia and Bulimia.* New York: Basic Books.

Campaigne, B.N. (1994). *Exercise in the Clinical Management of Diabetes.* Champaign, Ill.: Human Kinetics.

Cheung, W.Y. & Richmond, J.B. (Eds.) (1995). *Child Health, Nutrition, and Physical Activity.* Champaign, Ill.: Human Kinetics.

Christianse, C. (1993). Consensus Development Conference on Osteoporosis. *The American Journal of Medicine*, 95, 5a.

Clapp, J.F. (2002). *Exercise Through Your Pregnancy.* Omaha, Nebr.: Addicus Books.

Clark, J. (1992). *Full Life Fitness: A Complete Exercise Program for Mature Adults.* Champaign, Ill.: Human Kinetics.

Danneskiold-Samsoe, B. et al. (1987).The effect of water exercise therapy given to patients with rheumatoid arthritis. *Scandinavian Journal of Rehabilitation Medicine,* 19, 31–35.

Faigenbaum, A.D. & Westcott, W.L. (2001). *Youth Fitness*. San Diego, Calif.: American Council on Exercise.

Friesz, M.C. (2002). *Food, Fun 'n' Fitness: Designing Healthy Lifestyles for our Children.* Boca Raton, Fla.: Design for Healthy Lifestyles.

Frontera, W.R. et al. (1988). Strength conditioning in older men: Skeletal muscle hypertrophy and improved function. *Journal of Applied Physiology,* 64, 1038–1044.

Frymoyer, J.W. et al. (1980). Epidemiologic studies of low-back pain. *Spine,* 5, 419–423.

Gisolfi, C.V. & Lamb, D.R. (Eds.) (1989). *Perspectives in Exercise Science and Sports Medicine, Volume 2, Youth, Exercise and Sport.* Indianapolis, Ind.: Benchmark.

Gordon, N.F. (1992). *Arthritis: Your Complete Exercise Guide.* Champaign, Ill.: Human Kinetics.

Gordon, N.F. (1992). *Chronic Fatigue: Your Complete Exercise Guide.* Champaign, Ill.: Human Kinetics.

Gordon, N.F. (1992). *Diabetes: Your Complete Exercise Guide.* Champaign, Ill.: Human Kinetics.

Gordon, N.F. & Gibbons, L.W. (1990). *The Cooper Clinic Cardiac Rehabilitation Program: Featuring the Unique Heart Points Recovery System.* New York: Simon and Schuster.

Hanlon, T.W. (1995). *Fit for Two: The Official YMCA Prenatal Exercise Guide.* Champaign, Ill.: Human Kinetics.

Hiatt, W.R. et al. (1990). Benefit of exercise conditioning for patients with peripheral arterial disease. *Circulation,* 81, 602–609.

Hinson, C. (1995). *Fitness for Children*. Champaign, Ill.: Human Kinetics.

Holstein, B.B. (1988). *Shaping Up for a Healthy Pregnancy*. Champaign, Ill.: Life Enhancement Publications.

Institutes of Medicine (1995). *Weighing the Options: Criteria for Evaluating Weight Management Programs*. Washington, D.C.: National Academy Press.

Leppo, M. (1993). *Healthy from the Start: New Perspectives on Childhood Fitness.* Washington, D.C.: ERIC Clearinghouse on Teacher Education.

Miller, P.D. (Ed.) (1995). *Fitness Programming and Physical Disability*. Champaign, Ill.: Human Kinetics.

Nakamura, E., Moritani, T., & Kanetake, A. (1989). Biological age versus physical fitness age. *European Journal of Applied Physiology,* 58, 778–785.

Osness, W.H. (1990). *Functional Fitness Assessment for Adults Over 60 Years: A Field Based Assessment*. Reston, Va.: American Alliance for Health, Physical Education, Recreation, and Dance.

Paciorek, M.J. (1994). *Sports and Recreation for the Disabled* (2nd ed.). Carmel, Ind.: Cooper Publishing Group.

Pangrazi, R.P (1989). *Physical Fitness in the Elementary Schools: A Teacher's Manual* (2nd ed.). Reston, Va.: American Alliance for Health, Physical Education, Recreation and Dance.

Poehlman, E.T. et al. (1991). Influence of age and endurance training on metabolic rate and hormones in healthy men. *American Journal of Physiology*, 159, 66–72.

Pollock, M.L. & Schmidt, D.H. (Eds.) (1995). *Heart Disease and Rehabilitation*. Champaign, Ill.: Human Kinetics.

Rickers, R. (1986). *Seniors on the Move.* Champaign, Ill.: Human Kinetics.

Rowland, T.W. (1994). *Exercise and Children's Health.* Champaign, Ill.: Human Kinetics.

Sammann, P. (1994). *YMCA Healthy Back Book.* Champaign, Ill.: Human Kinetics.

Shephard, R.J. (1990). *Fitness in Special Populations.* Champaign, Ill.: Human Kinetics.

Sinaki, M. (1989). Exercise and osteoporosis. *Archives of Physical Medicine and Rehabilitation,* 70, 3, 220–229.

Skinner, J.S. (2005). *Exercise Testing and Exercise Prescription for Special Cases: Theoretical Basis and Clinical Application* (3rd ed.). Philadelphia: Lippincott Williams & Wilkins.

Smith, E.L. (1982). Exercise for prevention of osteoporosis: A review. *The Physician and Sports Medicine,* 10, 3, 72–83.

Tipton, C.M. (1991). Exercise, training and hypertension: An update. In: *Exercise and Sport Science*. 19, 447–505. Hollozy, J.O. (Ed.) Philadelphia: Lippincott Williams & Wilkins.

Van Norman, K.A. (1995). *Exercise Programming for Older Adults*. Champaign, Ill.: Human Kinetics.

Part VII

Legal, Professional, and Ethical Responsibilities

Chapter 19
Legal Responsibilities and Professional Ethics

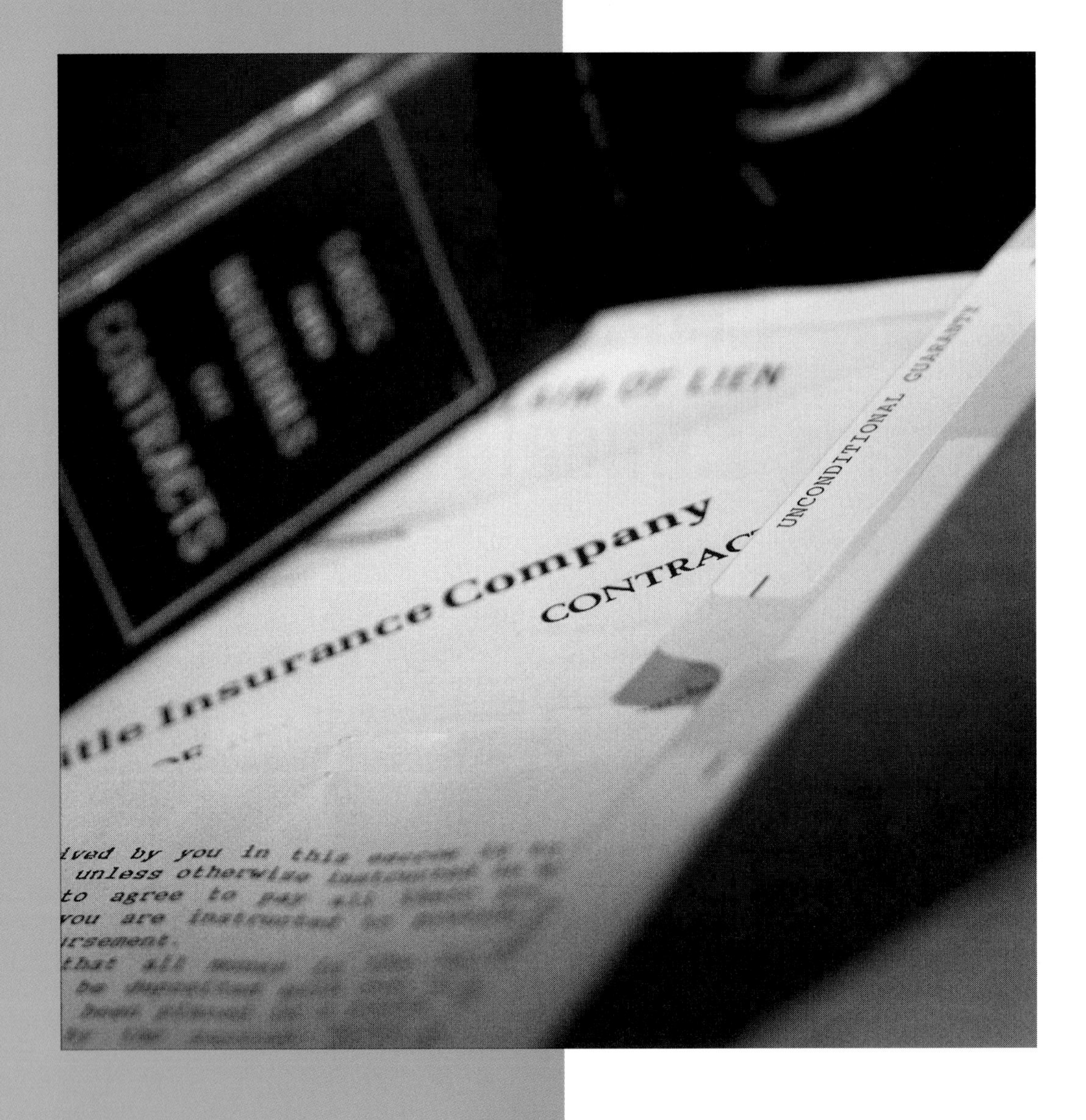

James A. Fein

James A. Fein, J.D., has been practicing law in Arizona for more than 30 years and is listed in the publication Best Lawyers in America. *He is also an ACE-certified Personal Trainer, an advisor to the American Council on Exercise, and is on the board of experts for* The Exercise Standards and Malpractice Reporter.

Chapter 19

Legal Responsibilities and Professional Ethics

IN THIS CHAPTER:

The number of individuals exercising in the United States has increased dramatically over the past several decades. This growth is expected to continue as members of the so-called "baby boomer" generation (born between 1946 and 1966) become more concerned about their health. Of course, as people age, their risk for illness and injury increases, which often causes them to more closely scrutinize the marketing tactics and service offerings of fitness professionals.

America is a highly litigious society. People are not afraid to file lawsuits to resolve conflicts, particularly those arising from personal injury. The best way fitness professionals or club owners can protect themselves from **liability** is to gain at least a basic understanding of the law in their particular state. It is incumbent on health-club operators and fitness professionals to recognize potential legal problems before they reach the litigation stage and force the health club or individual into court.

The Legal System

Lifestyle & Weight Management Consultants (LWMCs) are usually hoping to expand their practices and add clientele.

However, when money is tight, professionals may opt not to buy **liability insurance** in an effort to cut costs. Before making this decision, LWMCs should consider the following scenario: While working with a client, an LWMC turns his or her head to say hello to a coworker. At that moment, the client drops a weight on his foot, causing injury to himself. Before he knows it, the LWMC is served with legal papers and is being sued for the injury.

While this scenario may not directly apply to your practice, it is important to realize that anyone can be sued at any time. In fact, lawsuits arising from personal training in particular are becoming quite common. Anyone believing that he or she was injured through the fault of another person can bring a claim in court for money damages. These damages could include, but not be limited to, lost income, pain, suffering, and loss of enjoyment of life. The effect of a lawsuit on your practice can be enormous, both financially and emotionally. The good news is that there are ways to minimize the potential for being sued.

A basic knowledge of the legal system will improve your ability to conduct your business venture, whether you are a gym owner, work for a gym owner, or have your own practice. This chapter is intended to assist you in understanding some of the basic information you need to conduct a successful lifestyle- and weight-management business.

The legal system is divided into many facets, including **criminal law** and **civil law.** Criminal law involves someone being charged with a crime that can lead to incarceration. Civil law, which is much broader in scope, usually involves the payment of monetary damages for a committed "wrong" against someone. It usually involves a claim filed by one party against another party (including corporations and partnerships). A single act can sometimes involve components of both criminal and civil law.

Example:

John H. Jones is a fitness professional who thinks of himself as a bit of a ladies' man. He thinks that all of his female clients are physically attracted to him. One day, while training Lily, a 25-year-old woman, John inappropriately touches her. He is charged by the prosecuting attorney with criminal sexual assault. With this charge, he is facing prison time. He is later sued in civil court by Lily for assault and battery. For this lawsuit, he is facing financial damages.

Criminal Law

Hopefully, involvement in criminal law will never be a factor in your practice. Criminal charges can only be brought by a public government agency such as the Attorney General of a state or a prosecuting attorney, both state and federal. The penalties and procedures connected with charging, trying, sentencing, and imprisoning defendants convicted of crimes are governed by specific laws. Judges sometimes have latitude regarding the amount of time for which someone can be sentenced. Examples of such crimes include, but are not limited to, murder, theft, and criminal or sexual assault against another person.

Crimes are divided into misdemeanors and felonies. Misdemeanors are lesser crimes that usually carry a sentence up to one year in a municipal jail. A felony is a more serious charge that could cause a sentence of multiple years in a state or federal prison. However, a sentence upon conviction for a felony may sometimes be less than one year, at the discretion of the judge and within limits set by a particular statute. A judge can impose a financial penalty as well.

It was not so long ago that a personal trainer could face criminal charges as a result of simply practicing his trade. The charge could be made that the trainer was practicing medicine without a license. This has now changed in every state, as the importance of personal training has gained recognition for its health benefit to the public at large and is not viewed the same as the practice of medicine.

It is critical that you immediately seek legal counsel any time you believe that you are being accused of any type of criminal behavior. Never answer questions before obtaining competent legal advice.

Example:

Jill has been working as an LWMC in a health club for about a year. Recently, money disappeared from the club and Jill was accused of the theft. It would be best if Jill immediately retains a lawyer before answering any questions regarding the theft, regardless of whether she is guilty of the crime.

Civil Law

Contract Law

Contract law is one form of civil law. Contracts occur when a meeting of the minds takes place between two or more persons or entities during which there is a promise to do something in return for a valuable benefit, known as consideration. A contract can either be a verbal or written agreement, but verbal contracts are more difficult to prove. In some cases, a contract can consist of several documents, such as a series of letters, orders, offers, and counteroffers.

Example:

An agreement that says, "I promise to consult with you on Thursdays for a month and you promise to pay me $100.00 in return" is a contract.

Stated simply, there are five components to a valid contract:

- An offer to perform (a task) must be made.
- An acceptance of the offer must take place.
- Consideration must pass between the parties (usually some form of exchange of money or reliance upon the agreement).
- The contract must be for a legal purpose.
- All parties to the contract must be of a legal capacity to enter into the agreement.

An offer is basically a proposal to enter into a contract. Acceptance entails receiving an offer from another with the intent to consent. Consideration usually entails money being exchanged between parties. Consideration is a vital element in the law of contracts, as it is the result of bargaining between parties and the primary reason for a party to enter into a contract. Consideration must be of value (at least to the parties), and must be exchanged for the performance or promise of performance by the other party. Acts that are illegal or so immoral that they violate established public policy cannot serve as consideration for enforceable contracts.

Examples of nonenforceable contracts include gambling where it is outlawed, hiring someone to commit an illegal act, or inducing someone to breach an agreement (contracting with the intent to back out of a promise).

Finally, all parties to the contract must have the capacity to enter into the agreement.

Example:

An LWMC enters into a written agreement with a 16-year-old male to train him for a month. The contract is not enforceable, because a 16 year old is considered a minor and is unable to enter into a valid legal agreement. The agreement must be signed by the minor's parent or guardian if it is to be enforceable.

A contract can be oral rather than written. However, having a written document eliminates a lot of the ambiguity that could arise from a verbal agreement.

Example:

A fitness club offers you an opportunity to work for them. The club manager offers you $25.00 per hour, and you accept by shaking hands on the deal. After the first week, you receive a paycheck in which you were paid only $15.00 an hour. You inform the manager of the discrepancy and he responds by saying that you are mistaken, and that he agreed to pay you only $15.00 an hour. Without a written contract, it becomes your word against the manager's, and you are probably out of luck in enforcing your version of the agreement. If you had a written agreement that spelled out the complete terms, and the manager failed to honor the agreement, then you would have a valid, enforceable claim.

A contract should always be specific. Any agreements reached between the parties should be included in the written contract to eliminate the potential for conflict in the terms. Some fitness professionals choose to work as a team or in partnerships. Again, the terms of the partnership should be spelled out in clear language and be understood and agreed upon by all parties involved. Enforcing a contract can be very costly, which is a major reason why the terms of the contract should be in writing and very specific. Business matters are less likely to lead to costly lawsuits and hurt feelings if the specifics are set forth in a clearly understood written agreement that is signed by all parties. Usually, it is best that the contracts are drawn up by a lawyer who has an understanding of the law in the jurisdiction where the contract is to take place. Remember, contract law differs from state to state. What is valid in one state may be invalid in another.

Tort Law

Another area of civil law is known as **tort law.** The law in any state is usually developed by either statutory authority or **common law.** Tort law traditionally evolves from both **statutory law** and the common law that is developed in a particular state or jurisdiction. Statutory authority means that a law is passed by a legislative body and typically signed by the governor. Statutory law is also created by provisions in state constitutions and by a county or city ordinance. Common law is developed through interpretation of the law by judicial decisions, which means that a civil court of higher authority, usually a state appellate court, produces a legal opinion that seeks to interpret the existing law in a state.

Tort law includes both intentional torts, such as assault or battery, and **negligence** law. With an intentional tort, there is the mental desire and intent to act in a particular way.

Example:

John Jones gets into a dispute with another fitness professional and hits him in the face. This action constitutes the intentional tort of assault.

The term negligence describes the most common type of personal-injury claim brought against fitness professionals and health clubs. Negligence, which is defined as the failure to use the same care as an ordinary reasonable person would under similar circumstances, is accidental. By contrast, civil or criminal wrongs require intent. Negligence can result in all types of accidents that cause physical and/or property damage. In making a claim for damages based on an allegation of negligence, the injured party (plaintiff) must prove:

- That the party alleged to have been negligent had a legal "duty" (responsibility) to the injured party
- That the defendant's action (or failure to act) was not what a reasonably prudent person would have done under the same circumstances
- That the damages (injuries) were "proximately caused" by the negligence
- That the damages were "reasonably foreseeable" at the time of the alleged carelessness

Example:

An LWMC accidentally allows a barbell to fall on the knee of the client, causing him injury. The LWMC had a duty to the injured party; allowing the barbell to fall was not what a reasonably prudent fitness professional would have done; the injury to the client was caused by the acts of the LWMC; and it was foreseeable that an LWMC should have knowledge to prevent this type of injury from occurring.

Legal Concepts and Defenses

Standard of Care

The fulcrum of any legal civil claim of negligence is determined by whether the **standard of care** was breached. Standards of care are benchmark behaviors and actions that are universally exhibited by properly trained and experienced professionals. The standard of care becomes the minimally acceptable level of service owed to a client. The standard of care encompasses the watchfulness, attention, caution, and prudence that a reasonable person would exercise in the same circumstances. If a person's actions do not meet this responsibility, then his or her acts fail to meet the standard that people have toward one another. Failure to meet the standard is defined as negligence, and any damages resulting from this failure may be claimed in a lawsuit by the injured party. A problem is that the "standard" is often subjective, meaning that reasonable people can differ in their definition and understanding of the term.

As a general rule, professions and organizations that provide products or services to the public are expected to assure the public that they will deliver an acceptable level of quality and safety in their practice. What one person believes violates the standard of care may not agree with what another person believes. This disagreement can escalate into lawsuits. State and federal laws may be developed to regulate a profession that delivers important services that are considered potentially risky or harmful. For example, licensure of healthcare providers can set specific standards, such as minimum educational requirements and testing. To alleviate subjectivity, a uniform written standard of practice should be created for all professions. Responsible professionals and organizations issue practice recommendations and guidelines in part to help self-regulate their conduct to serve the overall public good and enhance their profession's reputation.

Example:

An orthopedic surgeon is accused of ***malpractice****. To determine if a valid claim exists, experts will look to the national standards of the American Orthopedic Association for guidance.*

The most common source documenting a standard of care comes from a national membership association, council, or commission that governs that particular profession. Unfortunately, in the fitness industry, there is not one written standard of practice that has gained universal acceptance. The guidelines and recommendations for exercise come from numerous associations and agencies. Currently, more than 50 organizations publish written standards for exercise, which often conflict with each other and are not entirely uniform. The most commonly accepted standards of practice for fitness professionals are published by the American College of Sports Medicine (ASCM). The American Council on Exercise (ACE) is among those organizations that play a prominent role in the fitness industry and implement standards by virtue of text books, articles, and other forms of written information.

Problems arise when a "standard" is a subjective issue upon which reasonable people can differ. This is where an expert witness will be employed to help interpret the standards of practice. An expert witness is a specialist in a particular subject—often a technical subject—who may present his or her expert opinion without having been a witness to any occurrence relating to the lawsuit or criminal case. This person's role is an exception to the rule against giving an opinion in trial, provided that the expert is qualified by evidence of his or her expertise, training, and special knowledge. If a criminal charge or civil lawsuit is brought, an expert may be employed to state an opinion, such as whether the standard of care has been breached.

Example:

Bill Budd has been sued for negligence after a client is injured. The client claims that he injured his back during a particular exercise. Bill employs a qualified expert (usually another fitness professional) to give an opinion that states that Bill did nothing below the standard of care. Bill's lawyer also employs a physician to give his opinion that the injury to the client's back is not related to the incident in question. The client's attorney will likely also employ experts to give their opinions on the same issues.

A fitness professional can be sued for being too aggressive with the rate of weight loss to the extent that it puts a client in danger. For example, if it can be shown that the recommendations for weight loss far exceed any standard norm and injury is caused to the client, this could be a basis for a claim.

Example:

Jason is an LWMC. He is very aggressive with his recommendations for weight loss while working with Lola. Lola becomes ill and anemic because of the recommendations made by Jason. It is demonstrated that Jason went well beyond the standard of care in his recommendations. Jason is sued for malpractice for the injuries suffered by Lola.

Contributory and Comparative Negligence

Generally, the defense to a claim of negligence involves either the act of contributory or **comparative negligence** on the part of the injured client. Another common defense, **assumption of risk,** is discussed later in this chapter. **Contributory negligence** is a doctrine stating that if a person was injured in part due to his or her own negligence (that is, his or her own negligence "contributed" to the accident), the injured party would not be entitled to collect any damages (i.e., money) from another party.

Example:

While Bill is training Jane, he looks away to say hello to a fellow trainer. While he isn't paying attention, a barbell falls on Jane's leg. Jane was asked not to lift the barbell until Bill gave her specific instructions. Jane, however, decided to try to lift the barbell anyway. Jane's actions could be considered contributory negligence and bar her from any recovery of damages against Bill. Even if Jane's actions were only minimally contributory to the accident, her action could bar her from recovering damages as part of a lawsuit.

Some states follow a variant of contributory negligence called the "doctrine of comparative negligence." This concept was developed because of the possibly unfair situations that have led some juries to deny recovery altogether, even when a person's comparative negligence is not as great as the negligent act itself. Most states have adopted a comparative negligence test in which the relative percentages of negligence by each person are used to determine damage recovery (i.e., how much money would be paid to the injured person).

Comparative negligence allows the jury to apportion responsibility to multiple parties, including the party bringing the claim. In that case, the injured party only recovers that percentage of the claim for which another person is found responsible. Stated another way, the party bringing the claim will have the damage recovery reduced by the percentage of his or her own failure to exercise reasonable care. Some states require the adverse party to the claim to be more than 50% comparatively responsible, or the party bringing the claim cannot prevail.

Ultimately, if a case goes to trial, a jury of ordinary citizens decides who is responsible and how much money should be paid to compensate a person for injuries. If a jury awards damages, they can include medical bills, loss of income, loss of family relationships, pain and suffering, and loss of enjoyment of life. The amount awarded is left for the jury to decide.

Example:

In the previous example, a jury hears evidence that Bill should not have looked away from Jane when she was sitting on the weight bench, but that Bill specifically asked Jane not to lift the weight. Jane's injuries are determined to be valued at $10,000. The jury decides that Bill is 50% responsible for the injury and that Jane is 50% responsible. Therefore, the judge orders Bill to pay $5000, or 50% of the total amount.

Assumption of Risk

Assumption of risk comes into play when a person takes a chance in a potentially dangerous situation and assumes the risk involved. Assumption of risk is a defense in which the defendant claims that in a given situation the injured plaintiff knew that a potential danger existed, but decided to act anyway. This usually occurs when an act is so inherently or obviously hazardous that the injured plaintiff should have known that there was danger, but took the chance despite knowing that he or she could be injured.

Example:

Sky diving, skiing on a restricted dangerous slope, and lifting unusually heavy weights knowingly beyond the exerciser's capacity are examples of situations in which the act was so inherently or obviously hazardous that as a general rule, in most states, a legal assumption-of-risk defense may be instituted by the party being sued.

Assumption of risk may operate to preclude or limit a person from recovering any damages in the personal-injury claim. This would also occur when evidence shows that the person making the claim voluntarily assumed a risk of harm by anticipating that the other party would be negligent in their conduct.

Releases, Hold-harmless Contracts, and Waivers

The issue of assumption of risk generally comes into play when a **waiver** or release document is signed prior to engaging in exercise. Most fitness professionals and health clubs try to protect themselves from liability by having a prospective client sign a waiver clause, also referred to as a "**hold harmless**" or exculpatory clause. This clause or agreement puts all risks associated with the training on the client. This segment of a written agreement is intended to relieve the trainer or health club from responsibility for injuries, including death or other losses that occur on someone else's property or as the result of someone's individual conduct.

Some states give these contractual clauses full recognition; others give them only partial recognition, or no recognition at all. It is a good idea to become familiar with the law in your particular state and the legal implication of these clauses. California appears to give considerable recognition to properly constructed waiver clauses in contracts. In other states, hold-harmless clauses are so frowned upon that there are statutory prohibitions against them. In Massachusetts, for example, a statute specifically prohibits a health club from releasing itself of negligent acts. An Arizona case declared that since the state had a constitutional provision requiring all assumption-of-risk issues to be left for the jury to decide, a hold-harmless clause was nonbinding (Phelps vs. Firebird Raceway, 2005). If the decision on the enforcement of the waiver clause is left to the **trier of fact** (usually a jury of ordinary people), it is then decided if the clause is enforceable under the conditions of how it was presented and signed. The jury then decides what effect the clause will have on the person bringing the lawsuit. The issue of whether contributory negligence, comparative negligence, or assumption of risk applies is considered by the jury. In some states, a jury, at its sole discretion, may give little or no weight to any hold-harmless clause if jury members decide that the participant was not properly informed of the legal implications.

Consider the following examples:

- In New York, a case was brought by a personal trainer's client, who was performing squats under the supervision of the trainer when he broke both of his ankles. The client claimed that, based upon his experience level, weight, size, and ability, the activity was not suited for him. He also claimed that the trainer was not properly spotting him. However, the client had executed a valid waiver. The court found the waiver enforceable and dismissed the case (Ciafalo vs. Vic Tanny Gyms).
- In Connecticut, a court held that a client could be barred from a claim because of a release, even though the release was destroyed in a fire, since there was no question that the release was signed (Corso vs. United States Surgical Corp., Connecticut Superior Court, 2005).

States that allow hold-harmless clauses usually have a general rule that the clause is valid and enforceable if it contains clear, express, and unambiguous language, and does not violate the public policy of the state. The first question, then, is whether the language of the waiver clause is clear enough that a reasonable signer would be aware that he is assuming the risk of any injuries that occur on the club's premises. The second question is whether the waiver clause violates public policy, either because it is too broad or because there is a statutory or constitutional prohibition against such clauses.

All states require that the language in the clause is clear and unambiguous, but the degree of clarity and ambiguity varies from state to state. The language of a waiver clause may cover an injury in one state, but that same language may not cover the same injury in another state. This distinction is usually based on the common law of each state and the degree of clarity the common law requires for the waiver clause. However, where states have adopted the express negligence doctrine, the language of the waiver must expressly list the act of negligence if it is to be effective. Some states require the term "negligence" to actually be in the clause so that the intent of the parties is spelled out with the greatest of particularity. In other states, the clause need not contain the word "negligence"—or any other magic words—to be valid.

In general, it is important to recognize that waiver clauses are not favored and are usually strictly construed against the drafter or presenter of the written document. Typically, this means that the health-club operator or fitness professional who presents a written agreement that contains any type of waiver or hold-harmless clause to a potential or existing client must ensure that the document states exactly what it is intended to purport. Whether any "magic words" are needed or not, the clause still only covers what is written in the agreement and nothing more. If the language only requires the applicant to attest to being physically sound and to having medical approval, the clause will not cover negligence by the facility. For the health-club operator's protection, the language in the agreement should be broad enough to cover any injuries that may occur on the premises, not just injuries that may occur while an individual is working out with a trainer. If the language is not broad enough, the defendant could still be held liable for unforeseeable injuries. The most effective waiver clauses clearly state that the client expressly assumes all risk, foreseeable or unforeseeable, while on the premises. This would include, but not be limited to, the negligence of the facility operator and all **employees.** The clause should clearly state that the signer (the client) is waiving and holding harmless any and all claims against the owners and employees of the facility.

Even the most unambiguously written waiver clause that meets the highest standards of clarity may not cover all injuries that may occur in a facility. Courts also analyze whether the clause is against public policy, which is defined as a system of laws or regulatory measures or courses of action promulgated by a governmental entity, to set the standard of what is accepted by the public at large. For example, most states will not enforce a contract made for illegal purposes (such as a contract based upon an illegal betting operation), because the **public policy** of the state does not allow that conduct to take place. Another way in which a clause can violate public policy is by being worded too broadly. Generally, a waiver clause cannot prevent a suit for **gross negligence** or for wanton recklessness or intentional misconduct. These actions are of a higher standard than normal negligence. These types of claims are less commonly made against fitness professionals and health clubs, because they involve a degree of misconduct that goes way beyond general negligence (such as an LWMC coming to work intoxicated or being sexually involved with a client).

The final way in which a clause can be void against public policy is if the signer of the contract has been misled, or is reasonably unaware of a clause in the contract that was not brought to his or her attention. Therefore, a thorough discussion explaining the details of the document increases the potential for the document to be enforced in court. In California, the burden is on the client to show that he or she was misled or unaware of the clause. However, in Ohio, the burden is on the health club or fitness professional to show that there was unambiguous intent. In Mississippi, the health club or trainer must show that the contract was negotiated fairly and honestly and understood by both parties.

Some states ensure that signers are not misled by requiring that a clause is distinguished from other sections. In other words, the clause cannot be buried in a lengthy document. One way to increase the validity of an exculpatory clause is to set it aside from other provisions, such as on its own page. At the very least, it should be placed in its own paragraph, preferably in different and larger print to stand out from the other provisions.

In another California case, a man joined a health club in February of 1997 and signed a release and waiver of liability as part of his membership agreement. The provision was printed in eight-point font and prefaced by a bold-faced heading that read "RELEASE OF LIABILITY AND INDEMNITY." Four years later, while in the club's steam room, the client squatted on a heated pipe and suffered a burn. He then brought suit for personal injuries. The California court upheld the validity of the waiver agreement (Frenzley vs. L.A. Fitness Sports Clubs, California Court of Appeals, 2003). A similar decision in 2005 also upheld the waiver clause in California (Fores vs. 24 Hour Fitness, California Appellate Court, 2005).

In summary, it is likely that a well-written waiver clause that seeks to hold a health club or trainer harmless may be enforceable if it stands out in the contract, is written clearly and conspicuously, and has been knowingly signed by a client. Such a clause may preclude a negligence action for injuries occurring on a health club's premises, unless a state has a specific constitutional statutory or common-law provision against a waiver or hold-harmless clause. Even in states that do not uphold a waiver clause as binding, it is still important that the trainer do everything possible to explain what a waiver clause is and document that the client understands what it does. Talking to and getting the client to understand the effect of the clause will go a long way in helping to minimize a fitness professional's exposure to adverse litigation results. If a court or jury does not uphold the waiver clause, a jury can award the injured client substantial damages. This could ruin an LWMC's practice and reputation in the community.

Lawyers always try to find ways to circumvent release clauses when they represent injured clients. The more information you give your client at the time the release is signed, the better your chances that the release will be upheld in court.

Employee vs. Independent Contractor

Are you the master of your work or do you have a master? That is a key question, because defining your employment plays a huge role in determining the various rights and responsibilities of fitness professionals and health-club operators. Many times, a fitness club may claim that it is using **independent contractors** when the law in fact defines these individuals as employees. It is important to understand the difference between an independent contractor and employee so that all parties have a correct interpretation of their duties and responsibilities.

An independent contractor is a person or business that performs services for another person or entity under a contract that specifies terms such as duties, pay, and the amount and type of work. An independent contractor is distinguished from an employee, who works regularly for an employer. The nature of the relationship between the independent contractor and the hiring party is vital, because the contractor pays his or her own social security and income taxes without payroll deduction, has no retirement or health-plan rights, and often is not entitled to worker's compensation coverage. Public agencies, particularly the Internal Revenue Service, scrutinize independent-contractor agreements when it appears that the contractor is treated like an employee. An independent contractor determines when and where to perform work, is able to work for other employers, provides his or her own equipment, and satisfies other factors indicative of true independence.

In contrast, an employee is hired for a salary to perform work for an employer. There are various elements to determine whether a person is an independent contractor or employee, but the key element is control over the person's employment.

Example:

Bill is an LWMC and works at Joe's gym. Bill has his own clients, comes and goes as he pleases, and is paid directly by his clients. Bill is considered an independent contractor.

Jill also works at Joe's gym. However, Joe dictates the hours that Jill has to be present at work and pays Jill directly on an hourly basis. Jill is clearly an employee. Joe may write a contract with Jill defining her role as an independent contractor, but by law she is considered an employee.

Responsibility for another person's actions can also arise from agency relationships. Liability arises under the legal doctrine of **respondeat superior** (Latin for "let the master answer"). In an agency relationship, one person (called the agent) acts on behalf of another person, known as a principal. Agency may arise when a principal expressly or implicitly asks an agent to do something for him or her.

The basic rule is that the principal becomes responsible for the acts of the agent, and the agent acts on behalf of the principal. If a potential claim arises, whether someone is an employee for a fitness club or an independent contractor may determine who can be held responsible. If someone is acting as an agent for a principal (such as working for a fitness club), the employer can also be held liable for any injury caused by the employee, as long as the employee is acting within the scope of his or her employment when the injury occurs.

In determining the validity of a claim against an employee, factual questions normally arise, such as, "Was the agent working within the scope of employment when he or she acted negligently?" There is also the problem of whether the principal acted in such a way as to make others believe that someone was his agent—this is known as "apparent" or "ostensible" authority. When someone uses company business cards or finance documents, or wears a shirt with the company logo, such use gives apparent authority as an agent and the company can be responsible for his or her actions.

Example:

Joe is an independent contractor and works with his clients at Adonis Fitness Club. Joe wears a shirt that says Adonis Fitness and has business cards that give Adonis Fitness as his business address. If Joe causes injury to someone, even though Joe is not an employee of Adonis Fitness, the club could be responsible for Joe's actions if the person injured believed that Joe was an employee of the fitness club. This is an example of an apparent agency relationship.

Example:

Dick is employed as an LWMC for A Better Way Health Club. While working at the club, Dick is negligent and collides with Victor, a club member, causing him injury. In addition to Dick being held responsible for damages to Victor, A Better Way Health Club is also responsible, since the accident occurred in the scope of Dick's employment. If Dick gets into an automobile accident while on a lunch break, A Better Way is probably not jointly responsible, because there is a strong inference that he was outside the scope of employment.

Scope of Practice

One of the greatest perils for professionals is to venture outside of the **scope of practice.** An internist would never perform heart surgery on a patient, because doing so is obviously outside the doctor's scope of medical practice. Likewise, fitness professionals who venture outside their scope of practice enter risky territory.

The most common example of this scenario is when a fitness professional starts prescribing a strict diet regimen when not trained as a dietitian. LWMCs must know their limits in terms of what their certification allows them to do and what scenarios necessitate referral. A good example is when a client begins exhibiting signs of an eating disorder, in which case the LWMC must refer the client to a specialist in this area. Another example is the issuance of exercise recommendations or programs without the completion of necessary prerequisites, such as a health screening. This action clearly exposes a fitness professional to liability in case of injury. Under some circumstances, the "prescription" of exercise may well be considered a medical procedure or practice that can only be issued by a physician. Fitness professionals who are not physicians can face serious charges, in some states potential criminal charges. When in doubt, LWMCs should exercise restraint and be conservative in their approach.

Similarly, LWMCs are not psychologists or marriage counselors and therefore should not provide advice or counseling on issues related to a client's emotional and/or psychological status. Participants should always be referred to licensed practitioners in these and related areas. A psychologist or therapist encourages their clients to go back and examine issues and look at their feelings in the context of their personal history. Such a discussion is outside the scope of practice of an LWMC, who must instead work with each individual as he or she currently exists and help him or her move forward. The line between an LWMC and a counselor or therapist must never be crossed.

LWMCs should also be careful when they get involved in providing nutrition advice. If the nutrition or dieting advice is too aggressive, it could place the client at risk. The matter is complicated if it can be shown that the fitness professional went beyond the scope of his or her practice in making the diet recommendations. Simply because a person calls him- or herself a fitness professional does not give that person the right to go into fields of practice that are not covered by his or her fitness credential. A family practice physician would be committing malpractice if he or she tried to attempt heart surgery. Similarly, a fitness professional who is only certified as a personal trainer or LWMC, for example, would be committing malpractice if he or she devises a specific diet plan for a client.

Other Legal and Professional Duties and Responsibilities

Malpractice

Malpractice, which is a form of negligence, is an act or an omission of an act by a professional that falls below the standard of care of a reasonably prudent professional of the same type and under the same circumstances. Such an error or omission may be the result of negligence, ignorance (when the professional should have known better), or intentional wrongdoing. However, malpractice does not include the exercise of professional judgment, even when the results are detrimental to the client or patient. In most cases, to prove malpractice, an expert in the same field of practice must provide testimony on the acceptable standard of care regarding the specific act or conduct claimed to be malpractice, and then establish that the professional did not meet that standard. The party accused of wrongdoing can then produce his or her own expert to counter that testimony. Many professions can be subject to lawsuits based on claims of malpractice, including lawyers, physicians, dentists, hospitals, accountants, and personal trainers. Many states have specific codified laws that define who can be held responsible for malpractice.

If a professional is found liable for professional malpractice, it would likely severely hurt his or her career. It becomes a record of professional conduct and can ruin a person's reputation for many years. Many legal observers believe that some malpractice claims can be avoided if the professional immediately deals with the situation rather than trying to cover it up. In some states, if a professional makes a mistake and says, "I'm sorry" or words to that effect, that statement cannot be used against him or her in a court of law. If you are accused of malpractice, immediately take action and get legal advice. Notify your malpractice insurance carrier of the complaint filed against you. Failure to notify your insurance carrier in a timely manner could cause the carrier to refuse to defend your claim.

Example:

During a workout with a client, Joey hears his client complain about hurting his back. Joey is so concerned that he agrees to personally pay the client's chiropractic bills, but does nothing further to inform his insurance carrier of the injury to the client. A year later, the client sues Joey. Joey's insurance company may refuse to accept the claim because Joey did not give the carrier timely notice.

Follow this simple rule if you feel that someone may file a claim against you: When in doubt, contact your insurance carrier and let them know of an expected or potential claim. Insurers often make attorneys available to provide advice free of charge. This is a right that fitness professionals purchase as part of their insurance policy. Contrary to public perception, substantial judgments in malpractice cases are rare. Studies show that only a small percentage of claims result in recovery for the allegedly aggrieved client. The principal reason is that most cries of malpractice are unfounded and are based on unhappiness with the result of the original services (no matter how well-handled), a breakdown in communication between the professional and the client, anger with the professional, or retaliation for attempts to collect unpaid fees.

Confidentiality and Maintenance of Proper Records

Like many professionals, LWMCs have a duty to maintain a degree of confidentiality. Obviously, if an LWMC works with a client in a fitness center, people often know of the client–professional relationship. However, the LWMC should never divulge personal information about the client without his or her written consent. Clients often entrust fitness professionals with sensitive information and assume that it remains confidential. This information is just as confidential as that given on signed forms, such as the fitness profile, medical history reports, and releases. A fitness professional enters a risk for liability when he or she uses the client's name as a referral without first getting the client's permission. Photos of the client, such as those used to measure success in an exercise regimen, should also be kept confidential. They should never be used in any form of advertising, even if the client's name is not divulged.

Example:

Alice trains regularly with Tom at Ultimate Fitness and has done so for the past year. During the year, Alice has lost 30 pounds. Tom starts bragging to other people that Alice is his client and tells of her success. Doing so violates the standard of confidentiality and subjects Tom to liability.

Maintaining meticulous records of clients is important for many reasons. First and foremost, it allows the fitness professional to review in an organized fashion the progress of any client without confusing that client's progress with someone else's. Secondly, it can help protect the fitness professional from liability should an incident occur in which the information maintained can play a role in determining if he or she is held responsible.

Example:

Jimmy has a serious heart condition. He intentionally fails to write down information about his heart condition when he fills out a medical profile at Art's Health Club. One day, during a training session with Art, Jimmy suf-

fers a heart attack and dies. Jimmy's estate sues Art for wrongful death and malpractice. Art is able to produce the health form on which Jimmy specifically omitted his history of heart problems. This document would help absolve Art of legal responsibility.

Records should be maintained and kept private and inaccessible to others. If maintained at a health facility, these records should be kept locked in a file drawer to maintain client privacy. If records are kept in computer-based spreadsheets or files, they should be kept under password protection.

Recommending Supplements

An area where a fitness professional or club owner can surely get into trouble and be subject to legal problems is when recommending supplements for clients. First of all, this could be construed as prescribing medication and subject the professional to severe civil, and perhaps criminal, penalties. Secondly, if the LWMC has a pecuniary interest (i.e., is making a profit) from the sale of the supplements and does not disclose this fact, this could subject the LWMC to claims of consumer fraud. There are certain professionals, such as properly credentialed nutritionists and physicians, who are specifically trained to recommend supplements. An LWMC or fitness facility can lose credibility with clients by trying to push certain products, especially if they make money from the sale of such items.

Avoiding Intimate Relationships With Clients

Any discussion about the responsibilities of fitness professionals must include a statement of the importance of maintaining an arm's length professional relationship with clients. In psychology, there is a phenomenon called **transference,** which is characterized by the unconscious redirection of feelings from one person to another. For instance, a person might mistrust somebody who resembles an ex-spouse in manners, voice, or external appearance, or be overly compliant to someone who resembles a childhood friend. Counter-transference is defined as the redirection of a therapist's feelings toward a client, or more generally as a therapist's emotional entanglement with a client. Transference was first described by Freud, who acknowledged its importance in psychoanalysis for better understanding of the patient's feelings. Transference is often manifested as an erotic attraction toward a therapist.

Many clients start to treat fitness professionals as confidants. Clients may disclose personal feelings about relationships with spouses or partners. The longer the fitness professional is involved with training the client, the more potential for the relationship to "cross over the line." Jokes about fitness professionals having sexual relationships with clients are abundant. At all costs, a fitness professional should keep a safe personal distance from a client so that the professional–client relationship does not become entangled with an intimate personal relationship. Fitness professionals sometimes touch clients in a very personal way and should always make sure that the client understands that he or she is acting only for professional reasons.

If a fitness professional becomes intimately involved with a client, the professional relationship should immediately cease. The professional should be up-front with the client to avoid misunderstandings that could lead to liability issues.

Sexual Harassment in the Workplace

Sexual harassment is a form of sex discrimination that violates Title VII of the Civil Rights Act of 1964. Title VII applies to employers with 15 or more employees, including state and local governments. It also applies to employment agencies and labor organizations, as well as to the federal government. Sexual harassment violates federal and state law. It is one of the most prevalent and offensive types of discrimination and exists in both small and large companies. Sexual harassment can occur in a variety of circumstances. It includes unwelcome sexual advances, requests for sexual favors, and other verbal or physical conduct of a sexual nature that affects an individual's employment, unreasonably interferes with an individual's work performance, or creates an intimidating, hostile, or offensive work environment. Either the victim or the harasser may be a woman or a man, and the victim does not have to be of the opposite sex. Also, harassment can be verbal or physical, and must be unwelcome.

A person who feels that he or she is a target of sexual harassment may file a complaint with a state or federal regulatory agency designed to protect against this unwelcome conduct. The harassed person may not need a lawyer to resolve the dispute and cannot lose his or her job for filing a complaint.

Use of Facilities and Equipment

Almost all fitness professionals use some type of equipment to assist in training. This equipment could be as simple as rubber straps or be as complex as a fully equipped gym. The use of equipment is a distinct and separate area in which liability can arise. Liability will usually arise because a piece of equipment becomes faulty. This may be due to the initial design, the manufacture, or the maintenance of the equipment. Lawsuits resulting from use of equipment are generally referred to as product-defect claims.

If a claim arises due to the manufacture or design of the equipment, it usually becomes an issue for the manufacturer and distributor of the equipment. A fitness club's direct liability usually results from improper maintenance. Many times, if the fitness club is sued, the manufacturer will be required to indemnify the fitness club owner, meaning that the manufacturer must cover any losses that the club might suffer.

Example:

Samantha is working out in Bill's Fitness Club. The belt on the treadmill that Samantha is using starts slipping, causing her to fall and suffer an injury. She ends up suing the fitness club, the manufacturer, and the distributor of the treadmill. It is determined that the belt was installed improperly on the treadmill. The fitness club's lawyer demands that the manufacturer protect the club and indemnify the club from the claim. The manufacturer agrees to do so.

In addition to the mechanism of the equipment, care should also be given to provide proper written instructions on the use of the equipment. Failure to provide such instructions could also be a basis for litigation. At minimum, instructions should include a detailed description of the function of the equipment, a step-by-step procedure on proper use, and adequate warnings of foreseeable risks in the use and misuse of the equipment. These instructions should appear on the equipment and be clearly visible to all equipment users.

It is extremely important that health-club operators document equipment maintenance to protect themselves. Maintenance is required on any safety equipment as well as **automated external defibrillators (AEDs).** Some states require certain equipment to be made available at all times in health clubs. For example, New York State law requires the availability of cardiopulmonary resuscitation (CPR) masks and gloves to protect rescuers. The New York City Department of Health developed regulations in response to this law. These regulations require operators of certain public places to have CPR equipment available in an accessible area. These regulations ensure that patrons and/or staff can access and reach the victim within three minutes of the onset of an incident. Cleanliness is always a consideration in the health-club environment. A health-club owner should create a maintenance-inspection sheet that is used throughout the day to document attempts to maintain and clean equipment and the facility. This document may become critical if a lawsuit is filed and questions arise regarding the frequency of equipment and facility maintenance.

Responsibility for Continuing Education

All respected licensed professions have continuing-education requirements. The purpose of continuing education is to help individuals maintain an understanding of the latest research and professional standards and guidelines and promote their professional development.

LWMCs, like personal trainers, are not yet licensed. However, there are many organizations, including ACE, that require professionals to complete continuing education to maintain their certification or membership. Continuing-education requirements can be met in multiple ways: completing distance-learning courses, attending seminars, writing articles, and lecturing in the field are a few options. Continuing education does not need to be expensive or laborious. Fitness professionals should view continuing education as a great opportunity to improve their professional knowledge and interact with their peers. Many fitness professionals use continuing education as an opportunity to travel to other locations and to network with like-minded members of the fitness industry.

For LWMCs, earning continuing education is a must, and no club should hire or retain LWMCs who do not make a commitment to meet their continuing-education requirements.

Copyright Compliance

Copyright compliance is not something that is familiar to many fitness professionals, but it could be the source of unneeded legal issues. Essentially, copyright is the exclusive right of the author or creator of a literary or artistic property (such as a book, movie, or musical composition) to print, copy, sell, license, distribute, transform to another medium, translate, record, or perform or otherwise use that property.

On any distributed and/or published work, a notice should be affixed stating the word copyright, copy, or ©, with the name of the creator and the date of copyright (which is the year of first publication). The notice should be on the title page or the page immediately following. On graphic arts, it should be in a clearly visible or accessible place. The work should also be registered with the U.S. Copyright Office. A copyright establishes proof of earliest creation and publication and is required for filing a lawsuit for infringement. Copyrights cover the following: literary, musical, and dramatic works; periodicals; maps; works of art (including models); art reproductions; sculptural works; technical drawings; photographs; prints (including labels); movies and other audiovisual works; computer programs; compilations of works and derivative works; and architectural drawings. The following items do not require copyrights: short phrases; titles; extemporaneous speeches or live unrecorded performances; common information; government publications; mere ideas; and seditious, obscene, libelous, and fraudulent work. For any work created from 1978 to date, a copyright is good for the author's life plus 50 years. There are a few exceptions, including work "for hire," which is owned by the commissioner of the work for a period of 75 years from publication. After that time period, the material is in the public domain. The United States is among the many countries that recognize international copyrights under the "Universal Copyright Convention."

In the fitness arena, copyright is important for two reasons. First, when you develop a program or write an article that you want to protect as an author, you need to submit the content for copyright. Secondly, you may not use another person's work without approval of the author/owner, including the use of music in group fitness instruction. An exception is usually made if the music is used in educational settings, such as a college course. Music companies have become more aggressive about enforcing copyright protection. Although two groups, the **American Society of Composers, Artists and Publishers (ASCAP)** and **Broadcast Music, Inc. (BMI),** issue licenses for the commercial use of recordings, their fees are probably prohibitive for most fitness professionals. It is more economical to use recordings designed and sold specifically for fitness programs. The most important thing is to make sure that permission for use has been granted before using any copyrighted material. The leading agency protecting consumers from misrepresentations is the Federal Trade Commission (FTC).

Consumer Fraud Issues and Advertising

Almost all states and the federal government have enacted consumer-protection laws and have set up agencies to protect the consumer (i.e., the retail purchasers of goods and services) from inferior, adulterated, hazardous, or deceptively advertised products, and deceptive or fraudulent sales practices. Federal statutes and regulations govern mail fraud, including false advertising. Mail fraud may include fake contests, "low-ball" price traps (e.g., the bait-and-switch approach), supposed credit for referrals of friends, phony home-improvement loans with huge final payments, and swamp-land sales.

Fitness professionals and fitness club owners should be aware that any representation that has even the tendency to deceive can be considered a violation of consumer-protection laws. Misrepresentations need not be in writing. Any oral statement that has a tendency to mislead the average consumer can constitute a violation if the consumer relies upon the statement. Fitness professionals and club owners should be very careful with the types of promises they make solely to win new clientele. Promises concerning weight loss or fitness improvements are particularly prone to scrutiny.

Example:

Carlie Mills owns a health studio and seeks new clients. She decides to put a flier in a local newspaper. The flier promises prospective clients that they will lose 25 pounds in six months. The flier also shows a "before and after" picture of a person who lost 25 pounds, and claims that the person achieved this result after training at the studio. In fact, the photo shows a person Carlie knows from her previous employment at another gym. The promise to lose 25 pounds and the use of the photo to induce clients into Carlie's studio both violate consumer-protection laws.

The Importance of Professional Liability Insurance

In real estate, it is often stated that the most important things to consider when purchasing property is location, location, location. In the fitness industry, the most important thing to consider in minimizing personal exposure to legal claims is insurance, insurance, insurance.

Essentially, insurance is a contract (insurance policy) in which the insurer (insurance company) agrees, for a fee (insurance premiums), to pay the insured party all or a portion of any loss suffered by accident or death. The losses covered by the policy may include property damage or loss from accident, fire, theft, or intentional harm; medical costs and/or lost earnings due to physical injury; long-term or permanent loss of physical capacity; and claims by others resulting from alleged negligence by the insured.

The most important insurance that any fitness professional or club owner can have is liability insurance, which protects against any claim brought by a client for personal injury. Cost of personal liability protection for a trainer is relatively inexpensive, considering the benefits that the coverage provides. Liability policies cover the amount of the claim (up to a certain amount), and offer the fitness professional or club owner the services of a skilled attorney to deal with claims. And remember, it is critical that any potential claims be immediately reported to the insurance company so that coverage cannot be denied.

Example:

Marquita is a club owner, LWMC, and personal trainer. She maintains $1,000,000 in liability insurance coverage. One day, a client has a heart attack and dies during his workout in the club. The relatives end up suing the club for wrongful death. Since Marquita bought liability coverage, the insurer will provide a lawyer, defend the case, and, if necessary, pay up to $1,000,000.

Marquita has another client who slips on a bar of soap and falls in the shower. The client breaks his femur and sues for damages. Again, Marquita's insurance coverage will assume responsibility for the claim and pay whatever damages are appropriate.

There are several other types of insurance that are important to fitness professionals, including disability and medical insurance. Table 19-1 summarizes these two forms and explains the difference between general liability insurance and professional liability insurance.

LWMCs working as independent contractors must pay special attention to their coverage. It is imperative that all aspects of any coverage that may be provided by the club or facility are understood and included in the written agreement for an LWMC's services. If insurance coverage is not provided by the club, it is in LWMCs' best interest—as well as that of their clients—to provide themselves with adequate coverage.

How to Avoid Liability Claims

Fitness professionals and club owners should constantly be vigilant in attempting to avoid liability claims. As discussed earlier in this chapter, continuing education plays a vital role in helping to educate LWMCs and health-club operators on new techniques to avoid injuries. In fitness clubs, regularly scheduled and documented meetings should be held among staff members and others involved in the club to discuss any potential areas of concern and liability. Fitness professionals and club owners should keep abreast of trends and programs and how they may enhance the risk of harm to clients. The applicable standard of care should be discussed among peers.

Risk Management

Identifying risks before they occur is called **risk management.** The purpose of risk management is to identify and eliminate or reduce potential risks. Some liability

Table 19-1
Types of Insurance

General Liability	General liability insurance covers basic trip-and-fall injuries that occur in a nonbusiness environment. These policies will not provide coverage for accidents that occur at work.
Professional Liability	Professional liability insurance is designed to protect you against a broad spectrum of claims. This includes allegations claiming injury to students or clients as a result of improper supervision of fitness activities, failure to adequately instruct, improper use or recommendation of equipment, and exposure to injury from substandard facilities. This coverage should extend to acts of omission (things you did not do) as well as acts of commission (actual conduct). Most policies also extend coverage for violations of a client's civil rights, such as sexual harassment, an important element to consider in today's sensitive environment. Defense coverage should be extended even if the charges are groundless.
Disability	Disability insurance, which provides income protection should you become injured, may or may not be supplied by your employer. If it is not provided, you may want to consider purchasing this type of insurance for yourself. While worker's compensation covers you when you are injured on or by the job, disability insurance will provide income even if your injury occurs outside of work.
Medical Insurance	Individual medical insurance, which provides hospitalization and major medical coverage, is another type of coverage that may be supplied by your employer. These plans vary widely and, because of increasing costs, many clubs have reduced or eliminated these benefits as a cost-saving measure. Rarely are independent contractors granted benefits.

insurance carriers offer discounts to persons practicing appropriate risk management.

Periodically reviewing programs, facilities, and equipment to evaluate potential dangers to clients allows LWMCs to decide the best way to reduce costly injuries in each situation. Most authorities recommend a risk-management protocol that consists of the following five steps:

- Identification of risks—This step entails the specification of all risks that may be encountered by the LWMC in the areas of instruction, supervision, facilities, equipment, contracts, and business structure.
- Evaluation of each risk—The LWMC must review each risk with consideration given to the probability that the risk could occur, and if so, what the conceivable severity would be. Table 19-2 can be used to assess the identified risks.
- Selection of an approach for managing each risk—Several approaches are available to the LWMC for managing and reducing the identified risks, including the following common methods:
  - ✓ Transfer, as with insurance policies
  - ✓ Reduction (through continuing education)
  - ✓ Retention (by budgeting for minor emergencies)
  - ✓ Avoidance of certain activities or equipment

  The recommended approach for risks that are extreme is to avoid the activity completely or transfer the risk through appropriate insurance. Risks that fall into one of the high categories can be managed either through insurance or viable actions to reduce the likelihood of occurrence or severity of outcome. Reduction is also the preferred method for addressing risks in the medium category, while risks with low impact can be handled through retention.
- Implementation—This step entails putting plans into action.
- Evaluation—This final step involves assessing the outcome of the risk-management endeavors.

Table 19-2
Evaluating Risk Based on Frequency and Severity

	Frequency of Occurrence		
Severity of Injury or Financial Impact	High or often	Medium or infrequent	Low or seldom
High or vital	Avoid or transfer	Transfer	Transfer
Medium or significant	Transfer	Transfer or retain	Transfer or retain
Low or insignificant	Retain	Retain	Retain

LWMCs can also manage risk by examining procedures and policies and developing conduct and safety guidelines for their clients' use of equipment. Strict safety guidelines for each activity, accompanied by procedures for emergencies, are particularly important. LWMCs must not only develop these policies, but also become thoroughly familiar with them, mentally practicing their emergency plans. Several lawsuits have resulted in substantial judgments against fitness professionals who failed to respond to the emergency medical needs of clients. Once risks are identified, LWMCs should carry out the actions needed to reduce them.

Professional Ethics

Professional ethics involves the rules or standards governing the conduct of a person or the members of a profession. Ethical guidelines can also be the basis for determining liability. If properly followed, ethical guidelines can enhance a professional's reputation in the eyes of consumers. Licensed professionals have boards (such as the bar association for attorneys or medical society for doctors) that can strip a person of his or her license for ethical violations.

The fitness industry will keep thriving if the public perceives that it is doing a good job of policing professionals by encouraging them to adhere to meaningful standards. Perception does not necessarily have anything to do with truth. Instead, it is what the public perceives to be true. Information need not be factual or even pertinent to create or change a person's perception. For example, a common misperception is that personal training is strictly for muscle-bound individuals or Hollywood stars.

Ethics can overlap with legal claims. Ethical violations, such as misrepresenting the expected benefits of training or unlawfully touching clients, can lead to legal claims. Misrepresenting your educational experience, while not likely to bring legal action unless someone is injured, is a clear ethical violation.

It is well-established that fitness professionals need to keep their interactions with clients confidential. Fitness professionals should extend this obligation to keeping the names of all clients confidential, unless they consent to revealing their identities.

Appropriate behavior and common sense constitute the cornerstone of ethical behavior. Appendix A presents the American Council on Exercise's Code of Ethics.

Summary

The fitness industry is young, but rapidly evolving. The need to understand legal and ethical concerns is key to protect both fitness professionals and their clientele. How can fitness professionals and club operators protect themselves from liability? The obvious answer is to practice safe methods of training, be vigilant to avoid potentially harmful situations, and ensure ongoing continuing education.

Suggested Reading

American College of Sports Medicine (2007). *ACSM's Health/Fitness Facility Standards and Guidelines* (3rd ed.). Champaign, Ill.: Human Kinetics.

Cotton, D. & Cotton, M.B. (1997). *Legal Aspects of Waivers in Sport, Recreation and Fitness Activities.* Canton, Ohio: PRC Publishing.

Herbert, D. (Ed.) *The Exercise Standards and Malpractice Reporter.* Canton, Ohio: PRC Publishing.

Koeberle, B.E. (1998). *Legal Aspects of Personal Fitness Training* (2nd ed.). Canton, Ohio: PRC Publishing.

Urquhart, J.R. (1993). *The IRS Independent Contractors and You!* Irvine, Calif.: The Fidelity Publishing Company of America.

Appendices

Appendix A

ACE Code of Ethics

ACE-certified Professionals are guided by the following principles of conduct as they interact with clients/participants, the public, and other health and fitness professionals.

ACE-certified Professionals will endeavor to:

- ✔ Provide safe and effective instruction
- ✔ Provide equal and fair treatment to all clients
- ✔ Stay up-to-date on the latest health and fitness research and understand its practical application
- ✔ Maintain current CPR certification and knowledge of first-aid services
- ✔ Comply with all applicable business, employment, and intellectual property laws
- ✔ Maintain the confidentiality of all client information
- ✔ Refer clients to more qualified health or medical professionals when appropriate
- ✔ Uphold and enhance public appreciation and trust for the health and fitness industry
- ✔ Establish and maintain clear professional boundaries

Provide Safe and Effective Instruction

Providing safe and effective instruction involves a variety of responsibilities for ACE-certified Professionals. Safe means that the instruction will not result in physical, mental, or financial harm to the client/participant. Effective means that the instruction has a purposeful, intended, and desired effect toward the client's/participant's goal. Great effort and care must be taken in carrying out the responsibilities that are essential in creating a positive exercise experience for all clients/participants.

Screening

ACE-certified Professionals should have all potential clients/participants complete an industry-recognized health-screening tool to ensure safe exercise participation. If significant risk factors or signs and symptoms suggestive of chronic disease are identified, refer the client/participant to a physician or primary healthcare practitioner for medical clearance and guidance regarding which types of assessments, activities, or exercises are indicated, contraindicated, or deemed high risk. If an individual does not want to obtain medical clearance, have that individual sign a legally prepared document that releases you and the facility in which you work from any liability related to any injury that may result from exercise participation or assessment. Once the client has been cleared for exercise and you have a full understanding of the client's/participant's health status and medical history, including his or her current use of medications, a formal risk-management plan for potential emergencies must be prepared and reviewed periodically.

Assessment

The main objective of a health assessment is to establish the client's/participant's baseline fitness level in order to design an appropriate exercise program. Explain the risks and benefits of each assessment and provide the client/participant with any pertinent instructions. Prior to conducting any type of assessment, the client/participant must be given an opportunity to ask questions and read and sign an informed consent. The types and order of assessments are dictated by the client's/participant's health status, fitness level, symptoms, and/or use of medications. Remember that each assessment has specific protocols and only those within your scope of practice should be administered. Once the assessments are completed, evaluate and discuss the results objectively as they relate to the client's/participant's health condition and goals. Educate the client/participant and emphasize how an exercise program will benefit the client/participant.

Program Design

You must not prescribe exercise, diet, or treatment, as doing so is outside your scope of practice and implies ordering or advising a medicine or treatment. Instead, it is appropriate for you to design exercise programs that improve components of physical fitness and wellness while adhering to the limitations of a previous injury or condition as determined by a certified, registered, or licensed allied health professional. Because nutritional laws and the practice of dietetics vary in each state, province, and country, understand what type of basic nutritional information is appropriate and legal for you to disseminate to your client/participant. The client's/participant's preferences, and short- and long-term goals as well as current industry standards and guidelines must be taken into consideration as you develop a formal yet realistic exercise and weight-management program. Provide as much detail for all exercise parameters such as mode, intensity, type of exercise, duration, progression, and termination points.

Program Implementation

Do not underestimate your ability to influence the client/participant to become active for a lifetime. Be sure that each class or session is well-planned, sequential, and documented. Instruct the client/participant how to safely and properly perform the appropriate exercises and communicate this in a manner in which the client/participant will understand and retain. Each client/participant has a different learning curve that will require different levels of attention, learning aids, and repetition. Supervise the client/participant closely, especially when spotting or cueing is needed. If supervising a group of two or more, ensure that you can supervise and provide the appropriate amount of attention to each individual at all times. Ideally, the group will have similar goals and will be performing similar exercises or activities. Position yourself so that you do not have to turn your back to any client/participant performing an exercise.

Facilities

Although the condition of a facility may not always be within your control, you are still obligated to ensure a hazard-free environment to maximize safety. If you notice potential hazards in the health club, communicate these hazards to the client and the facility management. For example, if you notice that the clamps that keep the weights on the barbells are getting rusty and loose, it would be prudent of you to remove them from the training area and alert the facility that immediate repair is required.

Equipment

Obtain equipment that meets or exceeds industry standards and utilize the equipment only for its intended use. Arrange exercise equipment and stations so that adequate space exists between equipment, participants, and foot traffic. Schedule regular maintenance and inspect equipment prior to use to ensure it is in proper working condition. Avoid the use of homemade equipment, as your liability is greater if it causes injury to a person exercising under your supervision.

Provide Equal and Fair Treatment to All Clients/Participants

ACE-certified Professionals are obligated to provide fair and equal treatment for each client/participant without bias, preference, or discrimination against gender, ethnic background, age, national origin, basis of religion, or physical disability.

The Americans with Disabilities Act protects individuals with disabilities against any type of unlawful discrimination. A disability can be either physical or mental, such as epilepsy, paralysis, HIV infection, AIDS, a significant hearing or visual impairment, mental retardation, or a specific learning disability. ACE-certified Professionals should, at a minimum, provide reasonable accommodations to each individual with a disability. Reasonable simply means that you are able to provide accommodations that do not cause you any undue hardship that requires additional or significant expense or difficulty. Making an existing facility accessible by modifying equip-ment or devices, assessments, or training materials are a few examples of providing reasonable accommodations. However, providing the use of personal items or providing items at your own expense may not be considered reasonable.

This ethical consideration of providing fair and equal treatment is not limited to behavioral interactions with clients, but also extends to exercise programming and other business-related services such as communication, scheduling, billing, cancellation policies, and dispute resolution.

Stay Up-to-Date on the Latest Health and Fitness Research and Understand Its Practical Application

Obtaining ACE-certification required you to have broad-based knowledge of many disciplines; however, this credential should not be viewed as the end of your professional development and education. Instead, it should be viewed as the beginning or foundation. The dynamic nature of the health and fitness industry requires you to maintain an understanding of the latest research and professional standards and guidelines, and of their impact on the design and implementation of exercise programming. To stay informed, make time to review a variety of industry resources such as professional journals, position statements, trade and lay periodicals, and correspondence courses, as well as to attend professional meetings, conferences, and educational workshops.

An additional benefit of staying up-to-date is that it also fulfills your certification renewal requirements for continuing education credit (CEC). To maintain your ACE-certification status, you must obtain an established amount of CECs every two years. CECs are granted for structured learning that takes place within the educational portion of a course related to the profession and presented by a qualified health and fitness professional.

Maintain Current CPR Certification and Knowledge of First-aid Services

ACE-certified Professionals must be prepared to recognize and respond to heart attacks and other life-threatening emergencies. Emergency response is enhanced by training and maintaining skills in CPR, first aid, and using automated external defibrillators (AEDs), which have become more widely available. An AED is a portable electronic device used to restore normal heart rhythm in a person experiencing a cardiac arrest and can reduce the time to defibrillation before EMS personnel arrive. For each minute that defibrillation is delayed, the victim's chance of survival is reduced by 7 to 10%. Thus, survival from cardiac arrest is improved dramatically when CPR and defibrillation are started early.

Comply With All Applicable Business, Employment, and Intellectual Property Laws

As an ACE-certified Professional, you are expected to maintain a high level of integrity by complying with all applicable business, employment, and copyright laws. Be truthful and forthcoming with communication to clients/participants, co-workers, and other health and fitness professionals in advertising, marketing, and business practices. Do not create false or misleading impressions of credentials, claims, or sponsorships, or perform services outside of your scope of practice that are illegal, deceptive, or fraudulent.

All information regarding your business must be clear, accurate, and easy to understand for all potential clients/participants. Provide disclosure about the name of your business, physical address, and contact information, and maintain a working phone number and email address. So that clients/participants can make an informed choice about paying for your services, provide detailed information regarding schedules, prices, payment terms, time limits, and conditions. Cancellation, refund, and rescheduling information must also be clearly stated and easy to understand. Allow the client/participant an opportunity to ask questions and review this information before formally agreeing to your services and terms.

Because employment laws vary in each city, state, province, and country, familiarize yourself with the applicable employment regulations and standards to which your business must conform. Examples of this may include conforming to specific building codes and zoning ordinances or making sure that your place of business is accessible to individuals with a disability.

The understanding of intellectual property law and the proper use of copyrighted materials is an important legal issue for all ACE-certified Professionals. Intellectual property laws protect the creations of authors, artists, software programmers, and others with copyrighted materials. The most common infringement of intellectual property law in the fitness industry is the use of music in an exercise class. When commercial music is played in a for-profit exercise class, without a performance or blanket license, it is considered a public performance and a violation of intellectual property law. Therefore, make sure that any music, handouts, or educational materials are either exempt from intellectual property law or permissible under laws by reason of fair use, or obtain express written consent from the copyright holder for distribution, adaptation, or use. When in doubt, obtain permission first or consult with a qualified legal professional who has intellectual property law expertise.

Maintain the Confidentiality of All Client/Participant Information

Every client/participant has the right to expect that all personal data and discussions with an ACE-certified Professional will be safeguarded and not disclosed without the client's/participant's express written consent or acknowledgement. Therefore, protect the confidentiality of all client/participant information such as contact data, medical records, health history, progress notes, and meeting details. Even when confidentiality is not required by law, continue to preserve the confidentiality of such information.

Any breach of confidentiality, intentional or unintentional, potentially harms the productivity and trust of your client/participant and undermines your effectiveness as a fitness professional. This also puts you at risk for potential litigation and puts your client/class participant at risk for public embarrassment and fraudulent activity such as identity theft.

Most breaches of confidentiality are unintentional and occur because of carelessness and lack of awareness. The most common breach of confidentiality is exposing or storing a client's personal data in a location that is not secure. This occurs when a client's/participant's file or information is left on a desk, or filed in a cabinet that has no lock or is accessible to others. Breaches of confidentiality may also occur when you have conversations regarding a client's/participant's performance or medical/health history with staff or others and the client's/participant's first name or other identifying details are used.

Post and adhere to a privacy policy that communicates how client/participant information will be used and secured and how a client's/participant's preference regarding unsolicited mail and email will be respected. When a client/participant provides you with any personal data, new or updated, make it a habit to immediately secure this information and ensure that only you and/or the appropriate individuals have access to it. Also, the client's/participant's files must only be accessed and used for purposes related to health and fitness services. If client/participant information is stored on a personal computer, restrict access by using a protected password. Should you receive any inquiries from family members or other individuals regarding the progress of a client/participant or other personal information, state that you cannot provide any information without the client's/participant's permission. If and when a client/participant permits you to release confidential information to an authorized individual or party, utilize secure methods of communication such as certified mail, sending and receiving information on a dedicated private fax line, or email with encryption.

Refer Clients/Participants to More Qualified Health or Medical Professionals When Appropriate

A fitness certification is not a professional license. Therefore, it is vitally important that ACE-certified Professionals who do not also have a professional license (i.e., physician, physical therapist, dietitian, psychologist, and attorney) refer their clients/participants to a more qualified professional when warranted. Doing so not only benefits your clients/participants by making sure that they receive the appropriate attention and care, but also enhances your credibility and reduces liability by defining your scope of practice and clarifying what services you can and cannot reasonably provide.

Knowing when to refer a client/participant is, however, as important as choosing to which professional to refer. For instance, just because a client/participant complains of symptoms of muscle soreness or discomfort or exhibits signs of fatigue or lack of energy is not an absolute indication to refer your client/participant to a physician. Because continual referrals such as this are not practical, familiarize and educate yourself on expected signs and symptoms, taking into consideration the client's/participant's fitness level, health status, chronic disease, disability, and/or background as they are screened and as they begin and progress with an exercise program. This helps you better discern between emergent and non-emergent situations and know when to refuse to offer your services, continue to monitor, and/or make an immediate referral.

It is important that you know the scope of practice for various health professionals and which types of referrals are appropriate. For example, some states require that a referring physician first approve visits to a physical therapist, while other states allow individuals to see a physical therapist directly. Only registered or licensed dietitians or physicians may provide specific dietary recommendations or diet plans; however, a client/participant who is suspected of an eating disorder should be referred to an eating disorders specialist. Refer clients/participants to a clinical psychologist if they wish to discuss family or marital problems or exhibit addictive behaviors such as substance abuse.

Network and develop rapport with potential allied health professionals in your area before you refer clients/participants to them. This demonstrates good will and respect for their expertise and will most likely result in reciprocal referrals for your services and fitness expertise.

Uphold and Enhance Public Appreciation and Trust for the Health and Fitness Industry

The best way for ACE-certified Professionals to uphold and enhance public appreciation and trust for the health and fitness industry is to represent themselves in a dignified and professional manner. As the public is inundated with misinformation and false claims about fitness products and services, your expertise must be utilized to dispel myths and half-truths about current trends and fads that are potentially harmful to the public.

When appropriate, mentor and dispense knowledge and training to less-experienced fitness professionals. Novice fitness professionals can benefit from your experience and skill as you assist them in establishing a foundation based on exercise science, from both theoretical and practical standpoints. Therefore, it is a disservice if you fail to provide helpful or corrective information—especially when an individual, the public, or other fitness professionals are at risk for injury or increased liability. For example, if you observe an individual using momentum to perform a strength-training exercise, the prudent course of action would be to suggest a modification. Likewise, if you observe a fitness professional in your workplace consistently failing to obtain informed consents before clients/participants undergo fitness testing or begin an exercise program, recommend that he or she consider implementing these forms to minimize liability.

Finally, do not represent yourself in an overly commercial or misleading manner. Consider the fitness professional who places an advertisement in a local newspaper stating: Lose 10 pounds in 10 days or your money back! It is inappropriate to lend credibility to or endorse a product, service, or program founded upon unsubstantiated or misleading claims; thus a solicitation such as this must be avoided, as it undermines the public's trust of health and fitness professionals.

Establish and Maintain Clear Professional Boundaries

Working in the fitness profession requires you to come in contact with many different people. It is imperative that a professional distance be maintained in relationships with all clients/participants. Fitness professionals are responsible for setting and monitoring the boundaries between a working relationship and friendship with their clients/participants. To that end, ACE-certified Professionals should:

- Never initiate or encourage discussion of a sexual nature
- Avoid touching clients/participants unless it is essential to instruction
- Inform clients/participants about the purpose of touching and find an alternative if the client/participant objects
- Discontinue all touching if it appears to make the client/participant uncomfortable
- Take all reasonable steps to ensure that any personal and social contacts between themselves and their clients/participant do not have an adverse impact on the trainer–client or instructor–participant relationship.

If you find yourself unable to maintain appropriate professional boundaries with a client/participant (whether due to your attitudes and actions or those of the client/participant), the prudent course of action is to terminate the relationship and, perhaps, refer the client/participant to another professional. Keep in mind that charges of sexual harassment or assault, even if groundless, can have disastrous effects on your career.

Appendix B

Exam Content Outline

The Examination Content Outline is essentially a blueprint for the exam. As you prepare for the exam, it is important to remember that all questions are based on this outline.

Target Audience Statement

Lifestyle & Weight Management Consultants (LWMCs) develop and implement weight-management programs in cooperation with qualified health professionals, balancing the three critical components of nutrition, exercise programming, and behavior modification within the framework of current guidelines and standards.

The following eligibility requirements have been established for the LWMC certification examination:

- At least 18 years of age.
- Adult CPR certification, current at the time of the examination.
- Hold a current ACE Personal Trainer, Group Fitness Instructor, or Advanced Health & Fitness Specialist Certification; or an NCCA-accredited certification in health and fitness; or hold a four-year

(bachelor's) degree in Exercise Science, Nutrition, or a related field. Registrants holding degrees in Nutrition or Nursing must submit documentation supporting completion of Exercise Science–related coursework at the time of registration.
- Recommended: 300 hours of work experience designing and implementing weight management and exercise programs for overweight and obese individuals is recommended.

Domains, Tasks and Knowledge and Skill Statements

A Role Delineation Study completed for the Lifestyle & Weight Management Consultant certification first identified the major categories of responsibility for the professional. These categories are defined as domains. It was determined that the profession can be divided into four performance domains, or major areas of responsibility. These performance domains are:

Domain I: Client Assessment
Domain II: Program Development and Implementation
Domain III: Program Modification and Adherence
Domain IV: Professional Responsibility

The Lifestyle & Weight Management Consultant draws upon knowledge from three foundational sciences or content domains in their work. This content domain includes all topics important to the competence of the Lifestyle & Weight Management Consultant and applies primarily to the client assessment, program development and implementation, and program modification and adherence performance domains.

The content domains are:
- Nutrition
- Lifestyle Modification
- Exercise Science

Table 1: Exam Content Blueprint for Exercise Science Domain: Lifestyle & Weight Management Consultant Certification

	Test Blueprint	
Specific Topics Domain	Percentage of Items on Test	Number of Items on Test
Anatomy	4.03%	5
Exercise Physiology	6.18%	7
Kinesiology	4.38%	5
Total:	**14.59%**	**17**

Table 2: Exam Content Outline: Lifestyle & Weight Management Consultant Certification

Content Domain					
Performance Domain	Total Items	Nutrition	Lifestyle Modification	Exercise Science	Domain-specific Knowledge
Client Assessment	38	7	7	5	19
Program Development and Implementation	42	8	7	6	21
Program Modification and Adherence	36	6	6	6	18
Professional Responsibility	9	0			
Total:	**125**	**21**	**20**	**17**	**58**

The domain of Exercise Science was delineated further into three significant topics: anatomy, exercise physiology, and kinesiology (Table 1). Within each performance domain, there is additional domain-specific information referring to tests, procedures, and techniques.

Each domain is composed of Task Statements that detail the job-related functions under each domain. Each task statement is further divided into Knowledge and Skill Statements to further detail the scope of information required and how that information is applied in a practical setting for task statement.

The domains are presented in two dimensions (Table 2):

- Performance domains that exist vertically for Client Assessment, Program Development and Implementation, Program Modification and Adherence, and Professional Responsibility
- Content domains that exist horizontally for Nutrition, Lifestyle Modification, Exercise Science (Anatomy, Exercise Physiology and Kinesiology), and Domain-Specific Knowledge

Domain I: Client Assessment 30%

Task 1 - Establish an environment that fosters effective communication using appropriate interviewing techniques to obtain accurate, comprehensive information and establish rapport

Knowledge of:

1. Communication techniques (e.g., active listening, appropriate eye contact, reflecting, and other attending behaviors, nonverbal vs. verbal communication).
2. Effective interviewing techniques (e.g., open-ended questioning, clarifying, paraphrasing, probing, informing, summarizing).
3. Factors that build and enhance rapport (e.g., empathy, genuineness, nonjudgmental responses, client confidentiality).
4. Cultural, ethnic, and personal differences as they affect communication, lifestyle, dietary habits, and personal and interpersonal behavior (e.g., common assumptions, misconceptions, complicating factors).
5. Environmental factors that affect communication (e.g., location, noise, temperature, distractions, sense of privacy).
6. Psychological factors that influence an individual's self-image and their impact on the communication process.

Skill in:

1. Selecting an appropriate environment for consultation sessions.
2. Applying interviewing and communication techniques.
3. Respecting the client's personal characteristics (e.g., gender, age, cultural/ethnic background) in all communication.
4. Building rapport.
5. Avoiding behaviors that are detrimental to building rapport (e.g., prejudicial statements, negative body language, and unproductive assumptions with regard to client's body size, eating habits, past success/failures with weight management).
6. Interpreting body language and recognizing incongruities between verbal and nonverbal behaviors.

Task 2 - Interview the client using a health risk appraisal to make appropriate test selections and determine the need for referral to an appropriate health professional.

Knowledge of:

1. Components of a client screening and health history form that document the client's physical and psychological health status, such as age, gender, body weight, blood pressure, personal health risk factors, mental health treatment history, biomechanical injuries/limitations, medications, and supplements.

2. Effects of and appropriate precautions to take with respect to prescription and non-prescription drugs (e.g., beta blockers, diuretics, antihistamines, tranquilizers, antidepressants, anti-anxiety medications, thyroid medications, diet pills, cold medications, nicotine).
3. Primary and secondary cardiovascular risk factors and their significance relative to referral and appropriate application of assessment tools.
4. Significance and limitations of measurement data obtained from assessment screening and testing.
5. Applicable guidelines and position statements published by accepted organizations (e.g., American College of Sports Medicine, American College of Obstetricians and Gynecologists, American Heart Association, American Diabetes Association, Institute of Medicine, National Cholesterol Education Program, U.S. Department of Agriculture), and their implications for referral and weight management.
6. Physical and psychological conditions that may require referral to appropriate allied health professionals (e.g., cardiovascular disease, diabetes, anorexia, bulimia, chronic dieting, compulsive overeating, morbid obesity, hypertension, elevated lipids, pregnancy, HIV/AIDS, being underweight, asthma, COPD, stroke, arthritis, anxiety disorder, depression).
7. Appropriate allied health professionals to use as referrals (e.g., physicians, psychotherapists, registered dietitians).

Skill in:

1. Processing the client's health history and interview and observation data relative to accepted guidelines, and making safe and effective decisions regarding continuance and/or referral.
2. Identifying and taking appropriate precautions with respect to prescription and non-prescription drugs.
3. Recognizing the characteristics of physical and psychological conditions that may indicate the need for referral.
4. Initiating referrals to appropriate health professionals, as required.

Task 3 - Review the client's exercise, dietary, and lifestyle questionnaires using appropriate evaluation techniques to identify client goals, exercise preferences, areas for lifestyle modification, and referral to provide the basis for program development.

Knowledge of:

1. The components of a comprehensive client profile including current and past health conditions, readiness to change, health risks, experience with health and fitness lifestyle change, and personal weight-management goal.
2. The factors that indicate a client's readiness to change (e.g., intrinsic and extrinsic motivators, past success with lifestyle change and weight management, goal-setting experiences).
3. Genetic, psychological, and physiological factors related to obesity and how they affect approaches to weight management.
4. Methods used to identify client goals, perceived and unperceived needs, and expectations for change.
5. Cognitive, affective, and psychomotor factors and learning styles that influence progress and goal attainment.
6. When to de-emphasize the use of fitness testing and body-composition analysis.
7. The relationship of body mass index (BMI), waist-to-hip ratio (WHR), and circumference measurements to body weight, and the determination of appropriate body weight.

Task 4 - Conduct appropriate testing using accepted protocols in order to collect baseline information about the client's fitness, health, and dietary habits.

Knowledge of:
1. Appropriate physiological fitness testing protocols, purposes, inherent risks, and benefits associated with testing protocols (e.g. aerobic fitness, body composition, flexibility, muscular strength and muscular endurance).
2. Appropriate dietary assessments protocols, purposes, inherent risks, and benefits (e.g., 24-hour dietary recalls, food logs).
3. Warning signs and symptoms that necessitate intervention during testing.
4. Physiological effects of, and appropriate precautions required with respect to, medications.
5. The motivational and demotivational implications of fitness testing.

Skill in:
1. Assessing physical-fitness levels using appropriate testing protocols.
2. Recognizing warning signs and symptoms that necessitate intervention during testing.
3. Interviewing and data-collection techniques to collect nutritional data.

Domain II: Program Development and Implementation 34%

Task 1 - Determine baseline values by comparing the client's assessment data to industry standards and guidelines in order to develop an individualized program.

Knowledge of:
1. Applicable standards, guidelines, and position statements published by accepted organizations (e.g., ACSM, YMCA, ACOG, ADA, AHA, IOM, NCEP, USDA) to use in the formulation of program development.
2. Methods of interpreting the client's assessment data as it relates to established guidelines.

Skill in:
1. Gathering applicable standards and guidelines published by accepted organizations.
2. Applying acceptable standards and guidelines in the development of individualized programs.
3. Interpreting applicable standards, guidelines, and client health data.

Task 2 - Establish effective goals based on the client's needs, preferences, expectations, and potential barriers in order to create program direction and structure.

Knowledge of:
1. Principles of goal-setting.
2. Qualities of a well-stated goal (i.e., specific, measurable, attainable, relevant, and time-bound).
3. Potential obstacles and challenges that may interfere with goal-setting and goal achievement.
4. Biological, psychological, and social factors that impact goal-setting and the development of safe and effective programs.
5. Communication styles to ensure collaborative goal-setting based on client needs, preferences, and expectations.
6. Safe and effective weight-loss methods and quantities.
7. Behavior-change principles in goal-setting.

Skill in:
1. Setting goals collaboratively that are specific, measurable, attainable, relevant, and time-bound.
2. Applying principles and knowledge of exercise, nutrition, and weight management to the establishment of short- and long-term goals.
3. Using effective communication techniques to develop an understanding of client needs, preferences, expectations, and potential barriers for goal-setting.

Task 3 - Design appropriate program components consistent with industry standards and guidelines to modify behavior

and ensure a safe and effective path toward goal attainment.

Knowledge of:

1. Concepts of energy balance including dietary intake (caloric values of food) and expenditure (energy BMR, requirements of physical activities).
2. Relationship of physical activity and exercise to health, physical fitness, and weight management with respect to mode, intensity, frequency, and duration of activity.
3. Different approaches to weight management and/or body composition change and the associated efficacy of each.
4. Dietary guidelines emphasizing balance, variety, and moderation.
5. Common nutritional supplements and weight-loss products and their role in weight management.
6. Components of skill-related and health-related parameters of physical fitness.
7. Metabolic and physiological processes and aerobic and anaerobic physical activity.
8. Exercise programming concepts including mode, frequency, intensity, duration, and progression as applied to weight management.

Skill in:

1. Applying principles and knowledge of exercise, nutrition, and weight management.
2. Applying different approaches to weight-loss and/or body composition change safely and effectively.
3. Approximating caloric intake (including MyPyramid servings) and expenditure.
4. Using all components of an activity program (i.e., aerobic, strength, flexibility) and applying exercise programming principles (i.e., frequency, intensity, duration, and progression).

Task 4 - Empower the client through education about assessment information, program components, and the importance of long-term support systems in order to promote understanding, motivation, adherence, and self-efficacy.

Knowledge of:

1. Effective learning, teaching, and communication styles.
2. USDA Dietary Guidelines, macronutrients and micronutrients and their functions, nutrient and caloric content of common foods, and dietary choices related to health conditions.
3. Health, psychological, and performance benefits of physical activity and recommended dietary choices.
4. Importance of support for long-term adherence.
5. Relapse-prevention principles and maintenance strategies.
6. Selection and preparation of healthful foods and beverages at home, in restaurants, and at the grocery store based on food labels, method of preparation, and key words on menus.
7. Misinformation, misconceptions, and sources of reliable information related to exercise, nutrition, and weight management.
8. Supplements, weight-loss products, fad diets, and associated risks.
9. Proper hydration during physical activity.
10. Environmental factors related to physical activity and dietary intake.

Skill in:

1. Communicating the benefits of weight management and participation in physical-activity programs.
2. Assisting the client in developing and/or enhancing social support systems.
3. Preparing the client for lapses and plateaus and developing a plan of action to handle them.
4. Explaining client assessment information as it relates to program design.
5. Explaining the individual program components in relation to program success and long-term adherence.

Task 5 - Maintain rapport by employing effective interpersonal skills to encourage program adoption and adherence.

Knowledge of:

1. Communication styles.
2. Factors that build and enhance rapport.
3. Cultural, ethnic, and personal differences as they affect communication, lifestyle, dietary habits, and personal and interpersonal behavior.
4. Verbal and nonverbal communication.

Skill in:

1. Interpreting body language and recognizing differences between verbal and nonverbal behavior.
2. Applying effective communication skills.
3. Applying techniques that build rapport.
4. Modifying interaction style and content appropriate to the client's personal characteristics.
5. Selecting an appropriate environment for consultation services.
6. Avoiding prejudicial statements, negative, and/or unproductive assumptions with regard to the client's body size, eating habits, exercise habits, and past successes/failures with weight management.

Task 6 - Instruct the client by demonstrating techniques and explaining key concepts in order to impart the knowledge and skills necessary for safe and effective program participation.

Knowledge of:

1. Appropriate application, safety, and effectiveness of various weight-management techniques.
2. Effective learning, teaching, and communication styles.
3. Educational materials that are current, effective, and appropriate.
4. Selection of healthful foods and beverages at home, in restaurants, and at the grocery store based on food guidelines, food labels, method of preparation, and key words on menus.
5. Supplements, weight-loss products, and fad diets and the risks associated with each.
6. Nutritional requirements during physical activity (energy needs, hydration).
7. Components of activity programs (aerobic, strength, flexibility) in relation to mode, frequency, duration, intensity, and progression.
8. Appropriate, safe, and effective exercise techniques and spotting procedures.

Skill in:

1. Explaining concepts related to nutrition and weight management.
2. Recognizing the signs and symptoms of exercise termination criteria and overtraining.
3. Using appropriate spotting techniques for the client.
4. Explaining and demonstrating correct cardiorespiratory, resistance, and flexibility exercise techniques.

Task 7 - Facilitate client participation through observation, feedback, and the use of self-reported data in order to enhance program safety and progression toward goals.

Knowledge of:

1. Effective communication, feedback, and reinforcement techniques.
2. Accuracy of information obtained through client self-reported data and direct measurement.
3. Appropriate documentation procedures (SOAP notes) and their use.
4. Subjective and objective observation techniques.
5. Self-reported data-collection procedures.

Skill in:

1. Educating the client in the use of self-report techniques.
2. Communicating information and feedback to the client and the healthcare team.
3. Observing and documenting a client's progress toward program goals.

Domain III – Program Modification and Adherence 29%

Task 1 - Review and discuss the client's progress toward goals in order to acknowledge achievements and identify barriers to success.

Knowledge of:
1. Principles of goal-setting (i.e., specific, measurable, attainable, relevant, and time-bound).
2. Barriers to attaining goals (e.g., time restraints, weather changes, family obligations, financial issues) and strategies to overcome barriers.
3. Safe and effective weight-loss, lifestyle-change, and physical-fitness programs.
4. Effective communication and interviewing techniques.
5. Methods for evaluating progress and the impact of the client's previous attempts at weight management.
6. Complexity of issues related to obesity, body size, eating disorders, and related lifestyle factors.
7. Professional boundaries as they relate to the client/consultant relationship.

Skill in:
1. Evaluating progress toward goals.
2. Creating appropriate goals that are specific, measurable, attainable, relevant, and time-bound.
3. Identifying and implementing strategies to overcome barriers.
4. Applying principles and knowledge of exercise, nutrition, weight management, and lifestyle change to the collaborative establishment of short- and long-term goals.
5. Applying effective communication and interviewing techniques.
6. Maintaining appropriate professional client/consultant boundaries.
7. Providing appropriate feedback and reinforcement.

Task 2 - Consider the client's perceptions and attitudes by discussing the effectiveness of program components in order to determine areas that require modification.

Knowledge of:
1. The factors that influence an individual's self-image and their impact on communication and goal achievement.
2. Genetic, psychological, and physiological factors related to obesity and how they affect approaches to weight management.
3. Importance of emphasizing the development of healthful habits instead of body weight/composition.
4. Factors that build and enhance rapport (e.g., empathy, genuineness, nonjudgmental responses).
5. Common assumptions with regard to a client's body size, eating habits, and exercise habits, and the impact such assumptions have on the client.
6. Communication techniques (e.g., interviewing, active listening, appropriate eye contact, reflecting, other attending behaviors).
7. Effects of personal issues and biases related to communication, rapport, and program design.

Skill in:
1. Interviewing the client to identify perceptions and attitudes (e.g., listening, questioning, responding).
2. Overcoming personal issues and biases.
3. Recognizing factors that affect the client's self-image and self-acceptance.
4. Applying various behavior-modification techniques.
5. Modifying the client plan with respect to client progress and goals.
6. Differentiating between real and perceived barriers.

Task 3 - Determine the client's current fitness levels, dietary habits, and associated lifestyle behaviors by performing ongoing assessments in comparison with previous values in order to support adherence,

determine program modifications, and evaluate the need for referral.

Knowledge of:

1. Timing, selection, and procedures related to periodic assessments.
2. Significance of, limitations of, and incongruities in assessment data.
3. Appropriate physiological fitness testing protocols and their purposes, inherent risks, and benefits (e.g. aerobic fitness, body composition, flexibility, muscular strength and muscular endurance).
4. Appropriate dietary assessment protocols and their purposes, inherent risks, and benefits (e.g., 24-hour dietary recalls, food logs).
5. Warning signs and symptoms that necessitate intervention during testing.
6. Physiological effects of, and appropriate precautions required with respect to, medications.
7. The motivating and demotivating implications of fitness testing.
8. Scope of practice for relevant health professionals and when to make referrals.
9. Effective and confidential record-keeping methods.

Skill in:

1. Reassessment of physical fitness levels using appropriate testing protocols.
2. Recognizing warning signs and symptoms that necessitate intervention during testing.
3. Evaluating reassessment data with respect to the client's program.
4. Making effective referrals.
5. Maintaining client confidentiality.

Task 4 - Revise program goals collaboratively by revisiting client needs, expectations, and potential barriers in order to provide direction for program modification.

Knowledge of:

1. Principles of effective goal-setting (i.e., specific, measurable, attainable, relevant, and time-bound).
2. Potential obstacles and challenges as they affect communication, lifestyle change, dietary habits, and personal and interpersonal behavior.
3. Physiological, psychological, and social factors that impact goal-setting and the development of safe and effective programs.
4. Relevance and limitations of assessment data in establishing client profile and short- and long-term goals.
5. Facilitating change as it applies to the role of the weight management consultant (e.g., goal-setting, support, motivation).
6. Communication techniques that ensure collaborative goal-setting.
7. Factors that enhance rapport (e.g., empathy, genuineness, nonjudgmental responses).
8. Importance and application of feedback, reinforcement, acknowledgement, and encouragement.
9. Safe and effective methods and rates of weight-loss.

Skill in:

1. Using effective verbal and nonverbal communication techniques (e.g., interviewing, feedback, body language) while respecting the client's personal characteristics.
2. Avoiding behaviors that are detrimental to maintaining rapport (e.g., prejudicial statements, negative body language, inappropriate assumptions with regard to the client's body size, eating habits, and past success/failures with weight management).
3. Applying the principles of exercise, nutrition, and weight management to the collaborative establishment of short- and long-term goals.

Task 5 - Modify the client's existing program based on ongoing assessments, goal achievement, and perceived barriers to promote sustainable lifestyle change.

Knowledge of:

1. Exercise programming with respect to frequency, intensity, duration, and progression as applied to weight management.
2. Appropriate modes of physical activity (e.g., swimming, biking, walking, strength training) and their integration into a weight-management exercise program.
3. Cognitive, affective, and psychomotor factors and learning styles that influence progress and goal attainment.
4. Educational materials that are safe, effective, and appropriate for the client.
5. Strategies to facilitate change as it applies to the role of the weight management consultant (e.g., support systems, motivation).
6. Relapse-prevention principles and maintenance strategies.
7. Self-monitoring techniques.
8. Importance and application of feedback, reinforcement, acknowledgement, and encouragement.

Skill in:

1. Implementing appropriate program revisions with respect to frequency, intensity, duration, and progression as applied to weight management.
2. Using effective and constructive communication techniques.
3. Encouraging client independence and self-efficacy through education, coaching, and recognition of achievements in order to enhance program adherence and achieve long-term success.

Domain IV – Professional Responsibility 7%

Task 1 - Maintain a professional consultant/client relationship by adhering to legal and professional boundaries, standards of care, and the American Council on Exercise Code of Ethics in order to protect the client and minimize liability.

Knowledge of:

1. Professional boundaries as they relate to the client/consultant relationship.
2. American Council on Exercise Code of Ethics.
3. Process for reporting violations of the American Council on Exercise Code of Ethics.
4. Accepted standards of care.
5. Scope of practice.
6. Liability issues associated with acting outside the appropriate standard of care, scope of practice, and the Code of Ethics.

Skill in:

1. Assessing areas of risk (e.g., client, facilities).

Task 2 - Ensure continuing competence and professional growth by staying current with scientifically based research, theories, and practice in order to provide the most effective services for clients, the public, and other health professionals.

Knowledge of:

1. Available continuing education programs (e.g., conferences, workshops, college/university courses, tele-seminars, online courses, in-home study courses).
2. American Council on Exercise continuing education requirements.
3. Appropriate and relevant consumer and professional publications (e.g., journals, books, texts, videos, DVDs, CDs, online publications, and resources).

Skill in:

1. Recognizing credible resources.

Task 3 - Ensure the highest quality of service for clients by establishing a referral network in related disciplines and cooperating as a member of the client's health care team in order to uphold professional standards and maintain an appropriate scope of practice.

Knowledge of:

1. Appropriate health professions required for outside referral.
2. Appropriate forms and documents required to involve outside health professionals in order to maintain continuity of care.

Skill in:

1. Identifying and networking with appropriate health professionals.
2. Establishing a method for referrals.
3. Creating a means of ongoing communication and follow-up with appropriate professionals.

Task 4 - Treat all individuals with respect, empathy, and equality regardless of weight, ethnicity, nationality, sexual orientation, gender, age, disability, religion, marital status, socioeconomic status, and health status in order to maintain integrity in all professional relationships.

Knowledge of:

1. Personal issues and biases that may interfere with effectiveness.

Skill in:

1. Modifying interaction style and content appropriate to client's personal characteristics (e.g., gender, age, cultural/ethnic background).

Task 5 - Document client-related data, communications, and progress using a secure record-keeping system that is confidential, accurate, current, and retrievable in order to maintain continuity of care and minimize liability.

Knowledge of:

1. Implications of breaching client confidentiality.
2. All required paperwork and documentation (e.g., waivers, informed consent, medical history, health risk appraisal, client contracts).
3. Effective and confidential record-keeping.

Skill in:

1. Understanding the importance of confidentiality.
2. Differentiating between non-confidential and confidential documents.

Task 6 - Respond appropriately in emergency situations in accordance with emergency action plans in order to ensure client safety.

Knowledge of:

1. Cardiopulmonary Resuscitation and Automated External Defibrillator procedures.
2. Worksite emergency plan.
3. Appropriate Emergency Medical Service system activation.
4. First aid.
5. Occupational Health and Safety Administration guidelines regarding bloodborne pathogens.

Skill in:

1. Identifying emergency situations.
2. Identifying potential physical hazards.
3. Identifying warning signs that require intervention.
4. Staying calm in emergency situations.

Task 7 - Develop risk-management strategies using recognized guidelines (e.g., IHRSA, ACSM, OSHA) in order to protect the client, consultant, and other relevant parties.

Knowledge of:

1. Negligence laws (comparative and contributory) as they pertain to LWMCs.
2. Intellectual property laws as they apply to video, written materials, Internet, and trademarks.
3. Limitations of waivers and informed consent.
4. Characteristics, types of coverage, and appropriate professional and general liability insurance.
5. Sexual harassment and discrimination laws.

Skill in:

1. Completing appropriate incident reports.

2. Developing an appropriate risk-management program for a facility or business.

Content Domains

The Lifestyle & Weight Management Consultant draws upon knowledge from three foundational sciences or content domains in their work. These content domains include all topics important to the competence of the Lifestyle & Weight Management Consultant and apply primarily to the client assessment, program development and implementation, and program modification and adherence performance domains.

The content domains are:

- Nutrition
- Lifestyle Modification
- Exercise Science

The domain of Exercise Science was delineated further into three significant topics: anatomy, exercise physiology, and kinesiology. Within each performance domain, there is additional domain-specific information referring to tests, procedures, and techniques.

Nutrition

Knowledge of:

1. Macronutrients, micronutrients, hydration, supplements, engineered foods, and alcohol, drugs, and stimulants.
2. Current credible nutrition resources, nutrition guidelines, food labels, food safety, food selection and preparation, and human digestion and absorption.
3. Popular diets, eating disorders, and associated health risks.
4. Nutrition requirements for fitness and sport, stages of life, special populations, vegetarians, energy balance and weight control, and different cultural populations and ethnic groups.

Skill in:

1. Assisting clients with appropriate food selection and dining choices while staying within scope-of-practice boundaries.

Lifestyle Modification

Knowledge of:

1. Elements of lifestyle programming, including stages of change, goal-setting, motivation, problem-solving, responsibility/accountability, adherence/relapse, psychological benefits of participation, and support strategies.
2. Common assessment tools (e.g., attitudes, belief systems, behavior, and lifestyle).
3. Communication techniques including learning and leadership styles.
4. Environmental, individual/personal factors, and obesity and eating disorders.

Exercise Science

Knowledge of:

Anatomy

1. General anatomy of the following systems: musculoskeletal, cardiorespiratory, neuromuscular, digestive, and endocrine.
2. General anatomical terminology (e.g. landmarks, planes of movement, position, muscle roles, origin, insertion).

Knowledge of:

Kinesiology

1. Human movement as it relates to participant safety.
2. Functional range of motion of the different joints of the body, including joint mobility and flexibility.
3. Muscle function, types of muscular contraction, and factors affecting movement (e.g., neurological, proprioceptive, biomechanical, kinesthetic awareness).
4. Principles of balance, proper postural alignment, and appropriate exercise design to improve these parameters.
5. Biomechanical concepts of human movement, including the use of Newton's Laws

(i.e., inertia, acceleration, and reaction) as they apply to exercise.

6. Terminology as it applies to muscular fitness (e.g., training effect, resistance, overload, specificity, repetitions, sets, frequency, rest periods, progression, muscular atrophy and hypertrophy).
7. Various methods of resistance, cardiovascular, and flexibility training, and the risks and benefits associated with each.

Knowledge of:

Exercise Physiology

1. Components of physical fitness, principles of training, and acute and chronic responses to exercise programming.
2. Cardiorespiratory systems with respect to oxygen-carrying capacity, delivery, and extraction; and cardiorespiratory terms as they apply to training.
3. Metabolic terminology and physiology including macronutrient utilization, and anaerobic and aerobic metabolism and utilization.
4. Neuromuscular physiology, muscle fiber types and characteristics, and muscle proprioceptors.
5. Benefits of aerobic exercise and programming guidelines to improve cardiorespiratory fitness in both healthy and diseased individuals.
6. Guidelines to observe when exercising in various environmental conditions (e.g., heat, humidity, cold, high altitude, air pollution).
7. Physiology of common musculoskeletal and metabolic disorders (e.g., obesity, diabetes, thyroid, hypertension, hypercholesterolemia).

Natalie Digate Muth

Natalie Digate Muth, M.P.H., R.D., is currently pursuing a medical doctor degree at the University of North Carolina at Chapel Hill. In addition to being a registered dietitian, she is an ACE-certified Personal Trainer and Group Fitness Instructor, an American College of Sports Medicine Health and Fitness Instructor, and a National Strength and Condition Association Certified Strength and Conditioning Specialist. She is also an ACE Master Trainer and a freelance nutrition and fitness author.

Appendix C

Frequently Asked Questions

This section includes answers to some of the most common questions asked by both clients and Lifestyle & Weight Management Consultants themselves.

Frequently Asked Questions From Clients

Does exercise curb appetite?

Research suggests that appetite decreases for about the first hour after strenuous exercise and then normalizes. However, appetite regulation is a very complex process that relies on insulin, hormones, psychological factors, and blood sugar levels. This complexity makes it difficult to generalize the effects of exercise on appetite. Overall, people who participate in moderate exercise tend to eat about the same number of calories (or only slightly more) than they would if they did not exercise. Competitive athletes overall do consume a lot more food than usual after exercise, but they usually burn off much more than the excess calories they consumed (Blundell & King, 1999).

How long should I wait to exercise after eating?

It is generally recommended that exercisers wait about three hours after eating a full meal before engaging in a strenuous exercise program. That's about how long it takes for a balanced meal that includes some carbohydrate, protein, and fat to move from the stomach into the small intestines, where nutrients are absorbed and energy becomes available. Exercising before food has had time to empty from the stomach can cause cramps and abdominal discomfort. But people respond differently and there is no set amount of time to wait. If you exercise in the morning, a quick carbohydrate-dense snack might help to provide some energy during the workout without a lot of discomfort. Carbohydrates are generally digested in approximately an hour, while protein takes about two hours and fat about four hours. But remember, most foods are a combination of the three types of macronutrients.

What should I eat before my workouts?

In general, foods should be eaten about three hours before working out to give the body a chance to move the food out of the stomach and begin digestion and absorption. The food should be something that is relatively high in carbohydrate to maximize blood glucose availability, relatively low in fat and fiber to minimize gastrointestinal distress and facilitate gastric emptying, moderate in protein, and easy on the stomach. While the amount of food to eat varies from person to person, most people do well with approximately 2 grams (8 calories) of carbohydrate per pound of body weight. For morning workouts, eat a small amount of a rapidly digestible carbohydrate, such as a slice of bread or a banana, 30 to 60 minutes before exercise. If you exercise in the afternoon or evening, you may want to have a light snack right before a workout, especially if it's been more than three hours since your last meal.

What should I eat after a workout?

For optimal recovery after an endurance workout, it is important to eat carbohydrates to replace the stored energy (glycogen) that was utilized doing the workout. For best results, the American Dietetic Association (ADA) recommends aiming to eat approximately 1.5 grams of carbohydrate per kilogram of body weight within 30 minutes of finishing the workout and then every two hours for four to six hours (ADA, 2000). A little bit of protein will also help to repair muscles, which is especially important after a resistance-training workout. Of course, the amount of refueling needed depends on the intensity and duration of the workout.

Which is better for weight control: consuming three square meals or eating five to six small meals spread out over the day?

Weight control is achieved by balancing the number of calories consumed with the number of calories burned. Therefore, it doesn't matter if the calories come in the form of three larger meals or five to six smaller meals. However, some people find that they're better able to control their caloric intake in one way or the other. For instance, people who consume three or fewer meals per day may find that long periods between meals leave them feeling famished, which leads them to overeat to compensate. Eating smaller meals spaced throughout the day may help some individuals with calorie control. On the other hand, someone who eats five to six meals per day may forget to make them small meals and instead consume more calories than he or she would with three meals. In the end, it's a matter of preference. One strategy for effective meal planning is to determine the total number of calories (or, alternatively, the total number of servings from each of the food groups) and divide them somewhat equally throughout the day—whether that's three meals or six. It is important to note that people who have diabetes should consume five to six equally small-sized meals to maintain healthy blood sugar levels throughout the day.

How many calories should I eat and how often should I exercise for optimal weight loss?

Several formulas have been developed to estimate caloric needs for weight maintenance. One that is particularly useful is the Mifflin-St Jeor equation:

For men: RMR = 9.99 x weight (kg) + 6.25 x height (cm) – 4.92 x age (years) + 5
For women: RMR = 9.99 x weight (kg) + 6.25 x height (cm) – 4.92 x age (years) – 161

Multiply the RMR value derived from the prediction equation by the appropriate activity correction factor:
1.200 = sedentary (little or no exercise)
1.375 = lightly active (light exercise/sports one to three days per week)
1.550 = moderately active (moderate exercise/sports three to five days per week)
1.725 = very active (hard exercise/sports six to seven days per week)
1.900 = extra active (very hard exercise/sports and a physical job)

Moderately active people are generally advised to consume approximately 1.5 to 1.7 times the calculated resting metabolic rate (RMR). Convert pounds to kilograms by dividing by 2.2. Convert inches to centimeters by multiplying by 2.54.

The numerical caloric value derived from this formula represents how many calories an individual should eat to maintain his or her current weight. To lose 1 pound of fat, a 3,500-calorie deficit is required. This can come from decreasing caloric intake, increasing caloric expenditure or, ideally, both. But keep in mind that losing weight is not the hard part. The hard part is keeping the weight off. It is well-established that people who are most successful at maintaining weight loss are those who engage in regular physical activity.

The USDA 2005 Dietary Guidelines suggest that adults seeking to maintain weight loss accumulate 60 to 90 minutes of moderate physical activity most days of the week. This goal, which may seem overwhelming, can be reached gradually over time by starting with 15- to 30-minute bouts of enjoyable activity.

Is it true that food eaten late at night is more likely to turn into body fat?

Eating late at night does not necessarily lead to greater weight gain, which is dependent on caloric intake and caloric expenditure. If people eat more than they expend, then they will gain weight—regardless of whether the calories come from breakfast, dinner, or a late-night snack. However, in reality, people who eat a lot of food late at night tend to consume more calorie-dense foods and thus eat more calories, which can cause weight gain. Ultimately, it's not when you eat, but what and how much. For example, if you find yourself mindlessly eating chips at 10 o'clock at night while watching TV, then it might be helpful to reverse this fat-promoting behavior by making a behavioral plan that includes not eating after 8 o'clock p.m.

Do I have to stop eating all of the foods that I enjoy to lose weight?

The most successful approach to weight loss and weight-loss maintenance is to make permanent lifestyle changes that include a healthful eating plan and ample physical activity. A diet—which implies short-term and hard-to-adhere-to changes—is not the answer. Thus, while certain foods are prohibited by various diet plans, a healthy lifestyle allows for all foods in moderation. This means that less-healthy foods can be eaten, as long as they make up only a small portion of the total daily caloric intake. The government's MyPyramid plan (www.mypyramid.gov) calls these "discretionary calories."

Should I be taking a supplement to obtain adequate nutrition?

The science on multivitamins is inconclusive. In 2006, a National Institutes of Health (NIH) panel convened to evaluate all of the research on multivitamins and develop recommendations for the public. The panel concluded that insufficient high-quality research has been done to be able to assess whether vitamins help in chronic disease prevention (NIH, 2006). Two exceptions are the strong indications for folic-acid supplements for all women of child-bearing age to prevent neural tube defects in the developing baby, and fish oil/omega-3 fatty acid supplements for the prevention of heart disease in people who are at risk. In general, most dietitians recommend that people take a multivitamin as "insurance" and, more importantly, aim to get optimal nutrition, including vitamins and minerals, from whole foods such as fruits, vegetables, fish, and low- or nonfat dairy products.

I've tried a million diets and have lost a ton of weight, only to regain more back. How much weight should I lose? And how do I keep it off?

The key to permanent weight-loss success is to make lifestyle changes that include a healthy eating plan and ample physical activity. The changes need to be doable enough that you can maintain them indefinitely and not feel deprived or unhappy.

A realistic goal for someone who is overweight or obese is to aim to lose 7 to 10% of starting weight over a six-month to one-year period and then to keep the weight off for at least six months before trying to lose more. This amount of weight loss will provide significant health benefits, including decreases in blood pressure, cholesterol, and the risk of developing diabetes. Also, weight loss is more easily maintained when the weight is lost slowly (about 1 to 2 pounds per week).

I don't have a lot of time. How can I fit a healthy exercise and nutrition program into my busy schedule?

One could argue that the extra time invested each day to healthy meal planning and physical activity will, in the end, add years to one's life and, as such, is worth the effort. While this is true, in a practical sense it may not be enough to encourage someone to make the time for these changes—at least not right away. So it is also important to note that small changes that do not take much extra time, such as taking the stairs instead of the elevator and parking in one of the far away slots at the grocery store, can add up. Also, most fast-food and take-out restaurants now offer healthier choices, such as grilled chicken, salads, and kids meals (that adults can order, too) with fruit and milk. Visit www.smallstep.gov for numerous tips on how to incorporate healthy living into a jam-packed schedule.

Frequently Asked Questions From Lifestyle & Weight Management Consultants

Why do nutritional experts advise people not to skip breakfast if they are trying to lose weight?

Breakfast is considered the most important meal of the day for several reasons. From a weight-loss perspective, research demonstrates that people who eat breakfast weigh less than those who skip breakfast. In fact, one study showed that rates of obesity and metabolic syndrome were 35 to 50% lower among people who eat breakfast (Kircheimer, 2003). This may be because people who skip breakfast tend to overcompensate throughout the day by eating larger portions of food. Some experts suggest that hormonal, metabolic, and appetite factors may play a role. Or, it may be that people who eat breakfast tend to be healthier in general for a variety of other reasons. Regardless, breakfast provides a good opportunity to eat heart-healthy foods such as whole grains, fruits, vegetables, and dairy, which tend to be low-calorie but filling because of their high fiber content. Notably, other types of breakfast foods such as sausage and biscuits or sugary cereals do not provide the same benefits (Kircheimer, 2003).

Why do some people have a more difficult time losing weight than others?

Genetics clearly is a factor in how easily someone loses weight. Also, gender differences play a role in that when men lose weight they tend to lose abdominal fat first, while women generally have a more difficult time losing abdominal fat. However, there are additional, more controllable factors as well. First, the amount of muscle mass an individual has is directly proportional to his or her metabolism, and thus caloric expenditure. People who have a large muscle mass can more easily lose weight when they control caloric intake than someone who has a low muscle mass. Secondly, people who have more weight to lose are more successful in their weight-loss efforts when they decrease their caloric intake and increase physical activity, because their baseline is often a very high-calorie diet. For example, if a 250-pound man normally eats 3,000 calories per day and he cuts back to 2,000 calories per day and expends 200 more calories per day with exercise, he can easily lose more than 3 pounds in one week. On the other hand, if a 125-pound (57-kg) woman who normally eats 2,200 calories per day cuts back to 2,000 calories per day and expends 200 more calories per day with exercise she will lose less than 1 pound per week. Finally, behavioral factors cannot be ignored. Some people are more successful at weight loss because they are better able to adhere to a lower-calorie diet and regularly engage in physical activity.

Are carbohydrates bad? What proportion of carbs, fats, and protein should people eat for optimal weight loss and health?

As far as weight loss goes, the proportion of macronutrients consumed is not as important as the total caloric intake versus caloric expenditure. However, foods rich in fiber and protein tend to be the most filling, which in theory would lead to a reduced intake of food and calories compared to high-fat foods and low-fiber carbohydrates. It is important to remember that people often eat for reasons other than hunger, which means that they will occasionally continue to eat even when they are full. An effective weight-loss program addresses both the recommended food intake as well as the behavioral factors that sometimes get in the way of successful weight loss. From a heart-health perspective, the healthiest overall meal plan appears to be a Mediterranean-type eating plan, which is rich in fruits, vegetables, whole grains, and omega-3 fatty acids from fish, and low in saturated fat, trans fat, sodium, and added sugars.

What are the glycemic index and glycemic load, and how are they related to weight control (if at all)?

Glycemic index is a measure of the amount of increase in blood glucose levels after consuming a particular food. Carbohydrates (CHO) with a high glycemic index value are rapidly broken down into glucose and released into the bloodstream, which causes a rapid peak blood glucose. Some examples of high-glycemic foods are baked potatoes, white rice, most cookies and cakes, bananas, and white bread. Low-glycemic foods are slowly digested and glucose is slowly released into the bloodstream, which leads to a much smaller peak. Milk, sweet potatoes, oatmeal, and apples are low-glycemic foods.

Glycemic load is a measure of the glycemic index multiplied by the number of carbohydrates consumed divided by 100:

$$\text{Glycemic index} \times \text{CHO (g)}/100 = \text{Glycemic load}$$

The glycemic load is useful in that it represents how much a given amount of a food will affect blood sugar levels. The thinking behind glycemic index and glycemic load is that if blood sugar is rapidly increased, insulin levels will rise quickly and lead to increased fat deposition. Published research studies offer conflicting results and it is not certain if glycemic index influences weight loss.

What guidelines can I use to evaluate the quality of a diet?

When evaluating popular diets, ask the following questions:

- *How does the diet cut calories?* For any diet to work, calories consumed need to be less than calories expended. Recall that it takes a 3,500-calorie deficit to lose 1 pound of fat.
- *Is it healthy?* A healthy diet promotes a variety of foods and exercise to improve the six primary modifiable risk factors for cardiovascular disease: high cholesterol, elevated blood pressure, impaired fasting glucose, physical inactivity, obesity, and smoking.
- *What is the nutrient density of the diet?* The best diets advocate at least nine servings daily of a variety of fruits and vegetables, which are generally low-calorie foods that provide most of the body's needed vitamins and minerals, as well as phytochemicals that help ward off infection and disease. Fiber-containing whole grains and calcium-rich, low-fat dairy products should also be encouraged. If the diet relies primarily on a supplement to ensure adequate vitamins and minerals, it probably is not the healthiest choice.
- *Does the diet advocate exercise?* Nutrition is only one component in making a long-term lifestyle change. Exercise moderately accelerates weight loss by increasing caloric deficit and is essential in keeping the weight off.
- *Does it make sense?* To sell books and win over dieters who have "tried everything," diet plans tend to make unbelievable claims that may only be substantiated by dieters' personal testimony. From promises to lose 8 to 13 pounds (3.6 to 5.9 kg) in the first two weeks of a diet to promotion of magic supplements, diets are marketed as so easy and effective that they may seem irresistible, at least at first. Fitness professionals play a critical role in helping clients to see through the hype and misinformation.
- *Where is the evidence?* Research studies can be a rich source of information on the effectiveness and safety of different diets. When assessing research results, it is important to note both the study limitations as well as the results. For example, most diet research has focused on obese middle-aged men and women. Thus, the results may not apply to younger people or those who are only slightly overweight. Also, the duration of most diet studies is one year or less. Therefore, the differences between the diets or the apparent benefits may not hold true for the long term.
- *Does it meet the client's individual needs?* The most negligent diet is one that advocates the same plan to all people regardless of their health status and other individual factors. Clients, especially those with existing health problems such as diabetes or heart disease, should always be encouraged to obtain physician approval before starting a diet or exercise regimen.
- *How much does it cost?* While some people may be able to scrape together enough money to begin an expensive weight-loss program, they may not be able to sustain the cost for an extended period of time. A wiser approach is to plan ahead and assess the individual's readiness to change and commit to a program before making huge lifestyle adjustments and financial sacrifices.
- *What kind of social support does the individual have?* Social support is key to successful weight loss. If a diet requires that an individual eats different food than the rest of the family, he or she probably won't be successful on the diet. If the individual's family is not supportive, he or she may struggle to adhere to the lifestyle change.
- *How easy is it to adhere to the diet?* Long-term adherence to a program (i.e., lifestyle change) is the most important factor for lifelong weight-loss success. And the specific diet really doesn't

matter. Dansinger and his colleagues (2005) conducted a one-year randomized trial to assess the adherence rate and effectiveness of the Atkins,® Ornish,® WeightWatchers,® and Zone® diets. They found that all of the diets modestly reduced body weight and cardiovascular risk factors after the one-year trial. And, for each of the diets, people who adhered to the diet had greater weight loss and risk-factor reductions. Of course, most of the study participants struggled with adherence, which overall was poor for all of the diets. This once again drives home the point that permanent lifestyle change, not a quick-fix, time-bound diet, is essential for successful weight loss and sustainable health improvement.

- *What are the strengths and weaknesses of the following popular diets: South Beach,® Atkins, WeightWatchers, NutriSystem,® Jenny Craig,® and the Zone?* See Table 1 for an evaluation of these popular diets.

What can or should I do to help an individual I believe may have an eating disorder?

If you suspect that someone has an eating disorder, consider using the "CONFRONT" approach advocated by the National Association of Anorexia Nervosa and Associated Disorders (ANAD) (www.anad.org):

C—Concern. Share that the reason you are approaching the individual is because you care about his or her mental, physical, and nutritional needs.

O—Organize. Prepare for the confrontation. Think about who will be involved, where is the best place, why you are concerned, how you plan to talk to the person, and the most appropriate time.

N—Needs. What will the individual need after the confrontation? Have referrals to professional help and/or support groups available should the individual be ready to seek help.

Table 1
Strengths and Weaknesses of Popular Diets

DIET	STRENGTHS	WEAKNESSES
South Beach	Differentiates "good" and "bad" carbs and fats Generally considered healthy after the first phase	Restrictive first phase Encourages too much initial weight loss Studied inadequately
Atkins	Good short-term results Recipes simple to prepare	Nutritionally deficient (too much fat, not enough fiber and fruits) Poor long-term adherence
WeightWatchers	Good variety of foods Behavioral support Lots of education Not too restrictive	Appeals to a specific audience Too costly for some Counselors not health professionals
NutriSystem	Food preparation easy to follow Serving sizes prepackaged	Requires prepackaged foods Expensive Not conducive to long-term adherence Studied inadequately
Jenny Craig	Good nutrition Behavioral support	Expensive Dependence on prepackaged food Counselors not health professionals Studied inadequately
The Zone	Lower in fat than Atkins Recipes simple to prepare Good short-term results	Poor long-term adherence Restricts many nutrient-dense foods

F—Face the confrontation. Be empathetic but direct. Be persistent if the individual denies having a problem.

R—Respond by listening carefully.

O—Offer help and suggestions. Be available to talk and provide other assistance when needed.

N—Negotiate another time to talk and a timeframe in which to seek professional help, preferably from a physician who specializes in eating disorders as well as an experienced psychologist.

T—Time. Remember that the individual will not be "fixed" overnight. Recovery takes time and patience.

Remember that an LWMC plays an important role in helping to identify individuals who may be suffering from an eating disorder and referring them to the appropriate trained professional. It is outside the scope of practice of an LWMC to attempt to counsel and treat individuals with a suspected eating disorder.

What are some general nutrition guidelines for clients with diabetes?

It is especially important for people with diabetes to balance nutrition intake (particularly carbohydrate intake) with exercise and insulin or other diabetic medications to maintain a regular blood sugar level throughout the day. Because most people with diabetes have type 2 diabetes, which is linked to an increased risk for cardiovascular disease, a heart-healthy eating plan including vegetables, fruits, and whole grains is key. While advocates of popular low-carbohydrate programs such as the South Beach, Atkins, and Zone diets claim that consuming a carbohydrate-restricted diet is better for people with diabetes, to date research has not supported any long-term cardiovascular benefit of low-carbohydrate diets versus a MyPyramid-like, moderate- to high-carbohydrate diet. However, it is prudent to recommend that clients limit consumption of simple sugars and carbohydrates with little nutritional value (e.g., cakes, cookies, candy bars), as these foods cause a spike in blood sugar. However, people with type 1 diabetes (insulin-deficient by definition) should carry hard candy or other sugary items to eat if their blood glucose drops too low.

What are some general nutrition guidelines for clients with hypertension?

Research has demonstrated that the DASH (Dietary Approaches to Stop Hypertension) eating plan is effective for the treatment and prevention of hypertension. The DASH plan emphasizes a diet low in saturated fat, cholesterol, and total fat that consists largely of fruits, vegetables, and low-fat dairy products. Fish, poultry, nuts, and other unsaturated fats and whole grains are encouraged as heart-healthy foods, while red meat, sweets, sugar-containing beverages, and high-salt foods should be limited. Salt restriction is recommended for individuals who are salt sensitive, typically—but not always—African Americans and older adults. Unfortunately, there is not a simple test to determine if an individual is salt-sensitive, so the best precaution for all Americans is to limit salt intake to no more than 2,400 mg per day. For more information about the DASH eating plan, refer to www.nhlbi.nih.gov/health/public/heart/hbp/dash/.

References

American Dietetic Association (2000). Position of the American Dietetic Association, Dietitians of Canada, and the American College of Sports Medicine: Nutrition and athletic performance. *Journal of the American Medical Association,* 100, 12, 1543–1556.

Blundell, J.E. & King, N.A. (1999). Physical activity and regulation of food intake: Current evidence. *Medicine & Science in Sports & Exercise,* 31, 11 Suppl., S573–S583.

Dansinger, M.L. et al. (2005). Comparison of the Atkins, Ornish, Weight Watchers, and Zone diets for weight loss and heart disease risk reduction: A randomized trial. *Journal of the American Medical Association,* 293, 1, 43–53.

Kircheimer, S. (2003). Breakfast reduces diabetes, heart disease. *WebMD Medical News.* www.webmd.com/content/Article/61/71457.htm.

National Institutes of Health State-of-the-Science Panel (2006). National Institutes of Health state-of-the-science conference statement: Multivitamin/mineral supplements and chronic disease prevention. *Annals of Internal Medicine,* 145, 5, 364–371.

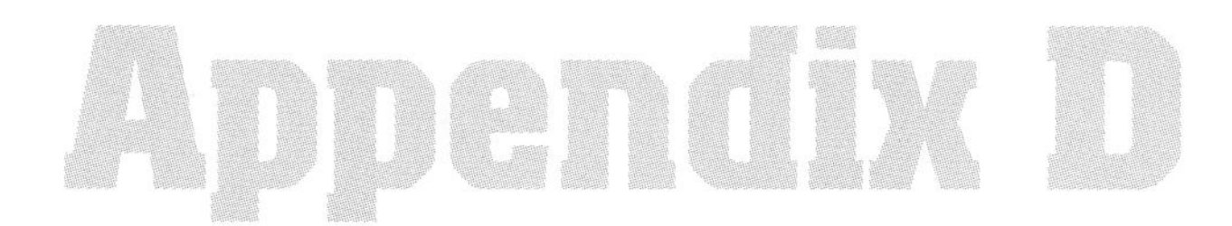

Cardiovascular Medications

GENERIC NAME	BRAND NAME	EXERCISE PRECAUTIONS
Antiarrhythmic		
Quinidine	Quinidex, Quinaglute Cardioquin	May increase HR and decrease BP
Disopyramide	Norpace	
Procainamide	Pronestyl, Procan SR	Little or no effect
Moricizine	Ethmozine	Little or no effect
Mexiletine	Mexitil	Little or no effect
Phenytoin	Dilantin	Little or no effect
Tocainide	Tonocard	Little or no effect
Flecainide	Tambocor	Little or no effect
Propafenone	Rhymol	May decrease HR
Amiodarone	Cordarone	May decrease HR
Beta-blockers Acebutolol Atenolol Betaxol Bisoprolol Carteolol Metoprolol Nadolol Penbutolol Pindolol Propranolol Timolol Sotalol	Sectral Tenormin Kerlone Zebeta Cartrol Lopressor, Toprol Corgard Levatol Visken Inderal Blocadren Betapace	Decrease resting and exercise heart rate, consider using RPE to monitor exercise intensity Decrease resting and exercise BP Decrease myocardial contractility Decrease maximum oxygen uptake May cause fatigue and limit exercise capacity in non-ischemic, hypertensive individuals May exacerbate asthma in individuals with hyperactive airways May worsen claudication in individuals with PVD
Alpha & Beta-blocker Carvedilol Labetalol	Coreg Trandate	Same as beta-blocker
Alpha-Adrenergic blocker Doxazosin Mesylate Prazosin Terazosin	Cardura Minipres Hytrin	No effect on HR Lower resting and exercise BP via peripheral vasodilation
Digitalis Digoxin	Lanoxin	May decrease HR in patients with atrial fibrillation No effect on BP May result in non-specific ST-T wave changes at rest and ST depression with exercise

GENERIC NAME	BRAND NAME	EXERCISE PRECAUTIONS
Diuretics *Thiazides* Chlorothiazide Hydorchlorathiazide (HTCZ Metolazone *"Loop"* Furosemide Ethacrynic Acid Torsemide	 Diuril Esidrex, Hyodrodiuril, Microzide Zaroxolyn, Mykrox Lasix Edecrin Demadex	No influence on HR May decrease BP Can cause hypovolemia (dehydration), reduced CO and PVC's due to hypokalemia, and/or hypomagnesemia.
Potassium Sparing Spironolactone Triamterene Amiloride *Combination* Triamterene & HTCZ Amiloride & HTCZ	 Aldactone Dyrenism Midamor Dyazide, Maxide Moduretic	
Calcium Channel Blockers Amlodipine Bepridil Diltiazem Felodipine Isradipine Mibefradil Nicardipine Nifedipine Nisoldipine Reserpine Verapamil Nimodipine	 Norvasc Vascor Cardizem, Dilacor, Tiazac Plendil DynaCirc Posicor Cardene Procardia, Adalat Sular Serpasil, Sandril Calan, Isoptin, Verelan, Covera Nimotop	Variable effects on HR: Diltiazem, Verapamil, and Bepridil may decrease resting and exercise HR; Nifedipine may increase HR Consider using RPE to monitor exercise intensity. Decrease resting and exercise BP.
Hyperlipidemic Cholestyramine Colestipol Clofibrate Dextrothyroxine Gemfibrozil Lovastatin Nicotinic Acid Pravastatin Probucol Simvastatin	 Questran, LoCholest Colestid Atromids Choloxin Lopid Mevacor Nicobid Pravachol Lorelo Zocor	Dextrothyroxine may increase HR and BP and along with Clofibrate can provoke arrhythmias. Nicotinic acid may decrease resting and exercise BP; be careful of hypotension following exercise.
Nitrates Isorbide Nitroglycerin Nitroglycerin Patch	 Isordil, Sorbitrate, Monoket, Ismo, Dilatrate Nitrostat, Nitro-bid Transderm Nitro, Nitrodisc, Nitro-Dur, Minitran, Deponit	May increase resting and exercise HR, decrease resting and exercise BP, and improve exercise capacity in individuals with angina.

GENERIC NAME	BRAND NAME	EXERCISE PRECAUTIONS
Vasodilators		May cause reflex tachycardia
Hydralazine	Apresoline	
Minoxidil	Loniten	Decrease resting and exercise BP
		May accentuate post-exercise hypotension
Other		Generally no effect on exercise, except Pentoxifylline, which may increase exercise capacity in patients with peripheral vascular disease
Dipyridamole	Persantine	
Warfarin	Coumadin	
Pentoxifylline	Trental	
Angiotensin-Converting Enzyme (ACE) Inhibitors		
Benazepril	Lotensin	Little or no effect on HR or BP
Captopril	Capoten	
Enalapril	Vasotec	
Fosinopril	Monopril	
Lisinopril	Prinivil, Zestril	
Perindopril	Aceon	
Quinapril	Accupril	
Rampril	Altace	
Trandolopril	Mavik	

Appendix E

ACE Position Statement on Nutritional Supplements

It is the position of the American Council on Exercise (ACE) that it is outside the defined scope of practice of a fitness professional to recommend, prescribe, sell, or supply nutritional supplements to clients. Recommending supplements without possessing the requisite qualifications (e.g., R.D.) can place the client's health at risk and possibly expose the fitness professional to disciplinary action and litigation. If a client wants to take supplements, a fitness professional should work in conjunction with a qualified registered dietitian or medical doctor to provide safe and effective nutritional education and recommendations.

ACE recognizes that some fitness and health clubs encourage or require their employees to sell nutritional supplements. If this is a condition of employment, fitness professionals should protect themselves by ensuring their employers possess adequate insurance coverage for them should a problem arise. Furthermore, ACE strongly encourages continuing education on diet and nutrition for all fitness professionals.

Glossary

Abduction Movement away from the midline of the body.

Absolute strength The maximal amount of weight an individual can lift one time.

Absorption The uptake of nutrients across a tissue or membrane by the gastrointestinal tract.

Abstinence violation effect The tendency to perceive lapses as indicators that one is no longer in a behavior-change program, and thus a rationalization for discontinuing one's behavior-change efforts.

Acceptable Macronutrient Distribution Range The range of intake for a particular energy source that is associated with reduced risk of chronic disease while providing intakes of essential nutrients.

Acclimatize To physiologically adapt to an unfamiliar environment and achieve a new steady state. For example, the body can adjust to a high altitude or a hot climate and gain an increased capacity to work in those conditions.

Acetylcholine A white crystalline neurotransmitter and derivative of choline that is released at the ends of nerve fibers in the somatic and parasympathetic nervous systems and is involved in the transmission of nerve impulses in the body.

Acromioclavicular (A/C) joint The junction of the acromion process of the scapula with the distal clavicle.

Actin Thin contractile protein in a myofibril.

Action *See* Action stage.

Action stage The stage of the transtheoretical model during which the individual started a new behavior less than six months ago.

Active listening Mode of listening in which the listener is concerned about the content, intent, and feelings of the message.

Active transport The energy-requiring transfer of a nutrient across a membrane.

Activities of daily living (ADL) Activities normally performed for hygiene, bathing, household chores, walking, shopping, and similar activities.

Adaptation-relapse process model A model developed as part of a theory of behavior change; specifically designed to promote exercise adherence. The three primary factors of this model are self-management and self-regulatory skills, ability to tolerate discomfort, and social support.

Adduction Movement toward the midline of the body.

Adenosine diphosphate (ADP) One of the chemical by-products of the breakdown of ATP during muscle contraction.

Adenosine triphosphate (ATP) A high-energy phosphate molecule required to provide energy for cellular function. Produced both aerobically and anaerobically and stored in the body.

Adequate intake A recommended nutrient intake level that, based on research, appears to be sufficient for good health.

Adipocyte A fat cell.

Adipose tissue Fatty tissue; connective tissue made up of fat cells.

Adrenocorticotropin hormone (ACTH) A hormone released by the pituitary gland that affects various important bodily functions; controls the secretion in the adrenal gland of hormones that influence the metabolism of carbohydrates, sodium, and potassium; also controls the rate at which substances are exchanged between the blood and tissues.

Aerobic With, or in the presence of, oxygen.

Aerobic glycolysis A metabolic pathway that requires oxygen to facilitate the use of glycogen for energy (ATP).

Agonist The muscle directly responsible for observed movement; also called the prime mover.

Air displacement plethysmography (ADP) A body-composition assessment technique based on the same body volume measurement principle as hydrostatic weighing; uses air instead of water.

Aldosterone One of two main hormones released by the adrenal cortex; plays a role in limiting sodium excretion in the urine.

Alpha cells Endocrine cells in the islets of Langerhans of the pancreas responsible for synthesizing and secreting the hormone glucagon, which elevates the glucose levels in the blood.

Alveoli The small membranous air sacs located at the terminal ends of bronchioles where oxygen and carbon dioxide are exchanged between the blood and air in the lungs.

Amennorhea The absence of menstruation.

American Society of Composers, Artists and Publishers (ASCAP) One of two performing rights societies in the United States that represent music publishers in negotiating and collecting fees for the nondramatic performance of music.

Amino acids Nitrogen-containing compounds that are the building blocks of proteins.

Anabolic Muscle-building effects.

Anaerobic Without the presence of oxygen.

Anaerobic glycolysis The metabolic pathway that uses glucose for energy production without requiring oxygen. Sometimes referred to as the lactic acid system or anaerobic glucose system, it produces lactic acid as a by-product.

Anaerobic threshold The point during high-intensity activity when the body can no longer meet its demand for oxygen and anaerobic metabolism predominates. Also called lactate threshold.

Anatomical position Standing erect with the feet and palms facing forward.

Androgenic Effects related to developing masculine characteristics associated with manhood.

Android obesity Abdominal obesity, or body fat distributed in the abdominal area (apple-shaped individuals). Associated with an increased risk of hypertension, coronary artery disease, type 2 diabetes, and all-cause mortality.

Anemia A reduction in the number of red blood cells and/or quantity of hemoglobin per volume of blood below normal values.

Angina Chest pain caused by an inadequate supply of oxygen and decreased blood flow to the heart muscle; an early sign of coronary artery disease. Symptoms may include pain or discomfort, heaviness, tightness, pressure or burning, numbness, aching, and tingling in the chest, back, neck, throat, jaw, or arms. Also called angina pectoris.

Anorexia *See* Anorexia nervosa (AN).

Anorexia nervosa (AN) An eating disorder characterized by self-starvation, distorted body image, and an intense fear of becoming obese.

Antagonist The muscle that acts in opposition to the contraction produced by an agonist (prime mover) muscle.

Antecedent The stimulus that precedes a given behavior, sometimes referred to as a cue or a trigger.

Antidiuretic hormone (ADH) A hormone released by the posterior pituitary gland during exercise; reduces urinary excretion of water and prevents dehydration.

Antioxidant A substance that prevents or repairs oxidative damage; includes vitamins C and E, some carotenoids, selenium, ubiquinones, and bioflavonoids.

Anus The end point of the gastrointestinal tract through which semisolid waste is passed from the body.

Anxiety A state of uneasiness and apprehension; occurs in some mental disorders.

Aorta The major artery of the cardiovascular system; arises from the left ventricle of the heart.

Applied force An external force acting on a system (body or body segment).

Arrhythmia A disturbance in the rate or rhythm of the heartbeat. Some can be symptoms of serious heart disease; may not be of medical significance until symptoms appear.

Artery A blood vessel that carries oxygenated blood away from the heart to vital organs and the extremities.

Arterioles Small-diameter blood vessels that extend and branch out from an artery and lead to capillaries; the primary site of vascular resistance.

Arteriosclerosis A chronic disease in which thickening, hardening, and loss of elasticity of the arterial walls result in impaired blood circulation; develops with aging, and in hypertension, diabetes, hyperlipidemia, and other conditions.

Arthritis Inflammation of a joint or a state characterized by inflammation of joints.

Articulation A joint.

Assertiveness Honest and straightforward expression of thoughts, feelings, and beliefs in a socially appropriate manner.

Assumption of risk A legal defense used to show that a person has voluntarily participated in a specific activity after being made aware of its known dangers.

Asthma A pulmonary condition caused by constriction of the bronchial tubes from allergies, physical activity, or other irritants; characterized by wheezing, coughing, and labored breathing (dyspnea).

Atherosclerosis A specific form of arteriosclerosis characterized by the accumulation of fatty material on the inner walls of the arteries, causing them to harden, thicken, and lose elasticity.

Atrophy A reduction in muscle size (muscle wasting) due to inactivity or immobilization.

Autogenic inhibition An automatic reflex relaxation caused by stimulation of the Golgi tendon organ (GTO).

Automated external defibrillator (AED) A portable electronic device used to restore normal heart rhythms in victims of sudden cardiac arrest.

Autonomic nervous system The part of the nervous system that regulates involuntary body functions, including the activity of the cardiac muscle, smooth muscles, and glands. It has two divisions: the sympathetic nervous system and the parasympathetic nervous system.

Axis of rotation The imaginary line or point about which an object, such as a joint, rotates.

Axon A nerve fiber that conducts a nerve impulse away from the neuron cell body; efferent nerve fiber.

Balance The ability to maintain the body's position over its base of support within stability limits, both statically and dynamically.

Basal energy expenditure (BEE) The calorie expenditure in a fasting state; also called basal metabolism.

Basal metabolic rate (BMR) The energy required to complete the sum total of life-sustaining processes, including ion transport (40% BMR), protein synthesis (20% BMR), and daily functioning such as breathing, circulation, and nutrient processing (40% BMR).

Behavioral contracting A method for outlining an agreement to fulfill a specific set of behaviors within a specified timeframe.

Behavioral theory States that the internal processes (e.g., intentions, perceived need) that individuals go through are of minimal concern when attempting to predict, explain, and affect behavior change. Instead, consequences of behavior are the primary determinants of maintaining or terminating such a behavior over time.

Beta blockers Medications that "block" or limit sympathetic nervous system stimulation. They act to slow the heart rate and decrease maximum heart rate and are used for cardiovascular and other medical conditions.

Beta cell Endocrine cells in the islets of Langerhans of the pancreas responsible for synthesizing and secreting the hormone insulin, which lowers the glucose levels in the blood.

Beta oxidation Metabolic pathway involving the breakdown of fatty acids (digested dietary fat) for the production of ATP.

Bile A greenish-yellow or brownish emulsifier that prepares fats and oils for digestion; produced in and secreted by the liver, stored in the gallbladder, and released into the small intestine.

Binge eating disorder (BED) An eating disorder characterized by frequent binge eating (without purging) and feelings of being out of control when eating.

Bioelectrical impedance analysis (BIA)

A body-composition assessment technique that measures the amount of impedance, or resistance, to electric current flow as it passes through the body. Impedance is greatest in fat tissue, while fat-free mass, which contains 70–75% water, allows the electrical current to pass much more easily.

Bioavailability The degree to which a substance can be absorbed and efficiently utilized by the body.

Biomechanics The mechanics of biological and muscular activity.

Body composition The makeup of the body in terms of the relative percentage of fat-free mass and body fat.

Body density (BD) The relative "heaviness" of an individual in a constant volume of water; calculated by dividing body mass by body volume.

Body mass (BM) The total weight of a person expressed in pounds or kilograms.

Body mass index (BMI) A relative measure of body height to body weight used to determine levels of weight, from underweight to extreme obesity.

Bolus A food and saliva digestive mix that is swallowed and then moved through the digestive tract.

Bradycardia Slowness of the heartbeat, as evidenced by a pulse rate of less than 60 beats per minute.

Broadcast Music Inc. (BMI) One of two performing rights societies in the U.S. that represent music publishers in negotiating and collecting fees for the nondramatic performance of music.

Bronchi The two large branches of the trachea leading into the lungs.

Brush border The site of nutrient absorption in the small intestines.

Bulimia nervosa (BN) An eating disorder characterized by episodes of binge eating, followed by self-induced vomiting or the use of diuretics or laxatives.

Caloric deficit The state of caloric expenditure surpassing caloric intake.

Calorie A measurement of the amount of energy in a food that is available after digestion. The amount of heat required to raise the temperature of 1 kilogram of water 1 degree Celsius. Also called a kilocalorie.

Capillaries The smallest blood vessels that supply blood to the tissues, and the site of all gas and nutrient exchange in the cardiovascular system. They connect the arterial and venous systems.

Carbohydrate The body's preferred energy source. Dietary sources include sugars (simple) and grains, rice, potatoes, and beans (complex). Carbohydrate is stored as glycogen in the muscles and liver and is transported in the blood as glucose.

Cardiac cycle The period from the beginning of one heartbeat to the beginning of the next heartbeat; the systolic and diastolic phases and the interval in between.

Cardiac output The amount of blood pumped by the heart per minute; usually expressed in liters of blood per minute.

Cardiac reserve The work that the heart is able to perform beyond that required of it under ordinary circumstances.

Cardiac sphincter Sits at the upper portion of the stomach; prevents food and stomach acid from splashing back into the esophagus from the stomach; also called the esophageal sphincter.

Cardiovascular disease General term for any disease of the heart.

Cardiovascular endurance The capacity of the heart, blood vessels, and lungs to deliver oxygen and nutrients to the working muscles and tissues during sustained exercise and to remove metabolic waste products that would result in fatigue.

Cardiorespiratory endurance *See* Cardiovascular endurance.

Catecholamine Hormones (e.g., epinephrine and norepinephrine) released as part of the sympathetic response to exercise.

Cellulose An indigestible carbohydrate that comprises much of plants.

Center of gravity (COG) The location at which the body's mass is distributed evenly in all planes.

Central nervous system (CNS) The brain and spinal cord.

Cholecystokinin A hormone released when fat is present in the small intestine; slows digestion and absorption.

Cholesterol A fatlike substance found in the blood and body tissues and in certain foods. Can accumulate in the arteries and lead to a narrowing of the vessels (atherosclerosis).

Chronic disease Any disease state that persists over a certain period of time.

Chylomicron Large lipoprotein particles that transfer fat from food from the small intestines to the liver and adipose tissue.

Chyme The semiliquid mass of partly digested food expelled by the stomach into the duodenum.

Circuit training A form of training that takes the participant through a series of exercise stations, sometimes with brief rest intervals in between; can emphasize muscular endurance, aerobic conditioning, muscular strength, or a combination of all three.

Circumduction A biplanar movement involving the sequential combination of flexion, abduction, extension, and adduction.

Civil law A broad area of law that usually involves the payment of money damages for a wrong committed against another and a claim usually brought by one party against another party (including corporations and partnerships).

Claudication Cramplike pains in the calves caused by poor circulation of blood to the leg muscles; frequently associated with peripheral vascular disease.

Cofactor A substance that needs to be present along with an enzyme for a chemical reaction to occur.

Cognitive restructuring Intentionally changing the way one perceives or thinks about something.

Colon The lower portion of the large intestine, the primary function of which is to absorb water; its segments are the ascending colon, the transverse colon, and the sigmoid colon.

Common law A law that is developed through the interpretation of existing laws in a judicial decision.

Comparative negligence A system used in legal defenses to distribute fault between an injured party and any defendant.

Complete proteins Foods that contain all of the essential amino acids. Eggs, soy, and most meats and dairy products are considered complete protein foods.

Complex carbohydrates The starches or long chains of sugars (polysaccharides) that are found in whole grain breads and cereals, vegetables, fruits, and beans. Take more time to digest than simple carbohydrates.

Concentric A type of isotonic muscle contraction in which the muscle develops tension and shortens when stimulated.

Contemplation *See* Contemplation stage.

Contemplation stage The stage of the transtheoretical model during which the individual is weighing the pros and cons of behavior change.

Contingency contracting *See* Behavioral contracting.

Contract law A system of law governing relationships between those providing products or services to others.

Contributory negligence A legal defense used in claims or suits when the plaintiff's negligence contributed to the act in dispute.

Copyright The exclusive right, for a certain number of years, to perform, make, and distribute copies and otherwise use an artistic, musical, or literary work.

Core stability When the muscles of the trunk function in harmony to stabilize the spine and pelvis to provide a solid foundation for movement in the extremities. A key component necessary for successful performance of most gross motor activities.

Coronary artery disease (CAD) *See* Coronary heart disease.

Coronary heart disease The major form of cardiovascular disease; results when the coronary arteries are narrowed or occluded, most commonly by atherosclerotic deposits of fibrous and fatty tissue; also called coronary artery disease.

Correlates Variables associated with sustained physical activity and weight-loss behaviors; also called determinants.

Cortical bone Compact, dense bone that is found in the shafts of long bones and the vertebral endplates.

Cortisol One of two main hormones released by the adrenal cortex; plays a major role in maintaining blood glucose during prolonged exercise by promoting protein and triglyceride breakdown.

Creatine phosphate (CP) A high-energy phosphate compound found within muscle cells, used to resynthesize ATP for immediate muscle contraction.

Criminal law A system of law whereby certain defined conduct is statutorily prohibited under threat of criminal prosecution of those violating such laws. The unauthorized practice of medicine and other allied healthcare professional practices falls under this system.

Cross training A method of physical training in which a variety of exercises and changes in body positions or modes of exercise are utilized to positively affect compliance and motivation, and also stimulate additional strength gains or reduce injury risk.

Cyanosis A bluish discoloration, especially of the skin and mucous membranes, due to reduced hemoglobin in the blood.

DASH eating plan An eating plan designed to reduce blood pressure; also serves as an overall healthy way of eating that can be adopted by nearly anyone; may also lower risk of coronary heart disease.

Decisional balance One of the four components of the transtheoretical model; refers to the numbers of pros and cons an individual perceives regarding adopting and/or maintaining an activity program.

Dehydration The lack of adequate fluids for the body to function normally. May occur as a result of fluid loss or inadequate intake, or a combination. The most common causes of dehydration are vomiting, diarrhea, excessive urination, and excessive sweating.

Delayed onset muscle soreness (DOMS) Soreness that occurs 24 to 48 hours after strenuous exercise, the exact cause of which is unknown.

Dendrites The portion of a nerve fiber that transmits impulses toward a nerve cell body; receptive portion of a nerve cell.

Deoxyribonucleic acid (DNA) A large, double-stranded, helical molecule that is the carrier of genetic information.

Depression 1. The action of lowering a muscle or bone. 2. A condition of general emotional dejection and withdrawal; sadness greater and more prolonged than that warranted by any objective reason.

Desirable weight *See* Ideal body weight.

Determinants *See* Correlates.

DEXA scan *See* Dual energy x-ray absorptiometry.

Diabetes A disease of carbohydrate metabolism in which an absolute or relative deficiency of insulin results in an inability to metabolize carbohydrates normally; also known as diabetes mellitus.

Diaphysis The shaft of a long bone.

Diastole The period of filling of the heart between contractions; resting phase of the heart.

Diastolic blood pressure The pressure in the arteries during the relaxation phase (diastole) of the cardiac cycle; indicative of total peripheral resistance.

Dietary Reference Intake (DRI) A generic term used to refer to three types of nutrient reference values: Recommended Dietary Allowance (RDA), Estimated Average Requirement (EAR), and Tolerable Upper Intake Level (UL).

Dietary restraint Exerting high levels of control over food intake, so that one is eating more according to cognitive rules (e.g., following a very restrictive diet) rather than in response to physical cues such as hunger and appetite.

Dietary supplement A product or substance

(other than tobacco) that functions to supplement the diet and contains one or more of the following ingredients: a vitamin, mineral, herb or other botanical, amino acid, dietary substance that increases total daily intake, metabolite, constituent, extra, or some combination of the above ingredients.

Dietary Supplement and Health Education Act (DSHEA) A controversial bill passed by Congress in 1994 that sets forth regulations and guidelines for dietary supplements and reduces governmental regulation of dietary supplements.

Digestion The process of breaking down food into small enough units for absorption.

Disaccharide Double sugar units called sucrose, lactose, and maltose.

Diuretic Medications that produce an increase in urine volume and sodium excretion.

Downbeat The regular strong pulsation in music occurring in a continuous pattern at an even rhythm.

Dual energy x-ray absorptiometry (DEXA) An imaging technique that uses a very low dose of radiation to measure bone density. Also can be used to measure overall body fat and regional differences in body fat.

Duodenum The top portion of the small intestine.

Dynamic stabilizers Muscles that actively contribute to core stability.

Dyslipidemia A condition characterized by abnormal blood lipid profiles; may include elevated cholesterol, triglyceride, or LDL levels and/or low HDL levels.

Eccentric A type of isotonic muscle contraction in which the muscle lengthens against a resistance when it is stimulated; sometimes called "negative work" or "negative reps."

Edema Swelling resulting from an excessive accumulation of fluid in the tissues of the body.

Eicosanoids Oxygenated fatty acids that the body uses to signal cellular responses; includes omega 3 and omega 6 fatty acids.

Electrolytes Minerals that exist as charged ions in the body and that are extremely important for normal cellular function.

Emotional eating Eating triggered by emotional states.

Empathy Understanding what another person is experiencing from his or her perspective.

Emphysema An obstructive pulmonary disease characterized by the gradual destruction of lung alveoli and the surrounding connective tissue, in addition to airway inflammation, leading to reduced ability to effectively inhale and exhale.

Employee A person who works for another person in exchange for financial compensation. An employee complies with the instructions and directions of his or her employer and reports to them on a regular basis.

Emulsify Mix together two unmixable substances (such as water and fat).

Encephalopathy Brain swelling; can result from hyponatremia.

Endosteum A soft tissue lining the internal surface of the diaphysis on a long bone.

Energy balance The balance between energy taken in, generally as food and drink, and energy expended through normal living and physical activity; when caloric intake equals caloric expenditure resulting in no change in body weight. A positive or negative energy balance will cause weight gain or weight loss, respectively.

Enzyme A protein necessary to bring about biochemical reactions.

Ephedra A naturally occurring amphetamine-like compound that can powerfully stimulate the nervous system and heart.

Ephedrine A synthetic derivative of ephedra.

Epiglottis The cartilage in the throat that guards the entrance to the trachea and prevents fluid or food from entering it when an individual swallows.

Epinephrine A hormone released as part of the sympathetic response to exercise. Also called adrenaline.

Epiphyseal cartilage Cartilaginous layer between the head and shaft of a long bone where bone growth occurs. Also called a growth plate.

Epiphysis The end of a long bone, usually wider than the shaft (plural: epiphyses).

Epithelial tissue Tissue that covers the surface of the body and lines the body cavities, ducts, and vessels.

Esophagus The food pipe; the conduit from the mouth to the stomach.

Esophageal sphincter *See* Cardiac sphincter.

Essential amino acids Eight to 10 of the 23 different amino acids needed to make proteins. Called essential because the body cannot manufacture them; they must be obtained from the diet.

Essential fat The amount of fat that is necessary for normal functioning of the body. Normal values are 3–5% for men and 8–12% for women.

Essential fatty acid A fatty acid that the body needs for proper growth, maintenance, and functioning but cannot synthesize; include linolenic, linoleic, and arachidonic acids.

Estimated Average Requirement (EAR) An adequate intake of a nutrient in 50% of an age- and gender-specific group.

Estrogen Generic term for estrus-producing steroid compounds produced primarily in the ovaries; the female sex hormones.

Excess postexercise oxygen consumption (EPOC) A measurably increased rate of oxygen uptake following strenuous activity. The extra oxygen is used in the processes (hormone balancing, replenishment of fuel stores, cellular repair, innervation, and anabolism) that restore the body to a resting state and adapt it to the exercise just performed. Also referred to as oxygen debt.

Exercise-induced asthma Intermittent labored breathing precipitated by exertion during exercise.

Expiration The act of expelling air from the lungs; exhalation.

External feedback Extrinsic reinforcement or encouragement.

Extracellular anion A negatively charged ion that is present primarily outside of the cell.

Extracellular cation A positively charged ion that is present primarily inside the cell.

Facilitated diffusion Transfer of a substance across a cellular membrane with the assistance of a protein carrier.

False-hope syndrome The tendency of people to set unrealistic goals.

Fartlek training A form of training during which the exerciser randomly changes the aerobic intensity based on how he or she is feeling. Also called speed play.

Fascia Strong connective tissues that perform a number of functions, including developing and isolating the muscles of the body and providing structural support and protection.

Fast-twitch (FT) muscle fiber One of several types of muscle fibers found in skeletal muscle tissue; also called type II fibers and characterized as having a low oxidative capacity but high a gylcolytic capacity; recruited for rapid, powerful movements such as jumping, throwing, and sprinting.

Fat An essential nutrient that provides energy, energy storage, insulation, and contour to the body. 1 gram of fat equals 9 kcal.

Fat mass (FM) The actual amount of essential and non-essential fat in the body.

Fat-free mass (FFM) That part of the body composition that represents everything but fat—blood, bones, connective tissue, organs, and muscle; also called lean body mass.

Fatty acids Clusters of carbon-chained atoms that are the building blocks of dietary fat and important for the production of energy during low-intensity exercise.

Feedback An internal response within a learner; during information processing, it is the correctness or incorrectness of a response that is stored in memory to be used for future reference. Also, verbal or nonverbal information about current behavior that can be used to improve future performance.

Ferritin The storage form of iron.

Fiber Carbohydrate chains the body cannot break down for use and which pass through the body undigested.

Flexibility The ability to move joints through their normal full range of motion.

Foramina Holes or openings in a bone or between body cavities.

Frontal plane A longitudinal section that runs at a right angle to the sagittal place, dividing the body into anterior and posterior halves.

Fructooligosaccharides A category of oligosaccharides that are mostly indigestible; may help to relieve constipation, improve triglyceride levels, and decrease production of foul-smelling digestive by-products.

Fructose Fruit sugar; the sweetest of the monosaccharides; found in varying levels in different types of fruits.

Functional food Any whole food or fortified, enriched, or enhanced food that has a potentially beneficial effect on human health beyond basic nutrition.

Galactose A monosaccharide; a component of lactose.

Ganglia A group of nerve cell bodies usually located in the peripheral nervous system.

Gastric-inhibitor peptide A hormone that slows motility of the intestine to allow foods that require more time for digestion and absorption to be absorbed.

Gastric emptying The process by which food is emptied from the stomach into the small intestines.

Gastrin A hormone that maintains the pH of the stomach by signaling the cells that produce hydrochloric acid whenever food enters the stomach.

Gastrointestinal (GI) tract A long hollow tube from mouth to anus where digestion and absorption occur; the principle organs are the stomach and intestines.

Ghrelin A hormone produced in the stomach that is responsible for stimulating appetite.

Glenohumeral (G/H) joint The ball-and-socket joint composed of the glenoid fossa of the scapula and the humeral head.

Glucagon A hormone released from the alpha cells of the pancreas when blood glucose levels are low; stimulates glucose release from the liver to increase blood glucose. Also releases free fatty acids from adipose tissue to be used as fuel.

Glucocorticoid An adrenocortical steroid hormone that increases gluconeogenesis, exerts an anti-inflammatory effect, and influences many bodily functions.

Gluconeogenesis The process of forming carbohydrates in the liver from molecules such as amino acids and fatty acids.

Glucose A simple sugar; the form in which all carbohydrates are used as the body's principal energy source.

Glycemic index (GI) A measurement of the impact on blood glucose levels after ingestion of particular carbohydrates.

Glycemic load (GL) A ranking system for carbohydrate content in foods based on their glycemic index (GI) and the portion size.

Glycogen The chief carbohydrate storage material. It is formed by the liver and stored in the liver and muscle.

Glycogenolysis Glycogen breakdown.

Glycolysis The breakdown of glucose or of its storage form glycogen.

Golgi tendon organ (GTO) A sensory organ within a tendon that, when stimulated, causes an inhibition of the entire muscle group to protect against too much force.

Gross negligence A form of negligence that is worse than normal negligence. Generally, a waiver clause cannot prevent a suit for gross negligence or for wanton or recklessness or intentional misconduct in any state or jurisdiction.

Growth hormone (GH) A hormone secreted by the pituitary gland that facilitates protein synthesis in the body.

Gynoid obesity Adipose tissue or body fat

distributed on the hips and in the lower body (pear-shaped individuals).

Health belief model A model to explain health-related behaviors that suggests that an individual's decision to adopt healthy behaviors is based largely upon their perception of susceptibility to an illness and the probable severity of the illness. The person's view of the benefits and costs of the change also are considered.

Health psychology A field of psychology that examines the causes of illnesses and studies ways to promote and maintain health, prevent and treat illnesses, and improve the healthcare system.

Heart rate (HR) The number of heart beats per minute.

Heart-rate reserve (HRR) The reserve capacity of the heart; the difference between maximal heart rate and resting heart rate. It reflects the heart's ability to increase the rate of beating and cardiac output above resting level to maximal intensity.

Heat index Guidelines regarding when exercise can be safely undertaken or when it should be avoided based on measures of heat and humidity.

Hemicellulose An indigestible fiber.

Hemoglobin The protein molecule in red blood cells specifically adapted to carry (by bonding with) oxygen molecules.

Hemopoiesis The formation of blood cells.

Herniated disc Rupture of the outer layers of fibers that surround the gelatinous portion of the disc.

High-density lipoprotein (HDL) A plasma complex of lipids and proteins that contains relatively more protein and less cholesterol and triglycerides. High HDL levels are associated with a low risk of coronary heart disease.

Hold harmless A form of waiver clause that places all risk associated with training on the client.

Hormone A chemical substance produced and released by an endocrine gland and transported through the blood to a target organ.

Human immunodeficiency virus (HIV) A retrovirus (family Retroviridae, subfamily Lentvirinae) that is about 100 nm in diameter and is the etiologic agent of AIDS.

Hydrostatic weighing An underwater test that measures the percentage of lean body weight and body fat, based on the principle that fat floats and muscle and bones sink (Archimedes principle); considered the gold standard of body-composition assessment due its accuracy.

Hypercholesterolemia An excess of cholesterol in the blood.

Hyperglycemia An abnormally high content of glucose (sugar) in the blood (above 100 mg/dL).

Hyperplasia Increased cell production in normal tissue. An excess of normal tissue.

Hypertension Elevated blood pressure generally defined as a systolic blood pressure reading greater than or equal to 140 mmHg or a diastolic blood pressure equal to or greater than 90 mmHg.

Hyperthyroidism A condition characterized by hyperactivity of the thyroid gland; the metabolic processes of the body are accelerated.

Hypertrophy An increase in the cross-sectional size of a muscle in response to progressive resistance training.

Hypoglycemia A deficiency of glucose in the blood commonly caused by too much insulin, too little glucose, or too much exercise. Most commonly found in the insulin-dependent diabetic and characterized by symptoms such as fatigue, dizziness, confusion, headache, nausea, or anxiety.

Hypokalemia A deficiency of potassium in the blood.

Hyponatremia Low blood sodium levels as a result of overconsumption of water; severe cases can lead to brain swelling and death.

Hypotension Low blood pressure.

Hypothermia Abnormally low body temperature.

Hypothyroidism Endocrine disease whereby there is an inadequate secretion of thyroid hormones causing a decreased basal metabolic rate and possibly accompanied by lethargy, fatigue and decreases in physical and mental ability.

Ideal body weight (IBW) A term used to describe the weight that people are expected to weigh for good health, based on age, sex, and height. Also called ideal weight or desirable body weight.

Ideal weight *See* Ideal body weight (IBW).

Ileum One of three sections of the small intestine.

Iliotibial band A band of connective tissue that extends from the iliac crest to the knee and links the gluteus maximus to the tibia.

Incomplete protein A protein that does not contain all of the essential amino acids.

Independent contractor People who conduct business on their own on a contract basis and are not employees of an organization.

Inorganic Non-carbon-containing compounds of mineral, not biologic, origin.

Insertion The point of attachment of a muscle to a relatively more movable or distal bone.

Insoluble fiber Fiber that does not bind with water and adds bulk to the diet (includes cellulose, hemicelluloses, and lignins found in wheat bran, vegetables, and whole-grain breads and cereals); important for proper bowel function and reduces symptoms of constipation.

Insomnia Inability to sleep; abnormal wakefulness.

Inspiration The drawing of air into the lungs; inhalation.

Insulin A hormone secreted into the bloodstream by the pancreas in response to elevated blood glucose and amino-acid concentrations in the blood; regulates carbohydrate metabolism.

Insulin-like growth factors Polypeptides structurally similar to insulin that are secreted either during fetal development or during childhood and that mediate growth hormone activity.

Internal feedback Encouragement or motivation provided by the clients themselves; the most important type of feedback for long-term adherence.

Interstitial fluid Fluid between the cells or body parts.

Interval training Short, high-intensity exercise periods alternated with periods of rest (e.g., 100-yard run, one-minute rest, repeated eight times).

Intracellular cation A positively charged ion that is present primarily inside the cell.

Ion A single atom or small molecule containing a net positive or negative charge due to an excess of either protons (positive) or electrons (negative).

Iron-deficiency anemia Anemia characterized by low levels of iron in the blood and decreased iron storage in the body.

Ischemia Lack of blood flow to the heart muscle.

Islets of Langerhans Irregular clusters of endocrine cells scattered throughout the tissue of the pancreas that secrete insulin (beta cells) and glucagon (alpha cells).

Isometric A type of muscular contraction in which the muscle is stimulated to generate tension but little or no joint movement occurs.

Jejunum One of three segments of the small intestine.

Kinematics The study of the form, pattern, or sequence of movement without regard for the forces that may produce that motion.

Kinesiology The study of the principles of mechanics and anatomy in relation to human movement.

Kinetics The branch of mechanics that describes the effects of forces on the body.

Knockouts Genetically manipulated animals that are made to lack specific genes and used to study the mechanisms of disease.

Kyphosis Excessive posterior curvature of the spine, typically seen in the thoracic region.

Kyphotic A type of curve of the spine; concave anteriorly and convex posteriorly.

Lactase An enzyme that is needed to break the bond between the glucose and galactose molecules in lactose so that they can be digested; a deficiency of this enzyme leads to lactose intolerance.

Lacto-vegetarian An individual who does not eat eggs, meat, fish, or poultry, but does eat dairy products.

Lacto-ovo-vegetarian An individual who does not eat meat, fish, or poultry, but does eat dairy products and eggs.

Lactose A disaccharide; the principal sugar found in milk.

Lactose intolerance A disorder that results from a deficiency in the enzyme lactase, which is required to digest lactose; symptoms include cramps, bloating, diarrhea, and flatulence.

Larynx The organ of the voice; located between the trachea and the base of the tongue.

Law of acceleration Newton's second law of motion stating that the force acting on a body in a given direction is equal to the body's mass times its acceleration in that direction.

Law of gravity Newton's theory stating that every object in the universe attracts every other object with a force that is proportional to the product of the masses of the two objects and inversely proportional to the square of the distance between them.

Law of inertia Newton's first law of motion stating that a body at rest will stay at rest and a body in motion will stay in motion unless acted upon by an external force.

Law of reaction Newton's third law of motion stating that for every applied force there is an equal and opposite reactive force.

Laxative Drugs that loosen the bowels.

Lean body mass (LBM) The components of the body including muscles, bones, nervous tissue, skin, blood, and organs.

Learning theory *See* Behavioral theory.

Leptin A hormone released from fat cells that acts on the hypothalamus to regulate energy intake. Low leptin levels stimulate hunger and subsequent fat consumption.

Liability Legal responsibility.

Liability insurance Insurance for bodily injury or property damage resulting from general negligence.

Ligament A strong, fibrous tissue that connects one bone to another.

Lignin An indigestible fiber.

Linoleic acid An unsaturated essential fatty acid found in corn, soy, and safflower oils. *See also* Essential fatty acids.

Linolenic acid Also known as Omega-3 fatty acid; an essential fatty acid that promotes a healthy immune system and helps protect against heart disease and other diseases; found in egg yolk and cold water fish like tuna, salmon, mackerel, cod, crab, shrimp, and oyster.

Lipolysis The release of triglycerides from fat cells.

Locus of control A generalized belief people have about whether the events in their lives are internally or externally caused.

Lordosis Excessive anterior curvature of the spine that typically occurs at the low back (may also occur at the neck).

Low-density lipoprotein (LDL) A plasma complex of lipids and proteins that contains relatively more cholesterol and triglycerides and less protein. High LDL levels are associated with an increased risk of coronary heart disease.

Lymph A clear yellowish fluid that resembles blood without the red blood cells; transports fat from the GI tract to the bloodstream via lymphatic vessels.

Lymphatic system A system of vessels carrying lymph from tissues to the circulatory system; closely related anatomically and functionally to the circulatory system.

Ma huang *See* Ephedra.

Macrocyle The longest timeframe in a periodized training program, usually a period of six months to one year. The goals of a macrocycle are long-term and require multiple steps to be achieved.

Macronutrient The three categories of nutrients (fats, carbohydrates, and protein) that supply energy to sustain life; needed in large quantities for normal growth and development.

Maintenance *See* Maintenance stage.

Maintenance stage The stage of the transtheoretical model during which the individual is incorporating the new behavior into his or her lifestyle.

Malpractice A form of negligence; an act or continuing conduct of a professional that does not meet the standard of professional competence and results in provable damages to his or her client or patient.

Maltose Two glucose molecules bound together; used to make beer.

Maximal oxygen uptake When the body's ability to take in oxygen from the atmosphere via the pulmonary system, transport it via the cardiovascular system, and utilize it via the muscular system reaches a point of little or no change with an additional workload; a direct measure of cardiorespiratory fitness. Also called maximal aerobic capacity, maximal oxygen consumption, or $\dot{V}O_2max$.

Mediastinum The portion of the thoracic cavity between the lungs.

Mesocycle The mid-length timeframe of a periodized training program, usually two weeks to a few months long. The goals of a mesocycle are designed to be steps on the way to the overall goal of the macrocycle.

Metabolic equivalents (METs) A simplified system for classifying physical activities where one MET is equal to the resting oxygen consumption, which is approximately 3.5 milliliters of oxygen per kilogram of body weight per minute (3.5 mL/kg/min).

MET *See* Metabolic equivalents (METs).

Micelles Aggregates of lipid- and water-soluble compounds in which the hydrophobic portions are oriented toward the center and the hydrophilic portions are oriented outwardly.

Microcycle The shortest timeframe in a periodized training program, usually one to four weeks long. The goals of a microcycle are short-term and are designed to be steps on the way to the overall goal of the mesocycle.

Micronutrient A nutrient found widely in foods that is needed in small quantities for normal growth and development.

Microvilli Tiny hairlike projections on each cell of every villus that can trap nutrient particles and transport them into the cells for absorption.

Mind/body vitality An individual's ability to minimize or alleviate unnecessary stress and tension from the body through the integration of physical exercise and mental focus.

Mineral An inorganic (non-carbon-containing) compound that the body requires and that must be provided in the diet.

Mitochondria Specialized cell structures that contain oxidative enzymes needed by the cell to utilize oxygen for metabolism.

Monosaccharide The simplest form of sugar; cannot be broken down any further.

Monounsaturated fatty acid A type of unsaturated fat (liquid at room temperature) that has one open spot on the fatty acid for the addition of a hydrogen atom (e.g., oleic acid in olive oil).

Motor end plate The location of the synapse of a motor neuron and muscle cell; also called the neuromuscular junction.

Motor neuron Nerve cells that conduct impulses from the CNS to the periphery signaling muscles to contract or relax, regulating muscular movement.

Motor unit A motor nerve and all of the muscle fibers it stimulates.

Muscle spindle The sensory organ within a muscle that is sensitive to stretch and thus protects the muscle against too much stretch.

Muscle stiffness The capacity of muscle tissues to resist internal and external loads.

Muscular balance The symmetry of the interconnected components of muscle and connective tissue.

Muscular endurance The ability of a muscle or muscle group to exert force against a resistance over a sustained period of time.

Muscular strength The maximal force a muscle or muscle group can exert during contraction.

Myelin The fatty insulation of nerve fibers that is important for the conduction of nerve impulses. These fibers are damaged in individuals with multiple sclerosis.

Myocardial infarction (MI) An episode in which some of the heart's blood supply is severely cut off or restricted, causing the heart muscle to suffer and die from lack of oxygen. Commonly known as a heart attack.

Myofibrils The portion of the muscle containing the thick (myosin) and thin (actin) contractile filaments; a series of sarcomeres where the repeating pattern of the contractile proteins gives the striated appearance to skeletal muscle.

Myoglobin A compound similar to hemoglobin, which aids in the storage and transport of oxygen in the muscle cells.

Myosin Contractile protein in a myofibril.

Myositis Inflammation of a muscle.

MyPyramid Food Guidance System An educational tool designed to help consumers make healthier food and physical-activity choices for a healthy lifestyle that are consistent with the 2005 USDA Dietary Guidelines.

Near infrared interactance (NIR) Body-composition assessment method that involves the use of light absorption and reflection to estimate percent fat and percent fat-free mass. It is based on the principle that body fat absorbs light while lean body mass reflects light.

Negative energy balance A state in which the number of calories expended is greater than what is taken in, thereby contributing to weight loss.

Negative reinforcement The removal or absence of aversive stimuli following an undesired behavior. This increases the likelihood that the behavior will occur again.

Negligence Failure of a person to perform as a reasonable and prudent professional would perform under similar circumstances.

Neuromuscular junction The region where a motor neuron approaches skeletal muscle plasma membrane.

Neuron The basic anatomical unit of the nervous system; the nerve cell.

Neutral spine position The balance of vertebrae in the three naturally occurring curves: two slight anterior curves at the neck and low back and one slight posterior curve in the thoracic region.

Norepinephrine A hormone and neurotransmitter released as part of the sympathetic response to exercise.

Nutrient Components of food needed by the body. There are six classes of nutrients: water, minerals, vitamins, fats, carbohydrates, and protein.

Obesity An excessive accumulation of body fat. Usually defined as more than 20% above ideal weight, or over 25% body fat for men and over 32% body fat for women; also can be defined as a body mass index of >30 kg/m^2, or a waist girth of >40 inches (102 cm) in men and >35 inches (89 cm) in women.

Oligosaccharide A chain of about three to 10 simple sugars.

Omega-3 fatty acid An essential fatty acid that promotes a healthy immune system and helps protect against heart disease and other diseases; found in egg yolk and cold-water fish.

Omega-6 fatty acid An essential fatty acid found in flax seed, canola, and soybean oils and green leaves.

One-repetition maximum (1 RM) The amount of resistance that can be moved through the range of motion one time before the muscle is temporarily fatigued.

Operant conditioning A learning approach that considers the manner in which behaviors are influenced by their consequences.

Organic A compound that contains carbon.

Origin The attachment site of a tendon of a muscle attached to the relatively more fixed or proximal bone.

Orthostatic hypotension A drop in blood pressure associated with rising to an upright position.

Osteoarthritis A degenerative disease involving a wearing away of joint cartilage.

This degenerative joint disease occurs chiefly in older persons.

Osteoblasts The bone-forming cells.

Osteoclasts The cells that reabsorb or erode bone mineral.

Osteomalacia Softening of the bone.

Osteopenia Bone density that is below average, classified as 1.5 to 2.5 standard deviations below peak bone density.

Osteoporosis A disorder, primarily affecting postmenopausal women, in which bone density decreases and susceptibility to fractures increases.

Overweight A term to describe an excessive amount of weight for a given height, using height-to-weight ratios.

Oxidative glycolysis *See* Aerobic glycolysis.

Oxygen consumption ($\dot{V}O_2$) The process by which oxygen is used to produce energy for cellular work; also called oxygen uptake.

Parasympathetic nervous system A division of the autonomic nervous system that governs the resting functions (i.e., the repair and repose response).

Partial pressure The pressure of each gas in a multiple gas system, such as air, which is composed of nitrogen, oxygen, and CO_2.

Pectin An indigestible fiber.

Percent body fat (%BF) The ratio of fat mass (FM) and fat-free mass (FFM) to total body mass (BM).

Percentage daily value (PDV) A replacement for the percent RDA on the newer food labels. Gives information on whether a food item has a significant amount of a particular nutrient based on a 2,000-calorie diet.

Periodization The systematic application of overload through the pre-planned variation of program components to optimize gains in strength (or any specific component of fitness), while preventing overuse, staleness, overtraining, and plateaus.

Periosteum A double-layered connective tissue sheath surrounding the outer surface of the diaphysis of a long bone; serves to cover and nourish the bone.

Peripheral nervous system (PNS) The parts of the nervous system that are outside the brain and spinal cord (central nervous system).

Peripheral vascular disease (PVD) A painful and often debilitating condition, characterized by muscular pain caused by ischemia to the working muscles. The ischemic pain is usually due to athero-sclerotic blockages or arterial spasms, referred to as claudication. Also called peripheral vascular occlusive disease (PVOD)

Peristalsis The process by which muscles in the esophagus push food to the stomach through a wavelike motion.

Pharynx The muscular, membranous tube extending from the base of the skull to the esophagus.

Phosphagen Adenosine triphosphate (ATP) and creatine phosphate (CP), two high-energy phosphate molecules that can be broken down for immediate use by the cells.

Phospholipid Structurally similar to triglycerides, but the glycerol backbone is modified so that the molecule is water soluble at one end and water insoluble at the other end; helps maintain cell membrane structure and function.

Photosynthesis Process by which plants turn radiant energy (sunlight) into chemical energy.

Physical fitness The physical components of well-being that enable a person to function at an optimal level.

Phytochemical Biologically active compound in plants thought to have beneficial health properties when consumed as part of a healthy diet.

Planning fallacy The tendency of people to underestimate the resources needed, in terms of time, effort, money, and so forth, to accomplish a given task or reach a certain goal.

Plasma The liquid portion of the blood.

Platelets One of the disc-shaped components of the blood involved in clotting.

Plyometrics High-intensity movements,

such as jumping, involving high-force loading of body weight during the landing phase of the movement.

Polypeptide A linear chain of amino acids.

Polysaccharide A long chain of sugar molecules.

Polyunsaturated fat *See* Polyunsaturated fatty acid.

Polyunsaturated fatty acid A type of unsaturated fat (liquid at room temperature) that has two or more spots on the fatty acid available for hydrogen (e.g., corn, safflower, soybean oils).

Portal circulation The circulatory system that takes nutrients directly from the stomach, small intestines, colon, and spleen to the liver.

Positive energy balance A situation when the storage of energy exceeds the amount expended. This state may be achieved by either consuming too many calories or by not using enough.

Positive reinforcement The presentation of a positive stimulus following a desired behavior. This increases the likelihood that the behavior will occur again.

Postmenopausal Pertaining to the time after menopause.

Postpartum The period of time after childbirth.

Precontemplation *See* Precontemplation stage.

Precontemplation stage The stage of the transtheoretical model during which the individual is not yet thinking about changing.

Prehypertensive A blood pressure greater than 120/80 mmHg.

Premenopausal Pertaining to the time before menopause.

Preparation *See* Preparation stage.

Preparation stage The stage of the transtheoretical model during which the individual is getting ready to make a change.

Prime mover A muscle responsible for a specific movement. Also called an agonist.

Progesterone Hormone produced by the corpus luteum, adrenal cortex, and placenta, the function of which is to facilitate growth of the embryo.

Proprioception Sensation and awareness of body position and movements.

Proprioceptors Somatic sensory receptors in muscles, tendons, ligaments, joint capsules, and skin that gather information about body position and the direction and velocity of movement.

Protection motivation theory A health-risk-reduction theory that emphasizes action based on the severity of a threatened event.

Protein A compound composed of a combination 20 amino acids that is the major structural component of all body tissue.

Protein complementarity Combinations of incomplete plant proteins that together provide all of the essential amino acids.

Protraction Scapular abduction.

Provitamin Inactive vitamins; the human body contains enzymes to convert them into active vitamins.

Psychotropic medication Drugs that affect the mental state; capable of modifying mental activity.

Public policy A system of laws or regulatory measures, or courses of action promulgated by a governmental entity to set the standard of what is accepted by the public at large. Laws that are contrary to the public policy are not enforceable.

Pulmonary circuit The circulatory vessels of the lungs; involved in the circulation of blood from the right ventricle of the heart to the lungs and back to the left atrium of the heart.

Pulmonary ventilation The total volume of gas inspired or expired per minute.

Punishment The presentation of aversive stimuli following an undesired behavior. Decreases the likelihood that the behavior will occur again.

Pyloric sphincter Separates the stomach from the small intestines.

Range of motion (ROM) The number of

degrees that an articulation will allow one of its segments to move.

Rapport A relationship of trust and mutual understanding.

Rating of perceived exertion (RPE) A scale, originally developed by noted Swedish psychologist Gunnar Borg, that provides a standard means for evaluating a participant's perception of exercise effort. The original scale ranged from 6 to 20; a revised category-ratio scale ranges from 0 to 10.

Reciprocal inhibition The reflex inhibition of the motor neurons of antagonists when the agonists are contracted.

Recommended Daily Allowance (RDA) The amount of selected nutrients that adequately meet the known nutrient needs of most healthy Americans.

Relapse In behavior change, the return of an original problem after many lapses (slips, mistakes) have occurred.

Relative strength The ratio of the amount of weight lifted to the total body weight of the person. It can be used to compare the strength of different individuals.

Relaxin A hormone of pregnancy that relaxes the pelvic ligaments and other connective tissue in the body.

Respiratory exchange ratio A ratio of the amount of carbon dioxide produced relative to the amount of oxygen consumed.

Respondeat superior A legal doctrine; Latin for "Let the master answer."

Resting metabolic rate (RMR) The number of calories expended per unit of time at rest. Often used to approximate basal metabolic rate (BMR). It is measured early in the morning in a lab after an overnight fast and at least eight hours of sleep at home.

Retraction Scapular adduction.

Rheumatoid arthritis An autoimmune disease that causes inflammation of connective tissues and joints.

Risk management Minimizing the risks of potential legal liability.

Sagittal plane The longitudinal plane that divides the body into right and left halves.

SAID principle A training principle that states that the body will adapt to the specific challenges imposed upon it, as long as the program progressively overloads the system being trained; SAID stands for specific adaptation to imposed demands.

Saliva The water, salt, and enzyme secretion from the salivary glands that begins digestion.

Sarcomere The basic functional unit of the myofibril containing the contractile proteins that generate skeletal muscle movements.

Satiety A feeling of fullness.

Saturated fat *See* Saturated fatty acid.

Saturated fatty acid A fatty acid that contains no double bonds between carbon atoms; typically solid at room temperature, very stable, and usually of animal origin.

Scapulohumeral rhythm Combined action of scapular and humeral movement.

Scapulothoracic (S/T) articulation The articulation of the scapula with the thorax beneath it.

Scoliosis Excessive lateral curvature of the spine.

Scope of practice The range and limit of responsibilities normally associated with a specific job or profession.

Screw-home mechanism A phenomenon that increases knee joint stability by locking the femur on the tibia (or vice-versa) when the knee is fully extended.

Secretin A hormone that signals the pancreas to produce and secrete bicarbonate to neutralize the stomach acid.

Sedentary Doing or requiring much sitting; minimal activity.

Self-control The control people exert over their thoughts, feelings, and behaviors.

Self-efficacy One's perception of his or her ability to change or perform specific behaviors (e.g., exercise).

Self-efficacy theory An explanatory model for predicting initiation and maintenance of health behaviors. This model hypothesizes that all sustained changes in behaviors are mediated by the common mechanism of self-efficacy.

Self-regulation *See* Self-control.

Sensory neuron Nerve cells that convey electrical impulses from sensory organs in the periphery (such as the skin) to the spinal cord and brain (CNS).

Serotonin A neurotransmitter; acts as a synaptic messenger in the brain and as an inhibitor of pain pathways; plays a role in mood and sleep.

Shaping The use of positive reinforcement to gradually reach a behavior modification.

Shoulder girdle The articulation of the scapula with the thorax beneath it.

Shoulder joint complex The three segments of the shoulder: the scapula, clavicle, and humerus.

Simple carbohydrate Single sugars (monosaccharides) and double sugars (disaccharides) that are rapidly digested.

SITS A pneumonic device for naming the rotator cuff muscles: the supraspinatus, which abducts the arm; the infraspinatus and teres minor, which externally rotate the arm; and the subscapularis, which internally rotates the arm.

Slow-twitch (ST) muscle fibers A muscle fiber type designed for use of aerobic glycolysis and fatty acid oxidation, recruited for low-intensity, longer-duration activities such as walking and swimming.

Small intestine The part of the gastrointestinal system that is the site of the majority of food digestion and absorption.

SMART goal A properly designed goal; SMART stands for specific, measurable, attainable, relevant, and time-bound.

SOAP note A communication tool used among healthcare professionals; SOAP stands for subjective, objective, assessment, plan.

Social support The perceived comfort, caring, esteem, or help an individual receives from other people.

Social-cognitive theory A behavior-change theory that posits that all health behaviors are goal-driven through anticipation of outcomes.

Soluble fiber A type of fiber that forms gels in water; may help prevent heart disease and stroke by binding bile and cholesterol; diabetes by slowing glucose absorption; and constipation by holding moisture in stools and softening them.

Specificity Exercise training principle explaining that specific exercise demands made on the body produce specific responses by the body; also called exercise specificity.

Spondylolisthesis Forward displacement of one vertebra over another; usually occurs at the 4th or 5th lumbar vertebrae.

Stability limits Boundaries of an area of space in which the body can maintain its position without changing the base of support.

Stages-of-change model A lifestyle-modification model that suggests that people go through distinct, predictable stages when making lifestyle changes; precontemplation, contemplation, preparation, action, and maintenance. The process is not always linear.

Standard of care Appropriateness of an exercise professional's actions in light of current professional standards and based on the age, condition, and knowledge of the participant.

Starch A plant carbohydrate found in grains and vegetables.

Static stabilizer Bony configuration of joints, fibrocartilages, and ligaments that contribute to core stability.

Statutory law Created by provisions in state constitutions and by a county or city ordinance.

Steady state Constant submaximal exercise below the lactate threshold where the oxygen consumption is meeting the energy requirements of the activity.

Stepped care model A model of treatment for obesity based on the premise that treatment can be cumulative or incremental.

Sternoclavicular (S/C) joint The junction of the sternum and the proximal clavicle.

Stimulant A substance that activates the central nervous system and sympathetic nervous system.

Stimulus control A means to break the connection between events or other stimuli and a behavior; in behavioral science, sometimes called "cue extinction."

Stroke The sudden death of brain cells in a localized area caused when blood flow is interrupted to part of the brain.

Stroke volume The amount of blood pumped from the left ventricle of the heart with each beat.

Sucrose Table sugar; a disaccharide formed by glucose and fructose linked together.

Sympathetic nervous system A division of the autonomic nervous system that activates the body to cope with some stressor (i.e., the fight or flight response).

Synapse The region of communication between neurons.

Synergist A muscle that assists another muscle in function.

Systemic circuit The circulatory vessels of the body.

Systole The contraction phase of the cardiac cycle.

Systolic blood pressure The pressure exerted by the blood on the vessel walls during ventricular contraction.

Tendon A band of fibrous tissue forming the termination of a muscle and attaching the muscle to a bone.

Testosterone The steroid hormone produced in the testes; involved in growth and development of reproductive tissues, sperm, and secondary male sex characteristics.

Thermic effect of food (TEF) An increase in energy expenditure due to digestive processes (digestion, absorption, metabolism of food). Also called thermic effect of feeding.

Thorax The portion of the trunk above the diaphragm and below the neck.

Thyroid hormones Hormones secreted by the thyroid gland and responsible for controlling the metabolic rate.

Tidal volume The amount of air inspired or expired per breath.

Tolerable Upper Intake Level (UL) The maximum intake of a nutrient that is unlikely to pose risk of adverse health effects to almost all individuals in an age- and gender-specific group.

Tort law A system of law that governs the management and disposition of personal injury and wrongful death lawsuits.

Total energy expenditure (TEE) Amount of energy expended in a 24-hour period, which includes basal metabolism, physical activity, and dietary-induced thermogenesis.

Trabecular bone Spongy or cancellous bone composed of thin plates that form a honeycomb pattern; predominantly found in the ends of long bones and the vertebral bodies.

Trachea The cartilaginous and membranous tube extending from the larynx to the bronchi; windpipe.

Trans fat An unsaturated fatty acid that is converted into a saturated fat to increase the shelf life of some products.

Transference The unconscious redirection of feelings from one person to another.

Transtheoretical model (TTM) A theory of behavior that examines one's readiness to change and identifies five stages: precontemplation, contemplation, preparation, action, and maintenance. Also called the stages-of-change model.

Transverse plane Anatomical term for the imaginary line that divides the body, or any of its parts, into upper (superior) and lower (inferior) parts. Also called horizontal plane.

Trier of fact A person who determines facts in a legal proceeding.

Trigger *See* Antecedent.

Triglyceride The principal storage form of fat consisting of three molecules of fatty acid and a glycerol molecule.

Type 1 diabetes Form of diabetes caused by the destruction of the insulin-producing beta cells in the pancreas, which leads to little or no insulin secretion; generally develops in childhood and requires regular insulin injections; formerly known as insulin-dependent diabetes mellitus (IDDM) and childhood-onset diabetes.

Type 2 diabetes Most common form of diabetes; typically develops in adulthood and is characterized by a reduced sensitivity of the insulin target cells to available insulin; usually associated with obesity; formerly known as non-insulin-dependent diabetes mellitus (NIDDM) and adult-onset diabetes.

Unsaturated fatty acid Fatty acids that contain one or more double bonds between carbon atoms and thus are capable of absorbing more hydrogen; liquid at room temperature and usually of vegetable origin; fairly unstable, making them susceptible to oxidative damage and a shortened shelf life.

Upbeat The deemphasized beat in a piece of music.

Valsalva maneuver A strong exhaling effort against a closed glottis, which builds pressure in the chest cavity that interferes with the return of the blood to the heart; may deprive the brain of blood and cause lightheadedness or fainting.

Vascularity An increase in the number and size of blood vessels enhancing blood supply and oxygen delivery to muscle cells.

Vasoconstriction Narrowing of the opening of blood vessels (notably the smaller arterioles) caused by contraction of the smooth muscle lining the vessels.

Vasopressin Hormone released by the posterior pituitary gland during exercise; reduces urinary excretion of water and prevents dehydration.

Vegan A pure vegetarian who excludes all animal-derived foods from the diet.

Vegetarian A person who does not eat or does not believe in eating meat, fish, fowl, or, in some cases, any food derived from animals, such as eggs or cheese, but subsists on vegetables, fruits, nuts, grain, etc. *See also* Vegan, Lacto-vegetarian, *and* Lacto-ovo-vegetarian.

Veins Blood vessels that carry deoxygenated blood toward the heart from vital organs and the extremities.

Ventilatory threshold Point of transition between predominately aerobic energy production to anaerobic energy production; involves recruitment of fast-twitch muscle fibers and identified via gas exchange exercise testing.

Venules Smaller divisions of veins.

Very-low-calorie diet A weight-loss program that consists only of liquid meals, and a calorie content that usually ranges between 420 and 800 kcal/day. VLCDs should only be used when under the care and supervision of a physician.

Villi Finger-like projections from the folds of the small intestines.

Visceral fat The fat located deep in the abdomen that surrounds the vital organs. Its accumulation is associated with insulin resistance, glucose intolerance, dyslipidemia, hypertension, and coronary artery disease.

Vitamins Organic compounds that function as metabolic regulators in the body and are essential for normal physiologic function; classified as water soluble or fat soluble.

$\dot{V}O_2$max *See* Maximal oxygen uptake.

Waist circumference Abdominal girth measured at the level of the umbilicus; values greater than 40 inches (102 cm) in men and 35 inches (89 cm) in women are strong indicators of abdominal obesity and associated with an increased health risk.

Waist-to-hip ratio A useful measure for determining health risk due to the site of fat storage. Calculated by dividing the ratio of abdominal girth (waist measurement) by the hip measurement.

Waiver Voluntary abandonment of a right to file suit; not always legally binding.

Wolff's Law A principle stating that bone is capable of increasing its strength in response to stress (e.g., exercise) by laying down more bone.

Index

A

B

C

D

E

F

L

M

N

O

P

Q

R

T

U

V

W

Y

Z